Radionuclide Therapy

Recep Bekiş • Berna Polack
Murat Fani Bozkurt
Editors

Radionuclide Therapy

Springer

Editors
Recep Bekiş
School of Medicine
Dokuz Eylül University
izmir, Turkey

Berna Polack
Dokuz Eylül University
Izmir, Turkey

Murat Fani Bozkurt
School of Medicine
Hacettepe University
Ankara, Turkey

Translation from the Turkish language edition.
Original title: Radyonüklit Tedavi
Name of the originator: Prof. Recep Bekiş, MD

ISBN 978-3-030-97219-6 ISBN 978-3-030-97220-2 (eBook)
https://doi.org/10.1007/978-3-030-97220-2

This Springer imprint is published by the registered company Springer Nature Switzerland AG
The registered company address is: Gewerbestrasse 11, 6330 Cham, Switzerland

Preface

Cancer, which is the disease of our age, continues to threaten human health at an increasing rate every day. Although standard methods such as surgery, chemotherapy, radiotherapy, and hormone therapy are among the ways to deal with this threat, newly developed biological treatments, targeted treatments, personalized treatments, external beam radiotherapy, and targeted radionuclide therapies have begun to take their place in professional practice. Therefore, cancer treatment is increasingly requiring special expertise. Nuclear medicine, in addition to its role as a tracer of cancer, also assumes the role of attack and treatment with radioactive molecules directed to the cancer it traces. These traceable next-generation radionuclide therapies, whose efficacy and reliability have been proven and where diagnosis, treatment, and follow-up are carried out together, are increasingly included in oncology practice with the new radiopharmaceuticals developed with each passing day. Traceable next-generation radionuclide therapies targeting cancer ensure a high rate of damage to cancer cells while protecting the surrounding normal tissues. Molecular cancer treatment will become more effective with individualized next-generation traceable radionuclide therapies, which will be shaped by genetic studies in the future.

Radionuclide therapies include treatment of hyperthyroidism and some joint diseases. Radioactive iodine therapy is a noninvasive treatment method that is an alternative to surgical and medical treatment in the case of hyperthyroidism and achieves good results. Radiosynovectomy is a minimally invasive radionuclide therapy method with a high treatment success used in patients with joint diseases who have not benefited from surgical and medical treatment.

This book was planned to be written due to the lack of sufficient resources in radionuclide therapies in Turkey. Radionuclide therapies for many cancer types and benign diseases were prepared and written by experienced nuclear medicine experts in the light of their own experience and case studies. Systemic treatments in common cancer types and side effect management of these treatments were summarized by medical oncologists. The main purpose of writing this book is to create a reference for the indications, contraindications, patient selection, treatment practice, treatment side effect management, and follow-up of radionuclide therapies.

We wish that the book will be beneficial to all physicians.
Best regards,

Izmir, Turkey Recep Bekiş
Izmir, Turkey Berna Polack
Ankara, Turkey M. Fani Bozkurt

Our Editorial Board

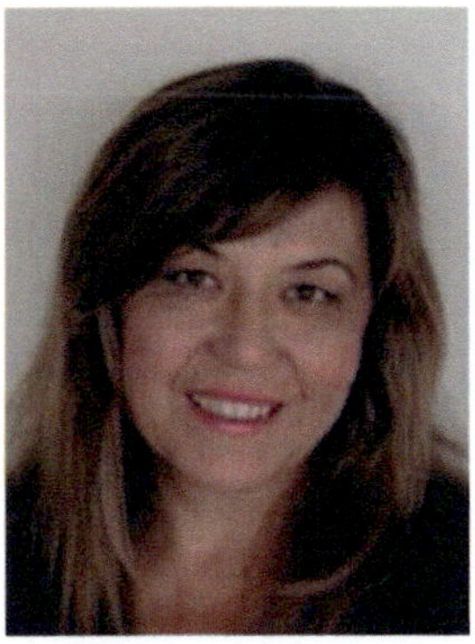

Berna Polack

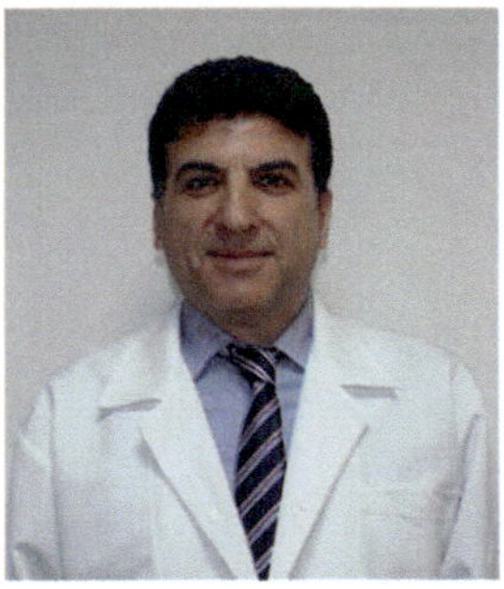

Recep Bekiş

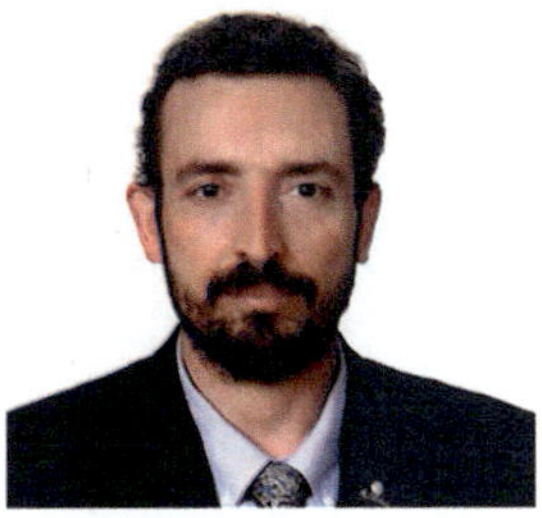

Murat F. Bozkurt

Our Authors

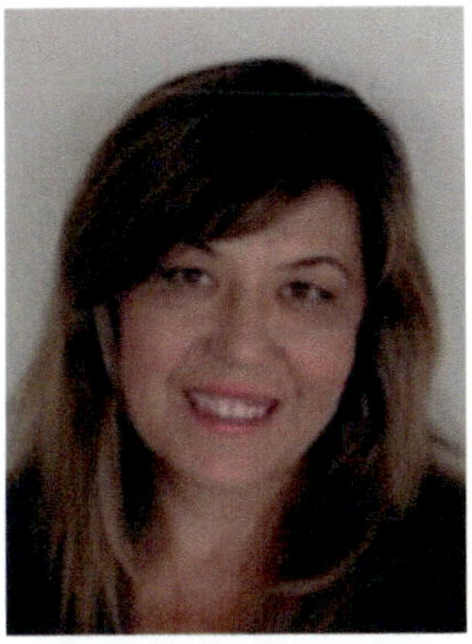

Berna Polack

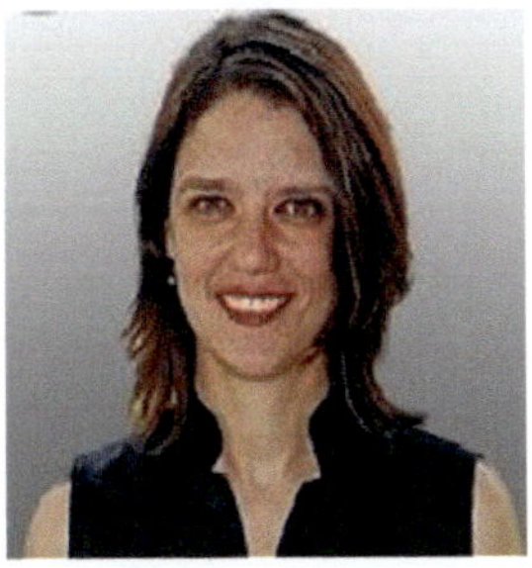

Bilge V. Salancı

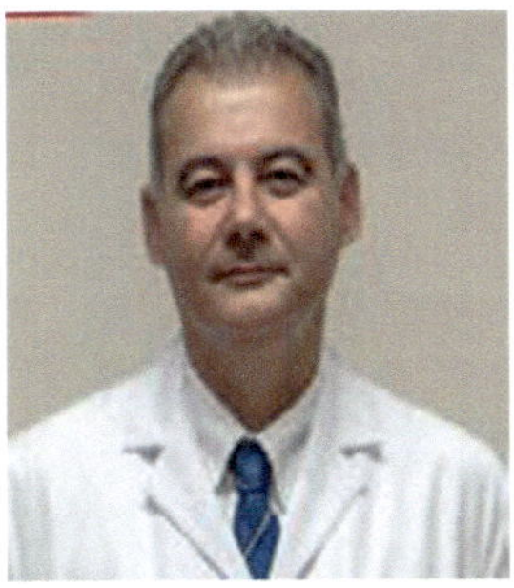

Cüneyt Türkmen

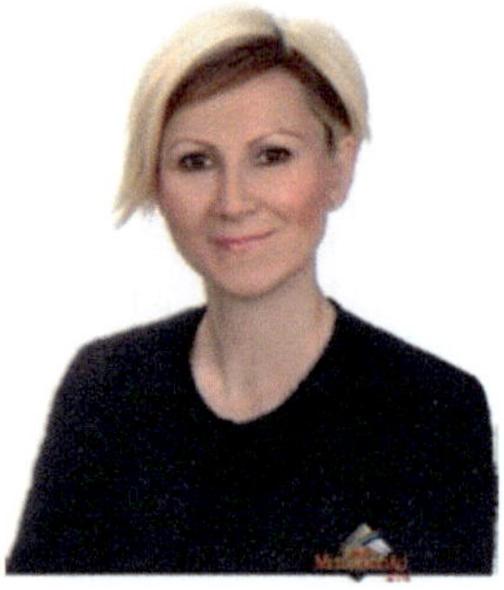

Çiğdem Soydal

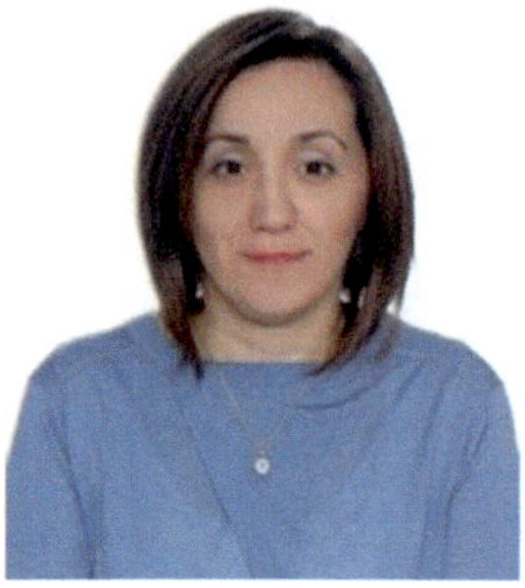

Elgin Özkan

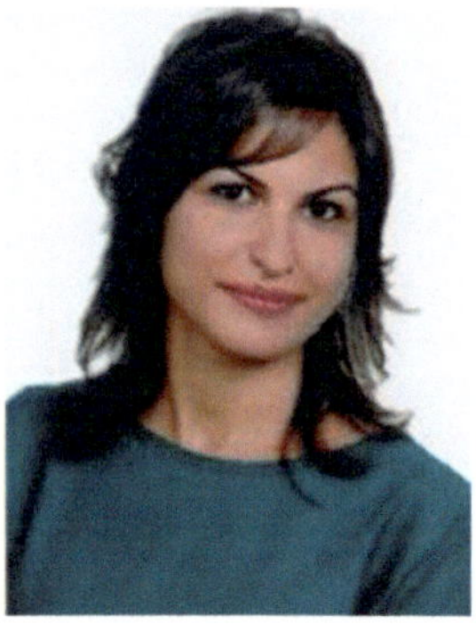

Emine Acar

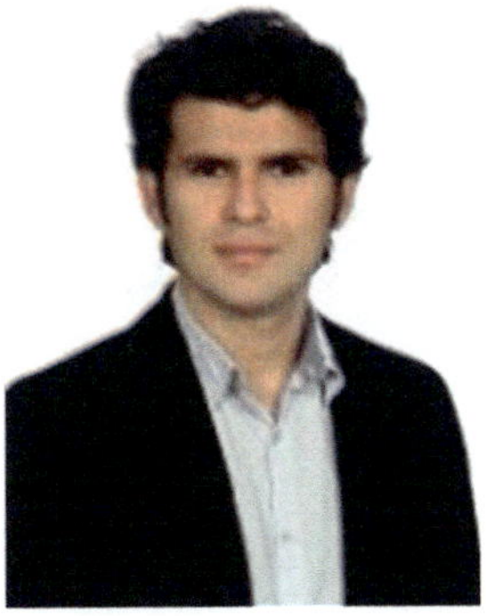

Emre Demirci

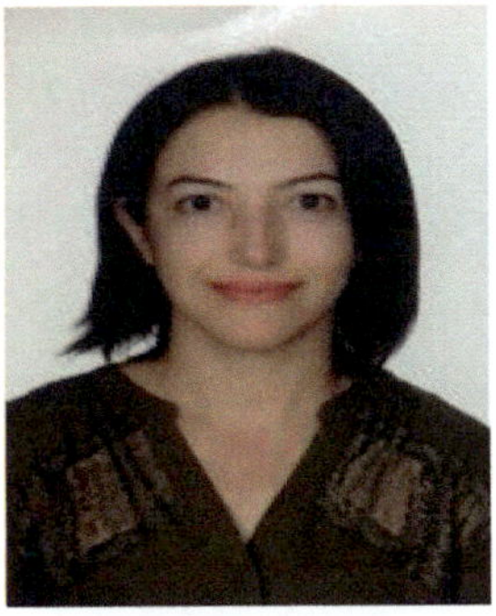

Evrim S. Budak

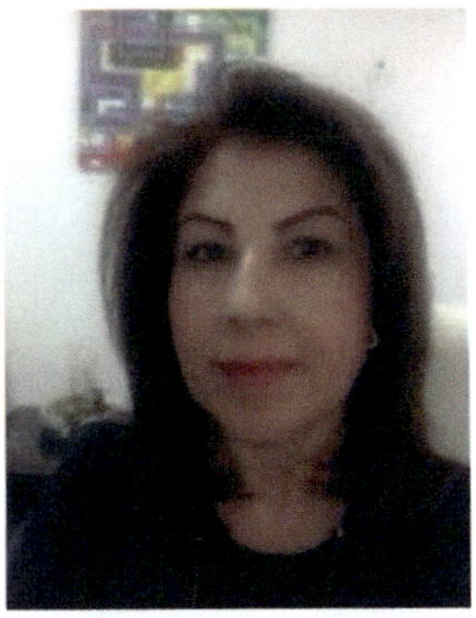

Funda Aydın

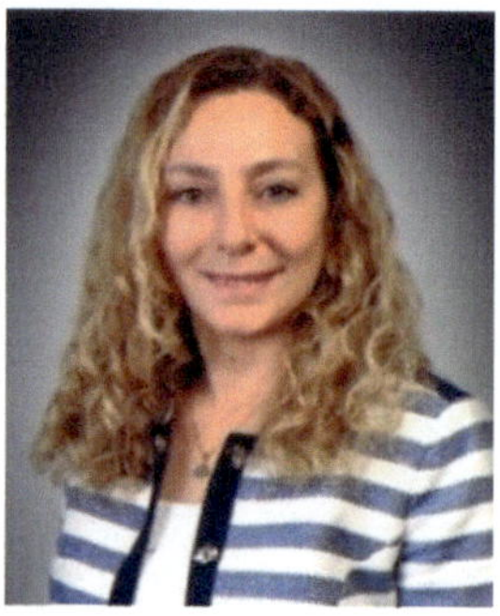

Gülin Uçmak

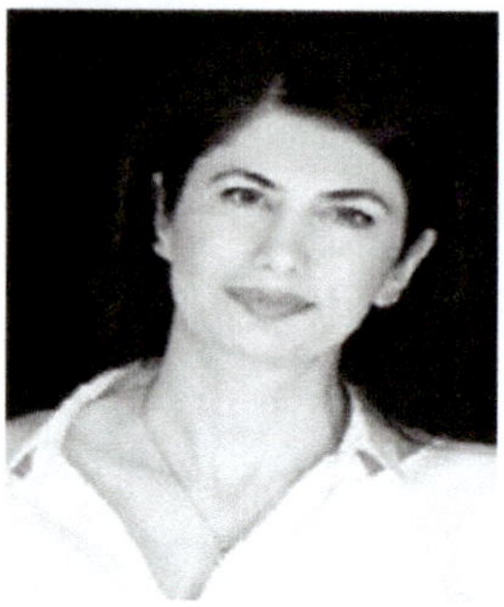

Handan Tokmak

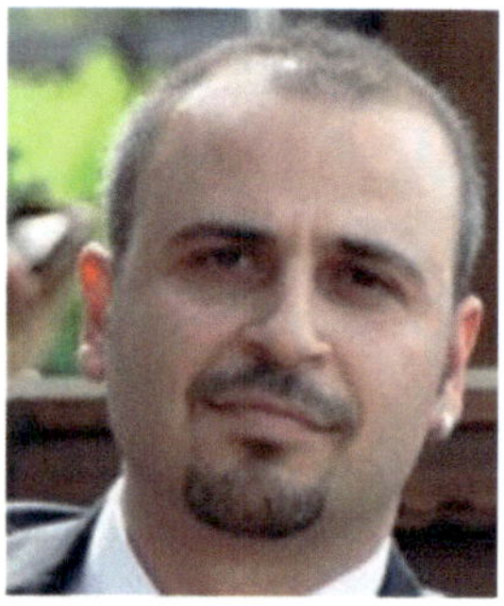

Hüseyin S. Durmaz

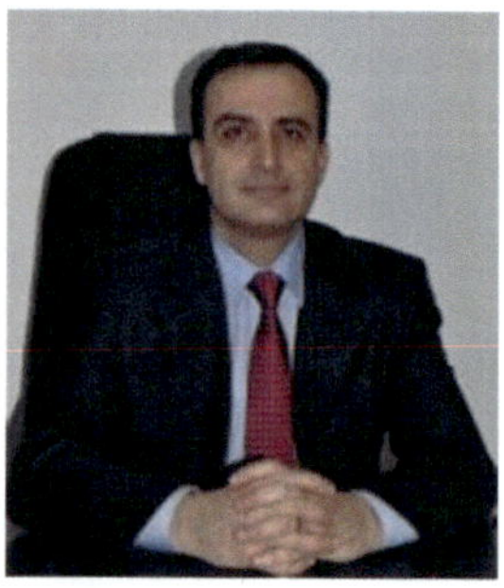

İlhan Öztop

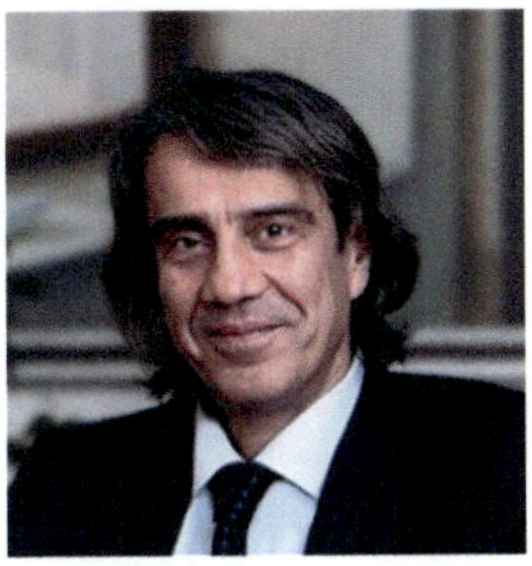

Levent Kabasakal

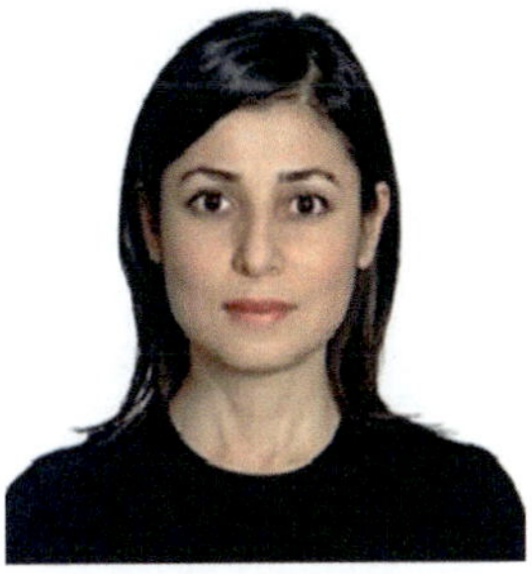

Meltem O. Demirci

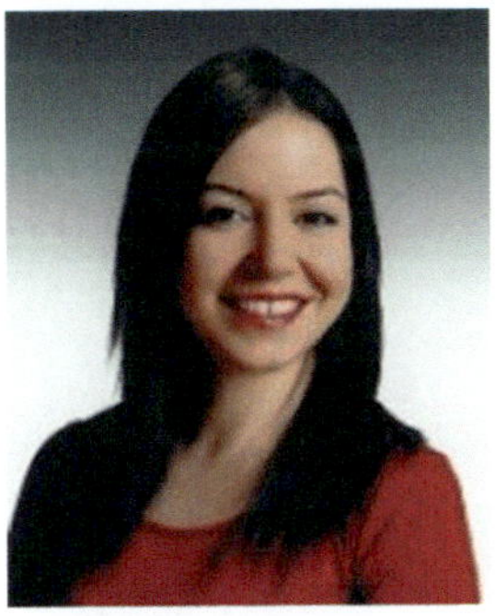

Mine Araz

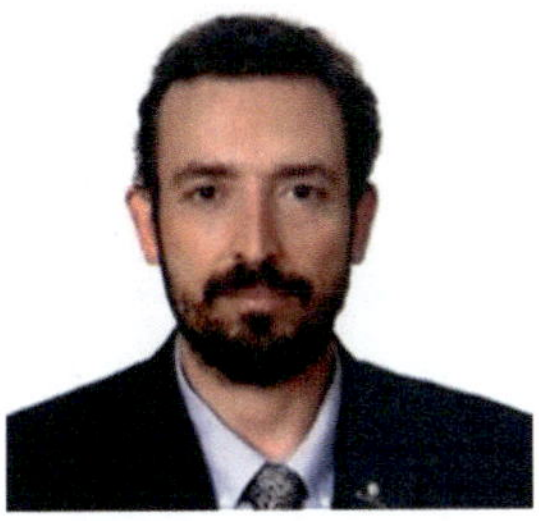

Murat F. Bozkurt

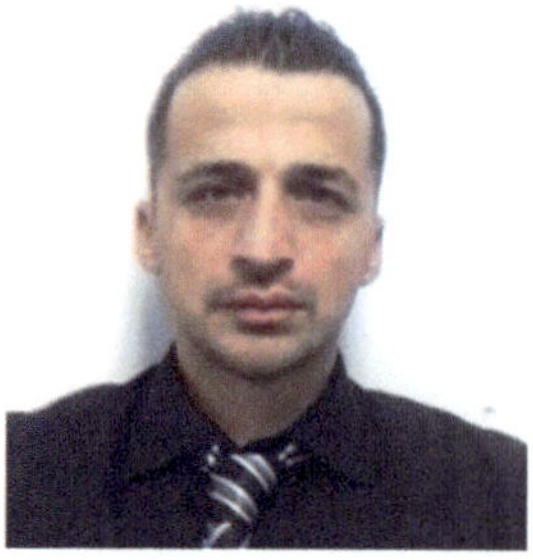

Murat Tuncel

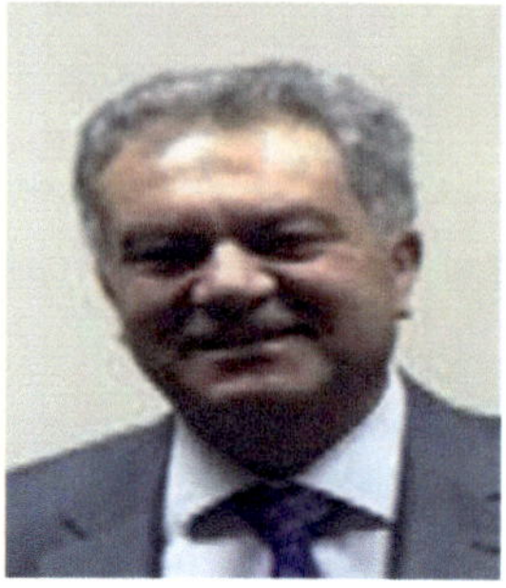

Mustafa Demir

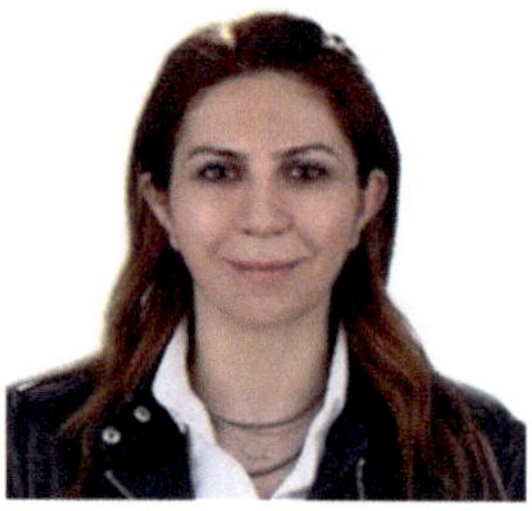

Nalan Alan

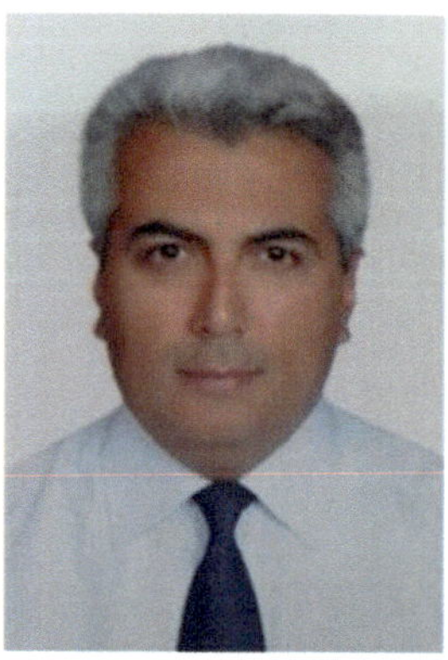

Özgür Karaçalıoğlu

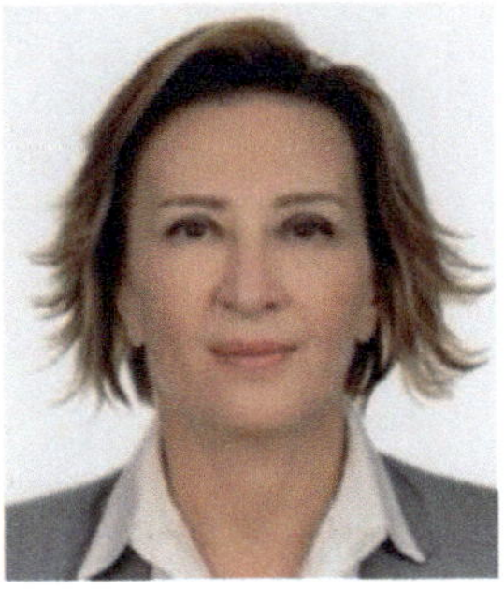

Özlem L. Atay

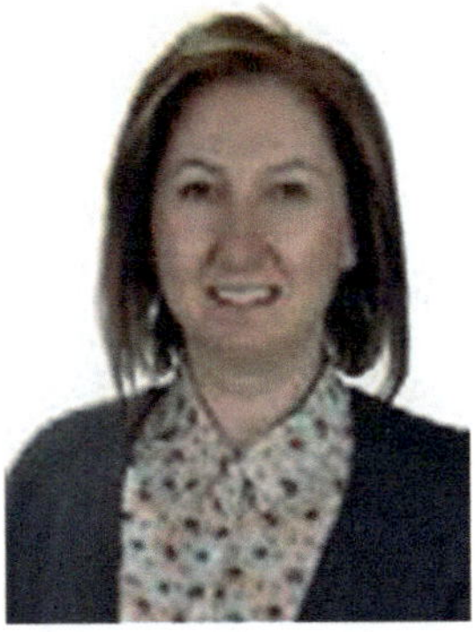

Özlem N.Küçük

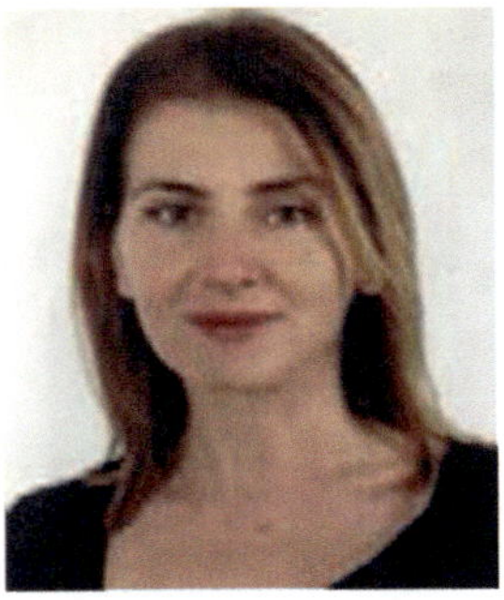

Pınar Ö. Kıratlı

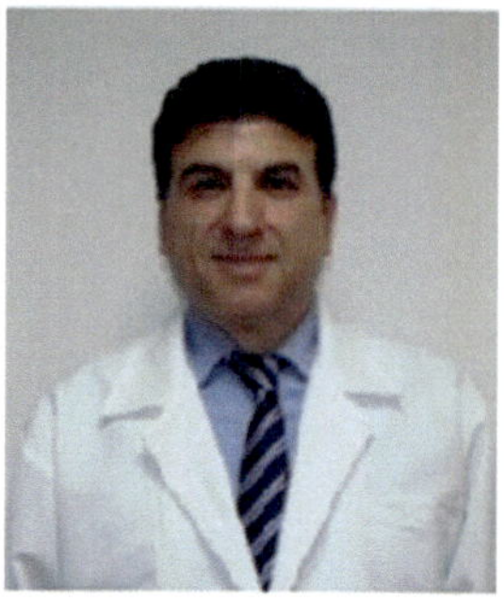

Recep Bekiş

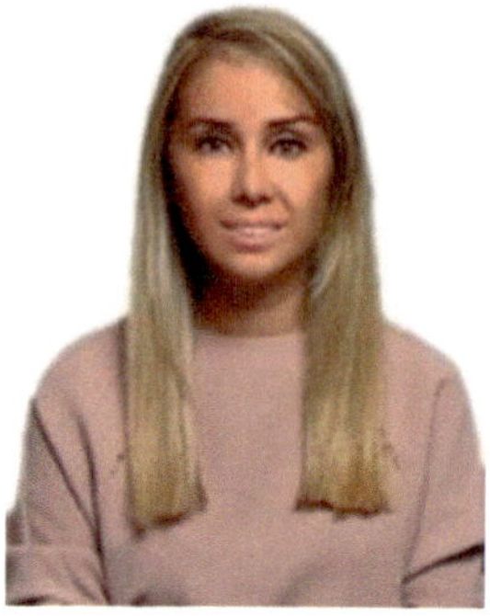

Seher N. Kazaz

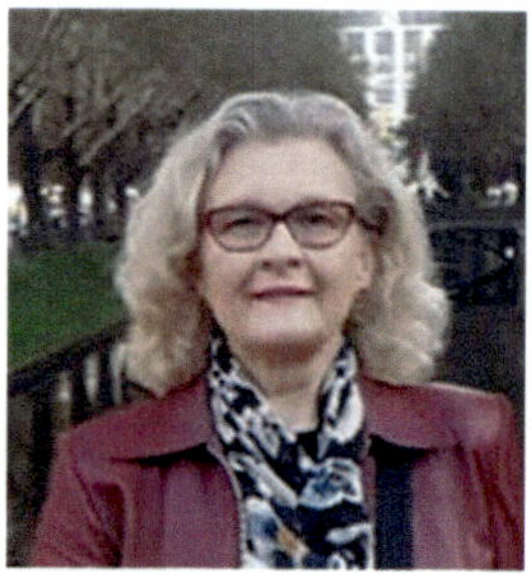

Suna Kıraç

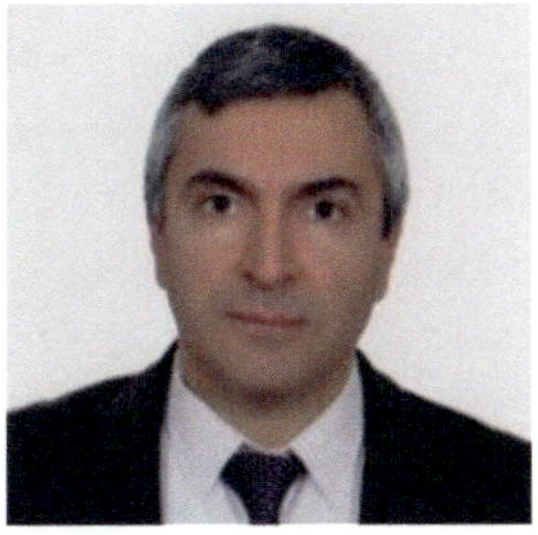

Ümit Ö. Akdemir

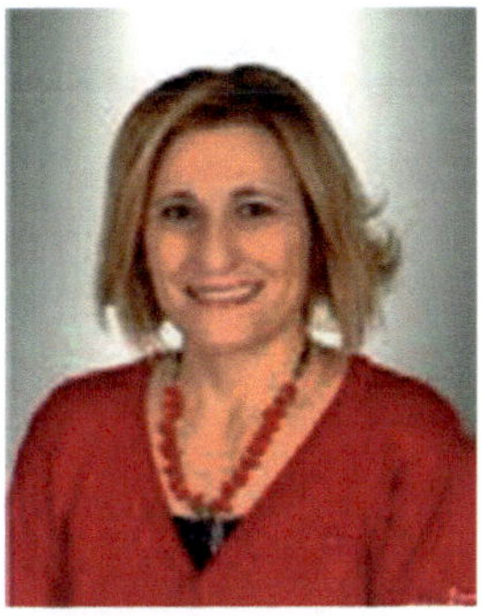

Zeynep Burak

Photographs of our physicians are sorted alphabetically.

Acknowledgments

We wish to express our deepest gratitude to the authors who contributed to this textbook. Many of them are our nuclear medicine colleagues at universities in Turkey. We are grateful to them for devoting their precious time to this book.

We wish to express our gratitude to Medical Oncology Department at Dokuz Eylul University for contributing to this book.

We are very thankful for the O'tip publishing house for the design of figures and graphs required.

As editors and writers, we'd like to express our gratitude to Eczacıbaşı-Monrol for their generous support in translating our book from Turkish to English.

Contents

Part I

Basic Information

Basic Properties and Preparation of Radiopharmaceuticals Used in Radionuclide Therapy

1

Meltem Ocak

In nuclear medicine therapy, therapeutic radiopharmaceuticals are given to the patient and a therapeutic dose of ionizing radiation is sent to the disease areas in the body, thus providing treatment, control, or pain palliation of the disease. Damages caused by ionized radiation such as single or double-strand breaks in DNA play a role in the effectiveness of treatment. A therapeutic radiopharmaceutical is a drug that contains a radionuclide emitting particle radiation such as beta (β^-), alpha (α), and auger electron, which will provide the necessary ionization for bond breakdown [1]. Therapeutic radiopharmaceuticals may be present in ionic form, such as Iodine-131 (I-131) or Strontium-89 (Sr-89), or radiolabeled forms of ionic radionuclides with carrier molecules (non-radioactive part) such as peptides, proteins, and particles. The non-radioactive part is administered a small amount therefore they usually have no pharmacological effect. Therapeutic radiopharmaceuticals should have high specific activity (radioactivity/unit mass) and can be orally, intraarterially, intravenously, intratumorally, and intracavitary administered. Therapeutic radiopharmaceuticals should be specific to the disease (target), show high involvement in the target, have a high target/non-target tissue ratio, be quickly discarded from non-target tissues, and be able to stay long enough to provide effective treatment in the target.

Nuclear medicine therapy applications first started in 1936 with the use of Phosphor-32 (P-32), a cyclotron product, in the treatment of leukemia [2]. Toward the 1940s, the treatment of thyroid cancers started with ^{131}I-NaI. Today, all countries have access to radioactive iodine (^{131}INaI) treatment. With recent studies, the biochemistry of diseases started to be better understood therefore therapeutic radiopharmaceuticals targeted to different mechanisms are developed and their use is becoming common in clinical applications.

1.1 Development of Therapeutic Radiopharmaceuticals

The process of developing therapeutic radiopharmaceuticals includes multidisciplinary studies in many fields such as molecular biology, microbiology, chemistry, physiology, pharmacology together with some radiation physics. And chemists, pharmacists, microbiologists, veterinarians, radiation physicists, and nuclear medicine doctors should work together.

1.1.1 Target

The first step in the development of a new therapeutic radiopharmaceutical involves determining

M. Ocak (✉)
Faculty of Pharmacy, Department of Pharmaceutical Technology, Istanbul University, İstanbul, Turkey
e-mail: melocak@istanbul.edu.tr

R. Bekiş et al. (eds.), *Radionuclide Therapy*, https://doi.org/10.1007/978-3-030-97220-2_1

the target in the diseased area with appropriate biochemical mechanisms. The target could be a receptor or groups of receptors or antigens, or enzymes that are densely located in the diseased area. Ideally, the target should never be found in normal tissues. However, this is not the case in reality.

Therefore, the statistically high concentration of the target in the diseased area (tissues) compared to normal tissues increases the success of therapeutic radiopharmaceuticals.

1.1.2 Carrier Molecule

Once the appropriate target is identified, the selection of carrier molecules that carry the therapeutic radionuclides to the target (target-specific) should be defined-. Carrier molecules could be target-specific peptides, antibodies, small drug molecules, or enzyme inhibitors.

1.1.3 Radionuclide

The characteristics of therapeutic radionuclides can be evaluated according to their physical and biochemical properties [3]. While physical half-life, particulate radiation type and emitted energy, production method, radionuclide impurities, and decomposition products constitute the physical properties, biochemical properties consist of the capability of being targeted, staying on target, in vivo stability, and toxicity [4]. These features will be discussed in more detail in the following sections.

1.1.4 Radiolabeling

The chemical properties of the selected radionuclide play a major role in labeling the carrier molecule. Non-metallic radionuclides such as I-131 can be directly bound to the carrier molecule. Metallic radionuclides bind to the molecules by forming complexes with bifunctional chelates (DTPA, DOTA, NOTE, DOTAGA, etc.) conjugated to the molecule in a way that does not change the interest of the molecule in the target [5, 6]. The ionic state and size of radionuclide are very important in complex formation with bifunctional chelates. Concentration, chemical impurities, reaction pH, duration, and temperature of reactions are important parameters to obtain radiopharmaceuticals in high radiochemical purity and radiolabeling efficiency. Table 1.1 summarizes the ideal labeling conditions for radiometals used in DOTA-chelated therapeutic radiopharmaceuticals [6]. It should also be noted that the molecule (deterioration of the structure of DOTA-antibodies at high temperatures, etc.), which is in complex form with DOTA chelate, plays a major role in determining the radiolabeling conditions. Radiolabeling efficiency and radiochemical purities can be calculated using physicochemical techniques such as TLC (thin-layer chromatography) and HPLC (high-pressure liquid chromatography). Radiochemical purity tests to be performed for a certain period of time after radiopharmaceutical preparation also provide information about the stability of the radiopharmaceutical. Therapeutic radiopharmaceuticals are intended to remain stable in vitro and in vivo.

Table 1.1 Radiolabeling conditions of DOTA chelate with therapeutic radionuclides used in clinical applications (In-111: Indium-111, Lu-177: Lutetium-177, Y-90: Yitrium-90, Ac-225: Actinium-225, Bi-213: Bismuth-213)

Chelate	Radiometal	Radiolabeling conditions
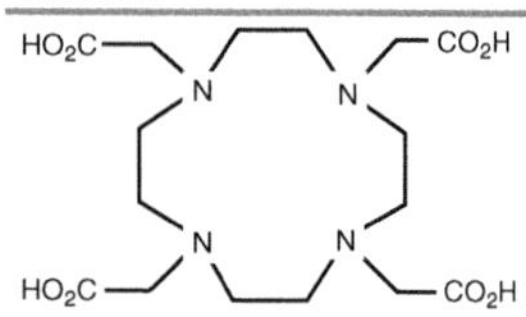	$^{111}In^{+3}$	37–100 °C, 15–60 min, pH 4.0–6.0
	$^{177}Lu^{+3}$	25–100 °C, 15–90 min, pH 4.0–6.0
DOTA, 1,4,7,10 Tetraazacyclododecane	$^{90}Y^{+3}$	25–100 °C, 15–90 min, pH 4.0–6.0
1, 4, 7, 10-tetraacetic acid	$^{225}Ac^{+3}$	37–60 °C, 30–100 min, pH 6.0
	$^{213}Bi^{+3}$	95–100 °C, 5 min, pH 4.0–6.0

1.1.5 Biological Assessment

Biological evaluation of therapeutic radiopharmaceuticals can be performed by in vitro and in vivo tests. In vitro tests often include serum stability studies and cell studies. Within the scope of cell studies, radioligand binding studies, radioligand internalization, and externalization studies are frequently performed. In addition, cytotoxic properties are also examined. Cytotoxic properties are frequently determined by cell viability studies. In vivo tests mostly include biodistribution and imaging (if the properties of radionuclide are appropriate). Appropriate therapeutic radiopharmaceuticals obtained as a result of in vitro studies are examined in healthy and diseased animal models. Therefore the pharmacokinetic properties of the therapeutic radiopharmaceutical and the radiation doses that different organs are exposed to are determined.

1.1.6 Toxicity Studies

Therapeutic radiopharmaceuticals may exhibit toxic properties due to both their radiation and carrier molecule. Radiation-induced toxic property is an important requirement in therapeutic radiopharmaceuticals. Radiopharmaceutical toxicity studies include both general toxicity studies (for the carrier molecule) and radiotoxicity studies. Radiotoxicity studies should be conducted for the target and other organs and tissues, usually involving studies to determine damage or necrosis occurring at the cellular dimension of radiation emitted from radionuclides. Since the general purpose of radiotoxicity studies is to determine the amount of live/dead cells, there are many methods applied to determine cell viability. These methods can be generally colorimetric, luminescent, and enzymatic.

1.2 Physical Properties of Therapeutic Radionuclides

In the preparation of therapeutic radiopharmaceuticals, radionuclides emitting various particular radiation (alpha, beta, auger electron) with different chemical properties, specific activities, and different physical half-lives are used. The success of therapy depends on the use of the suitable radionuclide for treatment. Although there are many radionuclides that can be used in treatment applications, very few of them are suitable in terms of nuclear, physical, and biological properties [7].

1.2.1 Particulate Radiation Emission

In nuclear medicine therapy, radionuclides emitting particular radiation such as beta, alpha, or auger electron, which cause cytotoxic effects due to their high LET (linear energy transfer) value, are used. The choice of radionuclide to be used for treatment depends on its LET value and the distance of progression within the tissue. Therapeutic radionuclides commonly used in nuclear medicine applications and their properties are shown in Table 1.2 [8–10]. Effective distance and relative biological activity of each particle emitted from radionuclide within the tissue are different from each other. The distance in the tissue of the radionuclide to be used in the treatment should be consistent with the size of the tumor or area to be treated.

1.2.1.1 Radionuclides Emitting Beta Particles

The maximum kinetic energies of radionuclides that undergo radioactive decay by emitting beta particles are between 0.3 and 2.3 MeV, and the distance is approximately 0.5–12 mm in soft tissue depending on their energy [11].

Their LETs are approximately 0.2 keV/μm [8]. The distance of beta particles in tissue is effective up to approximately 10–1000 cell distances compared to cell sizes. In addition, crossfire effects can also cause cytotoxic effects in non-target areas. This provides an advantage especially in the treatment of heterogeneous tumors [12]. Radionuclides emitting beta particles are effective in the treatment of medium and large masses, but the radionuclides to be used differ according to the size and localization of the mass [11].

Table 1.2 Frequently used therapeutic radionuclides (I-131: Iodine-131, Cu-67: Copper-67, Re-186 (188): Renium-186 (188), Ho-166: Holmium-166, Ga-67: Galium-67, Ac-225: Actinium-225, Th-227: Thorium-227, Ra-223: Radium-223)

Radionuclide [β^-], (LET:0.2 keV/μm)	$T_{1/2}$	Max β^- energy (keV)	Max. distance (μm)	Emission type
Y-90	2.7 days	2280.0	11.300	β^-
I-131	8.02 days	606.31	2300	β^-, γ
Lu-177	6.65 days	498.3	1800	β^-, γ
Cu-67	61.8 h	577	2100	β^-, γ
Re-186	3.7 days	1069.5	4800	β^-, γ
Re-188	17.01 h	2120.4	10.400	β^-, γ
Ho-166	26.6 h	1854.9	8700	β^-, γ
Radionuclide [auger], (LET:4-26 keV/μm)	**$T_{1/2}$**	**Max auger energy (keV)**	**Max. distance (μm)**	**Emission type**
In-111	2.80 days	26	17	Auger, γ
Ga-67	3.26 days	9.6	3	Auger, β^-, γ
I-125	59.4 days	32	20	Auger, γ
Radionuclide [α], (LET: 50–230 keV/μm)	**$T_{1/2}$**	**Max α energy (keV)**	**Max. distance (μm)**	**Emission type**
Bi-213	45.6 min	8400	90	α, β^-, γ
Bi-212	60.5 min	7800	100	α, β^-, γ
At-211	7.2 h	7500	80	α, EC
Ac-225	9.9 days	8400	90	α, β^-, γ
Th-227	18.7 days	7400	70	α, β^-, γ
Ra-223	11.4 days	5640	80	α, β^-, γ

1.2.1.2 Radionuclides Emitting Alpha Particles

Alpha particles progress at 50–100 μm levels in the tissue and their LET values are higher than those of beta particles (50–230 keV/μm) [8]. Cytotoxic properties are 100 times higher than beta particles. They are effective on small tumors and micro metastases. As long as auger electrons can pass through the cell membrane, they can only be effective on a cell-based basis. Few of the alpha particle emitting radionuclides among approximately 100 alpha particle emitting radionuclides can be used in nuclear medicine clinical applications. Many parameters such as half-life, decomposition products, chemical properties, energies, and availability play a role in the selection of alpha radiation emitting radionuclides [13]. Among the alpha radiation emitting radionuclides summarized in Table 1.3, Ac-225 is the most interesting radionuclide due to its successful applications in prostate cancer treatment in recent years [14].

Another feature to keep in mind regarding alpha radiopharmaceuticals is that other alpha-emitting radionuclides (defined as daughter radionuclides) formed by the decay of alpha radionuclides have different chemical properties and thus form unstable bonds with carrier molecules. As a result, alpha-emitting daughter radionuclides are quickly separated without binding to bifunctional chelates conjugated to carrier molecules [12]. In cases where the recoil energy exceeds 100 keV, the binding energy of radionuclide to the targeting molecule is exceeded and these released alpha radionuclides unnecessarily cause non-target organs to receive radiation and can cause serious problems in the long term. This issue is important for radionuclides that are decay by emitting multiple alpha particles, such as Ra-223 and Ac-225.

Table 1.3 Characteristics of alpha particle emitting radionuclides and decay products

Radionuclide	$T_{1/2}$	Main decomposition form	Energy (MeV)	Daughter radionuclides	$T_{1/2}$	Mode of decomposition	Energy (MeV)
Th-227	18.7 days	α	6	Ra-223	11.4 days	α, β⁻, γ	
Ac-225	9.9 days	α	5.8	Fr-221	4.8 min	α, γ	7, 0.218
				At-217	32.3 ms	α	7
				Bi-213	45.6 min	α, β⁻, γ	6, 0.444
				Po-213	4.2 μs	α	0.440
				Tl-209	2.2 min	β-	8
				Pb-209	3.5 hours	β-	0.659
				Bi-209	Stable		0.198
Ra-223	11.4 days	α	5.7	Rn-219	3.96 s	α	6.8
				Po-215	1.78 ms	α	7.4
				Pb-211	36.1 min	β-	
				Bi-211	2.13 min	α, β⁻	
				Pb-207	Stable		
Bi-213	45.6 min	α, β⁻, γ	6,0.444, 0.440	Po-213	4.2 μs	α	8
				Tl-209	2.2 min	β-	0.659
				Pb-209	3.5 hours	β-	0.198
				Bi-209	Stable		
At-211	7.2 h	α	5.9	Bi-207 Po-211 Pb-207	33.7 year 0.516 h Stable	β- α	

Radiolysis generally refers to the decay of the molecule due to radiation. Radionuclide emitting alpha particles during radiolabeling has a very high potential to produce radiolysis compared to beta-emitting radionuclides such as Y-90 or I-131. In order to prevent radiolysis, antioxidants such as ascorbic acid can be added to the reaction vial during or after radiolabeling [15].

Three different main strategies are mentioned in the preparation of alpha radiopharmaceuticals [16]. The first approach involves loading radionuclides into nano-carrier systems such as liposomes and nanoparticles. Small nanoparticles are rapidly removed from the body after involvement in the target, allowing non-target organs to be exposed to less radiation. The second approach involves rapid uptake of alpha radiopharmaceuticals into the tumor cell and rapid removal from non-target organs. This strategy ensures the administration of radiolabeled antibodies (radioimmunotherapy) and peptides (peptide receptor radionuclide therapy). The final approach is to administer alpha radiopharmaceuticals locally [16].

1.2.2 Physical Half-Life of Radionuclide

The physical half-life of radionuclide should be consistent with the biodistribution and clearance times of the radiopharmaceutical [17]. If the half-life of the radionuclide is too short, the radiopharmaceutical begins to decay before reaching the target tissue or cannot stay for the necessary time to provide effective treatment in the target tissue. On the contrary, when the half-life is too long, normal tissues are unnecessarily exposed to radiation. Radionuclides with a half-life of 1-14 days are generally considered appropriate for treatment [11].

1.2.3 Radionuclide Decay Products

Ideally, the decay product of therapeutic radionuclides is expected to be non-radioactive or a low-energy short half-life product [11].

1.2.4 Radionuclide Purity/Specific Activity

Radionuclides to be used for treatment purposes should be of high purity in terms of radionuclide, radiochemical, elemental, or chemical impurities. Production reactions and post-production purification methods are important factors in the purity of radionuclides. Low-specific radionuclides may be sufficient in the preparation of radiopharmaceuticals to be used in pain palliation in radiosynovectomy and bone metastases, while high-specific activity radionuclides should be used in the development of radiolabeled peptides or antibodies targeting limited amounts of receptors or antigens in the target region [18]. Thus, adequate treatment doses can be delivered to the target region without saturating the receptor or antigens in the target area. Non-carrier added (NCA) radionuclides are generally preferred in the preparation of radiolabeled peptides targeted at the receptor. Most NCA radionuclides are directly obtained from non-direct nuclear reactions in rectors or by the creation of a generator system of radionuclides with long half-lives [17].

1.2.5 Gamma Radiation

The fact that therapeutic radionuclides emit gamma radiation at optimal energy and abundance is advantageous in that it enables targeted radioactivity uptake and biokinetic calculations and contributes to the monitoring of treatment response and the determination of patient doses. In this case, although the use of radionuclides containing low density and appropriate energy gamma radiation is advantageous in terms of obtaining images, therapeutic radionuclides containing high energy and high-density gamma radiation cause unnecessary radiation to the patient [11].

1.2.6 Radionuclide Chemistry

Chemical properties of radionuclide such as its specific activity, radiochemical purity, and metal contamination content should be suitable for complex formation with a large number of molecules [11].

1.2.7 Economic Factors

Economically sustainable production of radionuclides suitable for radionuclide therapy is an important factor in the development and widespread applicability of therapeutic radiopharmaceuticals.

1.3 Production of Radionuclides

Radionuclides used in nuclear medicine therapy can be artificially produced by various nuclear reactions based on neutron bombardment in nuclear reactors or bombardment of particles loaded in accelerators (usually cyclotron). Alternatively, some therapeutic radionuclides can also be obtained from radionuclide generator systems. Today, research on the production and purification technologies of therapeutic radionuclides is ongoing intensively. According to the production method, carrier-added (CA) or NCA radionuclides are obtained.

1.3.1 Radionuclides Produced in Reactors

Since most radionuclides used in nuclear medicine therapy are rich in neutrons, they undergo beta decay and are generally produced in research reactors. Radionuclide production in nuclear reactors takes place by fission, fusion, neutron capture or activation and transmutation methods. Mo-99, I-131, and Xe-133 radionuclides are obtained by fission method and I-131 radionuclides are used for treatment purposes. Most other radionuclides used in nuclear medicine therapy are obtained by neutron activation or cap-

Table 1.4 Therapeutic radionuclides produced by different methods in reactors and potentially used in nuclear medicine applications

Radionuclide	T1/2	Target material	Mode of decomposition	Production method
Er-169	9.4 days	Er-168	β-	(n, γ)
Lu-177	6.65 days	Lu-176	β-, γ	(n, γ)
Lu-177	6.65 days	Yb-176	β-, γ	(n, γ) → β−
Ho-166	1.1 days	Ho-165	β-, γ	(n, γ)
Ho-166	1.1 days	Dy-164	β-, γ	(n, γ) (n, γ) → β−
P-32	14.3 days	P-31	β-	(n, γ)
P-32	14.3 days	S-32		(n, p)
Re-186	3.72 days	Re-185	β-	(n, γ)
Re-188	17 h	Re-187	β-	(n, γ)
Sm-153	2 days	Sm-152	β-	(n, γ)
Y-90	2.7 days	Y-89	β-	(n, γ)
Y-90	2.7 days	U-235	β-	(n, *f*)
Sr-89	53 days	Sr-88	β-	(n,γ)
I-131	8 days	Te-130	β-, γ	(n, γ) → β−
I-131	8 days	U-235	β-	(n, *f*)
Cu-67	2.4 days	Zn-67	β-, γ	(n, p)
Ac-225	10 days	U-233	α	U-233 decomposition product

ture method in nuclear reactors. Most commonly, the direct (n,γ) method is used. This reaction is based on the principle that the neutron sent to the nucleus is captured by the nucleus and a photon is emitted. The atomic number of the resulting radionuclide does not change, only the mass number increases, the main radionuclide has an isotope (CA radionuclide). In another used (n, p) reaction, the neutron emits a target nucleus proton and while the mass number of the newly formed radionuclide remains unchanged, a different product is obtained from the main nuclide (NCA radionuclide). The most known radionuclide obtained by this method is Cu-67 [19]. Table 1.4 summarizes the therapeutic radionuclides potentially used in nuclear medicine treatment applications.

1.3.2 Radionuclides Produced in Accelerators, Cyclotrons

In cyclotrons, radionuclides are neutron-deficient and thus degraded by electron capture (EC) or positron (β^+). In cyclotron, a positive charge is usually added to charged particles, and adding a positive charge to the nucleus changes the atomic number. Therefore, cyclotron products are usually NCA. Apart from electron capture or positron (β^+) emitting radionuclides in cyclotron centers, therapeutic radionuclides that emit alpha or beta can also be produced in some cases. Table 1.5 summarizes radionuclides that can be produced in cyclotron or accelerators and potentially used in nuclear medicine applications [20]. High-specific activity radionuclides are usually obtained using accelerators. Production of therapeutic radionuclides from cyclotrons is generally more costly than reactors due to reasons such as power requirement, operational costs, and obtaining products in low activities per production.

1.4 The Most Frequently Used Radionuclides for Therapy

Examples of radionuclides emitting beta or alpha particles that have recently been preferred for therapeutic use include Re-186, Re-188, Y-90, Ho-166, Lu-177, and Ac-225.

Table 1.5 Therapeutic radionuclides produced in accelerators or cyclotrons and potentially used in nuclear medicine applications

Radionuclide	T1/2	Mode of decomposition	Production method
Cu-67		EC	$^{70}Zn(p,\alpha)^{67}Cu$ $^{68}Zn(p,2p)^{67}Cu$ $^{78}Se(p,2n)^{67}Cu$
Rb-81	4.6 h	EC	$^{82}Kr\ (p,2n)^{81}Br$
In-111	2.8 days	EC	$^{112}Cd\ (p,2n)^{111}In$
Ga-67	78.3 h	EC	$^{66}Zn(p,n)^{67}Ga$
At-211	7.2 h	α	$^{211}Bi\ (\alpha,2n)^{211}At$
Ac-225	10 days	α	$^{226}Ra\ (p,2n)^{225}Ac$

1.4.1 Re-186

Re-186 can be produced in nuclear reactors or particle accelerators. They are obtained by Re-185 (n,γ) Re-186 reaction in nuclear reactors. Re-186 obtained by this method is CA. There are difficulties in obtaining Re-186 in high specific activity for use in antibody or peptide labeling in low neutron flux reactors. However, Re-186 obtained like that may be sufficient for the preparation of phosphonate derivatives and bone metastases for pain treatment, radiopharmaceutical preparation for use in radiosynovectomy or radioembolization. Since very few reactors in the world operate with high neutron flow, it is also desirable to obtain Re-186 with high specific activity in other ways. Although radionuclide production with nuclear reactors is appropriate in terms of quantity and unit price, cyclotrons remain the most suitable source for radionuclide production today. It is also possible to obtain NCA-added radionuclide in cyclotrons. In Re-186 cyclotrons, the proton or deuteron bombardment of the target material tungsten (W-186) is usually obtained by [W-186 (p, n) Re-186 or W-186 (d,2n) Re-186] [21].

1.4.2 Re-188

Re-188, unlike Re-186, can be produced in relatively higher specific activities by Re-187 (n,γ) Re-188 reaction in nuclear reactors, while W-188/Re-188 can be obtained in the center where it will be used more practically and economically than radionuclide generator systems. The biggest advantage of the generator system with a shelf life of more than 6 months is that it can give Re-188 without carrier in the form of Re-188-perrhenate and contribute to the development of various therapeutic radiopharmaceuticals [22]. These are summarized in Table 1.6 [23].

Table 1.6 Commercially available Re-188 generators and general specifications

Generator provider	Column material	W-188 Specific activity
ORNL,TN,USA	Alumina	148–185 GBq (4-5 Ci)/g
Dimitrovgrad, Russia	Alumina	185 GBq (5 Ci)/g
IRE, Belgium	Alumina	185 GBq (5 Ci)/g
ITG, Germany	Alumina	185 GBq (5 Ci)/g
Polatom, Poland	$^{99}Mo/^{99m}Tc$ generator column system	185 GBq (5 Ci)/g
IDB, Netherlands	Alumina	Unknown

1.4.3 Y-90

Y-90 is a radiometal that is widely used in treatment and is a pure beta emitter in +3 oxidation state [24]. To date, we find that it has most commonly been used in the treatment of hepatocellular carcinoma, radiosynovectomy, peptide receptor radionuclide therapy, and non-Hodgkin's lymphoma in nuclear medicine clinical applica-

Table 1.7 Radionuclide generator systems used and studied in clinical applications

Generator system	Production site of the main radionuclide		Parent radionuclide		Daughter radionuclide	
			$T_{1/2}$	Main decomposition	$T_{1/2}$	Main decomposition
^{188}W/^{188}Re	Reactor		69.4 days	β⁻	17 h	β⁻
^{90}Sr/^{90}Y	Reactor		28.5 year	β⁻	2.7 days	β⁻
^{166}Dy/^{166}Ho	Reactor		3.4 days	β⁻	1.1 days⁻	β⁻
^{225}Ac/^{213}Bi	Decay chain		10 days	α	45.6 days	β⁻, α
^{227}Ac/^{223}Ra	Reactor chain	Decay	21.7 year	β⁻, then Th-227 via α	11.4 days	α

tions. Y-90 is obtained via direct neutron activation of Y-89 in the reactor. Usually, this method yields Y-90 with high radionuclide purity. However, it is not always possible to obtain Y-90 in high specific activities according to the characteristics of the reactor used. Alternatively, production based on the Zr-90 (n, p) Y-90 reaction is also carried out in the reactor to obtain a non-carrier added Y-90. One of the most important limitations in this type of production is the problems encountered in obtaining Zr-90 in the long term. Apart from the reactor, Y-90 is also obtained from Sr-90/Y-90 radionuclide generators [25]. The critical situation in the use of this system is that there are no reliable methods for purifying the mother radionuclide (Sr-90) loaded on the column material from the final product obtained. Sr-90 is a radionuclide that shows involvement in bones and is allowed to be administered to patients up to a maximum of 2μci to keep the radiation received by the bones at low levels [26]. Therefore, it is necessary to know the amount of Sr-90 in Y-90 content obtained from the generator. However, since both Y-90 and Sr-90 radionuclides emit pure beta and overlap in the beta spectrum, the methods that can be used today are insufficient in terms of sensitivity.

1.4.4 Ho-166

Ho-166 is a therapeutic radionuclide emitting two gamma radiations, one is 1379 keV (1.13%) and the other one is 80.6 keV (6.2%), with a maximum of 1854 keV (50%) beta particles. Gamma radiation at 80 keV is suitable for imaging with gamma cameras. Ho-166 is produced by two different methods. One method includes direct neutron activation of Ho-165 (n, γ), while the other includes non-direct neutron activation of Dy-164, i.e. Dy-164 (n,γ) Dy-165 (n, γ) Dy-166 (beta decay). The first method yields Ho-166 in low specific activity. Even if radiolabeled peptides or antibodies can be obtained with Ho-166 obtained by this method, there is a need for molecules labeled with Ho-166 with higher specific activity in high-dose therapies [9].

The shortness of Ho-166's half-life ($t_{1/2}$: 1.1 days) is a limiting factor in the distribution from the production site. As a solution to this situation, the prototypes of the Dy-166/Ho-166 generator system have been developed and further studies on more practical versions for use in clinical applications have not yet been carried out [27]. Table 1.7 summarizes the radionuclide generator systems used in clinical applications [27].

1.4.5 Lu-177

Although the use of Lu-177 in nuclear medicine therapy has become widespread with the treatment of neuroendocrine tumors for the last 15 years, we see that many antibodies labeled with Lu-177, enzyme inhibitors (Lu-177-PSMA, prostate cancer) are involved in clinical applications. The physical half-life of Lu-177 is similar to I-131, which is commonly used in radionuclide therapies. The biggest advantage of Lu-177 is that it can be produced in high amounts and transported to remote sites without losing too much activity due to their long half-life. Lu-177

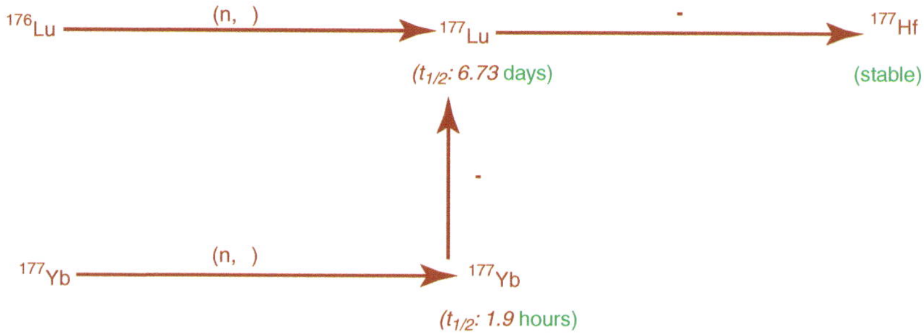

Fig. 1.1 Methods of obtaining Lu-177 radionuclide

can be directly produced by neutron activation of target material Lu_2O_3 in reactors or indirectly produced from target material Yb_2O_3 (Fig. 1.1). Indirectly manufactured Lu-177 has high specific activity, not including long-life Lu-177m radionuclide, which is even low in the directly generated Lu-177. In addition to this advantage, purification of Lu-177 from irradiated Yb-177 target includes complex analytical purification steps [28].

1.4.6 Ac-225

Ac-225 radionuclide, which decays by emitting 4 alpha particles, are primarily derived from the build up of Th-229 ($t_{1/2}$ 7340 y) and Ra-225 ($t_{1/2}$ 14.9 days).

The half-lives of both main radionuclides are very long and available in very limited amounts. Th-229 ($t_{1/2}$: 7340 years) is obtained by isolating Np-237 ($t_{1/2}$ 2.14 × 10^6 years) or U-233 ($t½$ 1.6 × 10^5 years) in limited quantities in stock. Ra-225, which is the breakdown product of Th-229, is isolated from Th-229 every 6-8 weeks [29]. In this way, <2 Ci Ac-225 is obtained by America, Russia and Germany in total annually, and Ac-225 radionuclide is obtained from Ra-225 [30]. As the use of Ac-225 in clinical applications has become widespread in recent years, studies have accelerated to obtain Ac-225 by different methods. Ra-226 (p, 2n) Ac-225, Ra-226 (γ, n) Ac-225, or Th-232 (p,x) Ac-225 nuclear reactions are produced in accelerators and reactors other than Th-229 [30].

1.5 Therapeutic Radiopharmaceutical Applications

Therapeutic radiopharmaceuticals are used in nuclear medicine therapy in various applications such as primary cancer treatment, pain treatment due to bone metastases, or treatment of non-cancerous diseases such as rheumatoid arthritis.

1.5.1 Primary Cancer Therapy

It does not seem possible for therapeutic radiopharmaceuticals to replace any operation, chemotherapeutic application or radiation treatment or to be used in the treatment of all types of cancer in today's conditions. Nowadays, some types of cancer and disease can be successfully treated with radiopharmaceuticals, but for most of them, appropriate radiopharmaceuticals have been developed yet. Using high-dose I-131 in the treatment of thyroid diseases in nuclear medicine is an example of the most successful radionuclide therapy applications. Na-I-131-capsule or Na-I-131 solution formulations are administered orally in the treatment of thyroid diseases. Both forms can be obtained in various activity amounts on the day of calibration [31].

1.5.2 Radioimmunotherapy

Radioimmunotherapy (RIT) refers to targeted cancer therapy with antibodies labeled with ther-

Table 1.8 The most used peptide derivatives and related receptors in nuclear medicine clinical applications

Peptide	Receptor	Types of tested malignancies	Intended use
Somatostatin analogs	Somatostatin 1-5	Neuroendocrine tumors	Imaging/treatment
GLP-1/Exendin	GLP1/R	Insulinoma	Imaging
Bombesin/gastrin releasing peptide	GRPR	Breast cancer, prostate cancer, gastrointestinal stroma	Imaging
CCK/gastrin	CCK-2R	Medullary thyroid cancer, small cell lung cancer, stromal ovarian cancer	Imaging
Substance-P	NK-1R	Glioblastoma	Treatment
RGD	$\alpha v\beta 3$	Melanoma, lung cancer, breast cancer, glioblastoma	Imaging/treatment
α-MSH	MC1R	Melanoma, glioblastoma, small cell lung cancer	Imaging
CXCR4	CXCR4-ligand	Multiple myeloma, glioblastoma, small cell lung cancer	Imaging/treatment

apeutic radionuclides [32]. Scientific studies on RIT have been ongoing for approximately 30 years and very important gains have been achieved to date. It has been repeatedly demonstrated that RIT can be an effective treatment method by administering radiolabeled monoclonal antibodies in various animal tumor models. As a result of successful applications in preclinical applications, CD-20 antigen-targeted Y-90 and I-131-tagged antibodies have been approved for use in the clinical treatment of hematological malignancies, especially in the treatment of non-Hodgkin's lymphoma (Bexxar: I-131-tocitumomab, Zevalin: Y-90-ibritumomab).

Finally, encouraging results have been obtained that RIT may also be effective in the treatment of solid tumors, and difficulties in the spread of routine clinical practices have been revealed [33].

1.5.3 Peptide Receptor Radionuclide Therapy

With the targeting feature of the receptors on the surface of cancer cells, the use of radiolabeled peptides in nuclear medicine imaging and treatment applications has begun. Due to the low molecular weights, radiolabeled peptides are expected to better penetrate tumor tissue and exhibit faster clearance from normal organs. When radiolabeled peptides bind with receptors on the cell, these receptors are internalized and they allow the radiation to remain in the cell. Vascular clearance is high from non-target tissues, so they show a high target/non-target tissue ratio. The radiolabeled octreotide derivatives used in the treatment of neuroendocrine tumors are the most successful example of the use of radiopeptides in nuclear medicine. Table 1.8 summarizes the most important peptides and related receptors used in nuclear medicine clinical applications to date [34].

1.5.4 Advantages of Peptides in Treatment Applications

Radiolabeled peptides have many advantages over other biologically active molecules (protein, antibody, etc.) used in treatment applications. First of all, they enter the target cell rapidly due to their small and low molecular weight and move away from non-target organs rapidly due to their high vascular clearance [35]. They are suitable for chemical and molecular modifications to increase *in vivo* stability and affinity to target receptors. They can be easily synthesized in automatic peptide synthesis devices or manually. Automatic synthesis devices are preferred in the rapid synthesis of simple sequenced peptides, while manual synthesis is preferred in the synthesis of time-consuming difficult sequenced and modified peptides. Peptides can be radiolabeled via commercially available or developed chelates that are conjugated to peptides with various radionuclides. They are resistant to chemical conditions (pH, heat, etc.) used during radiolabeling [36]. The development of radiopeptide-based radiopharmaceuticals to be used for therapeutic purposes is a complex process including the determination of the biological target, the presence of a molecule with high affinity for the target, chemical and radiochemical characterization, pre-clinical and clinical studies. Radiometals and radiolanthanides are mostly used in the preparation of therapeutic radiopeptides. Since different radionuclides will be used for therapeutic purposes, the most important criterion in chelate selection is that the cavity size of the bifunctional chelate forms stable complexes *in vitro/in vivo* in accordance with the ionic radius of the radionuclide to be used.

1.5.5 Treatment of Bone Pain

Bone metastases are one of the most common complications experienced by advanced prostate, breast, and lung cancer. Clinical management of bone pain due to bone metastases includes analgesic drugs, chemotherapy, hormone, radiotherapy applications as well as radionuclide therapy [37]. The aim of radionuclide therapy of bone metastases is to eliminate pain, prevent local tumor growth, and prevent pathological fracture development. The most important criterion to be considered in the development of radiopharmaceuticals is that the ionized radiation to be sent to the lesions creates minimal bone marrow suppression. Bone metastases can be osteoblastic, osteolytic, and mixed. Radiopharmaceuticals used in the palliative treatment of bone metastases can be divided into two groups. The first group consists of inorganic radiopharmaceutical formulations of calcium analog (Ca^{+2}) such as Sr-89-Cl_2. Sr-89^{+2} acts as Ca^{+2} in regions where mineralization occurs and joins hydroxyapatite crystals. The second group contains radiolabeled phosphonic acid compounds and they are localized by chemical adsorption to hydroxyapatite crystals or by direct binding to the organic matrix [38]. Table 1.9 summarizes the beta-emitting radiopharmaceuticals used in the palliative treatment of bone metastases in routine nuclear medicine applications.

Table 1.9 Radiopharmaceuticals used in the palliative treatment of bone metastases in routine nuclear medicine applications

Radiopharmaceutical	Dose administered
$^{89}SrCl_2$ (strontium chloride)	150–220 MBq
^{153}Sm-lexidronam (^{153}Sm-EDTMP)	37 MBq/kg
^{186}Re-ethydronate (^{186}Re-HeDP)	1.30 MBq

Apart from radiopharmaceuticals prepared with beta-emitting radionuclides, ^{223}Ra-CI_2 radiopharmaceuticals that emit alpha (α) have also begun to be used in the palliative treatment of osteoblastic bone metastases in recent years. Ra-223 acts as Ca^{+2} in regions where mineralization occurs just like Sr-89^{+2} and joins hydroxyapatite crystals. In treatments with ^{223}Ra-CI_2, lower radiation dosage and lower hematotoxicity to bone marrow are reported [39].

1.5.6 Radioembolization

It is used in the treatment of primary and/or metastatic tumors of the liver that cannot be resected. The blood supply of intrahepatic tumors is largely (at a rate of 80–100%) caused by the hepatic artery. Tumor vascularization is mostly concentrated in the periphery of the tumor. Radioactive microspheres applied from the hepatic artery concentrate in the peripheral region of the tumor and give high doses of radiation to the tumor [40]. Radiation is lethal for cancer cells when given at the appropriate dose. Radiation tolerance of hepatocyte cells is less than that of cancer cells, so tumor dosimetry is very important in this kind of treatment application. Table 1.10 shows the general characteristics of commercially available microsphere-based radiopharmaceuticals used in routine nuclear medicine applications [41, 42].

Table 1.10 Radiopharmaceuticals used in routine applications of radioembolization

Features	QuiremSpheres®	TheraSphere®	SIR-Spheres®
Material	PLLA (polylactic acid)	Glass	Resin
Radionuclide	Ho-166	Y-90	Y-90
γ energy (keV)	81	None	None
β-energy (MEV)	1.77	2.28	2.28
Diameter (μm)	30 ± 5	25 ± 10	32 ± 10
Activity (Bq)/microsphere	≤450	~2500	~75
Number of particles	33 million	4 million	50 million
Density (g/ml)	1.4	3.3	1.6
Biodegradability	PLLA, biodegradable	Glass, non-biodegradable	Resin, biodegradable

Table 1.11 Radiopharmaceuticals commonly used in routine applications of radiosynovectomy

Radiopharmaceutical	Application site	Applied activity (MBq)	Particle size (nm)
^{90}Y-silicate/citrate	Knee	185	10–100
^{186}Re-sulfite	Hip, shoulder & elbow, ankle	74–185 & 74	5–10
^{32}P-colloid	Knee, elbow, ankle	11–74	500–2000
^{169}Er-citrate	Foot-hand joints	37	10

1.5.7 Radiosynovectomy

Radiosynovectomy is a treatment method applied by intraarticular injection of radiopharmaceuticals in colloidal (particular) form [43]. When radiopharmaceutical reaches joint space in the colloidal form, it is perceived as a foreign body by the upper layer of the synovial membrane rich in cells and phagocytized by the cells. This means selective irradiation of inflammatory cellular cells. Because of this inflammatory cellular cell proliferation decreases and necrosis occurs [44]. The particulate radiopharmaceuticals to be used in radiosynovectomy should be small enough to be phagocytes and not too large to easily exit the joint (2–10 μm), the energy of the radionuclide to be used should be suitable for the treatment of the inflamed area and should not damage the lower layer of the articular cartilage and the skin. Radionuclide+particle binding should be stable and radioactive particles should not be toxic. Applied radioactive particles should be distributed homogeneously within the joint [45]. Table 1.11 summarizes the radiopharmaceuticals commonly used in routine applications of radiosynovectomy [44].

References

1. Ercan MT, Caglar M. Therapeutic radiopharmaceuticals. Curr Pharm Des. 2000;6:1085–121.
2. Doan CA, Wiseman BK. Radioactive phosphorus, p32; a six-year clinical evaluation of internal radiation therapy. J Lab Clin Med. 1947;32:943–69.
3. Hoefnagel CA. Radionuclide therapy revisited. Eur J Nucl Med. 1991;18:408–31.
4. Yeong C-H, Cheng M, Ng K-H. Therapeutic radionuclides in nuclear medicine: current and future prospects. J Zhejiang Univ Sci B China. 2014;15:845–63.
5. Brechbiel MW. Bifunctional chelates for metal nuclides. Q J Nucl Med Mol Imaging. 2008;52:166–73.
6. Price EW, Orvig C. Matching chelators to radiometals for radiopharmaceuticals. Chem Soc Rev. 2014;43:260–90.
7. Srivastava SC. Therapeutic radionuclides: making the right choice BT. In: Mather SJ, editor. Current directions in radiopharmaceutical research and development. Dordrecht: Springer Netherlands; 1996. p. 63–79. https://doi.org/10.1007/978-94-009-1768-2_4.
8. Martins CD, Kramer-Marek G, Oyen WJG. Radioimmunotherapy for delivery of cytotoxic radioisotopes: current status and challenges. Expert Opin Drug Deliv Engl. 2018;15:185–96.
9. Vosoughi S, Shirvani-Arani S, Bahrami-Samani A, Salek N, Jalilian AR. Production of no-carrier-added Ho-166 for targeted therapy purposes. Iran J Nucl Med. 2017;25:15–20. Available from: http://irjnm.tums.ac.ir/article_23655.html

10. Rubini G, Nicoletti A, Rubini D, Asabella AN. Radiometabolic treatment of bone-metastasizing cancer: from 186rhenium to 223radium. Cancer Biother Radiopharm. 2014;29:1–11.
11. Knapp FF, Dash A. Therapeutic radionuclides decay with particle emission for therapeutic applications BT. In: Knapp FF, Dash A, editors. Radiopharmaceuticals for therapy. New Delhi: Springer India; 2016. p. 25–35. https://doi.org/10.1007/978-81-322-2607-9_2.
12. Dekempeneer Y, Keyaerts M, Krasniqi A, Puttemans J, Muyldermans S, Lahoutte T, et al. Targeted alpha therapy using short-lived alpha-particles and the promise of nanobodies as targeting vehicle. Expert Opin Biol Ther Engl. 2016;16:1035–47.
13. Lacoeuille F, Arlicot N, Faivre-Chauvet A. Targeted alpha and beta radiotherapy: an overview of radiopharmaceutical and clinical aspects. Méd Nucl. 2018;42:32–44. Available from: http://www.sciencedirect.com/science/article/pii/S0928125817303819
14. Geerlings MW, Kaspersen FM, Apostolidis C, van der Hout R. The feasibility of 225Ac as a source of alpha-particles in radioimmunotherapy. Nucl Med Commun Engl. 1993;14:121–5.
15. Pozzi OR, Zalutsky MR. Radiopharmaceutical chemistry of targeted radiotherapeutics, Part 3: Alpha-particle- induced radiolytic effects on the chemical behavior of (211)At. J Nucl Med. 2007;48:1190–6.
16. de Kruijff RM, Wolterbeek HT, Denkova AG. A critical review of alpha radionuclide therapy-how to deal with recoiling daughters? Pharmaceuticals (Basel). 2015;8:321–36.
17. Das T, Pillai MRA. Options to meet the future global demand of radionuclides for radionuclide therapy. Nucl Med Biol. 2013;40:23–32.
18. Srivastava S, Dadachova E. Recent advances in radionuclide therapy. Semin Nucl Med. 2001;31:330–41.
19. Volkert WA, Goeckeler WF, Ehrhardt GJ, Ketring AR. Therapeutic radionuclides: production and decay property considerations. J Nucl Med. 1991;32:174–85.
20. Srivastava SC, Mausner LF. Therapeutic radionuclides: production, physical characteristics, and applications BT. In: Baum RP, editor. Therapeutic nuclear medicine. Berlin, Heidelberg: Springer; 2014. p. 11–50. https://doi.org/10.1007/174_2012_782.
21. Argyrou M, Valassi A, Andreou M, Lyra M. Dosimetry and therapeutic ratios for Rhenium-186 HEDP. ISRN Mol Imaging. 2013;2013:1–6. Available from: http://www.hindawi.com/journals/isrn/2013/124603/%0Ahttps://www.hindawi.com/archive/2013/124603/
22. Argyrou M, Valassi A, Andreou M, Lyra M. Rhenium-188 production in hospitals, by w-188/re-188 generator, for easy use in radionuclide therapy. Int J Mol Imaging. 2013;2013:290750.
23. Pillai MRA, Dash A, Knapp FFJ. Rhenium-188: availability from the (188)W/(188)Re generator and status of current applications. Curr Radiopharm. 2012;5:228–43.
24. Bhattacharyya S, Dixit M. Metallic radionuclides in the development of diagnostic and therapeutic radiopharmaceuticals. Dalton Trans. 2011;40:6112–28.
25. Wike JS, Guyer CE, Ramey DW, Phillips BP. Chemistry for commercial scale production of yttrium-90 for medical research. Int J Rad Appl Instrum A. 1990;41:861–5.
26. Ely TS. Maximum permissible body burdens and maximum permissible concentrations of radionuclides in air and in water for occupational exposure: recommendations of the National Committee on Radiation Protection. J Occup Environ Med. 1960:2. Available from: https://journals.lww.com/joem/Fulltext/1960/09000/MAXIMUM_PERMISSIBLE_BODY_BURDENS_AND_MAXIMU M.15.aspx
27. Knapp FF, Dash A. Radionuclide generator systems represent convenient production systems to provide therapeutic radionuclides BT. In: Knapp FF, Dash A, editors. Radiopharmaceuticals for therapy. New Delhi: Springer India; 2016. p. 131–57. https://doi.org/10.1007/978-81-322-2607-9_7.
28. Pillai MRA, Chakraborty S, Das T, Venkatesh M, Ramamoorthy N. Production logistics of 177Lu for radionuclide therapy. Appl Radiat Isot Incl Data, Instrum Methods Use Agric Ind Med. 2003;59:109–18.
29. Boll RA, Malkemus D, Mirzadeh S. Production of actinium-225 for alpha particle mediated radioimmunotherapy. Appl Radiat Isot INCL Data Instrum Methods Use Agric Ind Med. 2005;62:667–79.
30. Engle JW. The production of Ac-225. Curr Radiopharm. 2018;11:173–9.
31. Marzo K. Radiopharmaceuticals for therapy of thyroid diseases BT. In: Bombardieri E, Seregni E, Evangelista L, Chiesa C, Chiti A, editors. Clinical applications of nuclear medicine targeted therapy. Cham: Springer International Publishing; 2018. p. 19–23. https://doi.org/10.1007/978-3-319-63067-0_2.
32. Larson SM, Carrasquillo JA, Cheung N-K V, Press OW. Radioimmunotherapy of human tumours. Nat Rev Cancer. 2015;15:347. Nature Publishing Group, a division of Macmillan Publishers Limited. All Rights Reserved. https://doi.org/10.1038/nrc3925.
33. Aghevlian S, Boyle AJ, Reilly RM. Radioimmunotherapy of cancer with high linear energy transfer (LET) radiation delivered by radionuclides emitting alpha-particles or Auger electrons. Adv Drug Deliv Rev. 2017;109:102–18.
34. Opalinska M, Hubalewska-Dydejczyk A, Sowa-Staszczak A. Radiolabeled peptides: current and new perspectives. Q J Nucl Med Mol Imaging. 2017;61:153–67.
35. Reubi JC, Macke HR, Krenning EP. Candidates for peptide receptor radiotherapy today and in the future. J Nucl Med. 2005;46(Suppl 1):67S–75S.

36. Okarvi SM. Peptide-based radiopharmaceuticals: future tools for diagnostic imaging of cancers and other diseases. Med Res Rev. 2004;24:357–97.
37. Pandit-Taskar N, Larson SM, Carrasquillo JA. Bone-seeking radiopharmaceuticals for treatment of osseous metastases, Part 1: alpha therapy with 223Ra-dichloride. J Nucl Med. 2014;55:268–74.
38. Das T, Banerjee S. Radiopharmaceuticals for metastatic bone pain palliation: available options in the clinical domain and their comparisons. Clin Exp Metastasis. 2017;34:1–10.
39. Henriksen G, Fisher DR, Roeske JC, Bruland OS, Larsen RH. Targeting of osseous sites with alpha-emitting 223Ra: comparison with the beta-emitter 89Sr in mice. J Nucl Med. 2003;44:252–9.
40. Kim H-C. Radioembolization for the treatment of hepatocellular carcinoma. Clin Mol Hepatol. 2017;23:109–14. The Korean Association for the Study of the Liver. https://doi.org/10.3350/cmh.2017.0004.
41. Sangro B, Inarrairaegui M, Bilbao JI. Radioembolization for hepatocellular carcinoma. J Hepatol. 2012;56:464–73.
42. Smits MLJ, Nijsen JFW, van den Bosch MAAJ, Lam MGEH, Vente MAD, Mali WPTM, et al. Holmium-166 radioembolisation in patients with unresectable, chemorefractory liver metastases (HEPAR trial): a phase 1, dose- escalation study. Lancet Oncol Engl. 2012;13:1025–34.
43. Cwikla JB, Zbikowski P, Kwiatkowska B, Buscombe JR, Sudol-Szopinska I. Radiosynovectomy in rheumatic diseases. J Ultrason. 2014;14:241–51.
44. Ahmad I, Nisar H. Dosimetry perspectives in radiation synovectomy. Phys Med. 2018;47:64–72.
45. Melichar F, Kropacek M, Srank J, Beran M, Mirzajevova M, Zimova J, et al. Labelled compounds as radiopharmaceuticals for radiosynoviorthesis. J Radioanal Nucl Chem. 2009;280:353–8.

2 Physical Bases of Radionuclide Therapy (Biological Effects and Properties of Particle Radiation)

Mustafa Demir

The use of radionuclides in cancer treatment is dramatically increasing day by day with effective and promising outcomes. Radionuclide treatment and dose planning usually start after scintigraphic imaging of primary or metastatic cancer foci in the entire body. Thus, both scintigraphy with gamma camera and positron emission tomography (PET) are of great importance to determine the treatment type and evaluate the success of therapy. The ongoing technological developments have played a key role in expanding variable scintigraphy procedures and radionuclide treatment. Nowadays, PET/CT, PET/MRI, and SPECT/CT are the most modern multidisciplinary systems used for lesions detection and staging cancer in nuclear medicine.

While the idea of scintigraphic imaging was being under research, I-131 radioisotope was early used in 1950s for thyroid cancer treatment. The idea of scintigraphy became real with the invention of gamma camera in 1957 named after Hall Anger. Anger's gamma camera was designed to display images from Tc-99 m with 140 keV gamma rays. Besides, further efforts were exerted to usefully detect gamma rays with high energy like I-131 (364 keV). Later, rectilinear scanners and special collimators were invented for the purpose of detecting high-energy photons with high-quality images. Improvement of the imaging techniques persistently continued in line with the production of high-capacity and fast computers until the second period of 1980s. Significant advances have been made since early 1990s in the radionuclide treatment of cancer. Thus, nuclear medicine has become an important stream in the diagnosis and therapy of diseases [1].

Radiopharmaceuticals in radionuclide treatment are demonstrated under three main headings. First,: the appropriate physical properties of the radionuclide, second: radiation-interacting cell sensitivity, third: is the molecule that carries any given radionuclide to the tumor, i.e., the biological agent. So, today's modern nuclear medicine is a multidisciplinary science joining these three features. Dosimetry-based therapy is usually performed by health physicists for more accuracy and specificity in radionuclide treatment and therapeutic activity determination. Identifying bioactive agents and labeling radiopharmaceuticals is the responsibility of the radiopharmaceutical department [2].

In this section, the basic radiobiological criteria used in radionuclide treatment will be discussed in addition to the mechanisms of radiation interaction with living cells and physical parameters.

M. Demir (✉)
Cerrahpasa Medical Faculty, Department of Nuclear Medicine, Istanbul University-Cerrahpasa, Istanbul, Turkey
e-mail: demirm@iuc.edu.tr

R. Bekiş et al. (eds.), *Radionuclide Therapy*, https://doi.org/10.1007/978-3-030-97220-2_2

2.1 Formation and Physical Properties of Particle Radiation

Radiation is defined as the energy released from the atom. Energy release from atoms is caused by the nucleus disintegration or/and changing the electrons' location through the energy levels around the nucleus. These rules are considered basic nuclear physics. The more stable atom is related to the closer number of proton and neutron numbers in the nucleus. As the number of neutrons or protons differs from each other, the stability in the atom is disrupted. Atoms are stable when the neutron/proton ratio is <1.5, the natural radiation occurs with neutron/proton ratio ≥2.5, while the artificial radiation occurs if the neutron/proton ratio is 1.5–2.5 [3].

Radionuclides used in diagnosis and therapy are produced by bombarding slowed down thermal neutrons toward a specific target (U-135) in the reactor core. This event leads to increasing the number of neutrons in the target and starting nuclear disintegration. As the neutron/proton ratio in the target increases, the energies of the resulting radiation increase.

Alpha (α) and/or beta (β) radiation are released from the nucleus as a result of nuclear decay. After releasing amount of energy, the core may or may not reach the rest point. In case that the atoms are still unstable following α or β emission, gamma (γ) radiation is emanated to bring the atom to the stable state. Briefly summarized; core instability leads to nuclear disintegration. In this event, α, β, and γ radiation are simultaneously released. β particles are divided into two types according to their charge; these are (−) charged betas (β^-) and (+) charged betas (β^+). β^- particles are negatively charged electrons commonly used in radionuclide treatment. The β^+ particle is a positively charged electron (positron) used for diagnostic purposes in positron emission tomography (PET). Gamma radiation is released rather than from the nucleus decay, but further emissions arise from the nuclear excitation. In this case, the proton within the nucleus or some of the neutrons are excited due to gaining new energy. Then, the excited particle moves from its basic energy level to higher energy levels. Here, the excess energy is emitted as gamma photons when the excited particle returns back to its basic energy level.

Two modes of energy release are noted in this case: (1) Mono-energetic, it occurs in a single transition between two energy states, and (2) multi-energetic gamma emissions occur with multiple transitions between different energy levels. α and β are emitted in radioactive disintegration due to proton and neutron imbalance within the nucleus. Only one or both of these particles may be released. However, these particles are associated with gamma photon emission. For example, Y-90 is a radionuclide that decays into stable isotope Zr-90. Meanwhile, monoenergetic β^- particles are released with average and maximum energy of 930 keV and 2284 keV, respectively. Lu-177 decays into stable Hf-177 by emitting monoenergetic β^- particles with maximum energy of 497 keV (76.8% yield) and two different gamma energies of 113 keV (6% yield) and 208 keV (11% yield) (Table 2.1). Overall, performing scintigraphy by detecting gamma rays controls the implementation of targeted radionuclide therapy (TRT).

2.2 Selection of Radionuclide in Targeted Radionuclide Therapy

1. *Properties of Particle Radiation:* Particle radiation such as α, β^-, and auger electrons is of great therapeutic efficacy in radionuclide treatment. Particularly, β^- particle is well known with the common use and highest effect. These particles create strong destruction to the biological systems at a certain dose. Therefore, particle radiation is widely used in cancer treatment. Commonly, β^- particles with energy <1 MeV are used for treating leukemia, lymphoma, and metastases, while β^- particles with energy >1 MeV are used for solid tumors therapy [4].

   The energy imparted from the radiation source at the path distance is called linear energy transfer (LET). α and β particles with

Table 2.1 Radioisotopes used in radionuclide treatment and some physical properties

	Main emissions (keV)			Half-life	
Radionuclide	Alpha	Beta	Gamma		Penetration in tissue
P-32	–	1710	14.3	14.3 d	8.7 mm
Sr-89	–	1212	–	1212 h	8.0 mm
Y-90	–	2284	–	2.67 d	11.3 mm
I-131	–	606	364	8.04 d	2.3 mm
Sm-153	–	805	103	1.93 d	3.0 mm
Ho-166	–	1850	81	1.13 d	8.5 mm
Er-169	–	340	–	9.3 d	1.0 mm
Lu-177	–	497	113, 208	6.7 d	1.8 mm
Re-186	–	1070	137	3.8 d	4.5 mm
Re-188	–	2120	155	0.7 d	5 mm
Au-198	–	960	411	2.7 d	3.6 mm
Bi-212	6000	2000	–	1.0 h	90 μm
Bi-213	5800	1400	–	0.7 h	84 μm
At-211	5900	–	–	7.21 h	60 μm
Ac-225	5700	–	–	11.4 d	–
Ra-223	5780	–	–	273.6 h	<0.01 mm
Tb-149	4000	–	–	4.1 h	–
Th-226	6000	–	–	0.5 h	–
Th-227	4488	–	–	6.0 h	–

mm: millimeter, μm: micro meter, d: day, h: hour

charge and mass have high LET, while X-rays and γ-rays with photon characteristic transmit energy with low LET.

In other words, α and β particles deposit their total energy in short range and disappear. α particles LET is ~80 keV/μm; 0.2–2.0 keV/μm for β particles; and 4–26 keV/μm for auger electrons. α particles have high energy transfer and causes enormous damage in the target. So, when it interacts with DNA molecule, double-strand breakage occurs and irreversibly 2–3 consecutive cells will be destroyed.

β^- particles have LET lower than α particles and density of 100–1000. β^- are required to achieve the same effect as α particles (Table 2.2). So, β^- particles are used in TRT to reach farther distances within the tissue. The range of β^- particles is usually 10 mm depending on the particle energy. Often, high-energy beta particles might escape from the tumor toward the surrounding healthy cells leading to a particular level of damage known as (Bystander effect). So, average energy of <1 MeV is preferentially applied in TRT to minimize the cells destruction related to Bystander effect [5].

2. *Tumor Size and Heterogeneity*: The extent of α particles in the biological tissues is generally 50–100 μm taking into consideration the radionuclide pharmacokinetics and biodistribution in the targeted organ. Thus, α particles provide effective treatment for micrometastases of medium-sized neoplasms [6]. Alpha particles have high LETs and emit 80–300 keV/μm energy on the paths. Due to the short range of α particles, further damage to the healthy tissue compartments is negligible. In contrast, β^- particles have relatively similar properties. That makes high ionization in the tissue at a distance of 2–3 mm with respect to the corresponding energy. As tumor size decreases, the impact of α and β^- particles increases in the treatment outcome.
3. *Half-life of Radionuclide:* Radionuclides with physical half-life between 6 h and 8 days are commonly used in TRT except Sr-89 (half-life 50 days). In clinical practice, radioisotope elimination from the organism or targeted tis-

Table 2.2 Radioactive decay properties of particle radiation used in TRT

Characteristic	Beta emission	Alpha emission	Low energy electron decay
Emission	Negatively charged electron	Helium nucleus	Auger electrons
Energy	0.05–2.5 Mev	2–10 MeV	10 ev–10 Kev
Range	0.2–15 mm	50–100 μm	Nanometer
Ionization	Low	High	Small intensity in tissue
LET	0.2 keV/μm	80–300 keV/μm	4–26 keV/μm
Mechanism	Crossfire effect	Nuclear transition	Breaking DNA (bystander effect)
Relative biologic effectiveness	Low	High	Low
requirement	Cell surface/near to target	Binding to cancer cells	Fusion with the cell nucleus
Crossfire effect	Yes	No	No

sue is accomplished through two important components, biological and physical decay. Both physical and biological elimination occur simultaneously.

The amount of time needed to eliminate the activity to the half involving physical (Tf) and biological (Tb) elimination is called effective half-life (Tef). These three variables are expressed in the following mathematical eq. 1/Teff = 1/Tf + 1/Tb. Physical decay of any given radionuclide is constant. For example, the physical half-life of Lu-177 radionuclide is 6.7 days. But the biological half-life varies between the organisms and the body organs making the effective half-life variable as well. Consequently, the variation in the effective half-life among the individuals stands beyond the necessity to determine the therapeutic activity in TRT according to patient-specific data [7]. The amount of radiopharmaceutical activity to be administered to patients should be based on the tolerated dose of the most critical organs. Red marrow and kidneys are deemed the basic organs at risk in radionuclide therapy. Therefore, dosimetry-based therapy usually implies red marrow <2 Gy and kidneys dose <23 Gy as limited safe doses. Red marrow dose can be estimated from blood samples, while organs dose can be calculated from multiple scintigraphic images (at least 4 consecutive days). Dosimetry calculations can be performed based on MIRD formulas. In MIRD formula;

$$D_h = \sum_k \tilde{A}_k S(h \leftarrow k)$$

(*D*) target organ dose, (*Ă*) cumulative activity: area under time-activity curve in the organs, and (*S*) dose values from the source to the target. There are some software programs developed to facilitate calculations via MIRD formula. The most common among these is OLINDA EXAM.

4. *Chemical Purity of Radionuclide:* Radionuclides used in TRT should be with high degree of chemical purity, free of contaminating isotopes and radiopharmaceutical, and absence of carrier molecules containing metal radionuclides during radiopharmaceutical labeling. Lu-177 is the most commonly used radionuclide in TRT. The ratio of heavy metals which cause impurities in Lu-177 like Cu and Pb should be <0.1 μg/GBq and also Fe and Zn <1.0 0.1 μg/GBq. Impurities of Y-90 is existent as Y-91 (<0.99 × 10^{-4} kBq/mg) and Y-88 (<6.3 × kBq/mg).
5. *Radionuclides with* β^- and Gamma Emission: Patient-specific dosimetry in TRT and t determination of the maximum safe activity ensure the effectiveness and safety of treatment. Organ dosimetry is calculated from scintigraphic images relying on γ rays detection.

The ideal gamma energy is 140 keV. However, wide energy range 70–300 keV is also used in nuclear medicine.

6. *The Ability of Radionuclide to Bind with Carrier Molecules*: The labeled radiopharmaceuticals should remain stable for a long time with the body fluids, and not be metabolized in a short time.
7. *Cost of Radiopharmaceutical Used in TRT*: Low prices are the desired priorities for common usage of radiopharmaceutical materials in the medical field.

   β^- emitting radionuclides such as I-131 and Y-90 account for around 90% of the daily TRT. The current methods of radionuclides production used in TRT are nuclear reactors, accelerators, and radionuclide generators.

2.3 Determination of Maximum Tolerable Dose in Targeted Radionuclide Therapy and Dosimetry

There is certain confusion in the literature about the concept of dose. The term dose refers to the radiation energy absorbed by the body, expressed in Gray units. However, the concept of dose is incorrectly expressed as the amount of administered activity to the patient. The unit of radionuclide activity administered to the patient is expressed as Ci (Curie) or GBq. To avoid this confusion, if the intended concept is radiation dose" or "absorbed dose, the unit to express is Gy (Gray), but if the amount of activity is the intended expression, it is appropriate to specify the unit as Ci or GBq.

Body organs and tissues have a certain level of radiosensitivity. Organs overexposure to above threshold dose may temporarily or permanently impair the organs function. Organs that relatively lose function at certain dose values are called "critical organs". The maximum amount of dose that organs can receive without degrading function is called the "maximum tolerable dose". Critical organs and maximum tolerable dose are determined in targeted radionuclide treatments as in external radiation therapy. For example, 2 Gy for red bone marrow, 23 Gy for kidneys, and 27 Gy for lungs [8–10].

The aim of computing the maximum tolerable dose in TRT is to deliver lethal effective dose to the tumor without exceeding the dose tolerance of the critical healthy organs. Biokinetics of radionuclide may vary from patient to patient, while the critical organs remain fixed. For instance, in radioiodine treatment of thyroid cancer, thyroid uptake values are variable among the patients and the effective half-life is therefore uneven. Uptake values are measured separately for each patient in both ablation and organ dosimetry. Scintigraphic images are required for organ dosimetry and blood samples are necessary for estimating red marrow self-dose. As a result, the obtained data are processed in dosimetric calculations to determine the maximum safe activity that can be safely applied to the patient without critical organs toxicity. Then the assigned activity is measured by the dose calibrator and finally administered to the patient.

The maximum tolerable dose is determined by a comprehensive statistical study [10]. In order to determine the maximum amount of safe activity in TRT, the patient is subjected to dosimetry by giving tracer activity of the required radionuclide. Routinely, there are two methods for determining the therapeutic activity, empirical method, and dosimetry-based method. Despite the empirical dose method is easy to apply, different results can be obtained when the same amounts of activity are applied to the patients with similar histopathological characteristics. In the dosimetry method, the maximum safe iodine activity can be determined by the patient's realistic data. The tolerated doses should be taken into consideration for safe and effective dosimetry such as: <2 Gy to bone marrow, 300–350 Gy to residual tissue, and 80–100 Gy to distant metastases. MIRD method is broadly used in dosimetric calculations.

The above-mentioned method (Lu-177 dosimetry) is also used for radioiodine dosimetry. As a result, the amount of radiopharmaceutical activity determined with individualized dosimetry is specifically applied for patient treatment. Organ doses can be estimated after quantifying many scintigraphic images at variable time marks. Therefore, gamma-emitting radionuclides are suitable for achieving accurate dosimetry. Some of the radionuclides used in TRT emit β^- particles and gamma rays. For example, I-131 has 606 keV β^- and 364 keV γ rays.

Lu-177 has been usefully used for therapy and dosimetry. Currently, it has been used to treat prostate cancer with respect to its beta emission, and gamma rays of 208 keV (11% yield) and 113 keV (6% yield). Furthermore, Y-90 is a radionuclide with only β^- emission and therefore another radioactive material with gamma rays and similar biodistribution and biokinetic should be employed for performing dosimetry. Tc-99 m MAA (macro aggregate albumin) is used in Y-90 dose planning and overall dosimetry for the treatment of liver tumors. Alternatively, Y-90 has very low yield (32/1,000,000) of annihilation photons that can be imaged with PET. So, PET scan is also suitable for imaging and dosimetric procedures after Y-90 therapy. Also, Y-90 has a maximum efficiency of 110 keV (range: 75–160 keV) Bremsstrahlung radiation (braking radiation), i.e., X-rays. Accordingly, Y-90 can be also acquired by gamma camera with bremsstrahlung radiation detection. This kind of imaging allows dosimetry after Y-90 therapy [11]. Whereas, dosimetry procedures are routinely carried out using Tc-99 m MAA before Y-90 treatment.

2.4 Physical Properties of Alpha (α) Particle

Alpha particles are same as helium atom (^4_2He) with 2 protons and 2 neutrons. The only difference between them is the presence of external orbital electrons in the helium atom and the neutral state. Since alpha has 2 protons, the particle is defined with +2 charge. Alpha particle can ionize an atom by pulling 2 electrons from the outer orbits creating strong ionization in the environment. α-particle is 7400 times heavier than electrons and it loses 34 eV energy per ionization in the air. In other words, 34 MeV α-particle leads to 100,000 ionization events in the air.

Kinetic energy emitted by alpha particles is generally between 4 and 8 MeV. This energy enables alpha particle to move around 4 cm in air. In tissue, this distance is so shorter about 0.003 mm. Thus, it is not possible for alpha particle to transmit through the skin. But, it leaves all of its energy creating strong ionization in the same place. Superiorly, the physical properties of alpha particles enhance their efficiency in the treatment of cancers especially with micrometastases [12].

After alpha decay, the mass number of the atom decreases by 4 and the atomic number decreases by 2 electrons. This event is schematically shown below

$$^{A}_{Z}Y \rightarrow {}^{A-4}_{Z-2}Y + {}^{4}_{2}\mathrm{He}$$

2.5 Physical Properties of Beta (β) Particle

Beta particles are classified into positron (β^+) and electron (β^-). In fact, these two particles have the same characteristics except opposite charges. β^- particle is used in TRT and generated during the disintegration of the nucleus due to the excess of neutrons. This disintegration involves transforming one neutron (n) into a proton (p), where β^- and neutrino particles are released sometime (Fig. 2.1). β^- particles are released from the nucleus with particular kinetic energy. The collision of electrons with atoms and/or molecules on its path causes removing electrons from the orbits. During this event, the energy of β^-particle gradually decreases, and eventually the electron oscillates and disappears with transferring the atom into another type.

Mathematical analysis of nuclear disintegration due to excess of neutrons;

$$n^0 \rightarrow p^+ + \beta^- + \nu + \text{energy}$$

As shown in the above relation, the atomic number and proton number increase in the disintegrated atom due to excess electron.

$$^{A}_{Z}X \rightarrow {}^{A}_{Z+1}Y + \beta^-$$

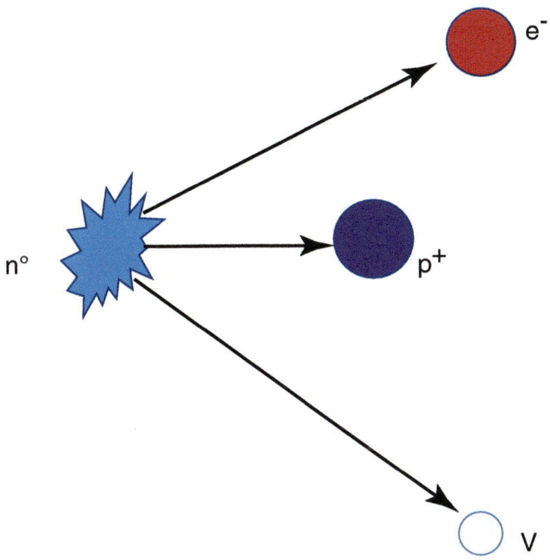

Fig. 2.1 Nuclear decay and (−) charged beta particle (e^-) release. n^o: neutron, p^+: proton, v: neutrino

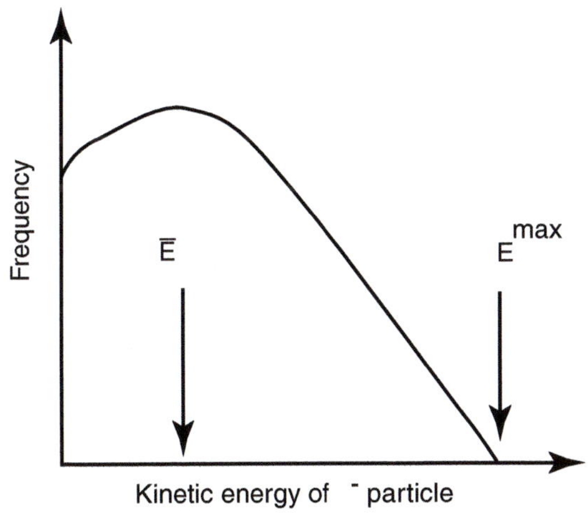

Fig. 2.2 β^- particle energy spectrum

Again, β^- particles released by the nucleus have dissimilar energies and the energy differences are represented by β^- energy spectrum (Fig. 2.2).

The average energy of β^- particle is approximately equal to one-third of the maximum energy ($1/3E^{\beta max}$). In practice, mean energy corresponding to about one-third the maximum energy of the β^- particle is the highest yield and energy. For example, the maximum β^- energy of Y-90 is 2286 keV and the emitted particles can travel about 11 mm in the tissue. The average energy of the same β^- particles is around 937 keV and roughly travel 2–3 mm through the tissue.

β^- particles can be classified into three groups according to the average energy:

(a) *Low energy β^- emitters*: Average energy of 80,180 keV with distance range 0.4–0.9 mm. These radionuclides are suitable for small tumors treatment. I-131 and Lu-177 are common examples with important clinical use. Rh-105 is another candidate radionuclide within this group.
(b) *Moderate energy β^- emitters*: Mean beta energy is about 180–500 keV and the average range in tissue is 0.9–3.0 mm. Those can provide ideal energy for the treatment of targets within 1–2 mm diameter, e.g., Sm-153, Re-186, Pr-143, As-77 radionuclides.
(c) *High-energy β^- emitters*: β^- average energies 500–1000 keV and average range in tissue is 2.2–5 mm. These radionuclides are effective in the treatment of tumors with diameter > 5 cm such as P-32, Sr-89, Y-90, and Re-188 radionuclides.

2.6 Physical and Biological Events in Particle Radiation Interaction with Living Cells

If β^- particle collides with living molecule, the targeted atoms lose electrons due to energy transfer and then turned into ionized atom. In this event, as β^- particle is high energy ionizing radiation, it binds to the living molecule and causes direct ionizations. Thus, the molecule that ejected atomic electron will lose its viability. Moreover, this event frequently occurs in the DNA molecule where a group of nucleotides (adenine, thymine, guanine, or cytosine) are formulating the DNA structure. Once a β^- particle hits nucleotide molecule, the links of the targeted nucleotide are broken down and electrons will be ejected in the interaction. If the energy of β^- particle is sufficient, the energy of the particle decreases slightly and continues striking and ejecting other electrons in the path of the atom. This chain of events per-

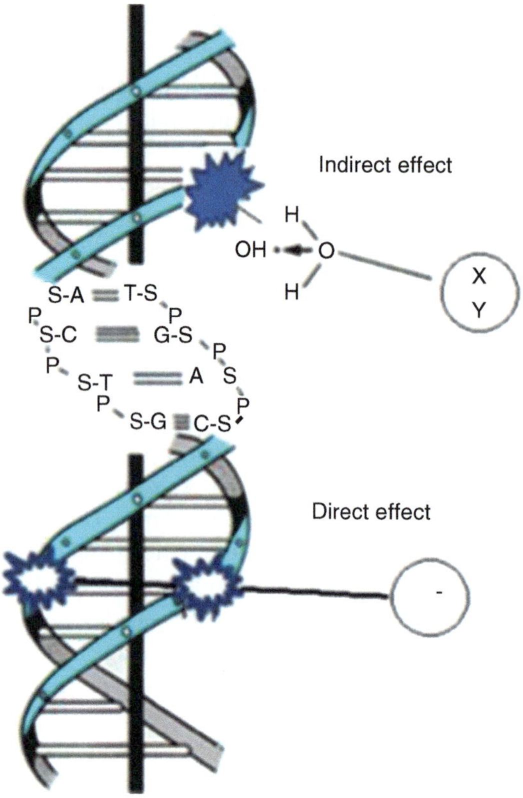

Fig. 2.3 Interaction of X-rays, gamma rays, and beta particles (e^-) with DNA. Electromagnetic radiation like X-ray or gamma interacts with the water molecules and hydrolyze them in an indirect process to dissociated OH^- and H^+. These ions are converted to free radicals with the effect of oxygen. Radical ranges are short and interact with DNA causing damage. Cell repair usually occurs after single-stranded DNA damage. In direct effect, the cell dies because of the broken double-stranded DNA

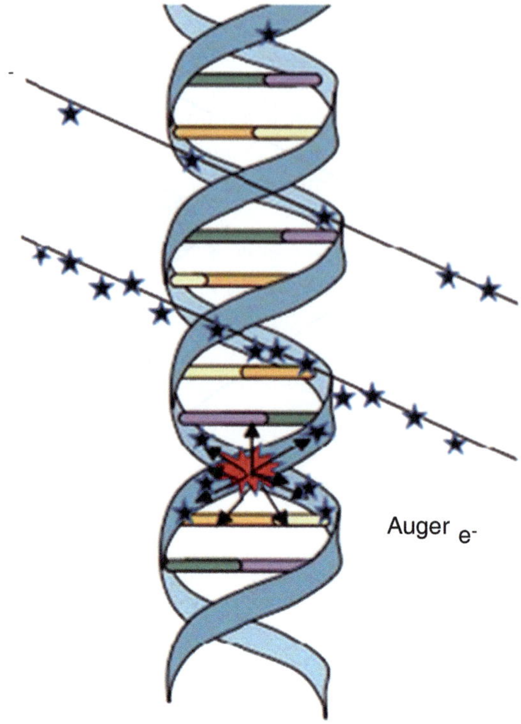

Fig. 2.4 Schematic representation of the ionization intensities of particle radiation along their pathways in DNA. Alpha ionization with high-intensity particles, low-intensity beta particles, and clustered Auger electrons

sists depending on the energy of β^- particle. I-131 is widely used in TRT with a maximum β^- energy of 606 keV. The emitted electrons move 2–3 mm in tissue transferring their energy to the atoms. This leads to ejecting electrons and the atom lacks electron is finally ionized. If the ionized atoms break both of the DNA strands, cell death is possible due to double-stranded DNA breakage. This event is the desired task of β^- particles released in the tumor, and this general concept stands beyond the principle of TRT (Fig. 2.3).

The damage created on the DNA structure depends on the ionizing radiation type and its energy. Linear energy transfers (LET) of alpha particles is high and intensive ionization is therefore produced in short distance after energy transfer to the atoms and electrons. LET of beta particles is less, and the range within the tissue is greater alpha. Therefore, when the electrons are released in tissue, less ionization is created by losing energy less than alpha. In addition, auger electrons regionally clustered causing further ionization in the medium (Fig. 2.4). The use of radionuclides with alpha (α) emission and radioactively labeled somatostatin analogs is a promising technique in TRT. Alpha-emitting radionuclides, such as Bi-213, have shorter range in tissue compared to β^- emitting radionuclides.

Alpha particles range in tissue is about 50–100 μm, which corresponds to approximately two or three cell diameters. The short range of (α) enables energy of the particle to be entirely absorbed within the targeted tissue. The absorbed dose leads to more DNA damage compared to β^- emitters. Another advantage is related to the healthy tissues protection as the corresponding absorbed is trivial. (α) emitting radionuclides have been tried in some studies, e.g., Arterial Bi-213-DOTATOC after Y-90/Lu-177-DOTATOC treatment in a pilot study conducted with seven patients. Promising results were manifested in terms of stability of the disease after 12 months follow-up for all patients. Acute hematotoxicity was less detected compared to β^- emitting radionuclides [13].

The events observed in the ionizing radiation interaction with the living cell are summarized in Table 2.3. X and gamma rays which are used for diagnostic purposes in nuclear medicine basically induce DNA single-strand break due to ionization, or excitations occurring at the atomic level. These events commonly occur in the cell biomolecules producing free radicals which are also produced from DNA, RNA, and proteins damage. These events might last from 10^{-12} s to hours and cancer may develop due to mutations in the next stages.

Ionization usually occurs during the interaction of particle radiation with the living cells and the expected events are given in Fig. 2.5. The

Table 2.3 Events causing radiation damage in living organisms

Initiative reaction (physical level)	Biomolecular damage (chemical level)	Biologic damage (biologic level)
– Radiation release to material – Ionization – Excitation	Free radicals Damage in the nucleic acids and proteins	Cell death, organism death, mutations, and cancer progression
10^{-18} to 10^{-12} s	10^{-12} s to hours	Hours, years

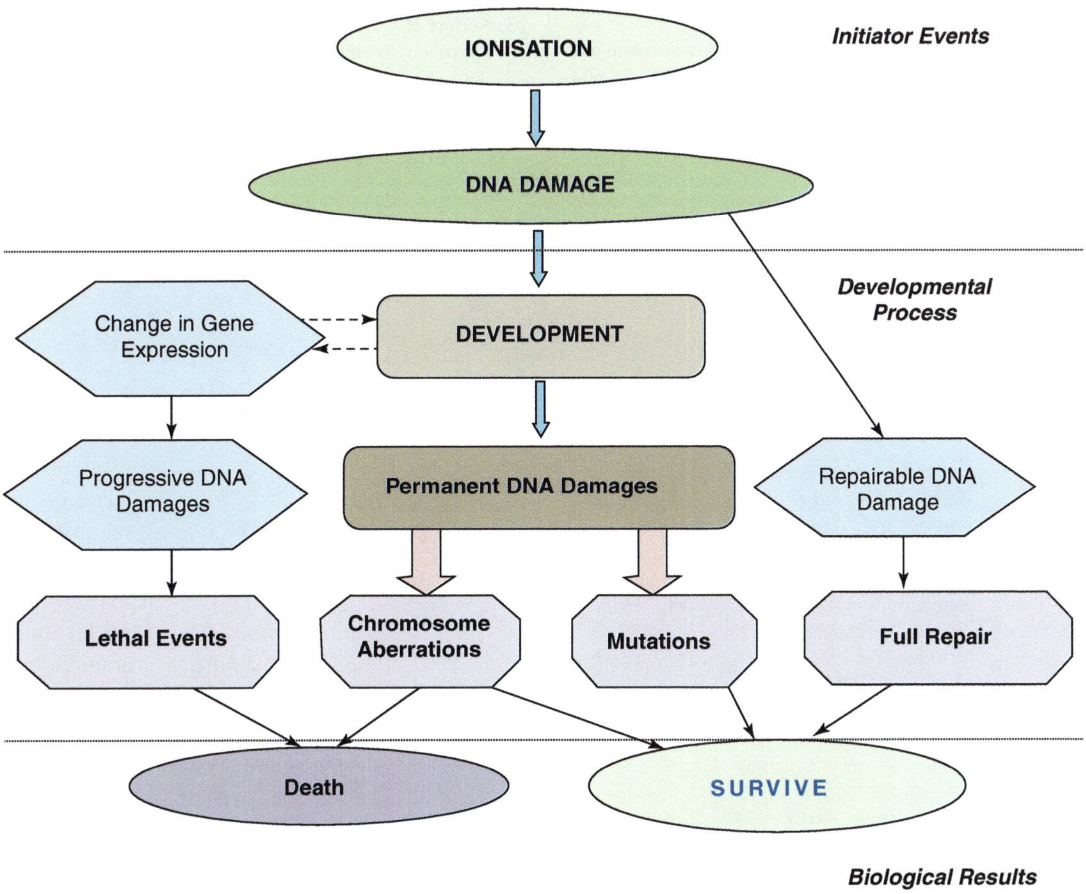

Fig. 2.5 The chain of events determining the cellular radiation sensitivity under the effect of radiation

energies of the utilized radionuclides in TRT mostly leads to DNA double-strand brake. This kind of interaction develops gene or chromosome aberrations as a result of permanent DNA damage and lastly cell death.

This phenomenon was beyond the emergence of TRT as an effective and successive route in cancer treatment.

References

1. Zukotynski K, Jadvar H, Capala J, Fahey F. Targeted radionuclide therapy: practical applications and future prospects. Biomark Cancer. 2016;8:35–8.
2. Kassas AI. Therapeutic radionuclides: biophysical and radiobiologic principles. Semin Nucl Med. 2008;38(5):358–66. https://doi.org/10.1053/j.semnuclmed.2008.05.002.
3. Cherry S, Sorenson J, Phelps M. Physics in nuclear medicine. In: Decay of radioactivity. 4th ed. Philadelphia: Elsevier; 2012. p. 31–43.
4. Jackson MR, Falzone N, Vallis KA. Advances in anticancer radiopharmaceuticals. Clin Oncol. 2013;25:604–9. https://doi.org/10.1016/j.clon.2013.06.004.
5. Kassis AI, Adelstein SJ. Radiobiologic principles in radionuclide therapy. J Nucl Med. 2005;46:4–12.
6. Barendsen GW, Beusker TL, Vergroesen AJ, Budke l. Effects of different radiations on human cells in tissue culture. II. Biological experiments. Radiat Res. 1960;13:841–9.
7. Emami B, Lyman J, Brown A, et al. Tolerance of normal tissue to therapeutic irradiation. Int J Radiat Oncol Biol Phys. 1991;21:109–22.
8. Boice JD, Inskip PD. Radiation-induced leukemia. In: Henderson ES, Lister TA, Greaves, editors. Leukemia. Philadelphia, PA: WB Saunders; 1996. p. 195–209.
9. Bernard BF, Krenning EP, Breeman WA, et al. D-lysine reduction of indium-111 octreotide and yttrium-90 octreotide renal uptake. J Nucl Med. 1997;38(12):1929–33.
10. Waldherr C, Pless M, Maecke HR. Tumor response and clinical benefit in neuroendocrine tumors after 7.4 GBq (90) Y-DOTATOC. J Nucl Med. 2002;43(5):610–6.
11. Shen S, Gerald L. De Nardo, et al. Planar Gamma camera imaging and quantitation of Yttrium-90 Bremsstrahlung. J NucI Med 1994; 35: 1381–1389.
12. Allen BJ. Future prospects for targeted alpha theraphy. Curr Radiopharm. 2001;4:336–42.
13. Seifert RP, Bulkeley W, Zhang L, et al. A practical approach to diagnose soft tissue myeloid sarcoma. Ann Diagn Pathol. 2014;18:253–60. https://doi.org/10.1016/j.anndiagpath.2014.06.001.

3 Fundamentals of Radiation Safety and Dosimetric Approach in Radionuclide Therapy Applications

Suna Kıraç

The use of radionuclides in the treatment coincides with the early 1900s after the discovery of radioactivity. After this date, radionuclides have been frequently used in the treatment of benign and malignant diseases. Henri Becquerel's discovery that the radium in his pocket which he carried for a short time caused inflammation of the skin has led to the development of the idea that radionuclides can be used in treatment. Radium was first used in the local treatment of tuberculous skin lesions and tumors and subsequently it was used systematically in 1921. With the development of new targeted radiopharmaceuticals in the following years, radionuclides have found a wide application area in the treatment of painful bone metastases, liver tumors, lymphomas, and neuroendocrine tumors (NET); and targeted radionuclide (RN) treatment has become one of the most preferred methods in cancer treatment. Many RNs such as Iodine-131 (I-131), Phosphorus-32 (P-32), Strontium-90 (Sr-90), and Samarium-153 (Sm-153) are successfully used in the treatment of benign and malignant diseases nowadays. The RNs for treatment are mostly administered in a fixed dose. However, sometimes therapeutic doses can be calculated according to the patient weight, body surface area, and clinical features. Radiation exposure of non-tumoral tissues is low in the RNT. RN treatment will be useful in the presence of widespread malignant lesions such as distant and diffuse metastases for which external radiation therapy is not possible. In targeted RN treatments, patient-specific treatment and dosimetric approach are essential [1–7].

Nowadays, radiopharmaceuticals that are used for specific targeted therapeutic purposes and also allow diagnostic imaging are called ***theranostics***. The term theranostic is derived from the combination of the words *therapy* and *diagnostic.* Theranostic agents use specific biological pathways in the human body [8]. Keeping it in high concentration in the target tumor tissue, it enables the selection of the effective therapeutic agent for the target and its administration at the appropriate dose. Targeted RN treatments can be co-administered with chemotherapy. For example, administration of Lutetium-177 (Lu-177) DOTATATE with capecitabine (5-fluorouracyl oral form) or capecitabine+temozolomide in gastrointestinal neuroendocrine tumors (NET) treatment will reduce side effects while increasing the effectiveness of therapy, especially in the high-risk cases [9, 10]. The clinical use of theranostics started with the application of I-131 in the diagnosis and treatment of thyroid cancer in the 1940s. In recent years, different theranostics were developed and started to be widely used in RN treatment. For example, Gallium-68 (Ga-68) octreotate in NETs, Lu-177 octreotate, and other Lu-177 somatostatin receptor analogs (SSRA) in the treatment of somatostatin receptor (SSR) carrying tumors, Lu-177 prostate-specific mem-

S. Kıraç (✉)
Faculty of Medicine, Department of Nuclear Medicine, Near East University, Nicosia, Turkey
e-mail: fskirac@yahoo.com

R. Bekiş et al. (eds.), *Radionuclide Therapy*, https://doi.org/10.1007/978-3-030-97220-2_3

brane antigen (PSMA) in the castration-resistant metastatic prostate cancer (CRPC) cases, Yttrium-90 (Y-90) microsphere selective internal radiation therapy (SIRT) for primary hepatic cancer or metastatic liver lesions, I-131 in thyrotoxicosis and thyroid cancer cases, Radium-223 (Ra-223) in the treatment of bone metastases, and Y-90 radiosynovectomy in benign joint diseases are commonly used [3, 5, 8, 10, 11–19]. Physical properties of agents used in radionuclide therapy are presented in Table 3.1. In this section, it is aimed to give information about the selection criteria of RNs used in the treatment of malignant diseases, their side effects, what to consider before and during treatment, radiation exposure dose, and radiation safety issues. General information about radionuclides and radiopharmaceuticals (RP) will be provided and dosimetric approaches will be discussed.

3.1 Factors Affecting Radionuclides and Radiopharmaceuticals Selection to be Used in the Treatment

RNs used in the treatment are effective through different mechanisms. For example, participation in metabolism, peptides, antibodies, and aptamers. Aptamers are single- or double-stranded RNA or DNA oligonucleotide ligands. They allow the combination of specific molecules with the relevant targets and to obtain stable compounds. Aptamers are 8–12 kDa in size and their transition to tumor tissue is fast [8]. I-131 NaI, P-32, and I-131 MIBG are effective by participating in the cell metabolism [2, 4, 9]. Bone-specific agents act like calcium and enter the hydroxyapatite molecule of the bone [3, 5]. In addition to physical properties such as half-life, decay type, radiation type and energy, production method, radionuclidic purity, biochemical properties such as tumoral uptake, toxicity, and preservation of in vivo stability are important features affecting RP selection [8, 12, 20]. The biological half-life of radionuclide is associated with the distribution, uptake, metabolism, and excretion of RN in the body. Effective half-life, which determines internal radiation exposure, can be calculated with the formula **1/te = 1/tp + 1/tb** by using physical and biological half-life. It is preferred that the physical half-life of the RN to be applied in the treatment is between 6 h and 7 days [7, 8]. RNs with very short or very long half-life are not preferred because they will lead to an inability to achieve the desired treatment efficacy or an increase in radiation exposure, respectively. Patient isolation time and length of hospital stay will be prolonged if treated with long-lived RN. If the biological half-life is too short, RP will be rapidly removed from the body and treatment effectiveness will be decreased.

For these reasons, it is desired that RNs to be used in treatment should have the optimum biological half-life [1, 4–8, 12, 15, 20–22]. Other important features that are desired in the RNs to be used in the treatment are to show alpha and beta decay providing short tissue travel (range) and high linear energy transfer (*LET*). Thus, the energy left in the short distance will be high and the destruction of tumor cells will be ensured. In addition, radiation will not be able to reach out of the body and special radiation safety precautions will not be required because the tissue range is very short. However, the treatment with some beta-emitting radionuclides (such as I-131, Sm-153, and Sr-89) should take into account external radiation exposure to the public by gamma rays or bremsstrahlung X-rays. Although tissue penetration rate of gamma and bremsstrahlung X-rays is high and adherence to radiation protection rules requires keeping the patient away from the public for a certain period of time, this feature is an important advantage since it enables post-treatment imaging and dosimetric studies [23–32].

Tumor size is another important factor affecting RN selection for treatment. While beta and alpha particle-emitting RNs are preferred in the treatment of large volume tumors, Auger electrons with very short range in the tissue are used in the treatment of small volume tumors. For example, Y-90 is preferred in the larger tumors due to its higher energy and longer travel distance of beta particles in the tissue. However, Lu-177

Table 3.1 Physical properties of radionuclides used in the radionuclide therapy

Radionuclide	$T_{1/2}$ p (day)	Type of radiation	Max. energy (MeV)	Gamma ray MeV (%)	Range (mm)	Daughter radionuclide
At-211	0.3	Alpha	5.87	0.570 (0.5%) 0.898 (0.5%)	<0.01	Bi-201 (unstable) Pb-207 (stable)
Ac-225	10	Alpha Beta	5.83 1.42	None	<0.01	Fr-221 (unstable) Bi-209 (stable)
Bi-212	0.04	Alpha Beta	10.55 2.25	None	<0.01	Po-212 (unstable) Tl-208 (unstable)
Bi-213	0.03	Beta (97%) Alpha (3%)	1.43	None	<0.01	Po-213 (unstable)
Ho-166	1.1	Beta	1.84	0.081	2.1	Er-166 (stable)
I-131	8.1	Beta	0.61	0.364 (82%)	0.8 (90%)	Xe-131 (stable)
In-111[a]	2.8	EC	None	0.245 (94%) 0.171 (90%) 0.023 (69%)	0.0005–0.0001	Cd-111 (stable)
In-114 m	50	Beta	0.19	0.190 (0.01%)	3.6	Cd-114 (stable)
Lu-177	6.7	Beta	0.50	0.113 (6.5%) 0.208 (11%)	1.7 - 0.23	Hf-177 (stable)
P-32	14.3	Beta	1.70	None	2.7	S-32 (stable)
Pb-212[b]	0.44	Beta	0.33	None	0.05–0.1	Bi-212 (unstable)
Ra-223	11.4	Alpha	5.78	0.154 (1.1%)	<0.01	Pb-207 (stable)
Re-186	3.8	Beta	1.07	0.137 (9%)	4.5	Os-186 (stable)
Re-188	0.7	Beta	2.12	0.155 (15%)	3.5	Os-188 (stable)
Sr-89	50.5	Beta	1.50	0. 910 (0.01%)	6	Y-89 (stable)
Sm-153	1.9	Beta	0.81	0.103 (29%)	2.5	Eu-153 (stable)
Y-90	2.7	Beta	2.27	None	2.5–11	Zr-90 (stable)

[a]It is involved in the treatment with Auger electron

[b]Pb-212 is considered an alpha-emitting agent. It is converted to Bi-212 by beta-negative decay. Bi-212 is an alpha-emitting agent

has a lower beta energy and a shorter range. Its efficacy will be lower than Y-90 in the large volume NETs with heterogeneous SSR distribution. Due to short-acting distance, it is used to treat small-volume NETs which have more homogeneous SSR. De Jong et al. [33] used Y-90 and Lu-177 labeled somatostatin analogs together in the animal model and showed that each RP had a better treatment response than its use alone. Afterward, Y-90/Lu-177 DOTATATE treatment [DUO peptide receptor RN treatment (PRRT)] was administered to 50 patients with diffuse NET disease. It has been shown that efficacy and life expectancy increased after treatment [34]. In the DUO PRRT protocol, Y-90 compound is administered when the tumor is in large volume, Lu-177 compound is used in the treatment after the tumor shrinks. While providing effective treatment, surrounding tissues will be protected from unnecessary radiation exposure.

Physical properties of the daughter product (nuclide) are also important in terms of the radiation dose to be exposed, and the RN used in the treatment should be decayed to the stable daughter nuclide in a short time. Otherwise, the radiation exposure dose will increase due to the radiation coming from the unstable daughter product. For example, the end-product of decay of Sm-153 ($t_{1/2}$ = 46 h; beta-gamma and X-ray emitter) used in the treatment of painful bone metastases is stable Europium-153 (Eu-153). Actinium-225 (Ac-225) decays to unstable Francium-221 (Fr-221) radionuclide via alpha decay (Table 3.1). However, the radiation exposure dose from daughter radionuclide is generally not too high and can be ignored [3, 7, 8, 22, 23, 28, 35–37]. The radiopharmaceutical uptake rate of the tumor cells and retention time in the tissue are other important features that determine the effectiveness of treatment. Tumor-specific agents will be retained less in normal tissues since their uptake rate in tumor cells will be high, and so circulating RP level will be low. Thus, whole-body radiation exposure will decrease while treatment effectiveness increases [4, 7, 8, 12, 19, 38, 39]. Characteristics such as chemical structure, molecular size, pH value, and clearance of the radiopharmaceutical are also important in the selection of the appropriate radiopharmaceutical for treatment [19, 20]. Protein-structured molecules should not be metabolized in the body before reaching the target tissue. Since small-sized molecules (<10 microns) easily enter into the capillary circulation, RPs administered must be of appropriate sized to remain for a long time in tumor cells. Thus, RP will remain within the tumor tissue and whole-body radiation exposure will be prevented. For example, Y-90 microspheres used in the treatment of liver tumors are 20–40 μm in size. It cannot enter the systemic circulation when applied locally (intratumoral) [39, 40]. Similarly, P-32 chromic phosphate, which is administered locally into the joint in the treatment of benign hemophilic arthropathy, cannot enter the systemic circulation. If P-32 sodium phosphate, which is used in the treatment of polycythemia vera, is applied instead of chromic phosphate for radiosynovectomy, it will enter the systemic circulation and lead to bone marrow suppression. Therefore, the selection of appropriate RP in the treatment is a very important issue in terms of therapeutic efficacy and radiation safety [2, 8, 12, 37, 39, 40].

3.2 Indications for Use and Characteristics of Radiopharmaceuticals

3.2.1 Theranostics in the Treatment of Thyroid Cancers

I-131 NaI has been used effectively since the 1940s in the treatment of differentiated thyroid cancers (DTC; papillary carcinoma, follicular carcinoma, hurthle cell carcinoma) with the aim of eliminating post-operative remnant thyroid tissue and metastases. Although its efficacy in treatment has been proven, discussions on the risk of developing beta radiation-related complications in the organs and tissues in which radioactive iodine is retained, metabolized, or excreted (especially bone marrow, salivary glands, lungs, and other organs) still continue. Medullary thyroid carcinoma (MTC; Euro-C-cell tumor) is another type of thyroid gland carcinoma, which is originated from thyroid parafollicular cells (C cells). Medullary thyroid carcinomas account for only 5% of all thyroid carcinomas. Parafollicular cells in the thyroid gland do not have any role in the iodine transport and metabolism. Consequently, unlike differentiated thyroid cancers, I-131 NaI is not an appropriate agent for the treatment of MTCs originating from C cells and considered in the neuroendocrine tumor (NET) group. Since medullary thyroid carcinomas, like other organ NETs, have SSRs especially SSR1 and SSR2 at a lower density, I-123/131 MIBG (metaiodobenzyl guanidine), radionuclide-labeled somatostatin receptor antagonists and agonists (In-111 octreotide, In-111/Y-90 DOTA-lanreotide, Y-90/Lu-177 DOTATATE) have been used in the diagnosis and treatment of MTC in recent years. However, since SSR2 density is low, the response to radiopeptide treatment will be less compared to gastrointestinal NETs [1, 17, 38, 41–48]. In this chapter, I-131 NaI administration in the treatment of DTC will be mainly mentioned and the treatment with radiopeptides will be discussed in detail in the NET section.

I-131 Sodium iodide (I-131 NaI) is the most commonly administered theranostic agent in capsule or liquid form. It is used in the treatment of benign or malignant thyroid diseases. Radioiodine therapy (RAIT) has proven to be a safe and effective method in the treatment of patients diagnosed with differentiated thyroid carcinoma (DTC) after total or near-total thyroidectomy. The efficacy of RAIT is related to the administered dose, the patient's pre-treatment preparation, tumor characteristics, and the stage of the disease. The probability of disease-free life for 10 years after I-131 treatment was reported as 90%. In the newly diagnosed DTC case, I-131 for ablation therapy is mostly administered at a fixed dose of 30–200 mCi (1.11 and 7.4 GBq) according to the risk group (low-risk, moderate-risk, or high-risk patients). In the presence of recurrent disease, the activity to be administered can be calculated to protect the red bone marrow as described in the relevant guidelines or a fixed-dose can be administered [4, 43, 47, 48]. The most important target organs in RAIT are bone marrow, salivary glands, and lungs. Especially in patients with diffuse bone metastases, the maximum reliable dose principle should be followed to ensure that the bone marrow dose does not exceed the allowed limits (<2 Gy). Care must be taken to ensure that the bone marrow dose is <2 Gy when planning to administer a high dose to the target tissue (300–350 Gy to the remnant thyroid tissue and 80–100 Gy to metastases) [47, 49]. Permanent gonadal dysfunction and the risk of developing second primary malignancy are possible severe adverse effects of RAIT. Salivary gland dysfunction, generally dry mouth syndrome, change or loss of taste, deterioration in oral hygiene, and dental problems are the most common complications. In radioactive iodine treatment, various methods such as providing adequate hydration, eating sour foods (lemon, lemon juice, sour candy, etc.), chewing gum, and cholinergic drug treatment are applied to protect the salivary glands from the undesired effects of radiation (radiation sialadenitis) through 24 h following oral radioiodine administration. These practices help to increase saliva secretion and prevent prolonged exposure of radioactive iodine in the salivary glands [20, 46, 47, 50]. However, there is still no definitely effective preventive or therapeutic method. Some studies have shown that chewing gum and sour foods have no significant effect on preventing the development of dry mouth in the late period [20, 51, 52]. Pilocarpine is a weak muscarinic agonist agent with low beta-adrenergic-effect and stimulates parasympathetic nerves in the exocrine glands; therefore, it is frequently used to reduce the symptoms of dry mouth occurring due to radiation sialadenitis [53, 54]. As well as there are publications showing that treatment has a protective effect in the early and late period (6 months later) [54], there are also studies reporting that it has no effect [53, 55]. It is thought that there is a difference in the results since different methods are used to calculate the accumulation of radioactive iodine in the salivary glands and the dose exposed. Further large case studies are needed for a definitive outcome. Lungs are other dose-limiting organs for RAIT in the patients with differentiated thyroid carcinoma. If the patient has diffuse lung metastases, the risk of developing radiation pneumonia and pulmonary fibrosis will increase [46, 56–60]. Rall et al. first reported in 1957 that radiation pneumonia and fibrosis developed due to I-131 treatment in DTC patients with diffuse lung metastasis [58]. In these cases, the threshold dose was reported as 80 mCi (2.96 GBq) for the development of inflammatory changes in the lungs by taking advantage of the retention of activity in the whole body 48 h after treatment [56, 58, 59, 60]. Increased TSH may cause diffuse inflammatory reactions and serious complications in these patients. Therefore, co-administration of I-131 therapy with corticosteroids is recommended [47].

The development of second primary malignancy after RAIT is an important side effect; and the nervous system, breast, prostate, kidney, bone marrow, salivary glands, urinary system, and gastrointestinal system are the most predisposed organs. Various factors such as age, genetic predisposition, smoking, race, radiation exposure, chemicals, and environmental causes also contribute to the increased risk of developing second primary malignancies [61–65]. The latent period ranges 5–10 years for the development of leukemia and 10–60 years for solid tumors. Single-dose RAIT is safe to avoid from the development of deterministic effects (tissue reactions). Even if administered at high doses, the absorbed dose does not exceed the *threshold* dose required for the development of important tissue reactions. Lower doses of RAIT in young patients will significantly reduce the risk of developing second primary cancer over a long life span [63, 64]. In published studies, the incidence of second primary cancer development within 7–13 years after RAIT was reported as 2.7% and 8.7%. Breast and digestive tract cancers are the most commonly occurred. Organs where RAI accumulates, such as breast tissue, digestive tract and urinary tract organs, or organs with NIS (Na/I-symporter) protein expression are predisposed to the development of malignancy. The incidence of second primary cancer development has been shown to increase significantly in patients with an administered I-131 dose of 1 Ci (37 GBq) and a cumulative dose of 1.08 Ci (40 GBq). The development of second malignancy after I-131 treatment and chemotherapy is not only dose-dependent, but genetic predisposition is also important [63–65].

The amount of radioactive iodine uptake in thyroid remnant tissue and metastases can be calculated from planar gamma camera images, SPECT, or SPECT/CT images which can provide more accurate quantification [60, 66–68]. PET/CT images with I-124 NaI can also be used. PET/CT images are more advantageous in detecting remnant tissue and tiny metastatic foci [32, 51]. Relevant publications recommend whole-body imaging and blood sampling for absorbed dose calculation in the bone marrow [1, 4, 49, 66–68]. The defined limiting dose for bone marrow is 2 Gy. In the blood sampling method, it is recommended to take 5 blood samples within the first 1 week following administration to monitor the time-related biokinetics of I-131 in the blood. Two milliliters of blood sample is taken into heparinized tube 2, 6, 24, 96, and 144 h after treatment and measurement is made in the well type counter. A time-activity curve is derived from I-131 measurements in the blood samples. Whole-body activity can be calculated from counts obtained by whole-body imaging or probes. After a low amount of I-131 is administered orally to the patients before the treatment, whole-body planar imaging is performed on the gamma camera at certain intervals. Region of interests (ROI) are drawn for lesion and non-lesion background activity on the acquired images ROI counts will define time-activity change and the area under the time-activity curve gives cumulative activity (A) [68]. Using these quantification methods, the absorbed dose in the remnant tissue and metastases has been reported to be between 10 Gy and 1000 Gy. Whole-body retention 48 h after radioactive iodine administration should not be exceeding 120 mCi (4.44 GBq) if there are no diffuse iodine-avid lung metastases or not to be higher than 80 mCi (2.96 GBq) if there is pulmonary metastasis [32, 46, 47, 58–60].

Since I-131 excretion from the thyroid gland is slower in the cases of hyperthyroidism (such as Graves' disease, toxic nodular goiter), the activity to be applied must be intended for the purpose and lower considering the risk of developing second primary malignancy. Formulas published by EANM can be used to calculate dosimetry in the hyperthyroidism cases in terms of avoiding the risk of developing second primary cancer (leukemia or solid tumor) [69].

3.2.2 Patient Preparation in I-131 Treatment of Differentiated Thyroid Cancer

In differentiated thyroid cancers, patient preparation before treatment plays an important role in the treatment effectiveness. First of all, pregnancy and breastfeeding are questioned in adult women. Women of childbearing age should be asked for a human chorionic gonadotropin-based pregnancy test (serum beta HCG) just a few days before RAIT. It should be explained that she cannot become pregnant for at least 6 months after treatment [1, 46–48]. If thyroid hormone replacement therapy has been initiated after the total thyroidectomy, the it should be discontinued. Before RAIT, waiting at least 3 weeks after thyroidectomy or discontinuation of long-acting L-T4 preparations for 3–4 weeks and short-acting L-T3 preparations for 2 weeks will be sufficient to increase TSH level (≥30 microU/ml). On the other hand, TSH can be increased to the desired level with recombinant TSH (rTSH) administration without long-term discontinuation of thyroid hormone therapy. It is preferred especially in the patients with metastatic or recurrent DTC cases. In addition, I-131 ablation therapy can be given with rTSH in selected cases with a disease (psychiatric problems, presence of dementia, etc.) that may increase in severity with hypothyroidism or in cases where it is thought that an adequate endogenous TSH response cannot be achieved [48, 70]. It has been reported that the success rate of ablation treatments administered under TSH elevation due to hypothyroidism induced by discontinuation of thyroid hormone drugs and due to rTSH administration is similar 12–18 months after treatment [47, 70]. Drugs used continuously by the patient should be questioned and if there is medication to block iodine uptake into the thyroid cells, it must be discontinued for an appropriate period of time before RAIT. The patient's serum thyroglobulin (Tg <10 ng/mL) and antithyroglobulin (AntiTg) levels should be measured. In order to detect the I-131 uptake rate in the remnant thyroid tissue, the patient can be administered a microCi dose of I-131 and thyroid uptake test can be performed in the first 24 h (expected value is <0.5%). Low-iodine diet should be initiated 2 weeks prior to treatment. If possible, it is recommended to check the iodine level in the patient's urine. Post-treatment patient follow-up should be performed in accordance with the national and international guidelines. Tg and TSH values measured during follow-up should be evaluated together with clinical findings [1, 43, 46–48].

3.2.3 Radiation Safety in I-131 Treatment

After I-131 treatment, radiation safety measures may vary between countries according to national radiation safety legislation. In our country, patients undergoing RAIT need to stay in a specially equipped room in the hospital until their whole-body radiation level reaches 30 microSv/h at a distance of 1 m [71]. According to the *International Atomic Energy Agency* (IAEA) guidelines, the discharge criterion for I-131 is a treatment dose of 30 mCi (1110 MBq) or radiation exposure of 0.05 mSv (50 microSv)/h radiation exposure rate 1 m away from the patient [1, 23]. The patient discharged from the hospital must comply with radiation safety measures to reduce radiation exposure of those around them and the public persons [23, 46–48, 50, 71, 72]. According to the ALARA principle, in order to protect the relatives of the patient who has received RAIT from unnecessary radiation exposure the directives released by *The Turkish Atomic Energy Authority* (TAEA; 72) and *International Commission on Radiological Protection* (ICRP; 23) should be followed. Since radioactive iodine is distributed in the patient's body, the patient cannot be considered as a point source and the inverse square law (the principle that the dose rate decreases as much as the square of the distance as one moves away from the patient) cannot be applied to a distance of >3 m from the patient [72]. The annual acceptable radiation exposure dose for family members should not exceed 5 mSv (500 mrem); however, it should not exceed 1 mSv (100 mrem) for pregnant women and children. Radiation safety precautions should be explained orally and written information form containing the radiation safety rules should be given when the patients are discharged. These rules should be applied to all patients receiving I-131 for the treatment of thyroid cancer, goiter, and hyperthyroidism. Patient-induced radiation exposure is caused by high-energytic gamma rays and bremsstrahlung X-rays (braking radiation) rather than by beta radiations. Radiation exposure of individuals close to the patient is related to the amount of radiation remaining in the patient's body, the distance from the patient and duration of contact. Although higher I-131 is administered in the thyroid cancer cases compared to hyperthyroidism cases, administered I-131 will be rapidly excreted through the kidneys since there is no thyroid gland and the remaining activity dose will be less. Excretion will be faster, especially in the euthyroid patients who are prepared for RAIT with rTSH since hypothyroidism does not occur. The effective half-life of I-131 in the treatment of hyperthyroidism cases was estimated to be approximately 5 days [1, 4, 23, 28, 29, 46, 47, 71, 72].

The patient who has received I-131 treatment can travel in their private car without any restriction. Only when using toilets in the resting areas, it should be recommended to pay attention not to contaminate around and to flush the reservoir at least 2 times. If the patient will not travel alone, they must follow the radiation safety rules of time and distance. The radioactive patient should be seated in the rear row in the opposite seat, not in the seat next to the driver. If the patient will use public transport, they have the right to travel between 1 h and 15 h according to the administered I-131 treatment dose and the time elapsed after treatment. For hyperthyroidism patients treated with I-131, the acceptable time on public transport is 30 min for 22 mCi (800 MBq) and 3.5 h for 5.4 mCi (200 MBq) [47, 71, 72].

Breastfeeding should be discontinued if the patient to be treated with radioactive iodine is lactating. Otherwise, I-131 will pass into the milk and destroy the baby's thyroid. In addition, radiation in the breast tissue will increase due to the increase in NIS (NaI symporter) expression during lactation. To reduce/prevent this, lactation suppressor medication should be administered 6–8 weeks prior to treatment and breastfeeding must be prohibited for 3 months following treatment. If RAIT needs to be given urgently, it should be checked with I-123 imaging whether there is a higher iodine uptake than normal (more than background activity) in the breast tissue; if there is a high uptake, treatment should be delayed as long as possible [43, 46, 47, 71].

Medullary thyroid carcinoma (**MTC**) is a rare neuroendocrine tumor which is originated from the thyroid C cells secreting calcitonin. The measurement of serum calcitonin and carcinoembryonic antigen (CEA), serum calcium and parathyroid hormone levels, urinary catecholamine, and normetanephrine (or free plasma normetanephrine) in 24-h urine are recommended in MTC cases before surgery. MTC develops both as a sporadic form and as a hereditary form which is a part of multiple endocrine neoplasia (MEN) type 2. Therefore, all patients diagnosed with medullary thyroid carcinoma should be examined for MEN2 before the operation [41, 43, 44]. In addition, RET proto-oncogene (a proto-oncogene tyrosine-kinase receptor) analysis should be performed after the operation [45].

I-131 MIBG and Y-90/Lu-177 labeled radiopeptide treatment are applied. In these treatments, the risky organ is bone marrow (the threshold dose is 2 Gy) [17, 45, 72–74]. Ga-68 SSR imaging is more sensitive than In-111 DOTATATE imaging and should be performed prior to radiopeptide therapy. Metastatic lesions can be detected by somatostatin receptor imaging in 70% of patients with advanced MTC. These cases will benefit from radiopeptide treatment. However, tumor heterogeneity is an important limiting factor for success of efficacy [17, 43, 45].

Anaplastic thyroid cancer (**ATC**) Several studies with PET/CT imaging of Ga-68 PSMA (prostate-specific membrane antigen) have shown prominent radiopharmaceutical uptake in primary tumor and metastatic lymph nodes in ATC cases. PSMA protein has been reported in the endothelium of the vessels in the tumor. Ga-68 PSMA PET/CT imaging based on the presence of neovascularization in anaplastic thyroid cancer paved the way for the use of 177 Lu-PSMA-DKFZ-617 in the treatment. However, there is a need for further large case studies [75–78].

3.3 Targeted Radionuclide Therapy in Neuroendocrine Tumors

3.3.1 Radiopeptide Treatments

Neuroendocrine tumors are epithelial neoplasms which show neuroendocrine differentiation and are characterized by the elevation of specific markers such as SSR, chromogranin A, CD53 protein, and neuron-specific enolase. Although it can develop from any part of the body, it develops from the gastroenteropancreatic system by 60–70%. NETs of the lungs are known as pulmonary carcinoid tumors; they account for 1–2% of all lung tumors and 30% of all NETs [9]. In-111 DTPA octreotide is the first radiopeptide agent used in the treatment of neuroendocrine tumors. In-111 radionuclide is used in treatment based on the high LET value of Auger electrons (0.005–0.025 MeV). Despite a marked regression in symptoms, a partial response is rarely seen. For cytotoxic effect, the In-111 labeled peptide compound must reach the nucleus. However, the tissue range for Auger electrons is very short (0.20–0.55 mm). It is a reliable agent for renal functions; however, leukemia or myelodysplastic syndrome due to bone marrow toxicity at high cumulative doses of 2.4–2.7 mCi (90–100 MBq) has been reported (estimated bone marrow radiation dose >3 Gy). In-111 DOTATOC with similar biokinetics has also been used in the treatment of NETs with a higher uptake ratio. However, recently developed beta-emitting Y-90 and Lu-177 bound peptides have replaced In-111-peptides [9, 11, 14, 79–81].

Y-90-bound peptides (DOTATOC, DOTATATE, lanreotide) are superior to In-111 compounds in destroying neuroendocrine tumor cells. Y-90 has a beta particle with high energy (maximum 2.28 MeV, 99.9% abundance) and a maximum range of 11 mm (2.5–11 mm) in tissue. Y-90 is considered a pure beta-emitting agent with a physical half-life of 64 h. Y-90 Dota-Tyr3-octreotide (DOTATOC) is the first developed SSR analog. In the treatment, 100 mCi (3.7 GBq)/m^2 dose is administered intravenously 2 times at 6–12 week intervals. It is preferred in the treatment of large volume tumors. The overall treatment response (complete, partial, and minimum response) was reported to be between 19–37% and stable disease was reported in the half of the patients [9, 38, 42].

Although the dose-limiting organs are kidneys in the treatment of DOTATOC, bone marrow and liver toxicities have also been reported. The reabsorption of the radiopeptide from the renal proximal tubules and its retention in the interstitium result in the increased radiation exposure to the kidneys. The presence of hypertension or diabetes mellitus will also result in an increase in the nephrotoxic effect. Positively charged amino acids such as L-arginine and L-lysine are administered by pre-treatment infusion to reduce the renal toxicity due to accumulation of radiopeptides in the kidneys. Reabsorption of the radiopeptide from the renal proximal tubules is prevented by competitive inhibition.

Thus, radiation exposure of the renal cortex will be reduced by 9–53%. Amino acid infusion should start 30–60 min before radiopeptide administration and last for 4 h. During infusion, the patient should be closely monitored for possible electrolyte imbalance (hyperkalemia and hypernatremia) and the development of metabolic acidosis. If these side effects are observed, an adequate hydration should be provided with 0.09 NaCl infusion, and also, antiemetic and corticosteroids should be administered [14, 37, 38, 42, 49].

Lu-177 DOTATATE is a somatostatin analog theranostic agent used in the treatment of neuroendocrine tumors. Since Lu-177 has both beta (maximum 0.498 MeV and average 0.133 MeV energy with 79% abundancy) and gamma rays (0.113 MeV with 6.5% abundancy and 0.208 MeV with 11% abundancy), it allows post-treatment imaging and volume-based dosimetric study with gamma camera. It is recommended to use medium-energy general-purpose collimators (MEGP) for imaging and to set an energy peak at 208 keV. Its physical half-life is 6.7 days. The traveling distance in tissue is shorter (1.7 and 0.23 mm) than Y-90. It is safely used in the treatment of small and medium-sized tumors without damaging the tumor surrounding tissue. The main route of excretion is the kidneys. An average of 46% of the administered dose is excreted in urine 4 h after administration and 65–70% in the first 24 h. In order to prevent accumulation in the kidneys, 150–200 mCi (5.55–7.4 GBq) dose is administered intravenously in 3 or 5 cycles at 6–12 week intervals together with amino acid infusion. The maximum reliable dose for bone marrow and kidneys is still unknown. Response to treatment is higher compared to Y-90 DOTATOC [14, 32, 38, 49, 80, 81]. An overall response rate has been reported as 46% in the treatment of diffuse and progressive NETs [12, 14, 81, 82]. The most important side effects are nephrotoxicity and acute bone marrow toxicity; however they are reversible. In addition to the kidney and liver toxicity at doses higher than 100 GBq (>3 Gy bone marrow radiation dose), severe bone marrow toxicity such as bone marrow suppression and even myelodysplastic syndrome may develop [14, 38, 80]. Previous studies have reported the amount of absorbed dose in the kidneys to be 0.2–2.0 Gy/GBq. Doses absorbed in tumor tissue when the standard-dose protocol is applied have been reported as 10–340 Gy using measurements obtained from SPECT/CT images [4, 14, 38, 80, 83–85].

As opposed to In-111-bound peptides and Lu-177 DOTATATE, post-treatment imaging and dosimetric study with Y-90-bound peptides, which is a pure beta-emitter agent, is not possible. A dosimetric study using Bremsstrahlung X-ray images will not be easy. For dosimetric studies, PET imaging with Y-86 (t ½p: 0.6 days) or Ga-68 (t ½p: 68 min) which are biochemically identical with Y-90, and gamma camera studies with Tc-99m (*t*½p: 6 h) or In-111 labeled peptides can be used [86–93]. Y-86 DOTATOC has the same chemical structure with Y-90 DOTATOC and provides important information in the biokinetic studies. It is a PET imaging agent. The fact that it is expensive and difficult to obtain limits its use. Y-86 DOTATOC biokinetics are also similar to In-111 DTPA octreotide; however, it has been shown in the published studies that its washout from tumoral tissue is slower than In-111 DTPA octreotide [79]. Tc-99m HYNIC-TOC and Tc-99m HYNIC-TATE compounds have been reported to be advantageous in the patients with lymph node and liver metastases [91]. The SSR2 affinity of Ga-68 DOTA-peptides is higher than that of In-111 DTPA octreotide. The sensitivity and specificity are high with the addition of the physical advantages of PET imaging in the detection of dense SSR2-containing tumors and metastases such as neuroendocrine tumors. Therefore, lesions with low or moderate SSR2 density, as well as smaller lesions, can be easily detected by Ga-68 DOTA-peptide PET imaging compared to In-111 DTPA-octreotide SPECT. Haug et al. showed that Ga- 68 DOTATATE PET/CT imaging may contribute to the detection of early progression of the disease and the determination of the prognosis in the well-differentiated NET patients undergoing PRRT [89]. Ga-68 DOTATOC, Ga-68 DOTATATE, and Ga-68 DOTANOC are commonly used in the clinical trials due to their rapid blood clearance and renal excretion, better visualization of the lesions, high image resolution and contrast, short imaging time, low radiation dose, and the possibility of accurate quantification [92]. However, being obtained from the Ge-68/Ga-68 generator and being expensive are the most important factors limiting its routine use [47, 80, 81].

3.3.2 Dosimetric Approach to the Treatment with Radiopeptides

While the absorbed dose in the radiopeptide treatments is high in the tumor tissue, it is acceptable in the critical organs. As explained in the previous paragraph, kidney and bone marrow toxicities are the most important dose-limiting side effects. In the Euratom Directive (1997), it was emphasized that the absorbed dose in the target organ should be calculated for the patient in radiation treatments and it is important to ensure as low radiation exposure as possible to non-tumoral tissues [94–96]. Important factors in a dosimetric study are the radiopharmaceutical administered, imaging method (PET, SPECT, planar, whole-body imaging), accuracy of activity measurement, and sampling time. The biological effective dose (BED) is considered to be the most reliable parameter in the evaluation of renal toxicity [38, 85]. Whole-body serial images are used to calculate the bone marrow toxicity, in accordance with the Guidance of the EANM Dosimetry Committee. However, since dosimetric studies cannot be performed in most nuclear medicine centers, fixed-dose treatment is applied. Appropriate imaging and sampling time are important in the accurate dosimetric evaluation. Minimum 3 times sampling (at 1, 3, and 5 effective half-lives) should be performed according to the MIRD guideline. Otherwise, the absorbed dose will be measured higher than 20%. Since the final imaging should be performed at 5 effective half-lives after radionuclide therapies applied, a dosimetric study with long (In-111) and very short half-life radionuclides (Ga-68) is not practical [13, 32, 49, 82, 93].

Radiopeptide agents are excreted by glomerular filtration; then they are reabsorbed by the renal proximal tubules and accumulate in the renal interstitial area. Therefore, kidneys are considered critical organs. Because the absorbed dose in the kidneys with Y-90 DOTATOC is higher than Lu-177 DOTATATE, treatment with Lu-177 DOTATATE is preferred in the patients with impaired renal function or requiring retreatment. In patients without a history of hypertension, diabetes mellitus, or prior chemotherapy, the BED threshold dose was defined as 40 Gy for the development of the radiopeptide-dependent nephrotoxicity in the late period. The recommended BED value in the patients with defined risk factors is 28 Gy [4, 38, 80, 85, 94, 95]. There are several methods for evaluating renal functions. However, serum creatinine measurement is generally recommended. Glomerular filtration rate (GFR) measurement has also been proposed by some authors. GFR measurement based on serum creatinine level can be performed. However, measurements using the gamma camera method with Tc-99m-diethylenetriamine pentaacetic acid (DTPA) are more useful in the risk determination and long-term follow-up in these cases. Infusion of positively charged amino acids, L-lysine and L-arginine together with radiopeptide agents will reduce the development of nephrotoxicity. Since accumulation of the radiopeptides in the interstitial area will decrease by inhibiting the reabsorption of the peptide in the renal proximal tubules, their infusion helps to prevent or reduce radiation-induced hazardous effects [94]. Administration of the total treatment dose in divided doses will also reduce the acute nephrotoxic effect. In the current guidelines, reliable dose limits for the development of radiotherapy-induced renal toxicity have been reported as 18 Gy in the cases treated with 2 Gy/fraction. The probability of developing radiation nephritis 5 years after 18 Gy external radiation therapy has been reported as 5% [83]. Individual dosimetric studies can increase the effect on the target tumor tissue and reduce complications. With the decrease in tumor volume, the absorbed dose in the tumor tissue has been shown to reach a substantial level of 200 Gy. However, individual dosimetric studies cannot be performed in every center and treatment with safe fixed doses is applied [14, 32, 38, 49, 79, 94, 96].

3.3.3 Radiation Safety in the Radiopeptide Treatments

Y-90 has little or no excretion from the body. Since it is a pure beta emitter, the risk of external radiation from bremsstrahlung rays around the patient is very low. Therefore, the patient can be discharged from the hospital for up to 4000 MBq activity; no special precautions are required after the patient is discharged, except for urgent clinical conditions. However, it is recommended to avoid pregnancy for up to 1 month [72]. Radiation safety measures in the treatment process with **Lu-177 compounds** vary according to the laws of the countries. For example, in Australia, Lu-177 radiopeptide treatment (200 mCi) is administered outpatient, while in European countries patients are required to stay in a specially equipped room for 1–3 days. In Turkey, similar to the practice in the European countries, according to the Directive on Discharge of Patients Receiving Radionuclide Therapy (RSGD-KLV-009. Rev 2) published by TAEA, patients should be hospitalized until the amount of activity in their bodies decreases to 1400 MBq [72]. It should be considered that the kidneys can receive doses up to 20 Gy since lutetium is retained at a high rate in the kidneys. The patient should be hospitalized for at least 24 h after receiving a treatment dose of 7400 MBq Lu-177. After discharge, the patients and their relatives should follow precautions against contamination. For the discharge procedure, the dose rate measured 1 m away the patient must be less than 20 μSv/h. Although the dose rate at a distance of 1 m from the patient receiving 7.4 GBq Lu-177 has been shown to be approximately 7.5 μSv/h after 24 h, isolation of the radioactive patient is recommended to protect the patient's relatives and the publics from external radiation exposure due to gamma rays and also bremsstrahlung-X rays which are originated from the high-energy beta particles. After Lu-177 treatment, provided that the amount of activity remaining in the patient's body and the dose rate 1 m away the patient do not exceed the permitted levels, the physician may discharge the patient if they are sure that necessary precautions will be taken and measures against radionuclide contamination will be followed by the patient and their relatives. However, it is recommended that the patients who are pregnant and/or close to young children should be kept in the hospital up to 48 h until the dose rate measured 1 m away from the patient decreases to 10 μSv/h. Patients must follow the measures to prevent contamination and general radiation safety precautions after discharge. Lu-177 may also contain a small amount of Lu-177m which is a metastable form with a long half-life (160.4 days). Therefore, caution should be exercised in disposing of contaminated waste. The total amount of radioactivity in wastes that a healthcare institution can give to the sewage system at once cannot exceed 2.5 times the ALImin value and 100 MBq level (ALImin value for Lu-177 3 × 103 μCi). Since 65–70% (approximately 5200 MBq Lu-177) of the activity administered to the patient is excreted in the urine in the first 24 h, liquid radioactive waste excreted from the patients' bodies should be kept in the special designed tank system in order not to exceed the limits of delivery to the sewage system. Wastes should be discharged into the sewer after waiting for 1–2 months [23, 49, 72, 82].

I-131 MIBG (meta-iodobenzylguanidine) is used to treat neuroendocrine tumors, especially inoperable pheochromocytoma, carcinoid tumor, metastatic MTC, and advanced neuroblastoma in children. Meta-iodobenzylguanidine is an analog of noradrenaline (norepinephrine). The treatment dose ranges between 100–300 mCi (3.7–11.2 GBq) and the standard dose is 5 GBq. The dose for children is approximately 666 MBq/kg. It is administered by slow injection for 1 h while checking vital signs (pulse and blood pressure). After administration, MIBG enters the cells in tissues with adrenergic innervation either by neuronal uptake-1 mechanism or by passive diffusion. Unlike noradrenaline, MIBG is not metabolized in the cells and is excreted unchanged. Pregnancy and breastfeeding, life expectancy less than 3 months, and renal failure are absolute contraindications. Relative contraindications are progressive hematological and/or renal toxicity resulting from the previously applied treatment, and presence of urinary incontinence and myelosuppression [41, 74].

Patients should have a definite diagnosis and staging just before I-131 MIBG treatment. To prevent free I-131 uptake in the thyroid gland, stable iodine should be administered orally 1–2 days before MIBG treatment and continued for 10–15 days after treatment. K-perchlorate is administered with stable iodine to accelerate free I-131 wash-out from the thyroid gland. Drugs that will interact with MIBG uptake by tumor cells should be discontinued for an appropriate period of time [74]. It is excreted primarily by the kidneys in the first 5 days after administration. Hospitalization, discharge, and radiation safety rules are the same as I-131 treatment. In pediatric cases, parents and caregivers should follow radiation safety rules and maintain contact with the patient as short time and long distance as possible. It is recommended that they wear a lead apron and should also carry a digital dosimeter [23, 72, 74].

3.3.4 Painful Bone Metastases and Radionuclide Therapy

Metastatic bone disease often occurs as a serious complication of many cancers. Breast, prostate, and lung cancers are the most common cancers that spread to bones and constitute approximately 80% of bone metastases. Vertebral column, pelvic bones, and ribs are affected at the earliest and 80% of metastatic lesions are located in the axial skeleton [3, 5, 6, 15, 31]. Radionuclide therapy is usually administered after non-steroidal anti-inflammatory drugs, morphine, chemotherapeutics, surgical treatment, biphosphonates, and external radiotherapy in the patients with painful bone metastases. Alpha (Ra-223, Bi-213) or beta radiation-emitting agents (P-32, Sr-89, Y-90, Sm-153, Re-188, Re-186, Lu-177) are used for bone pain palliation in the radionuclide therapy [3, 5, 6, 15, 16, 18, 24, 31]. The most important advantages of RN therapy are its positive effect on the quality of life, ease of administration, reproducibility, ability to treat common metastases, and administration with other treatment methods. In addition, studies have shown that it has a positive effect on the patient life expectancy. Considering that the palliative effect occurs in the period from a few days to 4 weeks after treatment, RN therapy will be very useful in the patients with relatively long life expectancy (>3 months) and with secondary bone involvement detected in early. It is not recommended in the patients with a life expectancy of less than 4 weeks. Bone-specific radiopharmaceuticals can also be used in the treatment of primary bone tumors with osteoblastic features such as osteosarcoma. Before treatment, bone scintigraphy should be performed to determine radiopharmaceutical uptake rate. However, use with this indication has not been approved yet [3, 6, 15, 97–100].

Patient preparation is not required before treatment. Patients should be informed about the possible side effects of RN treatment applied for pain palliation, that pain will increase especially in the early period, that RN treatment can be applied again if necessary and that pregnancy is forbidden for 6 months after the treatment. The patient should be asked to sign an informed consent form. Patients should receive supportive treatment with analgesics until the pain subsides. Sr-89 and Sm-153 solution at room temperature should be administered by slow infusion via an intravenous catheter (butterfly needle, triple catheter, or intracath line) by personnel qualified in the RN treatment. Then, the remaining activity in the catheter should be flushed with 0.9% NaCl solution. Before starting infusion, it should be checked whether the catheter is in the vein. Nonetheless, if an extravasation is detected, the infusion should be immediately stopped and a cold application should be made on the skin area negatively effected by the leakage. P-32 can be administered intravenously or orally [6, 15, 18, 31, 97].

Strontium-89 Chloride (Sr-89). Strontium is a divalent cation similar to calcium. Sr-89 chloride (Metastron®) is the first FDA-approved radiopharmaceutical for pain palliation in the painful bone metastases. It is also a licensed compound in Europe. Sr-89 binds into the hydroxyapatite molecule in the bone tissues after intravenous administration. Its physical half-life is 50.5 days and decays to stable yttrium-89. Its maximum beta particle energy (Emax) is 1.46 MeV; its range is 6–7 mm in the soft tissue, and 3–4 mm in the bone. There are gamma rays (910 keV) of 0.01% abundancy as well as high energy beta particles used in the treatment. Since the gamma-ray ratio is negligible, there is no risk of radiation exposure for people around the patient. Therefore, the patient receiving S-89 treatment does not need to be hospitalized. Plasma clearance is variable (1.6–11.6 L/day). Whole-body retention is 20% on 90 days after injection in the healthy group and the majority accumulate in the normal bone tissue. Radiopharmaceutical uptake in the osteoblastic lesions is 5 times greater than normal tissue (lesion/normal bone ratio is 5:1) and the retention time in the lesions is longer. The success rate of the treatment is high in the patients with osteoblastic lesions detected on the bone scintigraphy. Successful pain palliation has been reported with the administration of Sr-89 chloride in the cases with metastatic breast and prostate cancer which usually cause osteoblastic bone lesions [15]. The recommended standard treatment dose for Sr-89 chloride has been reported as 4 mCi (148–150 MBq; 1.5–2.2 MBq/kg). Relationship between the dose and response has not been documented for pain relief in the literature.

Biological half-life was examined in the measurements made with Sr-85 in urine and blood; previously published studies reported that trace amounts of Sr-85 were detected in urine on 148 days and blood on 80 days after injection [6, 15, 23, 24, 29, 72].

Samarium-153 ethylenediaminetetramethylenephosphonate (Sm-153 EDTMP; lexidronam) is a bone avid radiopharmaceutical that is retained particularly in the osteoblastic lesions with increased bone turnover rate. Sm-153 emits both beta particles (Emax 640, 710, and 810 keV) and gamma-rays (103.2 keV, 28% abundancy). Its physical half-life is 46.3 h and its average penetration range is 0.83 mm in the water. Sm-153 is produced from Sm-152 oxide by neutron bombardment. Contamination of Europium-154 (Eu-154), which has a physical half-life of 8.5 years, during Sm-153 production process and the retention of Eu-154 in the bone tissue after Sm-153 EDTMP treatment is important because it causes the system to alert when the patient is passing through patient safety checkpoints. Sm-153 is combined with the calcium salt of the EDTMP molecule to obtain the Sm-153 EDTMP theranostic. It has been approved for use in treatment in Europe and USA [3, 6, 22, 35, 97, 98].

Sm-153-EDTMP is localized in the skeleton via chemi-absorption of tetraphosphate by the hydroxyapatite molecule, and also, by the formation of samarium oxide containing an oxygen on the hydroxyapatite molecule. It is retained 5 times more in the metastatic areas in the skeleton than in the healthy bone tissue. It can be administered in the symptomatic and asymptomatic cases with bone metastasis. It is often administered at a dose of 0.5–2.5 mCi/kg in the treatment of diffuse bone metastases [3, 15, 98]. Generally, patients benefit from a single application, the pain relief begins within a few weeks and lasts for 2–8 months. Pain may not occur for a lifetime. However, if necessary, treatment can be repeated at short intervals such as 8–12 weeks or at long intervals such as 1 year [15, 97]. The total skeletal dose is associated with the prevalence of osteoblastic metastases, ranging from 15% to 95%. Radiation exposure of non-skeletal areas is negligible. Sm-153 EDTMP is rapidly cleared from blood (within 5.5 min after intravenous administration) and only 1% of the administered dose remains in the systemic circulation after an hour. The main route of excretion is the kidneys. It is completely excreted by the kidneys within 6 h after administration. The target organ is bone marrow. For Sm-153 EDTMP at a dose of 3 mCi/kg, the total absorbed radiation dose in the bone marrow has been reported to be 1.277–2.250 rad or 1.5 mGy/MBq. The recommended standard dose of Sm-153 lexidronam for effective treatment is 1 mCi/kg and is safe. It may cause a mild transient bone marrow suppression in the patients with normal hematological parameters prior to treatment [3, 6, 32, 49, 98, 101].

Phosphor-32 (P-32) is a pure beta-emitting agent. The maximum beta energy is 1.71 MeV, the average energy is 0.70 MeV, and the average range in the soft tissue is 3.0 mm. The physical half-life is 14.3 days [102]. P-32 is administered intravenously at the dose of 185–370 MBq and orally at 370–444 MBq.

The critical organ is the bone marrow (11.0 mGy/MBq). Myelosuppression may develop within 12–16 weeks post-treatment; however, it is transient. Due to the development of new bone-seeking radiopharmaceuticals for palliation of the cancer-induced bone pain, the frequency of administration has decreased [6, 28, 49].

Ra-223 dichloride is an alpha-decay radionuclide used in the treatment of bone metastases in patients with castration-resistant prostate carcinoma (CRPC) without known visseral metastasis. It has a half-life of 11.4 days. Radium is a calcium analog and is retained by osteoblasts in newly formed bone tissues with increased bone turnover. It is administered in divided doses (in 6 fractions) at a dose of 55 kBq/kg. Dosimetric imaging is difficult because it is an alpha emitter and is administered at low doses. Ra-223 uptake in the skeleton metastases is similar to Tc-99m MDP. Tc-99m MDP skeleton images were shown to be useful in treatment planning. However, it cannot be used for absorbed dose calculation [31, 32, 103, 104].

It is a bone-seeking agent and has been approved for use in the patients with CRPC with painful bone metastases but without visceral metastases in Europe and the USA. It is extremely safe because the penetration range in the soft tissue is very short (<100 μm; only 2–10 cell diameters). The likelihood of severe hematological effect is low. However, the patients with poor general condition (Karnofsky score <50% or ECOG performance status >2), limited bone marrow reserve (before the initial administration/cycle, absolute neutrophil count $<1.5 \times 10^9$/L, platelet $<100 \times 10^9$/L and hemoglobin <10.0 g/dL; prior to subsequent administrations/cycles, absolute neutrophil count $<1.0 \times 10^9$/L and platelet count $<50 \times 10^9$/L), and fecal incontinence (hospitalization is highly recommended in these cases) are relative contraindications. It has been reported that there is no synergistic interaction with chemotherapeutics. Ra-223 improves the quality of life as prolong as overall life expectancy (recommendation levels 7B and 8A) [12, 31, 49, 103]. Another type of cancer with the most common bone metastases is breast cancer. However, there is only one study (Phase IIa) on the use of Ra-223 in breast cancer cases. In this trial, Ra-223 (intravenous 50 kBq/kg/ cycle every 4 weeks, a total of 4 cycles) was administered to the patients with advanced breast cancer and progressive bone metastases who could not be treated with hormones for a longer period of time. Since it was shown that the metabolic activities of metastatic foci decreased, the results are promising [18]. However, large multicentric patient participation studies are needed for a definitive outcome.

Rhenium-188 hydroxyethylene diphosphonate (Re-188 HEDP) is another theranostic agent used in the palliative treatment of metastatic bone pain due to different types of malignant tumors. Its physical half-life is 16.8 h, its maximum beta energy is 2.1 MeV, and its gamma-rays energy is 155 keV (15% abundancy). The presence of gamma rays allows the evaluation of tissue distribution and to perform dosimetric measurements. The therapeutic dose ranges from 31 to 188 mCi (1.1–6.9 GBq). A single dose is administered by bolus injection. Its retention ratio is high in the skeleton and urinary excretion is rapid an hour after injection. 41% and 60% of the administered dose are excreted in the first 8 h and 48 h, respectively. The biological half-life in the bone is 60.9 h, 2.99 h in the muscle tissue, and 6.21 h in the blood. Liepe et al. [5] reported in their study that the average absorbed dose in the bone metastases was 3.8 mGy/MBq (with SPECT imaging method), 0.61 mGy/MBq in the bone marrow, 0.71 mGy/MBq in the kidneys, 0.99 mGy/MBq in the bladder, and 0.02–0.07 mGy/MBq in the whole body. Since the bone marrow dose is low, no severe hematological side effect is observed [5, 49].

Re-186 HEDP has both lower beta emissions (Emax = 1.1 MeV) suitable for RN treatment and gamma emissions (137 keV) allowing external imaging. It has a relatively short physical half-life of 3.6 days and the main route of excretion is the kidneys. Up to 45% is excreted in the first 5 h and 42% in the first 3 h after administration. Dosimetric results are similar to Re-188 [5, 49].

3.3.5 Patient Selection Criteria in the Palliation of Painful Bone Metastases

In case of extensive skeleton metastases, bone marrow toxicity, thrombocytopenia, and neutropenia development are the most important complications after radionuclide therapies [5, 6, 31, 49, 101]. The risk of bone marrow toxicity development will increase in the patients with evidence of compromised bone marrow reserve such as prior cytotoxic chemotherapy and/or external beam radiation therapy (EBRT) or with severe diffuse bone metastasis ("superscan finding" in the skeleton). Benefit-risk assessment should be performed before treatment in such patients and radionuclide therapy should be applied to the patients in whom it is thought to be clinically beneficial. Treatment should be given under close monitoring. Since the presence of superscan findings on bone scintigraphy indicates diffuse bone metastases, the risk of developing complications is high; RN treatment is contraindicated in these patients. Relatively low blood cell count is a relative contraindication due to the probability of myelotoxicity occurrence. In this case, treatment can be given together with granulocyte-colony-stimulating factor (GCSF) infusion [6, 31]. Patient selection criteria for RN treatment (except Ra-223) in the cases with bone metastases are presented in Table 3.2.

Table 3.2 The patient selection criteria for RN treatment (except Ra-223) in the cases with bone metastasis [6]

Hemoglobin <90 g/L, total white blood cell count (WBC) $<3.5 \times 10^9$/L, and platelet count $<100 \times 10^9$/L have been reported. Since disseminated intravascular coagulopathy (DIC) is a risk for severe thrombocytopenia after treatment, tests for the diagnosis of subclinical DIC should be performed prior to treatment	Recommendation level 1C
If there is bone marrow involvement, but the blood cells are at the acceptable limits and above the limit of possible severe myelotoxicity, radionuclide therapy can be applied	Recommendation level 2A
Blood cells counts should not change after bone pain receiving palliation treatment. If there is a suspicion or if treatment has been delayed due to low blood cell counts, blood count should be repeated immediately before treatment is administered	Recommendation level 3C
Poor renal function leads to a decrease in plasma clearance of bone-specific radiopharmaceuticals, resulting in an increased whole-body radiation dose and higher risk of myelotoxicity. Therefore, in patients with severe renal impairment, Cr >> 180 μmol/L and/or GFR <30 mL/min, radionuclide therapy is contraindicated	Recommendation level 4C
Palliative treatment with Sr-89, Sm-153, or P-32 is not appropriate in the patients with an expected life span of less than 4 weeks. The life expectancy should preferably be longer than 3 months	Recommendation level 5C
Radionuclide therapy may be recommended for the pain palliation in patients with painful bone metastasis of osteoblastic or mixed (osteoblastic/osteoclastic) pattern	Recommendation level 6A
It may be recommended to improve the quality of life in patients with bone metastasis osteoblastic or mixed (osteoblastic/osteoclastic) character	Recommendation level 7B
Treatment with Ra-223, which emits alpha particles, may be recommended to prolong survival in the patients with castration-resistant prostate cancer (CRPC) with osteoblastic or mixed (osteoblastic/osteoclastic) painful bone metastases but without visceral dissemination	Recommendation level 8A
Radionuclide therapy may be administered with or consecutively with external beam radiation therapy in the selected patients for the treatment of painful osteoblastic or mixed type (osteoblastic/osteoclastic) bone metastases	Recommendation level 9C
There is no contraindication for concomitant or sequential use of radionuclide therapy and bisphosphonates for the treatment of patients with painful osteoblastic or mixed type (osteoblastic/osteoclastic) bone metastases. Bisphosphonates do not negatively effect on Sr-89 and Sm-153 uptakes	Recommendation level 10B
Chemotherapy and radionuclide therapy should be carefully used due to possible hematological side effects. Current evidence on the effect of concomitant use of radionuclide therapy and chemotherapy on bone palliation is inconclusive.	Recommendation level 11D

3.3.6 Radionuclide Therapy in Bone Metastases and Radiation Safety

As with all radionuclide applications, patients should take plenty of fluids before and after treatment. No hospitalization is necessary after treatment. However, the patient should be kept in the nuclear medicine department for the first 4–6 h after RN treatment to observe if any early side effects develop. The permissible activity limit in the patient's body to leave from the hospital in outpatient treatment has been reported to be 300 MBq for Sr-89 due to its long half-life; <1200 MBq for P-32. The average dose rate measured 1 m away the patient 1–2 h after administration of 3700 MBq Sm-153-EDTMP was reported as 20–30 μSv/h. Similarly, the average dose rate 1 m away the patient with 4000 MBq Re-188 activity was 25 μSv/h and it was within acceptable limits according to radiation safety regulation.

The dose rate measured 1 m away a 70 kg patient who received 3.5 MBq Ra-223 treatment was reported as an average of 0.17 μSv/h [6, 23, 31, 71, 72]. Ra-223 is excreted from the body primarily by feces at a rate of 63–76% and in small amounts (2%) by urine within 7 days after treatment. Therefore, although the external radiation exposure is low, more attention should be paid to the risk of contamination than radionuclides emitting beta particles, as contamination may occur during urinary and feces excretion during this period. In outpatient treatments, the patient must not leave from the hospital without emptying the bladder at least once or twice. In general, urine contamination is important for the first 2–3 days. Patients should be informed orally about toilet use and good hygiene practices, and written information form should be provided to the patient, household members, or caregivers. General radiation safety precautions adviced in the radionuclide applications should be followed. In order to prevent contamination to the environment, urination should be done at sitting position, should flush 2–3 times before leaving the toilet, and patients should wash their hands. If hands are contaminated, patients should wash gently their hands with soap and plenty of water without rubbing and brushing. Patients should take contamination precautions for dishes and laundry, and must comply with radiation safety measures. Urethral catheters should be inserted in the patients with urinary incontinence just before application of radium-223. The catheter should remain for an appropriate time (4 days for Sr-89 and one day for Sm-153); the patient's urinary bag should be emptied frequently and with gloves. Radiation safety rules should be explained verbally in detail to the patients and caregivers and given in a printed form [23, 31, 72]. The treatment method of the patient should be determined according to the level of consciousness of the patient, his/her relatives and the caregiver, and also, the number, ages, and opportunities of people living at home. If the patient's cognitive abilities are weak and difficult to meet their needs, they may need to be hospitalized. However, hospitalization is strongly recommended in the patients with fecal incontinence. Patients should avoid pregnancy for 2 years after receiving Sr-89 treatment, 4 months following P-32 treatment, and 6 months after Ra-223 treatment [6, 31, 72].

3.3.7 Radioimmunotherapy in the Lymphomas and Dosimetric Approach

Non-Hodgkin's lymphoma (NHL) is the most common group among hematological malignancies, and chemotherapy, radiotherapy, and immunotherapy are used in the treatment. Radioimmunotherapy (RIT) is a new and an important alternative treatment method in the treatment of NHL. However, there is still no definitive consensus as to whether RIT is a first-line treatment in NHL cases or a secondary treatment to be applied in the cases refractory to other treatments. RIT with radionuclide-labeled monoclonal antibodies (antiCD20) was first used in 2002 in the treatment of patients with relapse or chemotherapy-resistant low grade follicular or transformed B-cell non-Hodgkin lymphoma.

Y-90 ibritumomab tiuxetan (Zevalin®) which is the first FDA-approved radiolabeled anti-CD20 mAb was used in RNT in 2002; whereas its use in the treatment in Europe has been approved since 2004. The ibritumomab tiuxetan compound is obtained by conjugation of the anti-CD20 murine IgG1 monoclonal antibody (ibritumomab) with tiuxetan which is a binding chelator agent. Conjugation with tiuxetan provides effectively binding of the ibritumomab molecule with In-111 for imaging and dosimetric studies, and with Y-90 for RIT. In 2003, **I-131 tositumomab (Bexxar®)** was the second radiopharmaceutical approved for use in the treatment of relapsed, refractory, and transformed indolent lymphomas. I-131 combines directly with monoclonal antibody tositumomab without the need for a chelating molecule [26, 27, 105–108].

CD20 antigen is an integral transmembrane, non-glycosylated protein that is expressed on all B-cell series from normal and neoplastic pre-B cells to mature B-cells. The CD20 antigen provides a suitable target for immunotherapy. Both rituximab which is a non-radioactive human/mice chimeric anti-CD20 antibody, and ibritumomab tiuxetan are bound to the CD20 receptors on the B-cells. Using this feature, rituximab is administered before Y-90 tiuxetan. Ibritumomab induces complement-dependent cytotoxicity, antibody-dependent cell-mediated cytotoxicity, and programmed cell death [25, 26, 107]. Similarly, non-radioactive tositumomab is administered to the patients who will receive I-131 tositumomab treatment for the same purpose [106]. Y-90 travels a longer distance in tissue than I-131 (5.3 mm and 0.8 mm, respectively). Higher linear energy transfer (LET) to the tissues at a longer distance provides an advantage in the treatment. It is more effective for both target cells and adjacent tumor cells with ***bystander effect*** (neighboring effect). Therefore, treatment with Y-90-bound antibodies should be firstly preferred in the large (≥5 cm) tumor masses with poor blood supply and expressed with heterogeneous CD20 receptors [1, 25, 26, 107]. Both radiopharmaceuticals used for radioimmunotherapy are stable. However, I-131 can be released from the carrier monoclonal antibody molecule by dehalogenization. In this case, free I-131 entering the bloodstream will increase the total body radiation dose and may cause hypothyroidism by being accumulated in the thyroid gland. Supersatured potassium iodide or Lugol solution is administered per oral to patients to prevent iodine uptake and retention in the thyroid cells. However, this risk is low as there will be no dehalogenation in the treatment of I-131 tositumomab which is a stable radiopharmaceutical [106]. Studies revealed a response rate of 67–83% in the treatment with these agents. Some considerations should be made when selecting Y-90 ibritumomab tiuxetan and I-131 tositumomab in treatment [25]. Radiation safety, treatment protocol, toxicity, clinical effectiveness, and quality of life differ for both radiopharmaceuticals. For example, I-131 tositumomab allows treatment, dosimetric studies, and imaging. Y-90 ibritumomab tiuxetan cannot be used except for treatment because Y-90 is a pure beta-emitting radionuclide. For dosimetric measurements and imaging, an In-111 labeled antibody study must be performed. However, since it was shown that there was no relationship between toxicity and the administered dose, fixed-dose administration was initiated without performing a dosimetric study [25, 27, 105–107].

Radiation dosimetry allows the determination of the radiopharmaceutical dose to be administered to each patient. This is particularly important in RIT agents whose urinary excretion varies from patient to patient, e.g., I-131 tositumomab. Kaminski et al. [106] reported urinary excretion in a wide range of 46–90% in the first 48 h after administration. 5 mCi I-131 tositumomab is administered one week before treatment. After a few days, whole-body serial images are obtained and the distribution of radiopharmaceutical and treatment dose are determined using obtained WB images. Variability between patients for urinary excretion of Y-90 ibritumomab tiuxetan has been reported at a very low rate of 5%. It has also been reported that urinary excretion is very low and does not exceed 11% in the first 7 days following administration. Since a dosimetric study with Y-90 is difficult to perform, a fixed-dose is preferred [25, 26]. Bone marrow is the target organ in radioimmunotherapies. Concerns about radiation-induced myelodysplastic syndrome (MDS) and AML have been frequently expressed. However, the incidence of MDS/AML that occurred following RIT is almost identical to the rates reported after treatment with many standard chemotherapeutic agents. Studies have shown that hematological toxicity is not linearly related to the administered dose. Patient-related factors (such as loss of bone marrow function due to previous chemotherapy and external radiotherapy or bone marrow involvement in NHL) have been reported to cause the bone marrow toxicity. In cases to whom radioimmunotherapy will be applied, a fixed dose of activity is mostly given without the need for a whole-body dosimetric study. However, compliance with patient selection criteria is recommended to reduce bone marrow toxicity. Bone marrow involvement must be less than 25% in bone marrow biopsy specimen; pre-treatment platelet count must be 150,000/mm^3 (at the dose of 15 MBq/kg [0.4 mCi/kg] Y-90 ibritumomab tiuxetan) or 100,000–149,000/mm^3 (at the dose of 11 MBq/kg [0.3 mCi/kg] Y-90 ibritumomab tiuxetan) and no autologous bone marrow or peripheral blood stem cell transplantation should have been performed before. The standard dose for I-131 tositumomab ranges between 50 and 160 mCi (1.85–5.92 GBq) in the patients with platelet counts of 150,000/mm^3 [25, 26, 32, 49, 106].

Since I-131 emits beta radiation as well as high-energy gamma rays, patients treated with I-131 tositumomab may need to stay in the hospital. However, Y-90 ibritumomab tiuxetan treatment can be administered outpatient. Since Y-90 is a pure beta-emitting agent and beta particles have a short penetration range in tissue (5.3 mm), the risk of radiation exposure to the persons near to the patient is low (<5 mSv). According to the Nuclear Regulatory Commission (NRC) guidelines (1997) [29] released from the USA, patients treated with Y-90 ibritumomab tiuxetan do not need to stay in the hospital. The new discharge criterion is based on the total effective dose equivalent (TEDE) limit for the maximum exposure dose, and TEDE <5 mSv (<500 mrem) allows outpatient treatment. Based on this rule, a minimum treatment dose is 38,500 mCi (1425 GBq) for Y-90 ibritumomab tiuxetan treatment in order for the patient to remain in the hospital. Accordingly, outpatient treatment is safe and within acceptable limits as the maximum standard dose ranges 20–30 mCi (0.74–1.11 GBq). In the guideline published by TAEA, the maximum activity level that patients can have in their bodies at the time of discharge is stated as 108 mCi (4000 MBq) for Y-90. Within the first week after Y-90 treatment, the patient should not be discharged until the measured external radiation dose from the patient or the activity of feces and body fluids has decreased to an acceptable level [72]. Again, the radiation dose that family members were exposed during the first week after Y-90 ibritumomab tiuxetan treatment was measured and the average exposure dose was reported to be 3.5 mRem. This value is the normal natural radiation level [23, 26, 108]. In the Directive on Release of Patients Receiving Radionuclide Therapy [72] published by TAEA, the acceptable activity level in the patient body for discharge after treatment with I-131 labeled theranostics was reported as 600 MBq and the acceptable radiation dose measured 1 m away from the patient was reported as 25–40 microSv/h.

(The permissible activity level in the Radiation Safety Regulation [71] is 600 MBq and the dose rate 1 m away from the patient is given as 30 microSv/h.) For Y-90, the dose rate measured 1 m away from the patient was defined as zero. Patients who receive 33 mCi (1.22 GBq) dose of I-131-labelled antibody therapy [or dose rate of 0.07 mSv/h (7 mrem/h) at a distance of 1 m] can be given outpatient treatment if there is no person in close contact to expose higher than 5 mSv of radiation dose around them [27, 72]. Since Y-90 is a pure beta-emitting radionuclide, the activity to be excreted with the patient's feces and body fluids gains importance. If the excretion of radionuclide from the body continues actively, more attention should be paid to the cleaning of laundry, dishes, and other items that are at risk of contamination used by the patient and especially toilet cleaning in order to protect people living at home [72]. Patient characteristics should also be taken into account when deciding on outpatient or inpatient treatment. The ability and desire of the patient to understand the radiation safety rules described verbally and given as a printed form, be able to meet their own needs, to avoid going back to work when necessary, the risk of radiation exposure for other people on their way home after treatment and urinary incontinence should be examined when deciding whether treatment with I-131-labelled antibodies (anti-B1-antibody) can be given outpatient. When preparing the patient for treatment, the questioning form should be filled in, then the nuclear medicine specialist and radiation safety officer should decide whether the patient should be sent home. Patients who are decided to be sent home should also be given a printed form containing the rules they should pay attention to in terms of radiation safety. This form, which contains the rules to be followed when sending home, should also be given to patients who have received Y-90 ibritumomab tiuxetan treatment. Urine contamination should be prevented in all radionuclide therapies. Personnel administering Y-90 ibritumomab tiuxetan treatment must definitely work with gloves and avoid direct contact with the patient's body fluids [27, 32, 49, 72, 108].

3.3.8 Theranostic Agents Used in the Liver Primary Tumors and Metastases

I-131 or Re-188 lipiodol (ethiodized oil) and radionuclide-labeled (Y-90, Ho-166, Re-188) microspheres (resin-based or glass) are used to create arterial embolization in the treatment of primary or secondary liver tumors. Since the properties of I-131 radionuclide are described in the previous sections, they will not be mentioned here. As known, Y-90 has a physical half-life of 2.67 days and is a pure beta-emitting agent with a high-energy. It has a maximum of 2.26 MeV and an average of 0.94 MeV beta energy. It travels a maximum of 11 mm and an average of 4 mm in the soft tissue. Microspheres used in intra-arterial treatment should have high mechanical and chemical stability and should be of equal size. **Y-90 resin-microspheres (SIR-Spheres®)** have an acrylic polymer structure with a diameter of 20–60 μm. Y-90 is bound to the carboxylic group of the polymer after microspheres are produced. **Glass microspheres (TheraSphere®)** are 20–30 μm in diameter. Y-89 embedded in the glass matrix is activated to Y-90 in a nuclear reactor. Microspheres are biocompatible; they do not decay in the body and Y-90 activity is not thrown into the sewer [19, 39]. **I-131 lipiodol** reaches to the tumor microvessels and is retained in the tumor tissue after being administered through the hepatic artery in the treatment of hepatocellular carcinoma (HCC). It is slowly cleared from the tumoral tissue as there are no lymphatic vessels, Kupffer cells, and endocytosis. The activity that is not retained in the tumor but remains in the circulation is distributed in normal liver tissue. It is administered at a standard dose of 60 mCi (2.22 GBq). Twenty-four hours after administration, 75–90% of the administered activity is retained in the liver; binding ratio of the tumoral to non-tumoral liver tissue is between 2.3 and 12. Effective half-life is 5.5 days in tumor tissue and 3.5 days in normal liver tissue. Pulmonary uptake is observed at 10–25% due to arteriovenous shunts in the liver. Lung activity slightly increases in the first 2 days but decreases within 4–5 days following administration. There is no recirculation. Excretion occurs mainly by the kidneys (30–50% in 7 days). The rate of excretion with feces is low (3% in 5 days). The urine contamination should be prevented for the first 2 days after treatment. The therapeutic effect of I-131 lipiodol is not due to an ischemia accompanied by chemo-embolization but alone results from direct radiation effect. Ninety percent of the radiobiological effect is caused by short-range beta irradiation. Patient relatives and caregivers must be informed about radiation safety rules. Patients should avoid pregnancy for at least 4 months after treatment [19, 109, 110].

Y-90 microsphere treatment results in the cell death due to free radicals. Optimal blood flow is required to increase treatment efficacy. Normal liver parenchyma is supplied from the portal vein by the rate of more than 80%, while more than 80% of blood supply of the tumors with a diameter of greater than 2 cm is provided by the hepatic artery. Radioactive compounds applied directly into the hepatic artery are firstly retained at a high rate in the arterial vascular structures in the tumor tissue. Thus, very high radiation doses are delivered to tumor tissue although tolerable radiation doses are delivered to normal hepatic tissue [40, 109]. Vascularization of liver metastatic lesions varies. Metastatic lesions may have avascular cystic structure as well as features of normal liver parenchyma. Less (i.e., colon, pancreas, breast cancer metastases) or more vascularized (i.e., renal, NET, thyroid carcinoma metastases) metastatic lesions may develop. Radiolabeled small diameter particles (lipiodol or sphere) will provide a highly effective treatment of liver metastatic lesions with a high absorbed dose without damaging normal parenchyma because of the relatively low absorbed dose [19, 40, 109, 110]. Before Y-90 microsphere treatment, quantification for possible hepatopulmonary shunt (must be <20%) should be performed using Tc-99m albumin macroaggregate (MAA) scintigraphy and whether the hepatic arterial flow is associated with the stomach, intestine, and pancreas should be examined by selective angiography. If a metastatic lesion is detected in the single lobe, the catheter should be selectively placed in the right or left lobe artery feeding the effected lobe. Thus, non-metastatic parenchymal tissue will be protected from radiation hazardous effects because the efficacy of treatment results from radiation rather than ischemia due to chemoembolization or pure embolization, such as I-131 lipiodol. The tumor cells surrounding the microvessels where the radioactive agent reaches at a high rate are destroyed by beta particles [27, 49, 109]. Each of the glass spheres has about 2500 Bq activity and 50 Bq activity in resin spheres at the time of production. Commercially available vials contain activities up to 20 GBq for the glass spheres and up to 3 GBq for the resin spheres. Since glass spheres are injected in a limited number, they may probably cause less embolism effect in microvessels and their dose distribution is heterogeneous. On the other hand, resin spheres can be applied in a higher number and show uniform dose distribution. Therefore, its biological effect (efficacy and toxicity) is higher than the glass ones [109]. Y-90 glass microspheres are used in the treatment of unresectable primary (hepatocellular carcinoma) and secondary (metastatic) lesions of the liver. Y-90 resin microspheres can be administered together with fluorodeoxyuridine in the treatment of liver metastases of the colorectal cancer. Y-90, which has a half-life of 2.7 days, has little or no elimination from the body. In addition, since it is a pure beta emitter, the dose of external radiation exposure around the patient resulting from X-rays will be very low. Therefore, the patient can be discharged from the hospital for up to 4000 MBq activity in the body. The radiation dose rate 1 m away the patient is 25 microSv/h. No precautions are required after discharge, except for urgent clinical situations. If an emergency develops after treatment (acute cerebral event, coma, etc.), precautions should be taken to prevent radioactive contamination and to minimize external irradiation as low as possible if the patient is admitted to the emergency care unit. Healthcare personnels should avoid direct contact with the patient's mouth and body secretions. All emergency staff should wear gloves for radioactive contamination protection and be informed about radiation safety rules. It is recommended to avoid pregnancy for up to 1 month after cancer treatment [32, 49, 72, 111]. The absolute contraindications for RN treatment in the liver malignancies are pregnancy and breastfeeding, life expectancy less than 1 month, hepatic encephalopathy, Child-Pugh score higher than B7, and iodine allergy. Relative contraindications are coagulation disorders, acute or severe renal failure (creatinine clearance < 30 ml/min) [32, 40, 49, 72]. Breastfeeding mothers constitute a special group. As a general rule, breastfeeding should be discontinued 2–3 weeks before and after RN treatments.

There are two possible radiation risks for the baby: (1) Ingestion of contaminated breast milk may cause significant internal radiation exposure in some organs of the nursing baby. If there is free Y-90, it will possibly pass into the systemic circulation of the treated mother. There is no such risk for glass microspheres. However, resin microspheres may have trace amounts of free Y-90 on their surface as low as 0.4% of the administered activity. Dosimetric studies have shown that the activity level detected in the maternal circulation during the first 24 h of treatment is less than 12 MBq when a 3 GBq treatment dose is administered. The rate of absorption of free Y-90 radionuclide in the breast milk from the baby's intestines is low (only 0.01% is absorbed from the intestine and enters into the systemic circulation). The descending colon wall of the baby is the target organ and is exposed to a dose of 0.1 mGy. This dose is much less than 1 mSv dose accepted for the interruption of breastfeeding. (2) Direct exposure of the baby to external radiation from the mother's body. Güleç et al. [39] found in their study that Y-90 microsphere treatments with administered activity less than 17 GBq dose could not reach 1 mSv radiation exposure dose in the baby; when 9 GBq glass microspheres were applied, the baby's radiation exposure from bremsstrahlung X rays was 0.53 mSv. Ultimately, they reported that external radiation exposure would be minimal as well as internal exposure. Therefore, they reported that advising patients to avoid close contact with children or pregnant women and even to stop breastfeeding would be highly conservative [39]. However, although external and internal radiation exposure is below the accepted level for babies, generally accepted rule is that the breastfeeding should be discontinued. Here, it is mainly aimed to avoid stochastic effects, to reduce the risk of developing cancer in the baby, and to reduce the radiation exposure of the mother's breasts [23, 29, 72].

Ho-166 polymer-based microspheres (20–50 μm) are administered through the hepatic artery in the treatment of liver malignancies. Ho-166 ($t_{1/2} = 26.8$ h) is a beta minus ($E\text{max} = 1.84$ MeV) and gamma ($E_\gamma = 81$ keV) emitter agent. It is an element belonging to the lanthanide group. It is obtained from neutron bombardment of Ho-165 microspheres [112]. Radioactive microspheres are located in the vessels around or inside the tumor and radiate the surrounding tissue. It has been shown in a Phase II study that radioembolization with Ho-166 microspheres is safe in the treatment of liver malignancies [113, 114]. Therapeutic dose is administered by a single injection; no more than 3 injections are recommended. Firstly, 250 MBq Ho-166 (approximately 3 million microspheres) is administered intraarterially as a scout dose; the vessels feeding the tumor or tumor foci are determined; extrahepatic activity and the absorbed dose are calculated. After the injection, SPECT/CT or MR (since it is a lanthanide element) imaging is performed. The total activity dose is determined by the absorbed dose in the target tissue as measured on CT images (the target absorbed dose is 60 Gy or 3.8 GBq/kg liver tissue, including the Ho-166 scout dose). Then, Ho-166 microspheres are administered intraarterially at the treatment dose; a total of 30 million microspheres are aimed to be administered. Since the most important side effect is observed in the gastrointestinal tract, proton pump inhibitors (6 weeks ago), antiemetic and steroid therapy should be initiated for patients before treatment [113, 114]. A patient-specific dosimetric study will increase effectiveness of the treatment. Unlike Y-90 microsphere treatment, Tc-99m MAA scintigraphy is not required. In Ho-166 microsphere therapy, scout imaging performed before the treatment dose ensures that the effective dose is determined with high accuracy. However, Tc-99m MAA can be used to predict the absorbed dose to the lungs which can be more accurately predicted with a scout dose. Studies have reported that the prescribed dose calculated from Tc-99m MAA decreases by 40% and consequently the risk of developing radiation pneumonitis will decrease. The presence of gamma rays partially increases the risk of radiation exposure when treatment with 7 GBq Ho-166 is administered. As the risk of exposure for the first 6 h after treatment is high, close contact with the patient should be prevented during this time. No restriction will be required in the cases with a treatment dose less than 7 GBq [113, 114].

Re-188 is a recently interesting theranostic agent because it is a generator product (W-188/Re-188 generator), has low cost and is easy to obtain, and also has low energy gamma rays. Re-188 has maximum beta energy of 2.2 MeV and has a physical half-life of 17.4 h. In addition, there is a 155 keV gamma-rays with 15% abundancy. **Re-188 HDD lipiodol** is the first form of various Re-188-labelled theranostic agents (lipiodol and microsphere) to be administered in clinical trials supported by the IAEA. The results of Phase I and II studies showed that intraarterial administration (1.8 and 9.8 GBq) was effective and cost-effective in the treatment of primary hepatocellular carcinoma [115–117]. Lipiodol injected intra-arterially weakly attaches to tumor capillaries and is poorly retained in them. It passes retrograde from hepatic sinusoids to portal venules and shows antegrade spread along the prebiliary vascular network. Radiation exposure secondary to Re-188 lipiodol molecules escaping outside the target tissue is low due to its short half-life. However, it has been reported that severe side effects (such as pneumonia) may sometimes occur due to Re-188 lipiodol entering the systemic circulation. 44.1% (±11.7) of the administered Re-188 lipiodol activity is excreted in the urine within 72 h following treatment [117, 118].

Re-188 microspheres remain highly stable without decaying in the in vivo and in vitro environment; 90% and 88%, respectively. Stability was reported to be 53% ± 4.5% for Re-188 microspheres. The rate of urinary excretion was lower (8.9 ± 3.8%) than Re-188 HDD lipiodol compound. No serious toxic effects have been identified. A mild transient liver toxicity may develop within 12 days after treatment. The development of hepatic toxicity is dose-dependent [119]. Further case studies are needed for clinical use. Strict precautions are not required except for urinary contamination and close contact with the patient in terms of radiation safety. Re-188 treatments require 784 mCi (29,000 MBq = 29 GBq) activity for 5 mSv and 157 mCi (5800 MBq) activity for 1 mSv absorption dose in the patient body [72]. The highest treatment dose in the studies is reported as 20 GBq [72, 119]. So that, it is suitable for outpatient treatment. Depending on the cognitive characteristics of the patient, inpatient treatment can be applied [72].

3.3.9 Lu-177 PSMA Treatment in Prostate Cancer Cases

The prostate-specific membrane antigen (PSMA) is a type II transmembrane glycoprotein. It is found at a high rate in metastatic prostate cancer and hormone-resistant prostate cancer (HRPC); same with the definition of castration-resistant prostate cancer (CRPC). It is not specific to the prostate gland; it is expressed in other normal tissues (salivary glands, duodenal mucosa, proximal renal tubular cells, and neuroendocrine cells in colonic crypts) and neoplastic tissues (transitional cell carcinoma, renal clear cell carcinoma, colon carcinoma and endothelial cells of the tumor-related microvessels or in "neo-angiogenesis") [104]. Different radioligands labeled with Lu-177 (small molecular inhibitors Lu-177 DKFZ-PSMA-617, Lu-177 DOTAGA-(I-y) fk(Sub-KuE), and Lu-177-Dota-J591 monoclonal antibody) other than Lu-177 PSMA-617 have been developed for use in the targeted treatment of PSMA [120, 121]. In addition, treatments with I-131 and Y-90 labeled radiopharmaceuticals are under investigation. Ga-68 PSMA PET/CT imaging is performed before targeted RN treatment in the prostate cancer cases. Although false-negative and false-positive results have been reported in the detection of small lesions and in the cases showing neuroendocrine differentiation, it is useful because the tumor tissue/background activity ratio is high in the prostate cancer cases. Ga-68 PSMA PET/CT imaging provides useful information on the efficacy and the patient follow-up not only PSMA-based RN therapy but also Ra-223 dichloride treatment [15, 104, 122].

Lu-177 PSMA-617 therapy is a reliable and safe treatment (mean activity administered is 5059 ± 1845 MBq, 1–4 cycles). It has a little toxic effect. It is excreted mainly by the kidneys. Biochemical response (decrease in sPSA level) to Lu-177 PSMA-617 treatment was reported in 50% of cases. Studies have shown that it prolongs life span expectancy. Salivary glands and lacrimal glands are critical organs and are exposed to radiation at doses of 0.72–1.4 Gy/GBq and 3.8 Gy/

GBq, respectively. Kidneys and bone marrow, which are the other risky organs, are exposed to radiation at a dose of 0.75–1 Gy/GBq and 12–48 mGy/GBq, respectively. Mild transient xerostomia may develop [104, 120, 121]. The absorbed doses in the organs are almost the same with Lu-177 DOTAGA-(I-y)fk(Sub-KuE). It was reported as 13 Gy/GBq for parotid, 0.8 Gy/GBq for kidneys, and 14 mGy/GBq for bone marrow. The radiation exposure to normal tissues is higher in Lu-177 DOTA-J591 treatment than other radiopharmaceuticals [32, 49]. The PSMA-617 molecule can be bound with I-125, Astatin-221 (Horse-221), Bi-213, Ac-225, and Scandium-44 (Sc-44).

Ac-225 PSMA-617 was administered every 2 months at a dose of 100 kBq/kg in the patients with metastatic CRPC; a prominent decrease in serum PSA levels was reported without hematological unwanted effects [36, 104]. Repeated treatments in the 8-week intervals can provide to continue the therapeutic efficacy. There is a low risk of developing bone marrow toxicity and salivary gland damage in the treatment with radionuclides emitting Auger electron or alpha particles with a short range in tissue. The risk of hematological toxicity has been shown to be significantly lower in the patients with prostate cancer with neuroendocrine differentiation during the treatment of bone metastases with Bi-213 DOTATOC, which is an alpha-emitter agent [123].

Lu-177 PSMA is excreted mainly by the kidneys after administration. It shows rapid clearance within 2 h following administration and then slow clearance within 41 h. It is excreted by about 70% in the first 12 h [120]. Lu-177 PSMA is a suitable agent for outpatient treatment. It has been reported that patients can be discharged 6 h after radiopharmaceutical application according to the radiation safety rule of 30 microSv/h at a distance of 1 m, which is an acceptable dose for discharge [30, 121]. In Australia, patient-specific radiation doses for patients receiving Lu-177 PSMA treatment at a standard dose of 6–8 GBq remain within acceptable outpatient doses (25 microSv/h at a distance of 1 m). Effective half-life for Lu-177 PSMA-617 has been reported as approximately 85 h in the dosimetric studies. Radiation exposure of people (personnel and patient relatives) around the patient 1 m away the patient was reported as 23 ± 6 microSv/h 4 h and 15 ± 4 microSv/h 6 h after administration of Lu-177 PSMA 617 at a dose of 7.5 GBq. The dose taken by family members close to the patient in 5 days following treatment has been reported as 202 ± 43 microSv [30, 32, 121]. However, since it is excreted in urine, it is considered that Lu-177 activity in the general sewer system has reached a significant level in many European countries and the patient should stay in the hospital. The Lu-177 level accepted in the sewage system is 100 kBq/ml in Germany. Patients receiving Lu-177 PSMA treatment should stay in the hospital for at least 48 h (3 days for Germany) according to local legislation in Austria and Italy, as well as Germany [23, 120, 121]. The main reason for this practice is that the Lu-177 level in the sewage fluid exceeds the annually accepted value (ALI) and the environment is more likely to be exposed to radiation higher than 1 mSv/year due to the increase in the number of prostate cancer cases treated with RN, and the repeated administration of treatment within one year (up to 4 cycles). According to the Directive on Discharge of Patients Receiving Radionuclide Therapy (RSGD-KLV-009.Rev 2) published by TAEA in Turkey, the amount of activity accepted in the body in order to send patients home is 1400 MBq and patients should be hospitalized for at least 24 h after Lu-177 treatment dose at 7400 MBq [72]. Twenty-four hours after treatment, the dose rate 1 m away the patient is approximately 7.5 μSv/h. However, isolation of the treated patient is recommended to protect the patient's relatives and publics from external radiation exposure caused by gamma rays and bremsstrahlung-X rays. The radiation safety measures for Lu-177 treatment discussed in the radiopeptides treatment section are also applied to the patients receiving Lu-177 PSMA treatment and their relatives. When calculating the radiation exposure dose, it is recommended to use effective half-life rather than physical half-life. Thus, unnecessary hospitalization will be avoided. Although the dose that family members are exposed to is within the acceptable limit (< 30 microSv/h and < 1 mSv/year for the public and 5 mSv/year for caregivers) [1, 70, 71], it is mandatory to comply with local legislation on outpatient treatment and discharge for the reasons we explained earlier [30, 72, 121].

3.3.10 Radiopharmaceuticals Used in the Treatment of Craniopharyngiomas

Craniopharyngiomas are a rare solid tumor of childhood. They are slow-growing benign epithelial tumors that arise from ectodermal residues, Rathke's cleft or other embryonal epithelial cells along the path of the craniopharyngeal duct. Craniopharyngiomas are most commonly observed in the supratentorial region. Localization and extension of the tumor are the most important factors effecting treatment and prognosis. Regardless of treatment, the 10-year survival rate exceeds 90%. Although tumors are benign, they should be treated due to their location.

Surgery is an essential treatment method. Total tumor resection increases morbidity and mortality, but does not eliminate the possibility of local tumor recurrence. In addition, radical resection negatively effects the patients' quality of life. Therefore, partial resection with or without postoperative radiotherapy or interstitial radiotherapy is recommended [124]. Interstitial radiotherapy can be applied after cyst fluid aspiration or drainage in the treatment of giant posterior fossa cystic craniopharyngiomas in the pediatric group, and phosphor-32 (P-32) in colloidal form can be used for this purpose (evidence level 2A). The most suitable group for this treatment is the patients with a simple cyst and a tumor volume of 3–40 ml. The therapeutic dose ranges between 50–1000 Gy, mostly 200–300 Gy. It has been reported that if the administered dose is less than 200 Gy, the efficacy of the treatment will decrease and the likelihood of recurrence will increase [125–127]. Bone tissue is a critical organ for P-32 compounds. The total dose to the skeleton system during treatment will be 160 mRem/Ci. Pure beta-emitting Y-90 colloids can also be successfully used in the RN treatment of craniopharyngiomas [128, 129].

3.3.11 Radionuclide Therapy in the Myeloproliferative Diseases

Myeloproliferative neoplasms (MPN) are the heterogeneous group of disorders characterized by the proliferation of one or more series of hematological cells in bone marrow. **P-32** was first used in the 1920s in the treatment of polycythemia vera (PV), essential thrombocythemia (ET) and chronic myeloid (CML) leukemia, and is still used in the treatment of PV and ET. It is a well-tolerated agent that can also be used in elderly patients (>65 years). It is a pure beta emitter (maximum beta energy 1.71 MeV). Its physical half-life is 14.3 days and is administered intravenously. There are reservations that it adversely effects bone marrow cells and causes leukemia development (5–14%). This risk increases when P-32 is administered alone at a cumulative dose of 1000 MBq and is used in combination with alkylating agents. However, it is known that there was no contact with P-32, hydroxyurea, or alkylating agent in 25% of patients who developed leukemia. Recently, its use has decreased with the development of new chemotherapeutic agents in the treatment of hematologic malignancies. However, it is still used today in the treatment of PV and ET. The absolute contraindications are pregnancy and breastfeeding. For the treatment of PV, relative contraindications are total white blood cell count (WBC) $<2.0 \times 10^9$/L and a rapid renal function loss. Relative contraindications for essential thrombocythemia are total WBC $<2.0 \times 10^9$/L and hemoglobin <90 g/L, and a rapid impairment in the renal function [37, 102].

In the treatment of polycythemia vera, venosection (phlebotomy) is performed with the patient's hematocrit until going down to 42–47% before administration to the patient. Most of the intravenously administered radionuclide rapidly accumulate in the bone marrow; a few days later, a lower uptake rate occurs in the liver, spleen, and lymph nodes. P-32 orthophosphate works by entering the nuclei of rapidly proliferating and protein-synthesizing cells. It is also retained by the hydroxyapatite molecule in the cortical bone. Chemotherapy should be discontinued for 1 week after P-32 administration. The use of estrogens or androgens may alter P-32 biodistribution [1, 6]. Since it is a pure beta emitter, the risk of radiation exposure of the personnel is ignored and no special protection measure is required for external irradiation around the patient. However, attention should be paid to the risk of contamination as P-32 is excreted in the large amounts in the urine within the first 48 h after administration. When leaving from the hospital, the level of activity remaining in the body is primarily taken into account (should be <1200 MBq) rather than external radiation dose rate measurements. If inpatient treatment is required, the personnel should be warned to avoid from contamination. Pregnancy is prohibited for 4 months after treatment [23, 37, 72, 102].

Holmium-166 (Ho-166) DOTMP (1,4,7,10-tetraazacyclo dodecane-1,4,7,10-tetraethylene phosphonic acid) is an agent used to treat multiple myeloma. The Ho-166 emits beta particles at high energy which are suitable for treatment, and also gamma rays for image acquisition. It is administered intravenously at a dose of 12.2–77.7 GBq. About 75–80% of the administered activity is excreted in the urine within 24 h. Therefore, attention should be paid to the risk of urinary contamination during this time. It is suitable for outpatient treatment. However, the patient should not be discharged from the nuclear medicine department without emptying the bladder at least once or twice. Urethral catheterization is required for patients with urinary incontinence. A special attention should be paid to toilet cleaning and contamination precautions should be taken for the patient's dishes (fork, spoon, plate, etc.) and laundries [23, 72].

3.4 Radionuclide Therapy in the Breastfeeding Mothers

Most radiopharmaceuticals can pass into the milk. In this case, the risk of radiation exposure on the baby will increase. Therapeutic RPs are potentially hazardous no matter which way they are administered. Breastfeeding should be definitely discontinued. The risk of cancer development is important for the children. Hypothyroidism may develop due to I-131 treatment or the risk of developing thyroid cancer in the future increases. It is generally accepted that intracavitary applications with Y-90-labelled radiopharmaceuticals or treatments through the hepatic artery are less harmful [23, 39]. However, in practice, the free radionuclide/theranostic agent may enter into the systemic circulation as described in the previous section. In addition, there will be external radiation exposure from close contact of the baby with the mother during breastfeeding. Reducing milk release from the breast tissue by terminating breastfeeding will reduce the radiation exposure of mother's breast tissue. It is recommended to decrease radiation exposure by discontinuing breastfeeding 2–3 weeks before the radionuclide therapy. Lactation suppressive medical treatment (bromocriptine) should be started 6–8 weeks prior to treatment with I-131-labelled theranostics and breastfeeding must be prohibited for 3 months following treatment [1, 49, 72].

3.5 Overview of Dosimetry Methods in the Radionuclide Treatments

The effectiveness of radionuclide therapy depends on the radiosensitivity of the tumor tissue and the amount of energy absorbed. The amount of radiation absorbed (=Gy) in a tumor or an organ is calculated by the following formula. The S value in this formula is specific to radionuclide and gives the level of linear energy transfer (LET).

$$\text{Gy} = \text{tumor volume in which activity distributes} \times \text{tumor retention time}(t) \times S(\text{mGy} / \text{MBq} / \text{s})$$

Patient-specific dosimetric studies are conducted to assess the risk of toxicity in critical organs such as kidney and bone marrow. Different methods can be used for this purpose. However, scintigraphic images and blood or urine samples are mostly used. Planar or SPECT imaging or PET imaging is performed. The amount of activity applied and residence time in the body should be known for the calculation of the absorbed dose. There are many programs used for absorbed dose calculation (such as MIRDOSE, OLINDA/EXM). Dosimetric analysis is usually based on the MIRD committee diagram [13, 49, 59, 67, 95, 130].

Dosimetric calculation can be performed more easily in the treatment of liver masses by radioembolization with Y-90 particles compared to systemic RN treatments. Because the tumor volume is obtained from CT images, total amount of the radionuclide administered intraarterially remains in the tumor tissue and *the residence time* is calculated with the following formula, *residence time= T1/2 eff ln2* by using the effective half-life. However, the dose of radiation exposure in systemic or local (intratumoral, intracavitary) RN treatments is difficult to determine. The amount of radioactivity accumulated in the target tissue in systemic treatment for radionuclides emitting gamma rays (e.g., I-131, Sm-153, Re-186, Re-188, Ho-166) can be detected by quantitative SPECT imaging or uptake measurements performed. However, this is not possible for pure beta-emitting therapeutic agents (e.g., Y-90, P-32).

The retention time of radionuclide in tumor tissue is related to metabolic activity and can be directly measured when gamma-emitting radiopharmaceuticals are used. Dosimetry in the radionuclide treatments should be directed at calculating the cumulative dose in bone marrow or critical organs to prevent the development of serious side effects, as noted in previous sections [1, 32, 49, 59, 60]. Anatomical tumor volume in the solid tumors can be measured by ultrasound, CT, MRI. However, it is difficult to calculate the target tumor volume in diffuse bone marrow involvement or intracavitary lesions. Quantitative SPECT and PET images enable the calculation of the target tumor volume with high accuracy [32, 49]. Volume calculation by scintigraphic methods is only possible with gamma-emitter or PET radionuclides, but is not possible with pure beta-emitters. In this case, [Volume (mL) = pixel vol (ml) × *n* pixels/ROI/cross section × n(sl) CF] equation is used [where *n = the number of pixels in the area where radionuclide is accumulated; n(sl) = the number of sections with marked pixels; CF= correction factor (a value determined for the system using the appropriate phantom*)] [1, 30, 131].

Although evaluating the maximum amount of radioactivity accumulation in tumor tissue by targeted RN treatment is easy in solid tumors, intracavitary and intraarterial treatments because the radionuclide administered is localized in the target lesion, it is difficult in a systemic treatment. In diffuse metastatic lesions, the relative maximum uptake value (% activity applied) of the radiopharmaceutical is calculated. Gamma counters or quantitative SPECT methods are used for this purpose. Local uptake or whole-body dose measurement can be performed with both gamma and beta-emitting radionuclides (I-131). For pure beta-emitting radionuclides, gamma-ray emitters or PET agents with similar chemical structure are used, e.g., In-111 DOTA-octreotide, In-111 DOTA-lanreotide, or PET-radiopharmaceutical

Y-86 Octreotide. For the whole-body dose calculation, urinary excretion within 48–72 h, clearance in serial blood samples, or whole-body ROI values obtained with gamma-emitting agents are used. Despite the use of advanced equipment and methods, there are still some problems in the calculation of dosimetry because applied radiopharmaceutical mostly will not distribute homogeneously within the lesion. As a result, some of the target tissue will receive a higher dose than the other (Gy/MBq) [32, 49, 95].

3.6 Advances in The Radionuclide Therapy

The results of studies on cancer genetics and cell structural molecules have led to the emergence of promising new targets for the "theranostic" concept. The idea that Lu-177 labeled theranostics will be used much more in the treatment in the coming years is not an overstatement. Since alpha emitters are highly effective on tumor tissue though almost no radiation exposure of normal tissue, their use will widen in the treatment of malignancies. There are a lot of studies on this subject. For example, Ra-223 dichloride, which is currently used in the treatment of painful bone metastases, has been reported to be effective in the brain metastases in patients with recurrent osteosarcoma with brain metastases at a dose of 75 kBq/kg administered as an infusion 3 times a month [100]. This finding is promising to use Ra-223 dichloride in the treatment of osteoblast-rich brain metastases. Ra-223 pazopanib or sorafenib treatment is also tried in the treatment of bone metastases in the advanced kidney cancers and in the radioactive iodine-resistant thyroid cancers. In addition, the opinion that Ra-223 dichloride administration will be effective in breast cancers with bone metastasis is getting stronger [18, 132]. Ra-223 dichloride has been approved in both the USA and Europe in the treatment of bone metastases in patients with castration-resistant prostate cancer [132]. It is also a licensed indication in Turkey. However, the potential role for Ra-223 in the detection of osteolytic bone metastases is much less certain due to the uptake of the osteolytic bone metastases may be suboptimal [18, 31, 132, 133]. There are studies on the use of docetaxel as well as other agents such as abiraterone, enzalutamide in the early stage of disease [18, 31, 132, 133].

Antibodies that inhibit immune checkpoints [ipilimumab (anti-CTLA4), nivolumab (anti-PD-1), and pembrolizumab (anti-PD-1)] have been of great interest in the treatment of many malignancies such as kidney cancer, malignant melanoma, lung cancer, and Hodgkin's lymphoma recently [134]. The initial results are promising. The immunotherapeutic compounds allow cytotoxic T cells to better recognize and destroy cancer cells. Binding of these antibodies with beta- or alpha-emitting radionuclides will increase the efficacy of treatment and reduce its toxic effects. Again, it is attempted to combine molecules developed for cell receptors (such as gastrin-secreting peptide receptor, integrins, melanocyte-stimulating hormone receptor, melanocortin-1 receptor, VCAM-1) with high-energy beta (Lu-177, Y-90) or alpha particle-emitting radionuclides (Bi-213, Bi-212, At-211, Ac-225, Pb-212) [36, 104, 130, 132, 134–139].

Another important development in the treatment is radiovirus therapy using oncolytic viruses in the treatment with RNs of infected cancer cells [140–143]. Miest et al. showed in the rats that the administration of NIS gene carrying measles virus (MV-NIS) together with I-131 was effective in the treatment of mantle cell lymphoma, which is an aggressive B-cell non-Hodgkin lymphoma [140]. However, further studies are needed on the effect in humans and the treatment dose to be administered. Similarly, studies on its efficacy in the treatment of ovarian cancer, glioblastoma multiforme, multiple myeloma, prostate cancer, and mesothelioma using the NIS gene carrying measles virus are ongoing [137, 141–143]. Li et al. have shown in their experimental study that cancer cells can be destroyed by using oncolytic herpes simplex virus type 1 (oHSV-1) in the treatment of radiovirus in prostate cancer cases. For this purpose, rats were administered systemic I-131 after intratumoral oHSV-NIS virus injection; it was detected that tumor-carrying rats had an extended life span after radiovirus treatment [143].

The effectiveness of targeted radionuclide therapies increases with the development of new target molecules, radionuclides, and unifying molecules that provide stable binding. Radiation exposure of normal tissues decreases while the effect on cancer cells increases. However, its use as the first-line treatment is still limited. In order to be widely used in treatment, it should be easily accessible and inexpensive, and its superiority over routine treatments should be demonstrated in the large case groups. The predisposition of oncologists responsible for the treatment and follow-up of cancer patients to administer these treatments will also contribute to the widespread use.

References

1. Therapeutic Applications of Radiopharmaceuticals IAEA, Vienna, 2001 IAEA-TECDOC-1228.
2. Zhen W, Yin Z, Yinghui G, Huijuan I, Yanhui L, Jiajun Z, et al. Therapeutic response of radiosynovectomy with P-32 colloid in 326 patients with hemophilic arthropathy. Chin J Hematol. 2017;38:39–43.
3. Resche I, Chatal JF, Pecking A, Ell P, Duchesne G, Rubens R, et al. A dose controlled study of ^{153}Sm-EDTMP in the treatment of patients with painful bone metastases. Eur J Cancer. 1997;33:1583–91.
4. Lassmann M, Hänscheid H, Chiesa Cİ, Hindorf C, Flux G, Luster M. EANM Dosimetry Committee series on standard operational procedures for pre-therapeutic dosimetry I: blood and bone marrow dosimetry in differentiated thyroid cancer therapy. Eur J Nucl Med Mol Imaging. 2008;35:1405–12.
5. Liepe K, Hliscs R, Kropp J, Runge R, Knapp FF, Franke WG. Dosimetry of ^{188}Re-hydroxyethylidene diphosphonate in human prostate cancer skeletal metastases. J Nucl Med. 2003;44:953–60.
6. Handkiewicz-Junak D, Poeppel TD, Bodei L, Aktolun C, Ezziddin S, Giammarile F, et al. EANM guidelines for radionuclide therapy of bone metastases with beta-emitting radionuclides. Eur J Nucl Med Mol Imaging. 2018;45:846–59.
7. Qaim SM, Tarkanyi F, Capote R. Nuclear data for the production of therapeutic radionuclides. Vienna, Austria: Int Atomic Energy Agency; 2011.
8. Kassis AI, Adelstein SJ. Radiobiologic principles in radionuclide therapy. J Nucl Med. 2005;46(S1):4S–12S.
9. Lee ST, Kulkarni HR, Singh A, Baum RP. Theranostics of neuroendocrine. Tumors Visc Med. 2017;33:358–66.
10. Kesavan M, Claringbold PG, Turner JH. Hematological toxicity of combined ^{177}Lu-octreotate radiopeptide chemotherapy of gastroenteropancreatic neuroendocrine tumors in long-term follow-up. Neuroendocrinology. 2014;99:108–17.
11. Valkema R, De Jong M, Bakker WH, Breeman WA, Kooij PP, Lugtenburg PJ, et al. Phase I study of peptide receptor radionuclide therapy with [In-DTPA] octreotide: the Rotterdam experience. Semin Nucl Med. 2002;32:110–22.
12. Gudkov SV, Shilyagina NY, Vodeneev VA, Zvyagin AV. Targeted radionuclide therapy of human tumors. Int J Mol Sci. 2015;17:E33.
13. Taïeb D, Garrigue P, Bardiès M, Abdullah AE, Pacak K. Application and dosimetric requirements for Gallium-68-labeled somatostatin analogues in targeted radionuclide therapy for gastroenteropancreatic neuroendocrine tumors. PET Clin. 2015;10:477–86.
14. Chalkia MT, Stefanoyiannis AP, Chatziioannou SN, Round WH, Efstathopoulos EP, Nikiforidis GC. Patient-specific dosimetry in peptide receptor radionuclide therapy: a clinical review. Australas Phys Eng Sci Med. 2015;38:7–22.
15. Jong JM, Oprea-Lager DE, Hooft L, de Klerk JM, Bloemendal HJ, Verheul HM, et al. Radiopharmaceuticals for palliation of bone pain in patients with castration-resistant prostate cancer metastatic to bone: a systematic review. Eur Urol. 2016;70:416–26.
16. Bianchi L, Baroli A, Marzoli L, Verusio C, Chiesa C, Pozzi L. Prospective dosimetry with ^{99m}Tc-MDP in metabolic radiotherapy of bone metastases with ^{153}Sm-EDTMP. Eur J Nucl Med Mol Imaging. 2009;36:122–9.
17. Kendler DB, Araújo ML, Renata Alencar R, de Souza Accioly MT, Bulzico DA, de Noronha Pessoa CC, et al. Somatostatin receptor subtype 1 might be a predictor of better response to therapy in medullary thyroid carcinoma. Endocrine. 2017;58:474–80.
18. Coleman R, Aksnes AK, Naume B, Garcia C, Jerusalem G, Piccart M, et al. A phase IIa, nonrandomized study of radium-223 dichloride in advanced breast cancer patients with bone-dominant disease. Breast Cancer Res Treat. 2014;145:411–8.
19. EANM Radionuclide Therapy Committee Guideline for 131 I - ethiodised oil [lipiodol] therapy. Eur J Nucl Med. 2003;30:B20–2. https://doi.org/10.1007/s00259-002-1060-6.
20. Haghighatafshar M, Nowshad R, Etemadi Z, Ghaedian T. The effect of chewing-gum on dose rate of salivary gland in differentiated thyroid carcinoma patients treated with radioiodine. Q J Nucl Med Mol Imaging. 2018; https://doi.org/10.23736/S1824--4785.18.03078-9. [Epub ahead of print]
21. Alexander C, Bader JB, Schaefer A, Finke C, Kirsch CM. Intermediate and long-term side effects of high-dose radioiodine therapy for thyroid carcinoma. J Nucl Med. 1998;39:1551–4.
22. Moro L, Fantinato D, Frigerio F, Shamhan G, Angelovski G. Europium-154 contamination levels in Samarium-153-EDTMP for radionuclide therapy. J Phys Conf Ser. 2006;41:535–7.

23. Release of patients after radionuclide therapy with contributions from the International Commission on Radiological Protection International Atomic Energy Agency Vienna, 2009 Safety Reports Series No 63.
24. Haquin G, Vexler A, Pelled O, Riemer T, Kaniun N, Datz H, et al. Biological half-life measurements of radioactive strontium in hormonal-resistant prostate cancer patients. Available from: http://www.iaea.org/inis/collection/NCLCollectionStore/_Public/35/066/35066098.pdf. Accessed March 12, 2018.
25. Brinker BT, Gordon LI. Radioimmunotherapy safety: radiation protection, administration guidelines, isotope comparison, and quality of life issues. In: Hillmen P, Witzig TE, editors. Immunotherapy of lymphoid malignancies. 1st ed. Clinical Publishing of Oxford. Atlas Medical Publishing Ltd; 2005.
26. Wiseman GA, Kornmehl E, Leigh B, Erwin WD, Podoloff DA, Spies S, et al. Radiation dosimetry results and safety correlations from ^{90}Y-Ibritumomab Tiuxetan radioimmunotherapy for relapsed or refractory non-Hodgkin's lymphoma: combined data from 4 clinical trials. J Nucl Med. 2003;44:465–74.
27. Rutar FJ, Augustine SC, Colcher D, Siegel JA, Jacobson DA, et al. Outpatient treatment with ^{131}I-Anti-B1 antibody: radiation exposure to family members. J Nucl Med. 2001;42:907–15.
28. Kocher DC Radioactive decay data tables: a handbook of decay data for application to radiation dosimetry and radiological assessments. DOE/TIC-11026, 1981.
29. United States Nuclear Regulatory Commission. Release of patients administered radioactive materials. Washington, DC: United States Nuclear Regulatory Commission; 1997. Regulatory guide 8.39
30. Demir M, Abuqbeitah M, Uslu-Besli L, Yildirim O, Yeyin N, Cavdar I, et al. Evaluation of radiation safety in (177) Lu-PSMA therapy and development of outpatient treatment protocol. J Radiol Prot. 2016;36:269–78.
31. Poeppel TD, Handkiewicz-Junak D, Andreeff M, Becherer A, Bockisch A, Fricke E, et al. EANM guideline for radionuclide therapy with radium-223 of metastatic castration-resistant prostate cancer. Eur J Nucl Med Mol Imaging. 2018;45:824–45.
32. Stokke C, Gabiña PM, Solný P, Cicone F, Sandström M, Gleisner KS, et al. Dosimetry-based treatment planning for molecular radiotherapy: a summary of the 2017 report from the Internal Dosimetry Task Force. EJNMMI Phys. 2017;4:27.
33. de Jong M, Breeman WA, Valkema R, Bernard BF, Krenning EP. Combination radionuclide therapy using ^{177}Lu- and ^{90}Y-labeled somatostatin analogs. J Nucl Med. 2005;46(Suppl. 1):13S–7S.
34. Villard L, Romer A, Marincek N, Brunner P, Mt K, Schindler C, et al. Cohort study of somatostatin-based radiopeptide therapy with [(90)Y-DOTA]-TOC versus [(90)Y-DOTA]TOC plus [(177) Lu-DOTA]-TOC in neuroendocrine cancers. J Clin Oncol. 2012;30:1100–6.
35. Joshi MC, Subbarao BN, Thosar BV. Decay of Samarium-153. Proc Indian Acad Sci Sect A. 1957;45:390–401.
36. Kratochwil C, Bruchertseifer F, Rathke H, Bronzel M, Apostolidis C, Weichert W, et al. Targeted α-therapy of metastatic castration-resistant prostate cancer with ^{225}Ac-PSMA-617: dosimetry estimate and empiric dose finding. J Nucl Med. 2017;58:1624–31.
37. Yeong CH, Cheng M, NG KH. Therapeutic radionuclides in nuclear medicine: current and future prospects. J Zhejiang Univ-Sci B (Biomed Biotechnol). 2014;15:845–63.
38. Zaknun JJ, Bodei L, Mueller-Brand J, Baum RP, Pavel ME, Hörsch D, et al. The joint IAEA, EANM, and SNMMI practical guidance on peptide receptor radionuclide therapy (PRRNT) in neuroendocrine tumours. Eur J Nucl Med Mol Imaging. 2013;40:800–16.
39. Gulec SA, Siegel JA. Posttherapy radiation safety considerations in radiomicrosphere treatment with ^{90}Y-Microspheres. J Nucl Med. 2007;48:2080–6.
40. Kennedy A, Brown DB, Feilchenfeldt J, Marshall J, Wasan H, Fakih M, et al. Safety of selective internal radiation therapy (SIRT) with yttrium-90 microspheres combined with systemic anticancer agents: expert consensus. J Gastrointest Oncol. 2017;8:1079–99.
41. Yin H, Wu H, Zhang Y, Tian W, Jiang X, Zhou X, et al. Diagnosis of multiple endocrine neoplasia type 2A in patients with positive thyroid imaging by iodine-131 metaiodobenzylguanidine scintigraphy. Clin Nucl Med. 2011;36:772–5.
42. Bodei L, Cremonesi M, Grana CM, Chinol M, Baio SM, Severi S, Paganelli G. Yttrium-labelled peptides for therapy of NET. Eur J Nucl Med Mol Imaging. 2012;39(Suppl. 1):S93–S102.
43. Mitchell AL, Gandhi A, Scott-Coombes D, Perros P. Management of thyroid cancer: United Kingdom National Multidisciplinary Guidelines. J Laryngol Otol. 2016;130(S2):S150–S160.
44. Kim BH, Kim IJ. Recent updates on the management of medullary thyroid carcinoma. Endocrinol Metab. 2016;31:392–9.
45. Nelkin B. Recent advances in the biology and therapy of medullary thyroid carcinoma. F1000 Res. 2017;6. (F1000 Faculty Rev): 2184 Last updated: 28 Dec 2017
46. Sisson JC, Freitas J, McDougall IR, Dauer LT, Hurley JR, Brierley JD, et al. American Thyroid Association Task Force on Radioiodine Safety. Radiation safety in the treatment of patients with thyroid diseases by radioiodine I-131: practice recommendations of the American Thyroid Association. Thyroid. 2011;21:335–46.
47. Luster M, Clarke SE, Dietlein M, Lassmann M, Lind P, Oyen WJG, et al. Guidelines for radioiodine ther-

apy of differentiated thyroid cancer. Eur J Nucl Med Mol Imaging. 2008;35:1941–59.

48. Yüksel D, Argon M, Atasever T, Çelen YZ, Kabasakal L, Karayalçın B, ct al. Guidelines for radioactive iodine (I-131) ablation and therapy in the differentiated thyroid cancers. Turkish Society of Nuclear Medicine, Endocrinology and Radionuclide Therapy Study Group. Turk J Nucl Med. 2001;10(suppl):S23–7.
49. Internal Dosimetry Task Force Report on. Treatment planning for molecular radiotherapy: potential and prospects. Eur Assoc Nucl Med. www.eanm.org. 2017;
50. Dehkordi FJ, Rasuli B, Mahmoud-Pashazadeh A. An evaluation of deviation from the international atomic energy agency-international commission on radiological protection proposed equation for calculation of radiation dose rate emanating from the patients with differentiated thyroid cancer undergoing radioiodine (I-131) therapy. World J Nucl Med. 2017;16:150–5.
51. Jentzen W, Richter M, Nagarajah J, Poeppel TD, Brandau W, Dawes C, et al. Chewing-gum stimulation did not reduce the absorbed dose to salivary glands during radioiodine treatment of thyroid cancer as inferred from pre-therapy (124)I PET/CT imaging. EJNMMI Phys. 2014;1:100.
52. Jentzen W, Richter M, Poeppel TD, Schmitz J, Brandau W, Bockisch A, Binse I. Discrepant salivary gland response after radioiodine and MIBG therapies. Q J Nucl Med Mol Imaging. 2017;61:331–9.
53. Haghighatafshar M, Ghaedian M, Etemadi Z, Entezarmahdi SM, Ghaedian T. Pilocarpine effect on dose rate of salivary gland in differentiated thyroid carcinoma patients treated with radioiodine. Nucl Med Commun. 2018;39:430–4.
54. Van Nostrand D. Sialoadenitis secondary to ^{131}I therapy for well-differentiated thyroid cancer. Oral Dis. 2011;17:154–61.
55. Silberstein EB. Reducing the incidence of ^{131}I-induced sialadenitis: the role of pilocarpine. J Nucl Med. 2008;49:546–9.
56. Chen L, Shen Y, Luo Q, Yu Y, Lu H, Zhu R. Pulmonary fibrosis following radioiodine therapy of pulmonary metastases from differentiated thyroid carcinoma. Thyroid. 2010;20:337–40.
57. Samuel AM, Unnikrishnan TP, Baghel NS, Rajashekharrao B. Effect of radioiodine therapy on pulmonary alveolar-capillary membrane integrity. J Nucl Med. 1995;36:783–7.
58. Rall JE, Alpers JB, Lewallen CG, Sonenberg M, Berman M, Rawson RW. Radiation pneumonitis. and fibrosis: a complication of radioiodine treatment of pulmonary metastases from cancer of the thyroid. J Clin Endocrinol Metab. 1957;17:1263–76.
59. Sgouros G, Song H, Ladenson PW, Wahl RL. Lung toxicity in radioiodine therapy of thyroid carcinoma: development of a dose-rate method and dosimetric implications of the 80-mCi rule. J Nucl Med. 2006;47:1977–84.
60. Song H, He B, Prideaux A, Du Y, Frey E, Kasecamp W, et al. Lung dosimetry for radioiodine treatment planning in the case of diffuse lung metastases. J Nucl Med. 2006;47:1985–94.
61. Dehghani M, Jangjoo S, Monabati A, Bandari DM, Namdari N. An unusual case report: occurrence of renal cell carcinoma, basal cell carcinoma and chronic lymphocytic leukemia in a case of papillary thyroid carcinoma treated with radioactive iodine. Iran J Med Sci. 2018;43:659–63.
62. Lim JW, Yeap FS, Chan YH, Yeoh AE, Quah TC, Tan PL. Second malignant neoplasms in childhood cancer survivors treated in a tertiary paediatric oncology centre. Ann Acad Med Singap. 2017;46:11–9.
63. Chow WH, Dong LM, Devesa SS. Epidemiology and risk factors for kidney cancer. Nat Rev Urol. 2010;7:245–57.
64. Corrêa NL, de Sá LV, de Mello RC. Estimation of second primary cancer risk after treatment with radioactive iodine for differentiated thyroid carcinoma. Thyroid. 2017;27:261–70.
65. Gandhi S, Abhyankar A, Basu S. Dual malignancies in the setting of differentiated thyroid carcinoma: their synchronous or metachronous nature, impact of radioiodine treatment on occurrence of second malignancy and other associated variables. Nucl Med Commun. 2014;35:205–9.
66. Brans B, Bodei L, Giammarile F, Linden O, Luster M, Oyen WJG. Clinical radionuclide therapy dosimetry: the quest for the "Holy Gray". Eur J Nucl Med Mol Imaging. 2007;34:772–86.
67. Stabin MG, Sparks RB, Crowe E. OLINDA/EXM: the second-generation personal computer software for internal dose assessment in nuclear medicine. J Nucl Med. 2005;46:1023–7.
68. Demir M, Yeyin N. Dosimetric approach in the treatment with theranostics: Dosimetry in I-131 therapies. Turkish Sci Nucl Med Special Top. 2018;4:11–5.
69. Hänscheid H, Canzi C, Eschner W, Flux G, Luster M, Strigari L, et al. EANM Dosimetry Committee Series on Standard Operational Procedures for Pre-Therapeutic Dosimetry II. Dosimetry prior to radioiodine therapy of benign thyroid diseases. Eur J Nucl Med Mol Imaging. 2013;40:1126–34.
70. Ak SI. Radioiodine treatment of differentiated thyroid cancer in current guidelines. Turkish Sci Nucl Med- Special Top. 2018;4:22–31.
71. Turkish Atomic Energy Authority. Regulation on radiation safety. Official Gazette date: 24.3.2000 / Number: 23999.
72. Directive on release of patients receiving radionuclide therapy (RSGD-KLV-009 Rev-2). Turkish Atomic Energy Authority. Publishing date: 18/09/2018.
73. Budiawan H, Salavati A, Kulkarni HR, Baum RP. Peptide receptor radionuclide therapy of treatment- refractory metastatic thyroid cancer using (90) Yttrium and (177)Lutetium labeled somatostatin analogs: toxicity, response and survival analysis. Am J Nucl Med Mol Imaging. 2013;4:39–52.

74. Francesco Giammarile F, Chiti A, Lassmann M, Brans B, Flux G. EANM procedure guidelines for I-131 meta-iodobenzylguanidine (I-131 mIBG) therapy. Eur J Nucl Med Mol Imaging. 2008;35:1039–47.
75. Damle NA, Bal C, Singh TP, Gupta R, Reddy S, Kumar R, et al. Anaplastic thyroid carcinoma on ^{68}Ga-PSMA PET/CT: opening new frontiers. Eur J Nucl Med Mol Imaging. 2018;45:667–8.
76. Bychkov A, Vutrapongwatana U, Tepmongkol S, Keelawat S. PSMA expression by microvasculature of thyroid tumors – potential implications for PSMA theranostics. Sci Rep. 2017;7:5202.
77. Lütje S, Gomez B, Cohnen J, Umutlu L, GotthardtM PTD, et al. Imaging of prostate-specific membrane antigen expression in metastatic differentiated thyroid cancer using ^{68}Ga-HBED-CCPSMA PET/CT. Clin Nucl Med. 2017;42:20–5.
78. Derlin T, Kreipe HH, Schumacher U, Soudah B. PSMA expression in tumor neovasculature endothelial cells of follicular thyroid adenoma as identified by molecular imaging using ^{68}Ga-PSMA ligand PET/CT. Clin Nucl Med. 2017;42:e173–4.
79. Förster GJ, Engelbach MJ, Brockmann JJ, Reber HJ, Buchholz HG, Mäcke HR, et al. Preliminary data on biodistribution and dosimetry for therapy planning of somatostatin receptor positive tumours: comparison of (86)Y-DOTATOC and (111)In-DTPA-octreotide. Eur J Nucl Med. 2001;28:1743–50.
80. Bodei L, Cremonesi M, Grana CM, Fazio N, Iodice S, Baio SM, et al. Peptide receptor radionuclide therapy with ^{177}Lu-DOTATATE: the IEO phase I–II study. Eur J Nucl Med Mol Imaging. 2011;38:2125–35.
81. Kam BLR, Teunissen JJ, Krenning EP, de Herder WW, Khan S, van Vliet EI, et al. Lutetium-labelled peptides for therapy of neuroendocrine tumours. Eur J Nucl Med Mol Imaging. 2012;39(Suppl. 1):S103–12.
82. Calais PJ, Turner JH. Radiation safety of outpatient ^{177}Lu-octreotate radiopeptide therapy of neuroendocrine tumors. Ann Nucl Med. 2014;28:531–9.
83. Bergsma H, Konijnenberg MW, van der Zwan WA, Kam BL, Teunissen JJ, Kooij PP, et al. Nephrotoxicity after PRRT with (177)Lu-DOTA-octreotate. Eur J Nucl Med Mol Imaging. 2016;43:1802–11.
84. Strosberg J, El-Haddad G, Wolin E, Hendifar A, Yao J, Chasen B, et al. and NETTER-1 Trial Investigators. Phase 3 Trial of ^{177}Lu-Dotatate for Midgut Neuroendocrine Tumors. N Engl J Med. 2017;376:125–35.
85. Cremonesi M, Botta F, Di Dia A, Ferrari M, Bodei L, De Cicco C, et al. Dosimetry for treatment with radiolabelled somatostatin analogues. A review. Q J Nucl Med Mol Imaging. 2010;54:37–51.
86. Hofman MS, Kong G, Neels OC, Eu P, Hong E, Hicks RJ. High management impact of Ga-68 DOTATATE (GaTate) PET/CT for imaging neuroendocrine and other somatostatin expressing tumours. J Med Imaging Radiat Oncol. 2012;56:40–7.
87. Pauwels E, Cleeren F, Bormans G, Deroose CM. Somatostatin receptor PET ligands—the next generation for clinical practice. Am J Nucl Med Mol Imaging. 2018;8:311–31.
88. Kratochwil C, Stefanova M, Mavriopoulou E, Holland-Letz T, Dimitrakopoulou-Strauss A, Afshar- Oromieh A, et al. SUV of [(68)Ga] DOTATOC-PET/CT predicts response probability of PRRT in neuroendocrine tumors. Mol Imaging Biol. 2015;17:313–8.
89. Haug AR, Auernhammer CJ, Wangler B, Schmidt GP, Uebleis C, Göke B, et al. 68Ga-DOTATATE PET/CT for the early prediction of response to somatostatin receptor-mediated radionuclide therapy in patients with well differentiated neuroendocrine tumors. J Nucl Med. 2010;51:1349–56.
90. Eberlein U, Cremonesi M, Lassmann M. Individualized dosimetry for theranostics: necessary, nice to have, or counterproductive? J Nucl Med. 2017;58:97S–103S.
91. Cwikla JB, Mikolajczak R, Pawlak D, Buscombe JR, Nasierowska-Guttmejer A, Bator A, et al. Initial direct comparison of ^{99m}Tc-TOC and ^{99m}Tc-TATE in identifying sites of disease in patients with proven GEP NETs. J Nucl Med. 2008;49:1060–5.
92. Velikyan I, Sundin A, Sörensen J, Lubberink M, Sandström M, Garske-Román U, et al. Quantitative and qualitative intrapatient comparison of ^{68}Ga-DOTATOC and ^{68}Ga-DOTATATE: net uptake rate for accurate quantification. J Nucl Med. 2014;55:204–10.
93. Josefsson A, Hobbs RF, Ranka S, Schwarz BC, Plyku D, de Amorim W, de Carvalho J, et al. Comparative dosimetry for ^{68}Ga-DOTATATE: impact of using updated ICRP phantoms, S values, and tissue-weighting factors. J Nucl Med. 2018;59:1281–8.
94. Erbas B, Tuncel M. Renal function assessment during peptide receptor radionuclide therapy. Semin Nucl Med. 2016;46:462–78.
95. Baechler S, Hobbs RF, Prideaux AR, Wahl RL, Sgouros G. Extension of the biological effective dose to the MIRD schema and possible implications in radionuclide therapy dosimetry. Med Phys. 2008;35:1123–34.
96. Council Directive 97/43/EURATOM, 1997.
97. Sasikumar A, Joy A, Nanabala R, Pillai MR, Thomas B. 68Ga-PSMA PET/CT imaging and ^{153}Sm-EDTMP bone pain palliation therapy. Clin Nucl Med. 2016;41:e353–4.
98. Anderson P, Nuñez R. Samarium lexidronam (^{153}Sm-EDTMP): skeletal radiation for osteoblastic bone metastases and osteosarcoma. Expert Rev Anticancer Ther. 2007;7:1517–27.
99. Yuan J, Liu C, Liu X, Wang Y, Kuai D, Zhang G, et al. Efficacy and safety of ^{177}Lu-EDTMP in bone metastatic pain palliation in breast cancer and hormone refractory prostate cancer: a phase II study. Clin Nucl Med. 2013;38:88–92.
100. Subbiah V, Anderson P, RohrenE. Alpha Emitter Radium-223 in high-risk osteosarcoma first clinical evidence of response and blood-brain barrier penetration. JAMA Oncol. 2015;1:253–5.

101. Pacilio M, Ventroni G, Basile C, Lalongo P, Becci D, Mango L. Improving the dose-myelotoxicity correlation in radiometabolic therapy of bone metastases with ^{153}Sm-EDTMP. Eur J Nucl Med Mol Imaging. 2014;41:238–52.
102. Lawless S, McMullin MF, Cuthbert R, Houston R. 32P in the treatment of myeloproliferative disorders. Ulster Med J. 2016;85:83–5.
103. Delgado Bolton RC, Giammarile F. Bone radionuclide therapy and increased survival with radium-223 is the way to go for nuclear medicine: the offer that oncologists cannot refuse. Eur J Nucl Med Mol Imaging. 2018;45:822–3.
104. Jadvar H. Targeted radionuclide therapy: an evolution toward precision cancer treatment. Am J Roentgenol. 2017;209:277–88.
105. Green DJ, Press OW. Whither radioimmunotherapy: to be or not to be? Cancer Res. 2017;77:2191–6.
106. Kaminski MS, Tuck M, Estes J, Kolstad A, Ross CW, Zasadny K, et al. I-131 tositumomab therapy as initial treatment for follicular lymphoma. N Engl J Med. 2005;352:441–9.
107. Witzig TE, Flinn IW, Gordon LI, Emmanouilides C, Czuczman MS, Saleh MN, et al. Treatment with ibritumomab tiuxetan radioimmunotherapy in patients with rituximab-refractory follicular non-Hodgkin's lymphoma. J Clin Oncol. 2002;20:3262–9.
108. Siegel JA, Kroll S, Regan D, Kaminski MS, Wahl RL. A practical methodology for patient release after Tositumomab and ^{131}I-Tositumomab therapy. J Nucl Med. 2002;43:354–63.
109. Giammarile F, Bodei L, Chiesa C, Flux G, Forrer F, Kraeber-Bodere F, et al. EANM procedure guideline for the treatment of liver cancer and liver metastases with intra-arterial radioactive compounds. Eur J Nucl Med Mol Imaging. 2011;38:1393–406.
110. Raoul JL, Bourguet P, Bretagne JF, Duvauferrier R, Coornaert S, Darnault P, et al. Hepatic artery injection of I-131-labeled lipiodol. Part I. Biodistribution study results in patients with hepatocellular carcinoma and liver metastases. Radiology. 1988;168:541–5.
111. Ayan A, Dönmez S, Aras F, Günalp B, Kıraç S, Alıç Ozaslan I, et al. Radiation safety process in case of changing medical condition of patients who received radionuclide therapy or radioactive substances: emergency medical procedures. Nucl Med Semin. 2016;3:168–71.
112. Geraldes AN, Miyamoto DM, Arivar de Lira R, Osso JA Jr, Nascimento N, de Burgos M, de Azevedo M. Microspheres of poly(e-caprolactone) loaded Holmium-165: morphology and thermal degradation behavior. 2011 International Nuclear Atlantic Conference—INAC 2011. Belo Horizonte, MG, Brazil, October 24–28, 2011. ASSOCIAÇÃO BRASILEIRA DE ENERGIA NUCLEAR—ABEN.
113. Prince JF, van den Bosch MAAJ, Nijsen JFW, Smits MLJ, van den Hoven AF, Nikolakopoulos S, et al. Efficacy of radioembolization with ^{166}Ho-microspheres in salvage patients with liver metastases: a phase 2 study. J Nucl Med. 2018;59:582–8.
114. Braat AJAT, Prince JF, van Rooij R, Bruijnen RCG, van den Bosch MAAJ, Lam MGEH. Safety analysis of holmium-166 microsphere scout dose imaging during radioembolisation work-up: a cohort study. Eur Radiol. 2018;28:920–8.
115. Liepe K, Kotzerke J, Lambert B. Advantage of ^{188}Re-radiopharmaceuticals in hepatocellular cancer and liver metastases. J Nucl Med. 2005;46:1407–8.
116. Lambert B, Bacher K, Defreyne L, Gemmel F, Van Vlierberghe H, Jeong JM, et al. 188Re- HDD/lipiodol therapy for hepatocellular carcinoma: a phase I clinical trial. J Nucl Med. 2005;46:60–6.
117. Bernal P, Raoul JL, Stare J, Sereegotov E, Sundram FX, Kumar A, et al. International Atomic Energy Agency-sponsored multination study of intra-arterial rhenium-188-labeled lipiodol in the treatment of inoperable hepatocellular carcinoma: results with special emphasis on prognostic value of dosimetric study. Semin Nucl Med 2008; 38: S40-S45.
118. Huang PW, Tsai SC, Luo TY, Kao CH, Lin WY. Therapeutic efficacy of ^{188}Re-MN-16ET lipiodol in an animal model of hepatocellular carcinoma. Ann Nucl Med. 2013;27:532–7.
119. Liepe K, Brogsitter C, Leonhard J, Wunderlich G, Hliscs R, Pinkert J, et al. Feasibility of high activity Rhenium-188-microsphere in hepatic radioembolization. Jpn J Clin Oncol. 2007;37:942–50.
120. Kurth J, Krause BJ, Schwarzenböck SM, Stegger L, Schäfers M, Rahbar K. External radiation exposure, excretion, and effective half-life in Lu-177 PSMA-targeted therapies. EJNMMI Res. 2018;8:32.
121. Emmett L, Willowson K, Violet J, Shin J, Blanksby A, Lee J. Lutetium-177 PSMA radionuclide therapy for men with prostate cancer: a review of the current literature and discussion of practical aspects of therapy. J Med Radiat Sci. 2017;64:52–60.
122. Ahmadzadehfar H, Azgomi K, Hauser S, Wei X, Yordanova A, Gaertner FC, et al. 68Ga-PSMA-11 PET as a gatekeeper for the treatment of metastatic prostate cancer with ^{223}Ra: proof of concept. J Nucl Med. 2017;58:438–44.
123. Kratochwil C, Giesel FL, Bruchertseifer F, Mier W, Apostolidis C, Boll R, et al. 213Bi-DOTATOC receptor-targetedalpha-radionuclide therapy induces remission in neuroendocrine tumours refractoryto beta radiation: a first-in-human experience. Eur J Nucl Med Mol Imaging. 2014;41:2106–19.
124. Yaşargil MG, Curcic M, Kis M, Siegenthaler G, Teddy PJ, Roth P. Total removal of craniopharyngiomas. Approaches and long-term results in 144 patients. J Neurosurg. 1990;73:3–11.
125. Maarouf M, El Majdoub F, Fuetsch M, Hoevels M, Lehrke R, Berthold F, et al. Stereotactic intracavitary brachytherapy with P-32 for cystic craniopharyngiomas in children. Strahlenther Onkol. 2016;192:157–65.
126. Yu X, Zhang J, Liu R, Wang Y, Wang H, Wang P, et al. Interstitial radiotherapy using phosphorus-32

for giant posterior fossa cystic craniopharyngiomas. J Neurosurg Pediatr. 2015;15:510–8.
127. Kickingereder P, Maarouf M, El Majdoub F, Fuetsch M, Lehrke R, Wirths J, et al. Intracavitary brachytherapy using stereotactically applied phosphorus-32 colloid for treatment of cystic craniopharyngiomas in 53 patients. J Neuro-Oncol. 2012;109:365–74.
128. Julow J, Backlund EO, Lányi F, Hajda M, Bálint K, Nyáry I, et al. Long-term results and late complications after intracavitary yttrium-90 colloid irradiation of recurrent cystic craniopharyngiomas. Neurosurgery. 2007;61:288–95. discussion 295-6
129. Julow J, Lányi F, Hajda M, Szeifert GT, Viola A, Bálint K, Nyáry I. Stereotactic intracavitary irradiation of cystic craniopharyngiomas with yttrium-90 isotope. Prog Neurol Surg. 2007;20:289–96.
130. Falzone N, Ackerman NL, Rosales LF, Bernal MA, Liu X, Peeters SG, et al. Dosimetric evaluation of radionuclides for VCAM-1-targeted radionuclide therapy of early brain metastases. Theranostics. 2018;8:292–303.
131. Falzone N, Fernández-Varea JM, Flux G, Vallis KA. Monte Carlo evaluation of Auger electron-emitting theranostic radionuclides. J Nucl Med. 2015;56:1441–6.
132. Takalkar A, Paryani B, Adams S, Subbiah V. Radium-223 dichloride therapy in breast cancer with osseous metastases. BMJ Case Rep. 2015;2015:bcr2015211152.
133. Nevedomskaya E, Baumgart SJ, Haendler B. Recent advances in prostate cancer treatment and drug discovery. Int J Mol Sci. 2018;19:E1359.
134. Ross K, Jones RJ. Immune checkpoint inhibitors in renal cell carcinoma. Clin Sci. 2017;131:2627–42.
135. Ferreira CA, Fuscaldi LL, Townsend DM, Rubello D, Barros ALB. Radiolabeled bombesin derivatives for preclinical oncological imaging. Biomed Pharmacother. 2017;87:58–72.
136. Dadachova E. Cancer therapy with alpha-emitters labeled peptides. Semin Nucl Med. 2010;40:204–8.
137. Norain A, Dadachova E. Targeted radionuclide therapy of melanoma. Semin Nucl Med. 2016;46:250–9.
138. Hagemann UB, Mihaylova D, Uran SR, Borrebaek J, Grant D, Bjerke RM, et al. Targeted alpha therapy using a novel CD70 targeted thorium-227 conjugate in *in vitro* and *in vivo* models of renal cell carcinoma. Oncotarget. 2017;8:56311–26.
139. Yong K, Brechbiel MW. Towards translation of ^{212}Pb as a clinical therapeutic; getting the lead in! Dalton Trans. 2011;40:6068–76.
140. Miest TS, Frenzke M, Cattaneo R. Measles virus entry through the signaling lymphocyte activation molecule governs efficacy of mantle cell lymphoma radiovirotherapy. Mol Ther. 2013;21:2019–31.
141. Msaouel P, Iankov ID, Allen C, Aderca I, Federspiel MJ, Tindall DJ, et al. Noninvasive imaging and radiovirotherapy of prostate cancer using an oncolytic measles virus expressing the sodium iodide symporter. Mol Ther. 2009;17:2041–8.
142. Aref S, Bailey K, Fielding A. Measles to the rescue: a review of oncolytic measles virus. Viruses. 2016;8(10):E294.
143. Li H, Nakashima H, Decklever TD, Nace RA, Russell SJ. HSV-NIS, an oncolytic herpes simplex virus type 1 encoding human sodium iodide symporter for preclinical prostate cancer radiovirotherapy. Cancer Gene Ther. 2013;20:478–85.

Part II

Clinical Information: Thyroid Diseases

Radionuclide Therapy in Benign Thyroid Diseases: Nodular Goiter Disease

4

Özgür Karaçalıoğlu

4.1 Thyroid Nodules

Thyroid nodules are very common and their prevalence is increased in older patients. Thyroid nodules can be palpated in about 5% of the population, and can be detected in up to 70% of people on ultrasound examination [1]. The majority of thyroid nodules derive from thyroid follicular cells. Benign follicular nodules, the most common mass lesions, can be single or part of a multinodular goiter. Benign thyroid nodules may tend to increase in size over time [2]. Therefore, the thyroid and cervical lymph nodes should be palpated for characterizing size, location, and texture during the routine physical examination. An ultrasonographic evaluation provides detailed information about the size and morphological structure of the gland and, if present, the thyroid nodules. In all patients with a thyroid nodule, serum thyroid-stimulating hormone (TSH) and free thyroxine (fT4) and/or free triiodothyronine (fT3) levels should be measured to determine thyroid gland function. A suppressed TSH level may be the biochemical sign of the presence of a hyperfunctioning nodule. In this case, information about the function of a thyroid nodule(s) can be detected from a technetium-99 thyroid scan. Correlating the thyroid ultrasonography and radionuclide scan can help to diagnose a toxic nodular goiter (TNG) or a toxic multinodular goiter (TMG). In cases with multinodular goiter, there may be tracheal compression and related respiratory distress symptoms. In this case, tracheal compression and tracheal deviation and, if any, retrosternal extension of the thyroid gland can be evaluated by non-contrast neck and upper mediastinal computed tomography [3].

In general, thyrotoxicosis can occur if:

(a) The thyroid gland is stimulated by trophic factors (e.g., Graves),
(b) Autonomous activation of thyroid hormone synthesis and secretion (TNG, TMG).
(c) Preformed hormone stores are passively released due to autoimmune, infectious, chemical, or mechanical insult (thyroiditis).
(d) Exposure to extrathyroidal sources of thyroid hormone (endogenous: struma ovarii, metastatic differentiated thyroid cancer, or exogenous: factitious thyrotoxicosis).

Hyperthyroidism is usually due to Graves' disease (GD) or toxic nodular thyroid disease, which is the subject of this chapter. A TNG or TMG with a persistently suppressed TSH can be treated with radioactive iodine, while surgery may be preferred for large toxic lesions, for those individuals with suspicious imaging characteristics. The aim of hyperthyroidism treatment is to correct hyperthyroid symptoms quickly and permanently, and the appropriate treatment approach is

Ö. Karaçalıoğlu (✉)
Gülhane Faculty of Medicine, Department of Nuclear Medicine, University of Health Sciences, Ankara, Turkey
e-mail: alperozgur.karacalioglu@sbu.edu.tr

R. Bekiş et al. (eds.), *Radionuclide Therapy*, https://doi.org/10.1007/978-3-030-97220-2_4

Table 4.1 Benign thyroid diseases that can be treated with I-131

Functional disorders (increased function)	Structural disorders (increased volume)
Diffuse toxic goiter (Graves' disease)	Non-toxic diffuse goiter (NTDG)
Toxic nodular goiter (TNG)	Non-toxic nodular goiter (NTNG)
Toxic multinodular goiter (Plummer's disease, TMG)	Non-toxic multinodular goiter (NTMG)

affected by some other factors such as the presence of other concomitant medical conditions and patient preference [4] (Table 4.1).

Although silent thyroiditis and subacute granulomatous thyroiditis have toxic episodes, these patients are not suitable candidates for I-131 therapy. The goal of I-131 treatment is to eliminate the thyroid's overproduction of hormones despite the risk of developing hypothyroidism. In addition, the volume of the nodules and the thyroid gland decreases after I-131 therapy. In addition to I-131 treatment, surgery and prolonged thionamide therapy are other options.

Thionamides reduce thyroid hormone production but do not usually cause remission in hyperthyroidism secondary to toxic nodular thyroid disease. Although thyroid hormone levels return to the normal range during antithyroid therapy, the majority of cases with toxic multinodular goiter will likely develop hyperthyroid symptoms at the end of treatment [5]. Moreover, antithyroid drugs consisting of propycil, methimazole, and its derivative carbimazole have serious side effects such as hepatitis and agranulocytosis. These drugs are generally used in patients with toxic nodular goiter to control hyperthyroid symptoms before a definitive treatment with I-131/surgery. In addition, Thionamides can also be used for the long term to treat hyperthyroidism due to toxic adenoma in patients at high surgical risk and/or unable to comply with radiation safety guidelines. Ultrasound-guided percutaneous ethanol injection, radiofrequency ablation (RFA), or interstitial laser photocoagulation are other options for patients with toxic nodular gout who do not want radioiodine therapy or surgery [6]. Lifelong thionamide therapy is also an alternative option. In a randomized controlled trial of older adult patients with subclinical hyperthyroidism, both RAI and long-term low-dose metimazole therapies have been reported to be effective and safe for the treatment of subclinical hyperthyroidism in the elderly [7].

Surgery provides rapid and definitive correction of hyperthyroidism. Surgery may be preferred in the presence of subsequent conditions: In the presence of neck compression, retrosternal extension, and insufficient I-131 uptake or the volume of the gland is too large (>80 g).

I-131 treatment can be preferred especially in the treatment of TNG or TMG in older patients with other systemic diseases. I-131 treatment is not an option in patients with toxic nodular thyroid disease in the presence of pregnancy, breastfeeding, and thyroid cancer risk. Contraception should be offered at least for 6 months after I-131 treatment. Other treatment options should also be considered for patients who will not comply with radiation safety rules. Before I-131 treatment, the possibility of pregnancy in women of childbearing age should be ruled out with biochemical tests.

Physiologically, iodine is naturally found in the structure of the hormones tetraiodothyronine (T4) and triiodothyronine (T3) produced by the thyroid gland. After oral administration of radioiodine, it is absorbed from the intestinal system and transferred to plasma and actively removed from plasma by the sodium-iodine transporter protein (NIS) found in the plasma membrane of thyroid follicle cells. The iodine accumulated in the follicle cells oxidizes and first, thyroglobulin is added to the T4 and T3 structure. 20–30% of the orally administered radioiodine is retained in a normally functioning thyroid gland, while this rate may increase to 90% in patients with hyperthyroidism [8].

I-131 which is used for the treatment of thyroid disorders decays to stable Xe-131 by beta emission. The physical characteristics of I-131 are as follows: $T_{1/2}$ phys = 8.02 days; β max = 0.807 MeV, β avg = 0.192 MeV; gamma ray range 80–723 keV, most abundant γ (82%) 364 keV. The average distance traveled by the beta particle of I-131 in soft tissue is 0.4 mm, and the maximum distance is approximately 3 mm [8].

I-131 is administered as oral or intravenous sodium iodide in the treatment of benign and malignant thyroid diseases.

Radiobiological effects of radioiodine on tissues are direct or indirect. Direct effects involve one-electron oxidation reactions, while indirect effects are mediated through water dissociation, leading to the production of reactive oxygen species, such as superoxide radicals and hydrogen peroxide, the precursors of the highly damaging hydroxyl radicals [9]. Radiation-induced oxidative DNA damage includes single-strand and double-strand DNA breaks, DNA base damage, and DNA–DNA or DNA–protein crosslinks [9]. The cell usually dies by going to apoptosis through the p53 protein secondary to irradiation [10]. Radiation causes structural changes in non-irradiated neighboring cells too. The first is genomic instability consisting of chromosomal aberrations and this can continue throughout the continuing generations of that cell [11]. The other is the "by-stander" effect, which occurs when damage markers released from irradiated cells are transmitted to a non-irradiated cell. In addition, hereditary damages on DNA repair mechanisms make individuals sensitive to the effects of radiation [12].

Before treatment, patients should be thoroughly examined and their history including contrast use, thyroid drugs used, other iodine-containing drugs such as amiodarone and iodine-containing foods should be taken in detail. Before I-131 treatment, the general uptake function of the thyroid gland and the nodules should be evaluated with Tc-99m pertechnetate or I-123 thyroid scintigraphy. In addition, if the calculated dose is planned to administer, iodine uptake testing should be performed at 4 and 24 h. If the 24-h iodine uptake value is <20%, I-131 treatment with rTSH or other treatment options should be considered. It is important to evaluate the morphological structure of the thyroid gland ultrasonographically and to calculate the volume of the thyroid gland before I-131 treatment. Since the possibility of malignancy is low in thyroid nodules with autonomic function, fine needle aspiration biopsy should be performed on nodules with suspicious sonographic findings. In a goiter extending to the mediastinum, the borders of the gland with other anatomical structures can be evaluated and the volume of the gland can be calculated by anatomical imaging methods such as computed tomography.

The aim of I-131 treatment in toxic nodular thyroid diseases is to destroy the autonomic nodules that produce excess hormone, to bring the hormone production to normal limits, and not to make the patients hypothyroid as much as possible by creating minimal damage to the remaining gland. High treatment success is associated with a high risk of developing hypothyroidism, and current treatment approaches are not ideal enough to include all factors that will affect the treatment process. There are two basic approaches to the radioiodine treatment of toxic nodular thyroid diseases: fixed dose and calculated dose administration.

In a calculated dose approach, approximately 100–150 Gy radiation absorption dose with 3.7–5.5 MBq/g-thyroid tissue is recommended in patients with toxic and non-toxic multinodular goiter, corrected for 24-h I-131 uptake [8]. The recommended formula (Marinelli's formula) to calculate the activity required to achieve the dose in the thyroid is as follows:

$$\text{I}-131\ \text{Therapeutic Activity}\,(\text{MBq}) = \left[25 \times \text{mass}\,(\text{g}) \times \text{Dose}\,(\text{Gy})\right] / \text{IU}_{24\text{h}(\%)} \times T_{\text{eff}}$$

In the formula, 25: unit conversion coefficient, mass: sonographically calculated mass of the thyroid gland, dose: absorbed dose of I-131, IU_{24h}: 24-h I-131 uptake, and T_{eff}: effective I-131 half-life in thyroid gland (days). The conversion factor converts the amount of ionization in the air (coulombs/kg) to the amount of dose (gray) absorbed in the tissue. The dose is I-131 absorption dose and is generally recommended as 150 Gy. While it is easy to calculate the volume of a single nodule in cases with TNG by ultrasonography, it is difficult or even not possible in some cases due to the interlocking of autonomous and non-autonomous nodules in cases with TMG.

Fixed-dose administration is based on estimating the size of the thyroid gland by ultrasonography, scintigraphy, or palpation. The range of activities currently used varies in the range 200–600 MBq [8]. It is more reasonable to plan I-131 treatment with dose calculation, especially in children and patients <45 years of age. A special condition is cases with end-stage renal disease. Since I-131 cannot be excreted by the kidneys, the dose can be reduced by one-fifth [13]. In a meta-analysis, it was reported that the two main methods, estimated and calculated, used to determine activity in the treatment of hyperthyroidism with radioiodine, resulted in an equally successful treatment outcome [14].

4.2 Toxic Multinodular Goiter

Antithyroid drugs are highly effective in controlling hyperthyroidism, but TMG rarely resolves with drug therapy. When surgery is not an option, I-131 treatment is a very safe and effective treatment approach in these cases, because the success rate with I-131 in the treatment of TMG cases is quite high in terms of treatment effectiveness. In a randomized controlled study, it was reported that 16.7 ± 2.7 mCi I-131 was given to 54 patients with TMG and these cases were followed for 60–100 months [15]. According to the results of this study, at the end of the follow-up, 22 (41%) of these patients were found to have hypothyroidism, 20 (37%) to have euthyroid, and 12 (22%) to have ongoing hyperthyroidism. In another study, 153 adult patients with TMG treated with constant activities of 15 mCi radioiodine (RAI) have been retrospectively analyzed with follow-up up to 12 years [16]. At the end of the follow-up, it has been reported that 61.6% of the patients were euthyroid, 11% of the patients had persistent hyperthyroidism, and 27.4% of the patients had hypothyroidism. According to the results of this study, it was reported that 89% of hyperthyroidism patients were treated. It has also been reported that the mean time to development of hypothyroidism after I-131 treatment was 2.7 ± 2.4 years, with a marked reduction in gland volume. The authors of the study have concluded that 15 mCi fixed-dose I-131 treatment in TMG cases resulted in a high success rate in the treatment of hyperthyroidism with significant volume reduction and low hypothyroidism rates.

The reported failure rate after I-131 therapy in TMNG varies from 12% to 20% and low uptake of I-131 or rapid clearance of I-131 from the thyroid gland are some possible mechanisms underlying treatment failure. The treatment failure rate of radioiodine in patients with TMNG has been reported to be reduced from 30% to 19% by withdrawing anti-thyroid drugs for a longer period (7–21 days) before radioablation [17]. Besides, it has also been reported that the failure rate of I-131 treatment in these cases was reduced by up to 12% by limiting the intake of iodine-rich foods and drugs and reducing the "cold" iodine pool in patients. Another solution to reduce treatment failure is to add lithium to the radioiodine treatment of patients with TMG, which may decrease I-131 clearance and increase the efficacy of the treatment [18].

I-131 treatment of patients with TMG also causes a decrease in the volume of the thyroid gland. In patients with TMG, the mean volume reduction of 50% or more at 3 years has been reported after I-131 treatment, with the greatest annual reduction has been observed in the first year ($30 \pm 17.8\%$) [16]. A proportion of patients with TMG have symptoms of compression to the trachea and this complaint disappears in almost all cases after surgery. However, about half of TMG patients with compression symptoms recover from these complaints, due to a 30-50% decrease in volume after I-131 treatment [19]. The development of hypothyroidism is a common side effect of I-131 treatment in patients with TMG. In the treatment of TMNG cases with I-131, the incidence of hypothyroidism increases depending on the initial dose [16]. In one study, overt hypothyroidism requiring replacement therapy with l-thyroxine has been reported to develop in 17.3% of patients with TMG and in

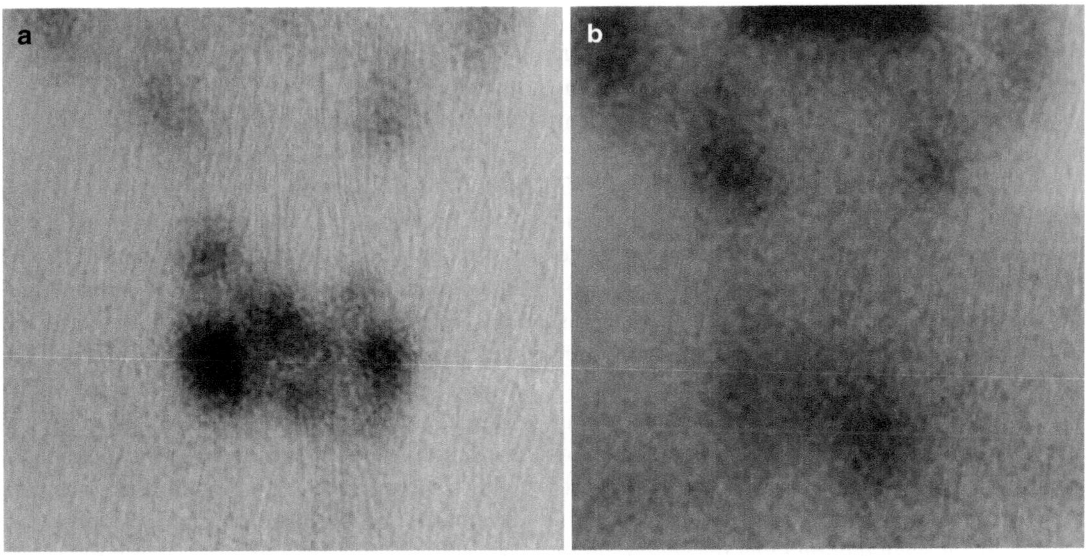

Fig. 4.1 Scintigraphic images of a patient with TMG before (**a**) and 3 months after 20 mCi I-131 treatment (**b**). Scintigraphic images show a marked reduction of I-131 uptake of hyperactive nodules after treatment

16.9% of patients with TNG during a 1-year follow-up [20]. Interestingly, approximately 4% of patients with toxic nodular goiter may develop Graves' disease after I-131 treatment [21]. The destruction of the thyroid gland after I-131 treatment appears to likely trigger the immune system. In some of these cases, elevated levels of thyroid receptor antibodies may be detected prior to I-131 treatment.

Scintigraphic images of a patient with TMG before and after 20 mCi I-131 treatment are shown in Fig. 4.1.

4.3 Toxic Nodular Goiter

Graves' disease and TNG are the most common causes of hyperthyroidism and radioiodine is considered as the first line of treatment for TNG. Fixed doses of iodine-131 (370–740 MBq) are usually preferred to administer. In one study, a calculated dose of I-131 was administered to patients with TNG and treatment efficacy has been evaluated 1 year after treatment. Accordingly, it has been reported that 94% of the cases were euthyroid, hypothyroidism developed in 3%, and hyperthyroid findings persisted in the remaining 3% [22]. In the follow-up of the patients in this study, the incidence of hypothyroidism has been reported to increase to 9% after 3 years and to 11% after 5 years. According to a retrospective clinical study investigating the first 6-month treatment results of 233 patients with TNG with I-131, the treatment success rate was reported as 93.9%. At the end of the 6th month, 74 (31.7%) of these patients had hypothyroidism, 145 (62.2%) had euthyroidism, and 14 (6%) had hyperthyroidism [23]. In another study, the cure rate and incidence of hypothyroidism of radioiodine treatment with a calculated dose regimen and an intended thyroid dose of 150 Gy in 265 consecutive patients with toxic nodular goiter during long-term follow-up (8 years) have been investigated [24]. According to their results, the cure rates at 3 months, at 1 year, and at the end of follow-up have been reported to be 85%, 98%, and 98% respectively. In addition, the incidence of hypothyroidism at 3 months, at 1 year, and at the end of follow-up have been reported to be 32%, 55%, and 73%, respectively. Similar results were reported in other studies. Due to low I-131 involvement in non-nodular areas, euthyroidism is achieved in 75-95% of cases within 3–12 months after the treatment of TNG cases with I-131, and therefore, I-131 therapy in patients with TNG is a highly effective treatment option [25].

Since it is different from temporary Graves's hypothyroidism after I-131 treatment, when hypothyroidism is detected after I-131 treatment in patients with TNG, replacement treatment should be started without delay [26].

Radioiodine treatment of patients with TNG leads to an increased incidence of hypothyroidism in the long-term follow-up. In a retrospective study with a 20-year follow-up, the prevalence of hypothyroidism has been reported to be such as 7.6% in the first year and 28% in 5 years, 46% in 10 years, and 60% in 20 years [27].

After radioiodine treatment of toxic nodular goiter cases, volumetric reduction is observed both in the hyperactive part and in the rest of the gland. In a clinical trial, after 12 months of follow-up, it has been reported that the sonographic volume of the diffuse parts of the glands decreased by 18% and the size of toxic adenomas by 54% [28]. Most of this volume reduction usually occurs as early as the first trimester of treatment.

In cases with TNG, thyroglobulin levels may be found to be high before I-131 treatment. The reduction in circulating thyroglobulin levels in these patients after treatment with I-131 is associated with a good response to treatment. In cases resistant to I-131 treatment, a significant decrease in thyroglobulin levels may not be observed [29]. This finding suggests a relationship between nodule activity and plasma thyroglobulin levels.

Graves' disease may develop after I-131 treatment of TNG cases whose antibody levels are negative before treatment. Although antibody levels before treatment are negative, thyrotropin receptor antibody and thyroid peroxidase antibody titers may tend to increase after treatment. In scintigraphic imaging, the appearance of toxic adenoma characterized by regional prominent activity uptake before treatment may turn into a Graves appearance characterized by diffuse activity uptake in the thyroid gland with decreased background activity [30, 31].

Scintigraphic images of a patient with TNG before and after 15 mCi I-131 treatment are shown in Fig. 4.2.

4.4 Non-Toxic Multinodular Goiter

NTMG is encountered frequently especially in areas of high/moderate iodine deficiency. Recurrent episodes of stimulation and involution of diffuse goiters result in irregularly enlarged multinodular goiters and can produce extreme thyroid enlargements. In addition, there are variations in follicular cell responses to hormonal stimulation [32]. An effective treatment is often required due to slow but continuous growth of the disease. NTMG causes symptoms of compression and cosmetic concerns due to enlargement in goiter size with time. Surgical resection is preferred especially in patients who have large goiters with compressive signs and symptoms, while levothyroxine (LT4) treatment is employed particularly in those with small and recently developed goiters. The incidence of NTMG increases with age and especially affects elderly patients accompanied by other diseases. Therefore, the benefits and harms of the surgical treatment of these cases should be well evaluated [33]. On the other hand, suppression treatment with LT4 is moderately effective. An overall beneficial response is average. Recurrence is a common finding with withdrawal of LT4 replacement therapy. Due to subclinical hyperthyroidism, LT4 replacement therapy carries risks such as atrial fibrillation and loss of bone tissue in elderly patients. Therefore, I-131 treatment seems to be a good alternative to reduce the volume of the thyroid gland in patients with NTMG. The main side-effect of I-131 treatment is alteration in thyroid function. Due to either radiation thyroiditis or development of thyroid receptor stimulating auto-antibodies, transient thyrotoxicosis appears a few days after treatment with a prevalence varying between 3 and 27%. Besides, hypothyroidism has been reported in 21–48% of treated patients after a follow-up of 1–2 years, depending on the dose of I-131 employed and on the thyroidal uptake [18].

I-131 leads to more thyroid volume reduction, when compared with levothyroxine suppressive

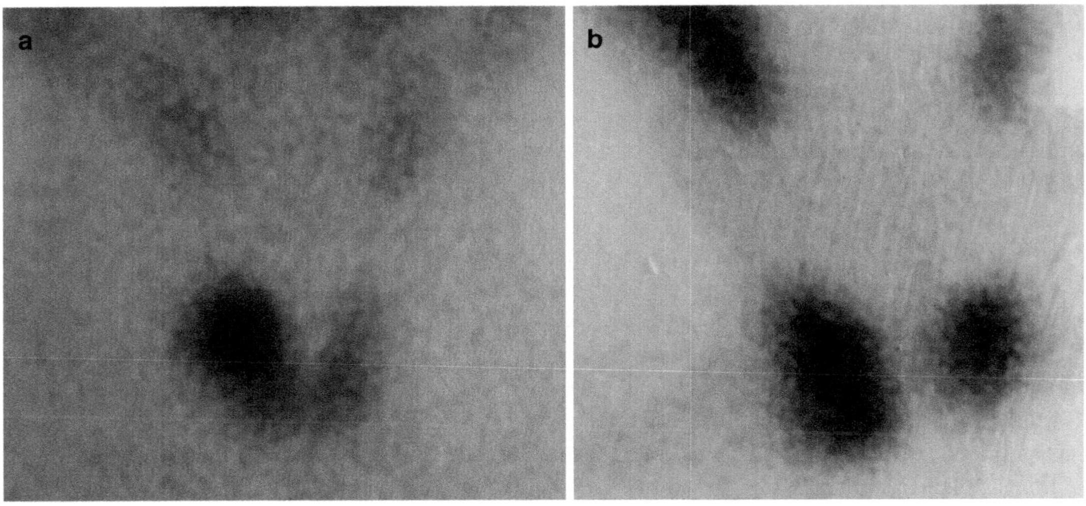

Fig. 4.2 Scintigraphic images of a patient with TNG before (**a**) and 3 months after 15 mCi I-131 treatment (**b**). Scintigraphic images show a marked reduction of I-131 uptake of hyperactive nodule after treatment. In addition, suppressed I-131 uptake by the rest of the thyroid gland became normal after treatment

therapy for the treatment of patients with NTMG. I-131 treatment has been reported to reduce the multinodular goiter volume by 40% after 1 year and by 50–60% after 2–5 years [34]. Retrosternal goiters can also be treated successfully. The success rate of I-131 treatment to reduce volume in large goiters depends on the administered dose and the homogeneous distribution of activity in the gland. With a total dose of 100-150 Gy with a dose of 3.7-5.5 MBq/g thyroid tissue corrected for 24-h I-131 uptake, there has been reported to be a 30-60% decrease in gland volume [35].

The repeating radioiodine therapy of patients with NTMG is also a safe and effective method. In a study, median thyroid volume of 145 cm^3 has been reported to decrease gradually to 76 cm^3 after 6 months and to 65 cm^3 after 12 months by repeating 22 mCi I-131 treatment every 3 months in the group of 7 female patients with NTMG [36].

The larger the radiation dose, the greater the volume reduction in the thyroid gland in patients with NTMG, but the goal here is to increase the radiation-absorbed dose in the thyroid gland without increasing the dose of I-131. Such an effect can be achieved by increasing the uptake of I-131 by using pretreatment with recombinant human TSH (rTSH) or increasing the retention of I-131 in the thyroid gland by lithium administration. However, rTSH pretreatment has been reported to be associated with a significantly higher percentage of I-131-induced hypothyroidism (36–65%) [37]. Since additional use of lithium may reduce transient subclinical hyperthyroidism caused by radioiodine, its use may be reasonable, especially in elderly patients with cardiovascular disorders [18]. Before I-131 treatment of NTMG patients, the administration of antithyroid methimazole can stimulate endogenous TSH secretion and increase the rate of I-131 uptake into the thyroid gland. It was reported that the rate of uptake of I-131 into the thyroid gland increased approximately twice in the methimazole patient group, the duration of treatment was reduced by half, and the occurrence of hypothyroidism did not differ significantly [38].

In summary, the volume of the thyroid gland in patients with NTMG can be effectively reduced by I-131 treatment. In order to increase the effectiveness of the treatment, endogenous TSH or rTSH can be applied to increase the uptake of

I-131 in the thyroid gland, or the retention time of I-131 in the thyroid gland can be prolonged by administration of lithium.

4.5 Non-Toxic Diffuse Goiter

Thyroid enlargement (goiter) is the most common manifestation of thyroid disease. It is caused by follicular hyperplasia to protect the euthyroid state against increased TSH production due to impaired synthesis of thyroid hormone [32]. Chronic TSH stimulation due to iodine deficiency has an important role in thyroid enlargement, and iodine supplementation for 8–12 months leads to a significant reduction in goiter size in patients with NTDG. LT4 replacement therapy for decreasing TSH stimulation may also decrease the volume of the thyroid gland of patients with NTDG. Although 50% or greater volume reduction was reported in 31% of patients after 6 months with LT4 suppression therapy, it has been reported that the volume of the goiter returned to its pre-treatment size after discontinuation of replacement therapy [33].

Radioiodine therapy can reduce pressure symptoms and relieve cosmetic complaints in patients with NTDG. In a study, the mean thyroid volume reduction achieved with a single dose of radioiodine within the first year has been reported to be 62%, and hypothyroidism has been reported to develop in 2 of the 11 patients (18%) [39]. In another prospective study, 34 patients with an NTDG have been treated with I-131 (200–600 MBq) due to compression symptoms and/or cosmetic discomfort [40]. In this study, after the median follow-up time of 36 months [12–82], goiter volume has been reported to reduce from 68 ml to 43 ml 3 months after the I-131 therapy and goiter has been reported to be no longer present in 76% of the patients at the end of follow-up. It has also been reported that 36% of patients developed hypothyroidism after 3 years of follow-up. The only problem in the treatment of I-131 cases is low radioactive iodine uptake rates and this problem can be solved with rTSH [41] or endogen TSH stimulation by using an antithyroid drug.

No significant swelling is generally expected in the gland after I-131 treatment, while in some cases there may be a 15–25% increase in the gland volume [42]. Therefore after I-131 treatment of patients with NTDG, It should be considered that this situation may increase the complaint of respiratory distress due to tracheal compression and this situation can be controlled with steroids.

A total of 70 mCi I-131 was administered to a middle-aged woman with right-sided low iodine intake and non-toxic goiter [43], and despite high-dose I-131 treatment, it has been reported that the size of the right lobe increased in the following years and compression symptoms developed. After histopathological examination, it has been reported that the right lobe contained a single large solitary adenoma instead of the normal thyroid parenchyma. As in this interesting case, it is of great importance that the thyroid gland be evaluated morphologically by an experienced physician before I-131 treatment.

In summary, the treatment of NTDG patients with I-131 leads to an increase in the quality of life of these patients, as it will reduce the compression symptoms and eliminate cosmetic problems [44].

4.6 Side Effects of I-131 Treatment

Although I-131 therapy, which is used to reduce thyroid function and volume, is well tolerated, this treatment approach has some undesirable side effects. I-131 therapy causes thyroidal and extrathyroidal irradiation. A transient rise in free T4 and free T3 levels can be detected 7–10 days following radioiodine treatment due to the release of possible stored hormones secondary to thyroid tissue destruction. Hence patients who have been poorly controlled before radioiodine therapy may experience cardiac problems such as heart failure and arrhythmia [8].

Since salivary glands express sodium iodide symporter and therefore, they naturally take up radioiodine, radioiodine-induced damage, inflammation, and dysfunction of the salivary glands are dose-dependent side effects of I-131 treatment. At the same doses, parotid glands appear to be more sensitive to I-131 radiation than submandibular glands. Slight discomfort of the salivary glands may accompany thyroid swelling but permanent injury is not usually observed. Salivary gland dysfunction has been reported to occur in 37 out of 108 glands (34.3%) treated with lower dose RAI (<30 mCi) whereas this effect has been reported to see in 53 out of 108 glands (49.1%) in the high-dose (30–100 mCi) group [45]. Hence sialadenitis, which is painful swelling of the salivary glands with concomitant reduction in salivary flow, is a common salivary gland complication of high-dose I-131 therapy for thyroid cancer.

Although radioiodine treatment of benign thyroid disorders results in an increase in parathormone levels, the condition does not influence the level of calcium and phosphorus concentration in any significant way [46].

Although thyroid storm after I-131 treatment is rare, patients with markedly elevated thyroid hormone concentrations at diagnosis may need to receive prolonged pre- and posttreatment with anti-thyroid drugs and beta blockers. Actually, it is safe to administer I-131 to patients who are severely hyperthyroid without fear of thyroid storm, provided beta blockade drugs are used to control the signs and symptoms [47]. In a case report, within 24 h of receiving I-131, an 11-year-old girl with newly diagnosed Graves' disease has been reported to diagnose with thyroid storm [48].

Hypothyroidism is the main side effect of radioiodine treatment. Its incidence continues to increase over time, and therefore, life-long follow-up is essential. LT4 replacement therapy is needed in all patients with elevated TSH after I-131 therapy [8]. The presence of pre-treatment autoantibodies increases the risk of developing hypothyroidism after treatment due to underlying autoimmune thyroiditis.

I-131 treatment may cause temporary swelling in the thyroid gland and this may increase compression symptoms in cases with large goiter.

I-131 treatment for Graves' disease was associated with increased risk of occurrence or progression of ophthalmopathy when compared with anti-thyroid drugs or surgery. On the other hand, development of ophthalmopathy post radioiodine treatment for toxic or non-toxic multinodular goiter has been very rarely reported. A 69-year-old male patient who developed ophthalmopathy after receiving 30 mCi of I-131 radioiodine treatment for a toxic nodule which was causing overt hyperthyroidism has been presented as a case report [49]. The clinical findings of ophthalmopathy may be unilateral, bilateral, symmetric, or asymmetric. Ophthalmopathy development can be prevented by prophylactic glucocorticoids in patients with preexisting suspicious symptoms of ophthalmopathy.

In a subset of predisposed individuals with benign toxic nodular disease of the thyroid gland, damage to the thyroid gland by I-131 may lead to the development of an immunological response which can be detected by seroconversion from negative to positive titers for anti-TPO and thyroid receptor antibodies. One potential mechanism is that necrosis of thyroid cells after I-131 treatment can cause the release of antigens, which in turn stimulates autoimmunity against thyroid and production of TSH-stimulating immunoglobulins. An alternative mechanism is that I-131 may kill the suppressor T cells in the thyroid gland during therapy, which in turn may cause an imbalance between T helper and suppressor cells resulting in autoimmunity [30]. While an increase in thyroid autoantibodies is detected 3-6 months after I-131 treatment [50], it returns to its basal levels within 1 year, but in some cases, it may continue to be detected in serum for years. Autoimmune thyroiditis is observed in 1% of the patients following radioiodine therapy of goiter/autonomous nodules. The risk has been reported to increase up to 10% in patients with preexisting thyroid peroxidase or thyroglobulin antibodies [8].

In radioiodine therapy for non-toxic goiter (adenoma or multinodular goiter), it has been reported that 5% of patients developed anti-thyrotropin receptor antibody-positive Graves' hyperthyroidism after 3 months, and 3% developed radiation thyroiditis at 1 month [51]. Therefore, patients with toxic nodular disease should be followed up for Graves' disease development after 3–12 months of RAI treatment [52]. In another study, it has been reported that there is an estimated 1.1% risk of developing post-radioiodine immunogenic hyperthyroidism/ Graves' disease in patients undergoing radioiodine therapy for autonomous thyroid disease and this increases approximately ten-fold when TPO antibody levels are elevated before radioiodine therapy [53]. In the same study, the estimated risk of a temporary increase of TSH receptor antibodies after radioiodine therapy for autonomous thyroid disease without development of clinically overt hyperthyroidism has been reported to be 1.3%. In cases with toxic or non-toxic nodular goiter, Graves and rarely thyroid-related ophthalmopathy due to newly developing autoantibodies after I-131 treatment have been reported [53], and new-onset Graves' disease has been reported in 4% cases after I-131 treatment [31]. If TSH-receptor antibodies are high before I-131 treatment, there is an increased possibility that post-treatment hyperthyroidism may be more severe.

Although a low rate of increased non-thyroid malignancy, especially hematological malignancies, after high-dose I-131 treatment has been reported in cases with thyroid cancer [54], the risk of developing cancer after low-dose treatment for benign thyroid diseases is not very clear. No increase in cancer diagnoses or deaths has been reported with therapeutic radioiodine-associated cancer for hyperthyroidism, except for a small increase in the risk of thyroid cancer, which may be associated with underlying thyroid disease [55, 56]. On the other hand, in RAI-treated patients with hyperthyroidism, greater organ-absorbed doses have been reported to appear to be modestly positively associated with risk of death from solid cancer, including breast cancer [57]. Serious criticisms of this last publication have been published and it has been claimed that the interpretation of this last publication is not valid [58]. Authors of the last reference insistently stated that "Radioactive Iodine Treatment was not associated with Cancer Mortality in Patients with Hyperthyroidism".

4.7 Other Issues Related to I-131 Treatment of Nodular Thyroid Diseases

Age and sex are controversial factors affecting the success of I-131 treatment. While nodule diameter and RAI dose are important factors for treatment efficacy; age, gender, underlying etiology, and antithyroid drugs have been reported not to affect the outcome of received radioiodine treatment [23]. Similarly, in a study, when the results of treatment with I-131 in cases with toxic nodular goiter were investigated, it has been reported that no relationship could be shown between treatment efficacy and age and gender [59–61].

After pre-therapeutic administration of iodine-131 for diagnostic purposes, reduced therapeutic iodine-131 uptake in the thyroid gland is defined as thyroid stunning. A reasonable underlying mechanism may be that the β-radiation of iodine-131 may lead to a decreased number of functioning thyroid cells and a reduced capability of viable thyroid cells to store iodine-131. Thyroid stunning has been shown to exist during fractionated I-131 treatments of benign thyroid diseases [62, 63]. Therefore to achieve the desired therapeutic radiation dose to the thyroid, administered radioiodine-131 therapy activity should be adapted depending on the dose in the radioiodine uptake test [64]. There is a waiting period after the I-131 dose for stunning to occur and the effect of stunning gradually increases over the days. In uptake studies conducted at 4-week intervals in cases with non-toxic goiter, no significant difference has been reported to detect, suggesting that the stunning effect disappeared over time [65]. Although stunning is clinically effective, the degree of this effect is uncertain and this effect seems to be more pronounced in vitro conditions than in vivo conditions.

Toxins in tobacco smoke adversely affect thyroid function. Thiocyanate in cigarette smoke has inhibitory effects on the synthesis of thyroid hormones by inhibiting the uptake and organification of iodide. Thiocyanate may cause a relative iodide deficiency state in the gland, and therefore, it may be responsible for the goitrogenic effect of cigarette smoking. Smoking has been reported to increase the incidence of multinodular goiter, especially in iodine-deficient areas and may cause goiter development [66, 67]. A strong evidence for a causal association between smoking and development of thyroid eye disease has been reported to provide by a systematic review, and current smokers have also been reported to be also more likely to experience disease progression or poorer outcome of treatment [68, 69]. The higher risk of non-toxic goiter has been reported to be higher in female smokers but in toxic nodular goiter, no significant relationship with smoking has been reported to be present, but the number of studies was limited [70].

The beta-adrenoceptors involved in the regulation of thyroid hormone secretion have been reported to be mainly of the beta 2-subtype in rats [71]. The principal mechanism of action of beta blockers is to antagonize beta-receptor mediated effects of catecholamines in hyperthyroidism. Hence beta blockers are effective in treating hypermetabolic symptoms in patients with toxic nodular goiters. They offer significant symptomatic relief and they are also useful adjuvants to antithyroid medications, surgery, and radioactive iodide treatment [72]. I-131 treatment may cause the clinical picture to deteriorate in the elderly or in sensitive cases with heart disease. Therefore, beta-blocker drug use should be recommended after I-131 treatment in cases >60 years of age, those with heart disease or severe hyperthyroidism [73].

Larger thyroid glands may cause severe compression on the trachea, and these compression symptoms may increase in severity after I-131 treatment. In one study, the efficacy of radioiodine therapy as an alternative to surgery in 19 elderly patients with large, compressive goiter was investigated and no exacerbation of compressive symptoms after I-131 therapy has been reported to observe [74]. However, adding steroids to I-131 treatment in cases with tracheal air clearance <1 cm due to tracheal compression has been reported to be beneficial in terms of preventing the development of severe respiratory distress after treatment [75].

Iodine is a trace element found in many substances such as seafood, salt, antiseptics, radiocontrast agents, etc. A pure allergic reaction to iodine does not exist, because simple atoms or molecules such as iodine or contrast material do not have the complexity required for antigenicity, although theoretically they might act as haptens [76]. Iodine may cause adverse reactions such as iododerma or iodide mumps. However, such reactions are usually related to large amounts of iodine and may not be allergic in nature. It is very rare that radioiodine administration causes hypersensitivity reactions because these preparations contain very low doses of active iodine compared to daily iodine intake (100–150 μg) such as 0.05–0.18 μg. For example, if the specific activity of I-131 is considered to be about 5Ci/mg, then it can be calculated that 100mCi of radioactive I-131 would contain ~20μg of sodium iodide [77]. In a case report, it was reported that a severe urticarial rash developed 30 min after ingestion of both radioactive I-123 and I-131 for thyroid screening and treatment of papillary thyroid carcinoma, but when liquid I-131 was administered to the patient, no allergic reaction developed. For this reason, it was thought that the content of the capsules containing radioiodine used in the previous treatment was the agent that triggered the allergic reaction [78]. I-131 can be safely administered even in patients with radioiodine contrast sensitivity and steroids may be required in suspicious cases.

In general, antithyroid drugs are administered in cases with hyperthyroidism before I-131 treatment since patients are desired to be euthyroid in order to prevent increased hyperthyroidism symptoms before I-131 treatment. The concomitant use of antithyroid drugs with I-131 reduces the treatment effectiveness in cases with TNG, since antithyroid drugs will increase the retention of I-131 involvement by non-nodular tissues rather than toxic nodules due to the increase in serum TSH levels in cases with TNG [79]. However, the use of antithyroid drugs before, during, or after I-131 treatment has been found to reduce the risk of hyperthyroidism treatment failure and hypothyroidism development [80]. In addition, it has been shown that administration of these drugs within 7 days of I-131 treatment does not change the treatment efficacy [81]. Besides discontinuation of carbimazole 3 days before I-131 treatment has been reported to increase the treatment effectiveness [82]. These drugs used with I-131 treatment can also reduce the risk of cardiac events. To summarize in the light of the information above, it is reasonable not to use antithyroid drugs before I-131 treatment in patients with mild hyperthyroidism and without concomitant disease, or to prefer thyramazole if antithyroid drugs will be used before I-131 treatment. It seems plausible to discontinue antithyroid drugs 3–7 days before treatment to increase I-131 uptake and restart 3–7 days after treatment to prevent temporary hyperthyroidism. In addition, it should be recommended that elderly patients with cardiovascular disease whose symptoms will worsen after treatment with I-131 in toxic nodular or multinodular diseases are given methimazole in addition to beta-blockers before treatment and continue to use antithyroid drugs after treatment.

I-131 uptake test shows wide differences between individuals. It is also affected by the levels of iodine taken with food and this rate decreases where iodine supplementation is given. It is associated with instantaneous iodine levels in urine and a 25% reduction in I-131 uptake rate has been reported to observe with a two-fold increase in urine [83]. Although the iodine restrictive diet is a standard practice in thyroid cancer patients to increase the efficacy of I-131 treatment, excess iodine rarely affects the treatment of hyperthyroidism with I-131. When the iodine load in the diet is increased, thyroid radioiodine uptake is decreased. This causes an increase in the dose of I-131 to achieve a similar effect. In a study, there has been reported to be significant negative correlation between higher iodine content in the diet and lower values of radioiodine uptake, which led to the application of the higher activity of I-131 during treatment [84]. Whereas to obtain the optimal target energy dose in the thyroid can only be achieved with a high level of uptake and a long effective half-life of radioiodine in the thyroid. The turnover of iodine in the hyperactive thyroid gland can increase and this usually results in a lowering of the effective half-life. Whereas administration of non-radioactive iodine-127, 2–3 days after radioiodine administration can also increase the effective half-life of radioiodine in the thyroid. It has been reported in a study that, the administration of non-radioactive iodine after the maximum level of thyroid uptake had been reached resulted in a 34% increase in the energy target dose in patients with toxic nodular goiter [85]. Thus, lower activities of I-131 could be administered with lower effective doses to the rest of the body, while achieving an equally effective target dose in the thyroid due to improved biokinetics of radioiodine. In the light of these data, reducing the body iodine pool before I-131 treatment of patients with toxic nodular goiter and adding iodine to the daily diet after I-131 treatment seems to increase the effectiveness of the treatment.

Lithium, which is used in psychiatric diseases, usually causes the development of hypothyroidism and goiter in some sensitive cases. While lithium does not affect the uptake of I-131, it inhibits its release from the follicle cells, and therefore, lithium enhances I-131 retention in the thyroid gland. In one study, 885 mg/day lithium carbonate has been reported to result in a 60% prolongation in the I-131 half-life and a 39% increase in the radiation dose applied to the thyroid without a change in I-131 uptake rate [86]. Although routine use is not recommended, it can be suggested to use for 7 days after I-131 treatment as 250 mg twice a day, especially in those with I-131 uptake rate < 20% [87]. In one study, it has been reported that RAI therapy combined with lithium showed a trend toward higher cure rate, safe and time to cure was less than RAI alone [88]. In a meta-analysis, it has been reported that observational and interventional trials showed a significant improvement in the cure rate of hyperthyroidism when lithium was added to the RAI, but interventional trials did not reach statistical significance [89].

Although diuretics reduce the body's iodine pool by increasing iodine excretion, they are not widely used because their side effects outweigh their benefits. In one study it was reported that diuretic administration led to a 58.4% increase in iodine uptake over the baseline value, compared to low-iodine diet (17.22%) in patients with non-toxic goiter [90].

The therapeutic efficacy of I-131 in patients with NTMG depends to some extent on the I-131 uptake and multinodular goiters frequently have a low and heterogeneous uptake of I-131. Therefore, the treatment with radioiodine requires relatively high I-131 activities. Whereas, the administration of rTSH before I-131 increases radioiodine uptake and homogenizes the uptake of I-131 in the thyroid gland [91]. Thus, the volume reduction of multinodular goiter can be enhanced at lower I-131 activities via rTSH administration. In a randomized, double-blind, placebo-controlled study, the mean goiter volume reductions obtained at 1 year and final follow-up in the rTSH group have been reported to be significantly greater than those obtained in the I-131-alone group [92]. On the other hand, the prevalence of hypothyroidism was also significantly higher in the rTSH group.

Benign thyroid disease requiring I-131 therapy is relatively rare in children and is almost exclusively limited to the treatment of Graves' disease, since Graves' disease accounts for approximately 96% of pediatric cases of thyrotoxicosis. Radioactive iodine therapy may be an option for children in the following conditions: poor adherence to antithyroid medication, not in remission after 1–2 years of antithyroid medication, and major adverse event while taking an antithyroid medication [93]. The rate of recurrence after antithyroid treatment and the risk of drug-related side effects are higher in children compared to adults [94]. I-131 treatment should be avoided in children under 5 years of age as the thyroid gland will be sensitive to radiation in the future due to cancer development [95, 96]. It should be remembered that radioiodine treatment leads to a significantly higher incidence of hypothyroidism as compared with both anti-thyroid drugs and thyroidectomy [97].

Graves' disease accounts for ~95% of cases of overt hyperthyroidism during pregnancy, hence the remaining etiologies of hyperthyroidism in pregnancy are all relatively uncommon [98]. I-131 therapy is absolutely contraindicated in pregnancy. Since I-131 may cross the placenta and the developing fetus can concentrate I-131 starting at 10 weeks which causes permanent hypothyroidism in the fetus. Besides, whole-body fetal irradiation can occur from both transplacental passage of I-131 and external radiation from maternal tissues, particularly the bladder [99].

If we evaluate the thyroid nodule and Graves' association, a thyroid nodule may also be present in the background of Graves' disease and the presence of at least one thyroid nodule in patients with GD has been reported to be associated with higher risk for thyroid cancer [100]. In a study, nodules and cancer have been reported to detect in 53% and 12.5% of cases, respectively in a cohort of 151 patients who have been retrospectively analyzed after total thyroidectomy for Graves' disease [101]. If >1 cm nodule is detected on the ground of Graves' disease, it is approached like a normal thyroid nodule. In patients with thyroid cancer <1 cm on a Graves background, the disease-free survival rate for 20 years is 99% [102].

4.8 Concluding Remarks

I-131 treatment has both structural effects on the thyroid gland, such as volume reduction, and functional effects, such as reducing hormone production. Therefore, it is an ideal radionuclide agent in toxic nodular thyroid diseases. I-131 treatment in cases with toxic nodular goiter is effective, safe, and the results are quite satisfactory despite the risk of development of hypothyroidism. Besides, I-131 treatment seems to be a good alternative to surgery in terms of reducing compression symptoms and eliminating cosmetic concerns, especially in elderly patients with non-toxic diffuse goiter and non-toxic nodular or diffuse goiter, as it causes a prominent decrease in thyroid volume. Considering the serious side effects of antithyroid drugs and potential surgical complications, I-131 comes to the forefront in the treatment of benign nodular thyroid diseases.

References

1. Burman KD, Wartofsky L. Clinical practice. Thyroid nodules. N Engl J Med. 2015;373:2347–56.
2. Angell TE, Vyas C, Medici M, et al. Differential growth rates of benign versus malignant thyroid nodules. J Clin Endocrinol Metab. 2017;102:4642–7.
3. Wong R, Farrell SG, Grossmann M. Thyroid nodules: diagnosis and management. Med J Aust. 2018;209:92–8.
4. Ross DS, Burch HB, Cooper DS, Greenlee MC, Laurberg P, Maia AL, et al. American Thyroid Association guidelines for diagnosis and management of hyperthyroidism and other causes of thyrotoxicosis. Thyroid. 2016;26:1343–421.
5. Freitas JE. Therapeutic options in the management of toxic and nontoxic nodular goiter. Semin Nucl Med. 2000;30:88–97.
6. Douglas S. Ross, Treatment of toxic adenoma and toxic multinodular goiter. *Up to date*, 2021.
7. Azizi F, Abdi H, Cheraghi L, Amouzegar A. Treatment of subclinical hyperthyroidism in the elderly: comparison of radioiodine and long-term methimazole treatment. Thyroid. 2021;31:545–51.
8. Stokkel MPM, Junak DH, Lassmann M, Dietlein M, Luster M. EANM procedure guidelines for therapy of benign thyroid disease. Eur J Nucl Med Mol Imaging. 2010;37:2218–28.
9. Pouget JP, Lozza C, Deshayes E, Boudousq V, Navarro-Teulon I. Introduction to radiobiology of targeted radionuclide therapy. Front Med (Lausanne). 2015;17:2–12.
10. Bourguignon MH, Gisone PA, Perez MR, Michelin S, Dubner D, Giorgio MD, Carosella ED. Genetic and epigenetic features in radiation sensitivity. Part I: Cell signalling in radiation response. Eur J Nucl Med Mol Imaging. 2005;32:229–46.
11. Bourguignon MH, Gisone PA, Perez MR, Michelin S, Dubner D, Giorgio MD, Carosella ED. Genetic and epigenetic features in radiation sensitivity. Part II: Implications for clinical practice and radiation protection. Eur J Nucl Med Mol Imaging. 2005;32:351–68.
12. Jorgensen TJ. Enhancing radiosensitivity: targeting the DNA repair pathways. Cancer Biol Ther. 2009;8:665–70.
13. Holst JP, Burman KD, Atkins F, Umans JG, Jonklaas J. Radioiodine therapy for thyroid cancer and hyperthyroidism in patients with end-stage renal disease on hemodialysis. Thyroid. 2005;15:1321–31.
14. de Rooij A, Vandenbroucke JP, Smit JW, Stokkel MP, Dekkers OM. Clinical outcomes after estimated versus calculated activity of radioiodine for the treatment of hyperthyroidism: systematic review and meta-analysis. Eur J Endocrinol. 2009;161:771–7.
15. Azizi F, Takyar M, Madreseh E, Amouzegar A. Treatment of toxic multinodular goiter: comparison of radioiodine and long-term methimazole treatment. Thyroid. 2019;29:625–30.
16. Roque C, Santos FS, Pilli T, Dalmazio G, Castagna MG, Pacini F. Long-term effects of radioiodine in toxic multinodular goiter: thyroid volume, function, and autoimmunity. J Clin Endocrinol Metab. 2020;1:105–7.
17. Mitra S, Muthu SG. Reduction in relapse rate of radioiodine therapy in patients of toxic multinodular goiter: a quality improvement project. Indian J Nucl Med. 2012;27:5–9.
18. Vannucchi G, Chiti A, Mannavola D, Dazzi D, Rodari M, Tadayyon S, Beck-Peccoz P, Fugazzola L. Radioiodine treatment of non-toxic multinodular goitre: effects of combination with lithium. Eur J Nucl Med Mol Imaging. 2005;32:1081–8.
19. Porterfield JR Jr, Thompson GB, Farley DR, Grant CS, Richards ML. Evidence-based management of toxic multinodular goiter (Plummer's disease). World J Surg. 2008;32:1278–84.
20. Finessi M, Bisceglia A, Passera R, Giaccherino RR, Pagano L, Castellano G, Ghigo E, Bisi G, Deandreis D. Predictive factors of a worse response to radioactive Iodine-I131 treatment in hyperthyroidism: outcome analysis in 424 patients. A single centre experience. Endocrine. 2021;73:107–15.
21. Meller J, Siefker U, Hamann A, Hufner M. Incidence of radioiodine induced Graves' disease in patients with multinodular toxic goiter. Exp Clin Endocrinol Diabetes. 2006;114:235–9.
22. Szumowski P, Rogowski F, Abdelrazek S, Kociura-Sawicka A, Sokolik-Ostasz A. Iodine isotope 131I therapy for toxic nodular goitre: treatment efficacy parameters. Nucl Med Rev Cent East Eur. 2012;24(15):7–13.
23. Şakı H, Cengiz A, Yürekli Y. Effectiveness of radioiodine treatment for toxic nodular goiter. Mol Imaging Radionucl Ther. 2015;24:100–4.
24. Kahraman D, Keller C, Schneider C, Eschner W, Sudbrock F, Schmidt M, Schicha H, Dietlein M, Kobe C. Development of hypothyroidism during long-term follow-up of patients with toxic nodular goitre after radioiodine therapy. Clin Endocrinol. 2012;76:297–303.
25. Schiavo M, Bagnara MC, Camerieri L, Pomposelli E, Giusti M, Pesce G, et al. Clinical efficacy of radioiodine therapy in multinodular toxic goiter, applying an implemented dose calculation algorithm. Endocrine. 2015;48:902–8.

26. Sheehan MT, Doi SAR. Transient hypothyroidism after radioiodine for graves' disease: challenges in interpreting. Thyroid Function Tests. 2016;14:40–5.
27. Ceccarelli C, Bencivelli W, Vitti P, Grasso L, Pinchera A. Outcome of radioiodine-131 therapy in hyperfunctioning thyroid nodules: a 20 years' retrospective study. Clin Endocrinol. 2005;62:331–5.
28. Erdoğan MF, Küçük NO, Anil C, Aras S, Ozer D, Aras G, Kamel N. Effect of radioiodine therapy on thyroid nodule size and function in patients with toxic adenomas. Nucl Med Commun. 2004;25:1083–7.
29. Bonefačić B, Crnčić TB, Tomaš MI, Girotto N, Ivanković SG. The significance of serum thyroglobulin measurement before and after the treatment of toxic nodular goiter with 131I. Nucl Med Commun. 2020;41:344–9.
30. Rehman A, Obici S, Yaqub A. Radioiodine therapy-induced conversion of toxic adenoma to graves' disease. Cureus. 2020;12:e8683.
31. Nygaard B, Faber J, Veje A, Hegedus L, Hansen JM. Transition of nodular toxic goiter to autoimmune hyperthyroidism triggered by 131I therapy. Thyroid. 1999;9:477–81.
32. Mitchell RN, Kumar V, Abbas AK, Aster JC. Pathologic basis of disease. Endocrine system. Philadelphia, USA: Elsevier; 2017. p. 661–703.
33. Knobel M. Which is the ideal treatment for benign diffuse and multinodular non-toxic goiters? Front Endocrinol (Lausanne). 2016;7:48.
34. Graf H. Recombinant human TSH and radioactive iodine therapy in the management of benign multinodular goiter. Eur J Endocrinol. 2015;172:R47–52.
35. Manders JMB, Corstens FHM. Radioiodine therapy of euthyroid multinodular goitres. Eur J Nucl Med. 2002;29(Suppl2):466–70.
36. Pisarek M, Baczyk M, Gryczyńska M, Sowiński J. The treatment of multinodular large non-toxic goiter using repeated doses of radioiodine (preliminary report). Endokrynol Pol. 2007;58:18–26.
37. Silva MN, Rubio IG, Romao R, Gebrin EM, Buchpiguel C, Tomimori E, et al. Administration of a single dose of recombinant human thyrotrophin enhances the efficacy of radioiodine treatment of large compressive multinodular goiters. Clin Endocrinol. 2004;60:300–8.
38. Szumowski P, Abdelrazek S, Sykała M, Mojsak M, Żukowski Ł, Siewko K, Maliszewska K, Adamska A, Popławska-Kita A, Krętowski A, Myśliwiec J. Enhancing the efficacy of (131)I therapy in non-toxic multinodular goitre with appropriate use of methimazole: an analysis of randomized controlled study. Endocrine. 2020;67:136–42.
39. Hegedüs L, Bennedbæk FN. Radioiodine for non-toxic diffuse goitre. Lancet. 1997;350:409–10.
40. Bonnema SJ, Nielsen VE, Hegedüs L. Long-term effects of radioiodine on thyroid function, size and patient satisfaction in non-toxic diffuse goitre. Eur J Endocrinol. 2004;150:439–45.
41. Fast S, Nielsen VE, Bonnema SJ, Hegedüs L. Time to reconsider nonsurgical therapy of benign non-toxic multinodular goitre: focus on recombinant human TSH augmented radioiodine therapy. Eur J Endocrinol. 2009;160:517–28.
42. Bonnema SJ, Nielsen VE, Boel-Jørgensen H, Grupe P, Andersen PB, Bastholt L, Hegedus L. Improvement of goiter volume reduction after 0.3 mg recombinant human thyrotropin- stimulated radioiodine therapy in patients with a very large goiter: a double-blinded, randomized trial. J Clin Endocrinol Metab. 2007;92:3424–8.
43. Hartoft-Nielsen ML, Rasmussen AK, Friis E, Blichert-Toft M, Buhl T, Hesse B, Rasmussen UF. Unsuccessful radioiodine treatment of a non-toxic goiter: a case report. Basic Clin Pharmacol Toxicol. 2004;95:72–5.
44. Kaniuka-Jakubowska S, Lewczuk A, Majkowicz M, Piskunowicz M, Mizan-Gross K, Zapaśnik A, Kaszubowski M, Lass P, Sworczak K. Nontoxic goiter (NTG) and radioiodine: what do patients think about it? quality of life in patients with NTG before and after 131-I therapy. Front Endocrinol (Lausanne). 2018;9:114.
45. Fard-Esfahani A, Fallahi B, Karimi M, Beiki B, Saghari M, Emami-Ardekani AR, Fard-Esfahani P, Ansari M, Eftekhari M. Changes in salivary gland function following radioiodine therapy of thyroid diseases: a comparison of high-dose therapy for thyroid cancer and low-dose therapy for benign thyroid disease. Iran J Nucl Med. 2015;23:1–7.
46. Szumowski P, Abdelrazek S, Mojsak M, Rogowski F, Kociura-Sawicka A, Myśliwiec J. Parathyroid gland function after radioiodine ((131)I) therapy for toxic and non-toxic goitre. Endokrynol Pol. 2013;64:340–5.
47. Vijayakumar V, Nusynowwitz ML, Ali S. Is it safe to treat hyperthyroid patients with I-131 without fear of thyroid storm? Ann Nucl Med. 2006;20:383–5.
48. Rohrs HJ, Silverstein JH, Weinstein DA, Amdur RJ, Haller MJ. Thyroid storm following radioactive iodine (RAI) therapy for pediatric graves disease. Am J Case Rep. 2014;15:212–5.
49. Ahmadieh HC, Salti I. Graves's eye ophthalmopathy developing following radioiodine therapy for toxic adenoma. Open J Endocrine Metabolic Dis. 2013;3:259–62.
50. Chiappori A, Villalta D, Bossert I, CeresolaEM LD, Schiavo M, et al. Thyrotropin receptor autoantibody measurement following radiometabolic treatment of hyperthyroidism: comparison between different methods. J Endocrinol Investig. 2010;33:197–201.
51. Nygaard B, Knudsen JH, Hegedus L, et al. Thyrotropin receptor antibodies and Graves' disease, a side-effect of 131I treatment in patients with nontoxic goiter. J Clin Endocrinol Metab. 1997;82:2926–30.
52. Roque C, Vasconcelos CA. 131 I-Induced Graves' disease in patients treated for toxic multinodular

goitre: systematic review and descriptive analysis. J Endocrinol Investig. 2018;41:1019–28.
53. Schmidt M, Gorbauch E, Dietlein M, et al. Incidence of postradioiodine immunogenic hyperthyroidism/ Graves' disease in relation to a temporary increase in thyrotropin receptor antibodies after radioiodine therapy for autonomous thyroid disease. Thyroid. 2006;16:281–8.
54. Molenaar RJ, Sidana S, Radivoyevitch T, Advani AS, Gerds AT, Carraway HE, Angelini D, Kalaycio M, Nazha A, Adelstein DJ, Nasr C, Maciejewski JP, Majhail NS, Sekeres MA, Mukherjee S. Risk of hematologic malignancies after radioiodine treatment of well-differentiated thyroid cancer. J Clin Oncol. 2018;36:1831–9.
55. Franklyn JA, Sheppard MC, Maisonneuve P. Thyroid function and mortality in patients treated for hyperthyroidism. JAMA. 2005;294:71–80.
56. Lucignani G. Long-term risks in hyperthyroid patients treated with radioiodine: is there anything new? Eur J Nucl Med Mol Imaging. 2007;34:1504–9.
57. Kitahara CM, de Gonzalez AB, Bouville A, Brill AB, Doody MM, Melo DR, Simon SS, Julie Sosa A, Tulchinsky M, Villoing D, Preston DL. Association of radioactive iodine treatment with cancer mortality in patients with hyperthyroidism. JAMA Intern Med. 2019;179:1034–42.
58. Greenspan BS, Siegel JA, Hassan A, Silberstein EB. There is no association of radioactive iodine treatment with cancer mortality in patients with hyperthyroidism. J Nucl Med. 2019;60:1500–1.
59. Ahmad T, Khoja A, Rashid NH, Ashfaq MA. Outcome of radioactive iodine therapy in toxic nodular goiter in Pakistan. Pak J Med Sci. 2018;34:1146–51.
60. Lu L, Gao C, Zhang N. Age moderates the associations between TRAbs, free T3 and outcomes of Graves' disease patients with radioactive iodine treatment. Clin Endocrinol. 2021;94:303–9.
61. Allahabadia A, Daykin J, Sheppard MC, Gough SC, Franklyn JA. Radioiodine treatment of hyperthyroidism-prognostic factors for outcome. J Clin Endocrinol Metab. 2001;86:3611–7.
62. Sabri O, Zimny M, Schreckenberger M, Meyer-Oelmann A, Reinartz R, Buell U. Does thyroid stunning exist? A model with benign thyroid disease. Eur J Nucl Med. 2000;27:1591–7.
63. Krohn T, Meyer PT, Ocklenburg C, Knollmann D, Nowak B, Schaefer WM. Stunning in radioiodine therapy of benign thyroid disease. Quantification and therapeutic relevance. Nuklearmedizin. 2008;47:248–54.
64. Happel C, Kranert WT, Ackermann H, Binse I, Bockisch B, Gröner D, Herrmann K, Grünwald F. Thyroid stunning in radioiodine-131 therapy of benign thyroid diseases. Endocrine. 2019;63:537–44.
65. Fast S, Nielsen VE, Grupe P, Bonnema SJ, Hegedu¨ sL. Optimizing 131I uptake after rhTSH stimulation in patients with nontoxic multinodular goiter: evidence from a prospective, randomized, double-blind study. J Nucl Med. 2009;50:732–7.
66. Brauer VF, Below H, Kramer A, Fu¨ hrer D, Paschke R. The role of thiocyanate in the etiology of goiter in an industrial metropolitan area. Eur J Endocrinol. 2006;154:229–35.
67. Sawicka-Gutaj N, Gutaj P, Sowiński J, Wender-Ożegowska E, Czarnywojtek A, Brązert J, Ruchała M. Influence of cigarette smoking on thyroid gland--an update. Endokrynol Pol. 2014;65:54–62.
68. Thornton J, Kelly SP, Harrison RA, Edwards R. Cigarette smoking and thyroid eye disease: a systematic review. Eye (Lond). 2007;21:1135–45.
69. Plazinska MT, Sawicka-Gutaj N, Czarnywojtek A, Wolinski K, Kobylecka M, Karlińska M, Prasek K, Zgorzalewicz-Stachowiak M, Borowska M, Gut P, Ruchala M, Krolicki L. Radioiodine therapy and Graves' disease – myths and reality. PLoS One. 2020;15:e0226495.
70. Vestergaard P. Smoking and thyroid disorders—a meta-analysis. Eur J Endocrinol. 2002;146:153–61.
71. Ahrén B, Rerup C. Effects of beta-adrenoceptor agonists and antagonists on thyroid hormone secretion. Eur J Pharmacol. 1983;88:383–7.
72. Geffner DL, Hershman JM. Beta-adrenergic blockade for the treatment of hyperthyroidism. Am J Med. 1992;93:61–8.
73. Ventrella S, Klein I. Beta-adrenergic receptor blocking drugs in the management of hyperthyroidism. Endocrinologist. 1994;4:391–9.
74. Huysmans DA, Hermus AR, Corstens FH, Barentsz JO, Kloppenborg PW. Large, compressive goiters treated with radioiodine. Ann Intern Med. 1994;121:757–62.
75. Papini E, Petrucci L, Guglielmi R, Panunzi C, Rinaldi R, Bacci V, et al. Long-term changes in nodular goiter: a 5-year prospective randomized trial of levothyroxine suppressive therapy for benign cold thyroid nodules. J Clin Endocrinol Metab. 1998;83:780–3.
76. Coakley FV, Panicek DM. Iodine allergy: an oyster without a pearl? AJR Am J Roentgenol. 1997;169:951–2.
77. Puchalski AR, Chopra IJ. Radioiodine treatment of differentiated thyroid cancer despite history of 'iodine allergy'. Endocrinol Diabetes Metab Case Rep. 2014;2014:130084.
78. Nunez R, Sellin RV, Fareau GG, Drucker CR. Images in thyroidology: skin rash after radioactive iodine caught on a cell phone camera. Thyroid. 2007;3:277–8.
79. Körber C, Schneider P, Körber-Hafner N, Hänscheid H, Reiners C. Antithyroid drugs as a factor influencing the outcome of radioiodine therapy in Graves' disease and toxic nodular goitre? Eur J Nucl Med. 2001;28:1360–4.
80. Walter MA, Briel M, Christ-Crain M, Bonnema SJ, Connell J, Cooper DS, et al. Effects of antithyroid drugs on radioiodine treatment: systematic review and meta-analysis of randomised controlled trials. BMJ. 2007;334:514.
81. Kung AW, Yau CC, Cheng AC. The action of methimazole and L-thyroxine in radioiodine ther-

apy: a prospective study on the incidence of hypothyroidism. Thyroid. 1995;5:7–12.
82. Walter MA, Crist-Crain M, Schindler C, Mueller-Brand J, Mueller B. Outcome of radioiodine therapy without, on or 3 days off carbimazole: a prospective interventional three-group comparison. Eur J Nucl Med Mol Imaging. 2006;33:730–7.
83. Meller B, Haase A, Seyfarth M, Wenzel BE, Richter E, BaehreM. Reduced radioiodine uptake at increased iodine intake and 131I-induced release of "cold" iodine stored in the thyroid. Nuklearmedizin. 2005;44:137–42.
84. Baczyk M, Junik R, Ziemnicka K, Sowiński J. Iodine prophylaxis intensification. Influence on radioiodine uptake and activity of 131I used in the treatment of hyperthyroid patients with Graves' disease. Nuklearmedizin. 2005;44:197–9.
85. Moka D, Dietlein M, Schicha H. Radioiodine therapy and thyrostatic drugs and iodine. Eur J Nucl Med Mol Imaging. 2002;29(Suppl 2):486–91.
86. Dunkelmann S, Künstner H, Nabavi E, Eberlein U, Groth P, Schümichen C. Lithium as an adjunct to radioiodine therapy in Graves' disease for prolonging the intrathyroidal effective half-life of radioiodine. Useful or not? Nuklearmedizin. 2006;45:213–8.
87. Bal CS, Kumar A, Pandey RM. A randomized controlled trial to evaluate the adjuvant effect of lithium on radioiodine treatment of hyperthyroidism. Thyroid. 2002;12:399–405.
88. Lingudu B, Bongi V, Ayyagari M, Venkata SK. Impact of lithium on radioactive iodine therapy for hyperthyroidism. Indian J Endocrinol Metab. 2014;18:669–75.
89. Kessler L, Palla J, Baru JS, Onyenwenyi C, George AM, Lucas BP. Lithium as an adjunct to radioactive iodine for the treatment of hyperthyroidism: a systematic review and meta-analysis. Endocr Pract. 2014;20:737–45.
90. Kapucu LO, Azizoglu F, Ayvaz G, Karakoc A. Effects of diuretics on iodine uptake in non-toxic goitre: comparison with low-iodine diet. Eur J Nucl Med Mol Imaging. 2003;30:1270–2.
91. Mojsak MN, Abdelrazek S, Szumowski P, Rogowski P, Sykała M, Kostecki J, Sawicka A, Jurgilewicz D, Myśliwiec J. Single, very low dose (0.03 mg) of recombinant human thyrotropin (rhTSH) effectively increases radioiodine uptake in the I-131 treatment of large nontoxic multinodular goiter. Nucl Med Rev Cent East Eur. 2016;19:3–11.
92. Fast S, Nielsen VE, Grupe P, Boel-Jørgensen H, Bastholt L, Andersen PB, Bonnema SJ, Hegedüs L. Prestimulation with recombinant human thyrotropin (rhTSH) improves the long-term outcome of radioiodine therapy for multinodular nontoxic goiter. J Clin Endocrinol Metab. 2012;97:2653–60.
93. Leung AKC, Leung AAC. Evaluation and management of children with thyrotoxicosis. Recent Pat Endocr Metab Immune Drug Discov. 2017;11:22–31.
94. Chao M, Jiawei X, Guoming W, Jianbin L, Wanxia L, Driedger A, et al. Radioiodine treatment for pediatric hyperthyroid Graves disease. Eur J Pediatr. 2009;168:1165–9.
95. Kaplowitz PB, Vaidyanathan P. Update on pediatric hyperthyroidism. Curr Opin Endocrinol Diabetes Obes. 2020;27:70–6.
96. Luster M, Pfestroff A, Hänscheid H, Verburg FA. Radioiodine therapy. Semin Nucl Med. 2017;47:126–34.
97. Chao M, Jiawei X, Guoming W, Jianbin L, Wanxia L, Driedger A, Shuyao Z, QinZ. Radioiodine treatment for pediatric hyperthyroid Grave's disease. Eur J Pediatr. 2009;168:1165–9.
98. Cuff RD. Hyperthyroidism during pregnancy: a clinical approach. Clin Obstet Gynecol. 2019;62:320–9.
99. Kobaly K, Mandel SJ. Hyperthyroidism and pregnancy. Endocrinol Metab Clin N Am. 2019;48:533–45.
100. Papanastasiou A, Sapalidis K, Goulis DG, Michalopoulos N, Mareti E, Mantalovas S, Kesisoglou I. Thyroid nodules as a risk factor for thyroid cancer in patients with Graves' disease: a systematic review and meta-analysis of observational studies in surgically treated patients. Clin Endocrinol. 2019;91:571–7.
101. Casella C, Morandi R, Verrengia A, Galani A, Molfino S, Cuka D, Groppo G, Cappelli C, Portolani N. Thyroid cancer and nodules in Graves' disease: a single center experience. Endocr Metab Immune Disord Drug Targets. 2021;21(1):2028–34.
102. Kikuchi S, Noguchi S, Yamashita H, Uchino S, Kawamoto H. Prognosis of small thyroid cancer in patients with Graves' disease. Br J Surg. 2006;93:434–9.

5 Radionuclide Therapy in Benign Thyroid Diseases: Graves' Disease

Mine Araz and Elgin Özkan

5.1 Epidemiology

Toxic diffuse goiter (Graves' disease) is more common in women, as in most autoimmune diseases, and is the most common cause of hyperthyroidism in young women (60–80%). The ratio of women to men is 10:1 [1]. Family history is found in close to 50% of patients [2].

5.2 Etiology and Pathogenesis

In 1964, a factor stimulating thyroid was found to play a role in the etiopathogenesis of the disease and this factor was found to be an immune globulin (TSH receptor antibody or TSH stimulating antibody) mimicking TSH [3]. With TSH stimulation, the thyroid gland grows and begins to produce excessive hormones. The same autoantibodies play a role in the physiopathology of the classic clinical picture by stimulating TSH receptors present in orbital and dermal fibroblasts and adipocytes. Thyroid-stimulating antibodies are believed to be involved in the pathophysiology of Graves' ophthalmopathy. TSH receptors are also found on orbital fibroblasts. It is thought that some other antibodies that can bind to some special non-TSH receptors on retroorbital fibroblasts and orbital muscles also constitute the secondary mechanism as stimulants [4].

5.3 Clinical Signs

Although the clinical signs of Graves' disease coincide with those of classic hyperthyroidism, some specific findings related to autoimmune-induced physiopathology of the disease are also observed. Typical patient profiles are females aged 20–30 years. Emotional lability, agitation and sleep disorders, and apathy can be observed. Fatigue, acceleration in gastrointestinal system activity, and weight loss despite increased appetite are observed. Oligomenorrhea or amenorrhea may be seen in premenopausal patients. On physical examination, the skin is warm and moist. The hairs are thin. Onycholysis is one of the common findings. Gynecomastia due to excessive estrogen production may occur in male patients. Tremor is observed in the hands; tendon reflexes are hyperactive. Among the eye findings, an increase in the distance between both eyelids due to increased sympathetic tonus (lid lag), vivid gaze, and continuous blinking are observed. These are not specific to Graves. Its effects on the cardiovascular system include sinus tachycardia, increased pulse pressure, and increased systolic blood pressure. Some cardiac arrhythmias, such as atrial fibrillation, may trigger or aggravate heart failure. Muscle atrophy and weakness may develop and hypokalemic periodic paralysis may

M. Araz · E. Özkan (✉)
Faculty of Medicine, Department of Nuclear Medicine, Ankara University, Ankara, Turkey
e-mail: maraz@ankara.edu.tr; eozkan@ankara.edu.tr

R. Bekiş et al. (eds.), *Radionuclide Therapy*, https://doi.org/10.1007/978-3-030-97220-2_5

be observed. Bone turnover is accelerated. Blood calcium levels may increase up to 12 mg/dL. Some biochemical abnormalities may include ALP elevation, hyperbilirubinemia, mild anemia, and neutropenia. Renal tubular acidosis may develop. Immune complex nephritis has been reported [5–12].

Diffuse hyperplasia is observed in the thyroid gland. In the examination, the gland is symmetrically enlarged and is generally soft and smooth on palpation. Rarely, it can be present with nodules. In advanced cases, murmur can be heard on the gland and thrill can be felt in palpation [10].

The incidence of severe ophthalmopathy in Graves' disease is less than 5%. Patients have complaints such as photophobia, tears in the eyes, and diplopia. Periorbital edema may occur due to a decrease in the drainage of the chemosis orbital veins. Swelling and fibrotic orbital muscles cause retraction. Proptosis in the eye sphere due to hypertrophy in the retroorbital connective tissue causes limitation of eye movements, dry eye, and keratitis. Optic nerve compression may develop due to retroorbital compression [13].

Thyrotoxic periodic paralysis is a rare clinical presentation of Graves' disease. Hypokalemic periodic paralysis occurs in extremities. While the myopathic pattern is observed in EMG during attacks, this pattern disappears when the disease enters remission. The difference from familial euthyroid periodic paralysis is that acetazolamide does not provide a benefit, or even cause worsening. Cardiac conduction anomalies such as grade 1–2 heart blocks and fibrillations can be observed [14]

Marine-Lenhart syndrome is typically a hypoactive nodule with diffuse increased uptake in thyroid scintigraphy (Fig. 5.1). This nodule is mostly benign adenoma and is dependent only on TSH. The thyroid is not affected by stimulating antibodies. Therefore, while the rest of the gland is active, the nodule is relatively hypoactive. However, when TSH increases again after RAI (radioactive iodine) treatment, the nodule regains its activity and this time it is hyperactive on scintigraphy [15].

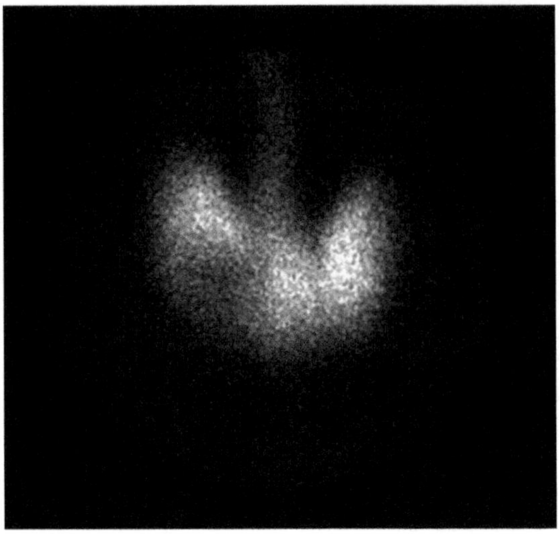

Fig. 5.1 Diffuse increased uptake in both lobes of thyroid gland and pyramidal lobe together with a hypoactive area located laterally in the mid-inferior of right lobe (Marine-Lenhart syndrome)

5.4 Laboratory Findings

In severe cases, it is easy to diagnose with specific clinical findings accompanying thyrotoxicosis. T3, T4 elevation, and undetectable TSH suppression are classic laboratory findings [16]. Although T4 is normal in regions with iodine deficiency, T3 elevation may be found (T3 thyrotoxicosis) [17]. T4 may remain normal as the production of T3 due to excessive stimulation of TSH receptors increases very much. It is more common in the first stage of Graves or in relapse cases. Today, TSH receptor antibody can give an idea among laboratory findings in the diagnosis and prognosis of Graves [3].

5.5 Thyroid Scintigraphy and Radioactive Iodine Uptake (RAIU)

In general, RAIU measurement in a patient with classic thyrotoxicosis findings and T3, T4 elevation and TSH suppression can distinguish roughly whether thyrotoxicosis is due to hyperthyroidism (increased hormone production and release from

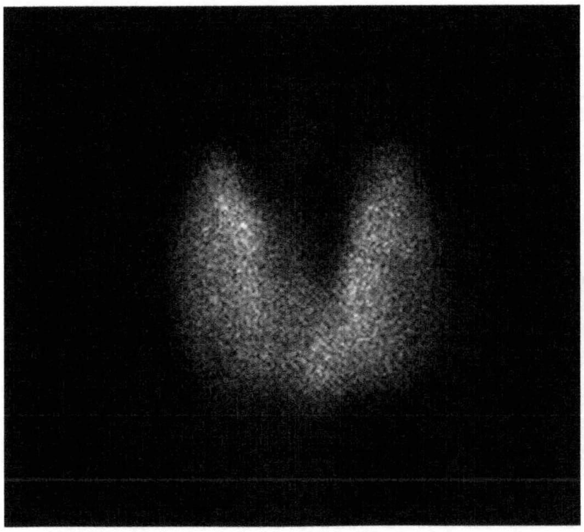

Fig. 5.2 Prominent hyperplasia and diffuse increased uptake in both lobes of the thyroid gland

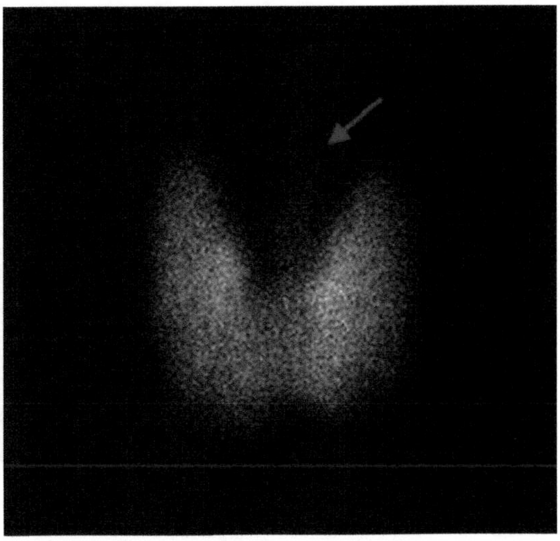

Fig. 5.3 Pyramidal lobe (blue arrow)

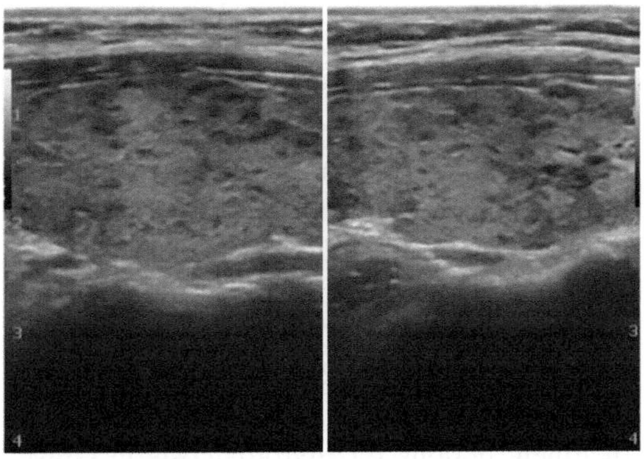

Fig. 5.4 Decreased thyroid echogenicity and heterogeneity in both lobes

the thyroid gland) or an increase in hormone production or release without an increase in thyroid gland activity.

Scintigraphy indicates that the thyroid usually expands. Uptake throughout the gland has increased compared to the background due to both stimulation and increased function of the gland (Fig. 5.2).

From time to time, such stimulation causes the pyramidal lobe (a remnant of the thyroglossal canal) to become visible (Fig. 5.3). Due to its relatively small size, the pyramidal lobe does not become visible unless the gland is overstimulated. The importance of thyroid scintigraphy in the demonstration of nodules that may develop on the background of Graves is that while diffuse increased uptake is observed around the nodule, scintigraphy will reveal the need for biopsy if the nodule is hypoactive [18, 19].

5.6 Thyroid Ultrasonography

Ultrasonography is the most commonly used method in radiological imaging of thyroid diseases. It plays an important role in the demonstration of goiter, especially nodular, in predicting the malignant-benign nature of the structure of the nodules according to the blood supply, size, and some other characteristics. Autoimmune thyroiditis forms a broad clinical spectrum with Graves at one end and Hashimoto at the other end, and there may be transitions within the spectrum.

Ultrasonographic findings are very similar in this general case of thyroiditis. There is a decrease in thyroid echogenicity and heterogeneity due to histopathologically observed lymphocytic infiltration and impaired tissue structure (Fig. 5.4). This is a common finding for both thyroiditis.

In Graves, the overall increase in blood supply can be easily demonstrated by doppler (Fig. 5.5a, b). This provides the differential diagnosis because in Hashimoto thyroiditis, either no blood supply is observed or a spectrum extending to normal blood supply is observed [20].

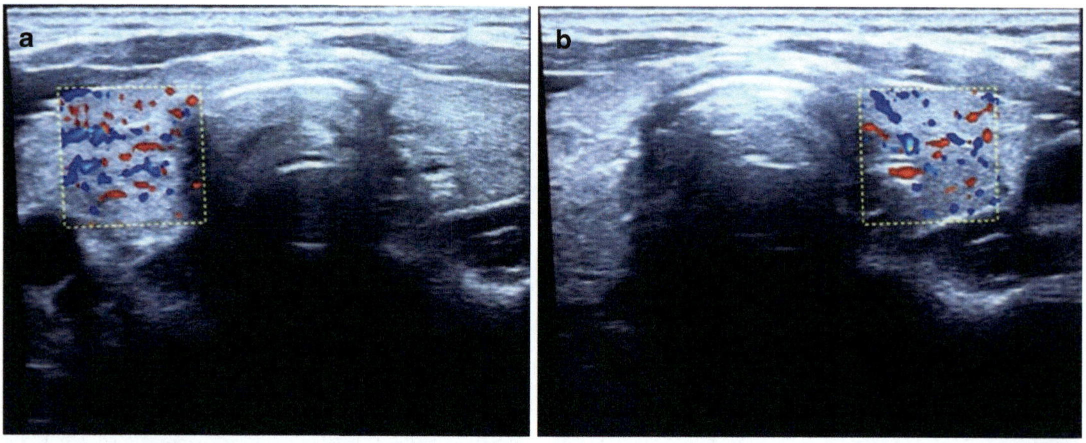

Fig. 5.5 (**a** and **b**) General increase in blood supply in both lobes of the thyroid gland (**a**: right lobe, **b**: left lobe)

5.7 Treatment Options

Lifetime follow-up is recommended as Graves' disease is a disease in which thyrotoxic symptoms increase and improve and autoimmune activity constantly changes. While spontaneous remission may occur in 10–20% of patients, hypothyroidism may develop in approximately half of the untreated patients after 20–30 years, possibly due to continuous autoimmune destruction. Of course, untreated follow-up and spontaneous remission are not recommended today. Treatment options for thyrotoxicosis in Graves' disease are antithyroid drug therapy, radioactive iodine therapy, surgical treatment, and alternative supportive treatments. Treatments targeting the autoimmune mechanism, which plays a major role in physiopathology, are not yet developed.

5.7.1 Antithyroid Medication Therapy

They target the production and release of thyroid hormones. It is the first treatment option in Graves' disease if there is no contraindication. Propylthiouracil (PTU), thionamide derivatives, methimazole (MMI), and carbimazole (then metabolized to MMI) reduce thyroid hormone synthesis during the stages of organification and iodothyrosine coupling as peroxidase inhibitors. It has mild immunosuppressive effects. They also indirectly reduce the level of thyroid-stimulating antibodies due to this partial immunosuppressive effect and possibly a decrease in the amount of thyroid hormone released after some time after starting treatment. PTU also reduces T4 ➔ T3 conversion in the periphery and provides an additional 10–20% reduction in T3 levels. MMI has no such peripheral effect, but is 10 times more potent than PTU and has a longer duration of action (MMI is sufficient at a single dose per day, while PTU has a half-life of 6–8 h). While thyrotoxic symptoms regress in 2–3 weeks, euthyroidism can be achieved after 4–6 weeks.

In patients with moderate thyrotoxic symptoms, the dose can be increased to 30–40 mg per day if MMI starts at 20–30 mg/day and does not improve in TFT follow-up after 4 weeks. When thyroid hormone levels return to normal, the dose is gradually reduced. However, if hormone levels and symptoms increase again when the dose is reduced, the previous dose can be started again. This can be maintained for 12–24 months unless side effects are seen.

PTU should be preferred over MMI as it reduces T3 levels more effectively in patients presenting with severe thyrotoxicosis findings. It is administered as 4 × 200–300 mg/day. With the improvement of clinical and laboratory findings, treatment can be continued for 12–24 months with low-dose MMI.

While most patients remain euthyroid after treatment discontinuation, the most common stage of relapse is the first 3–6 months after treatment discontinuation. In this case, a new course can be started, but there is little chance of permanent remission. The likelihood of recurrence after treatment in Graves' disease has been reported as 40–50% [21–23].

The most common undesirable effects of thionamide group drugs occur at 3–6 months after the start of treatment. Among these, allergic skin reactions are the most common (2–3%). A major toxic reaction is sudden agranulocytosis in 0.2–0.5% of patients. Although routine leukocyte follow-up is not required, a complete blood count should be performed before treatment. Patients should be warned to consult their physician in the presence of infection and fever [24]. Less rare side effects include hepatitis, which may extend to liver failure, cholestatic jaundice, hypoprothrombinemia, aplastic anemia, Lupus-like syndrome, vasculitis, hypoglycemia (due to insulin antibodies), urticaria, arthralgia, arthritis, diarrhea, and dysgeusia [25]. In case of serious side effects, the drugs should be discontinued immediately and supportive treatment should be initiated.

In this case, other options for the treatment of hyperthyroidism, especially radioactive iodine therapy, should be tried.

5.7.2 Surgical Treatment

Subtotal thyroidectomy is preferred in cases with gland size too large to be controlled by RAI, in patients with obstructive symptoms, in the presence of accompanying suspected nodules or nodules proven to be malignant with FNAB. Surgery may be performed in the second trimester in pregnant patients with severe thyrotoxicosis and symptoms that cannot be controlled by medication. In addition, thyroidectomy may also be attempted in young patients who do not respond to antithyroid therapy or whose treatment has been discontinued due to side effects, and in patients who do not accept the radioactive iodine treatment option [26]. However, the patient must be absolutely euthyroid in order to be taken to surgery. This can also be achieved by administering potassium iodide for 10 days before surgery in order to use PTU for up to 6 weeks before surgery and to reduce blood supply to the gland [27]. Postoperative complications include hypothyroidism, hypoparathyroidism, recurrent nerve injury, and hemorrhage. In addition, wound infection and keloid formation may occur.

5.7.3 Radioactive Iodine Therapy

5.7.3.1 Physical Properties of I-131 NaI

I-131 is a radiopharmaceutical obtained by sodium iodide (NaI), Uranium-235 (U-235) fission, or neutron bombardment. High gamma energy (364 keV) is used for diagnostic imaging and high beta energy (610 keV) is used for ablation and treatment. Beta radiation destroys cells within an average distance of 0.5-2mm.

Capsule or liquid forms of I-131 NaI are available for oral administration. It can also be administered intravenously in patients with oral intake problems. The iodine capsule is produced by evaporating no-carrier-added I-131 NaI alcohol solution and absorbing the gelatin into the inner surface of the capsule. The liquid I-131 NaI in isotonic serum physiological is colorless, tasteless, and odorless. The pH value may vary between 7.5 and 9. The physical half-life is 8.1 days and the shelf life is 4 weeks after calibration [28].

5.8 Pharmacokinetics and Pharmacodynamics

After oral administration, I-131 is absorbed from the intestines and reaches the highest level in the blood at 3 hours. Approximately 90% of the administered dose is excreted from the kidneys, while 10% is excreted by sweat and feces [29]. The average penetration of the beta particle is 0.8mm. It causes cell necrosis or DNA damage in surviving cells as a result of exposure to beta radiation from the thyroid follicle. This leads to inflammation and ultimately radiation fibrosis. Therefore, the thyroid cell either dies or its hormone synthesis capacity decreases [30–35].

5.8.1 Indications

It is the preferred treatment modality in elderly patients, in cases where antithyroid drug therapy is unsuccessful when regular drug use is considered impossible, when side effects to antithyroid drugs develop or euthyroidism cannot be achieved despite regular use, in patients with comorbidities that increase the risk of surgery, in patients with a history of periodic thyrotoxic hypokalemic paralysis, right heart failure, and pulmonary hypertension, or in the presence of congestive heart failure, in patients with a history of previous neck surgery or neck radiotherapy. There should be no pregnancy plan within 4–6 weeks [36].

5.9 Contraindications

Radioactive iodine therapy is contraindicated in pregnant or lactating patients, in the presence or suspected presence of concomitant thyroid cancer, in patients who cannot comply with radiation safety recommendations, and in patients with a pregnancy plan within 4–6 weeks [36].

It has been reported that ophthalmopathy may develop or aggravate in smoking, especially in male patients after radioactive iodine therapy [37, 38]. Therefore, radioactive iodine therapy is relatively contraindicated in smokers, thyroid receptor autoantibody (TRAb)-positive patients, and patients with a clinical activity score (CAS) >1 [39, 40].

Gland size also plays an important role in choosing the treatment method to be applied. It has been reported in the literature that higher doses may be required to make the thyroid gland over 60 g euthyroid. Since the success of I-131 treatment is known to be low especially in glands over 80 g, surgery should be considered as a priority in these patients [41, 42].

5.10 Patient Preparation and Cautions

Serum T3, T4, TSH, TPO, and TRAb titers should be known. Thyroid scintigraphy and especially 24-hour RAIU should be >20%. If iodine uptake is low, other treatments should be considered. It is important to distinguish between cases with an early washout at the 4th-hour uptake. Higher doses may be considered if uptake is higher at the 4th hour [43]. Thyroid target volume should be calculated by USG, and if intrathoracic extension is present, it should be confirmed by MRI or CT. CT should be noncontrast. Malignancy should be ruled out with FNAB in the necessary nodules [44–46].

The definitive contraindication is pregnancy and breastfeeding. The fetus has the capacity to capture iodine from weeks 10 to 12. In addition, bladder activity causes fetal irradiation. Therefore, a pregnancy test should be performed before treatment in female patients [47, 48]. In order to prevent the accumulation of radioactive iodine in breast tissue after lactation is discontinued in breastfeeding mothers, treatment should be suspended for at least 6 weeks, or even 3 months if possible to return sodium-iodine symporter activity to normal [49].

In some studies, Graves ophthalmopathy has been reported to worsen with RAI treatment. Radioactive iodine administration is relatively contraindicated, especially in smokers. Various steroid protocols have been tried as a precaution, and in randomized controlled clinical trials, steroid-assisted radioactive iodine treatment has been reported to be very useful in preventing the aggravation of ophthalmopathy when steroid-assisted cases are compared with patients without steroids.

However, there is no definitive dose concept in this regard. 40 mg prednisone/day steroid, started on the same day as RAI treatment, can be gradually reduced and discontinued within 2–3 months. In such a case, it would be useful to get the opinion of the ophthalmologist on a case-by-case basis [43].

The patient's history of antithyroid drug use, amiodarone, contrast, exposure to other foods with high iodine content should be questioned. Since thyroid hormone production and release will be reduced in patients using antithyroid drugs, on the one hand, the appropriate ground for radioactive iodine treatment is prepared, and on the other hand, the efficacy of radioactive iodine therapy decreases due to the reduction of iodine retention and effective half-life of drugs. Therefore, carbimazole and methimazole should be discontinued at least 2 days before treatment and PTU at least 2–3 weeks (8 weeks if possible) before treatment [22, 50–52]. In the period when antithyroid drugs are discontinued, ß-blocker group drugs can be tried for symptomatic control. Although it is not necessary to restart the use of antithyroid medication after radioactive iodine treatment, there is no harm in its use. Amiodarone or other iodine-containing drugs, foods, and contrast agents should be discontinued 6 months before treatment in patients using these. Lithium reduces iodine release from the thyroid gland but does not affect iodine uptake. It does not need to be discontinued in patients using routinely before treatment [43].

5.11 Radioactive Iodine Administration and Dosimetry

Radioactive iodine is usually used orally, but it can also be administered intravenously in patients with difficulty in swallowing or serious complaints such as vomiting [43]. While the superiority of liquid iodine over the capsule is that it is cheaper and can be easily stored and used as much as needed, contamination is more likely. In addition, the magnesium stearate present in the capsules may slow the release of iodine. Therefore, absorption of the solution form is better.

The aim of radioactive iodine treatment in Graves patients is hypothyroidism. However, the ways tried for this purpose are still a matter of debate. Although there is no definitive consensus on the administration of the dose to be recommended on a per-person basis based on various calculations with fixed-dose administration, it has been reported that their overall success is similar [53]. In cases where hypothyroidism cannot be fully achieved after RAI treatment, mortality due to cardiovascular and cerebrovascular diseases has been reported to be higher compared to patients with hypothyroidism and those receiving T4 [54, 55].

The dose to be administered can be formulated by taking into account the dose absorbed by the thyroid per gram of tissue. The optimal dose that will maintain euthyroidism in Graves' disease should be around 150Gy, while it should be higher (200–300 Gy) for total ablation [56]. The recommended formula for dose calculation is as follows [43]:

$$A[MBq] = \frac{F}{\ln 2} \cdot \frac{M[g] \cdot D[Gy]}{\int_0^\infty RIU(t)\,dt}$$

- *A: Dose to be administered.*
- *F: conversion factor (Coulombs/kg ➔ Gy), i.e., converting the amount of ionization* in the air to the dose absorbed in the tissue
- *M: mass of target volume.*
- *D: targeted dose.*
- *RIU: radioactive iodine uptake.*

More commonly used formula for dose calculation in Graves' disease (Marinelli formula) was obtained by placing the desired dose per gram of tissue in μ Ci [57].

$$\text{Dose}(\mu\,\text{Ci}) = \frac{\text{desired}\,\mu\,\text{Ci} / \text{g tissue} \times \text{gland weight}(\text{g}) \times 100\,\text{Dose}}{24 - \text{hour uptake}}$$

The dose to be administered per gram thyroid tissue is 0.08–0.12 mCi/g tissue for most clinicians. This corresponds to a total dose of approximately 5–15 mCi. Studies have shown that a dose of >150 μCi/g is required to achieve hypothyroidism [58–60]. Higher doses (>200 μCi/g) are not recommended in routine as there is no data indicating that they can provide hypothyroidism in more patients, and these doses can be used in relapsed cases and in patients with very large thyroid glands.

Fixed-dose approaches are generally based on measuring the size by ultrasonography or scintigraphy or palpation. Although the doses reported to be administered with this method in the literature vary between 200 and 800 MBq, they are mostly between 400 and 600 MBq [43].

Although dose reduction is recommended in patients undergoing high-dose radioactive iodine therapy such as thyroid cancer in case of renal failure, this is not true for low doses applied for the treatment of hyperthyroidism. In addition, since a very large fraction of the dose administered in the case of hyperthyroidism will be retained in the thyroid gland, the amount to be excreted from the kidneys decreases [61, 62].

The average blood and whole-body dose with 10 mCi I-131 is 8–16 rad, while the dose taken by the ovaries is around 2 rad [63].

5.12 Side Effects of Iodine Therapy

5.12.1 Acute Side Effects

Swelling, pain, difficulty breathing may be observed especially in patients with large thyroid glands within the first week. Hyperthyroidism symptoms may exacerbate due to free hormone release on days 7–10 (thyroid storm) [63–65]. Caution should be exercised especially in patients with a history of cardiac disease, and beta-blockers should be added to treatment if necessary [66, 67].

Hypersensitivity reaction due to radioactive iodine treatment is very rare, so it is very safe to administer. Even in patients known to have iodine hypersensitivity, radioactive iodine preparations can be used safely because their stable iodine concentration is 0.05–0.18 μg, which is less than daily iodine intake [68].

5.12.2 Hypothyroidism

The main side effect of radioactive iodine treatment is hypothyroidism. Its frequency is variable and its incidence increases over time. In the first year, 50% of patients may develop additionally in 2–3% of subsequent years. Lifetime follow-up is therefore recommended. It is very difficult to predict the possibility of hypothyroidism before treatment. The likelihood of developing Graves' disease is higher than nodular and multinodular goiters. Patients with transient hypothyroidism attacks in the early period are more likely to develop permanent hypothyroidism in the long term [69].

5.12.3 Ophthalmopathy

Ophthalmopathy may become more severe with radioactive iodine treatment and thus the treatment may need to be administered with the recommendations of the ophthalmologist and accompanied by steroid treatment. It has been shown that this condition may become more severe, especially in smoking patients and the male sex. Quitting smoking should be recommended in these patients. Steroid therapy is still not required in patients with inactive ophthalmopathy. However, steroid prophylaxis will be required before treatment in smokers and thyroid receptor autoantibody (TRAb)-positive patients and patients with active ophthalmopathy. Since TSH levels will increase in case of hypothyroidism that may develop after treatment, the condition may aggravate again. Therefore, patients should be under T4 replacement therapy [70].

5.13 Radiation-Related Cancers

Although extensive epidemiological studies in various countries have shown that the risk of developing thyroid cancer and the relative risk for thyroid cancer-related deaths is slightly increased in patients receiving radioactive iodine treatment, it is thought that the absolute risk is still low and is due to underlying diseases rather than radioactive iodine treatment [71–75]. In a meta-analysis, no statistically significant increase in cancer risk was reported after radioactive iodine therapy due to hyperthyroidism [76].

5.14 Infertility

The testosterone/luteinizing hormone (LH) ratio has been shown to temporarily decrease in some male patients [77]. Conception should be prevented for 3–4 months for male patients to have sperm production return to normal, and for women until euthyroidism is achieved (approximately 4–6 months). However, for both sexes, fertility function is considered the same as the general population after euthyroidism is achieved, and it is known that the likelihood of developing congenital anomalies in children of patients receiving RAI treatment due to hyperthyroidism is not increased [78].

5.15 Post-RAI Treatment Follow-Up

5.15.1 Radiation Safety

5.15.1.1 Recommendations

Although the doses used in the treatment of hyperthyroidism are not as high as the tumor dose, radiation safety is still important in these patients because the thyroid is intact and shows high iodine uptake.

Inpatient or outpatient treatment is still dependent on national legislation. In most countries, treatment is outpatient [79, 80]. However, in cases where contamination is likely, such as urinary incontinence, hospitalization may be recommended to be followed up with a urinary catheter if possible and to perform the necessary intervention in patients with concomitant severe diseases and serious complications. There is no clear information about the length of hospital stay.

After discharge, the duration of not approaching young children and pregnant women and whether they can continue their profession are regulated by national legislation. However, care is widely taken in Europe to ensure that the dose the patient can give to society before discharge is below 1 mSv, which is equivalent to the 1-year cumulative dose for one person. In general, patients are advised to stay as far away from those around them as possible and to reduce the duration of exposure as much as possible [43].

According to the recommendations of the International Atomic Energy Agency (IAEA), it is recommended that patients should be hospitalized or discharged strictly on a case-by-case basis and can be discharged when the dose given around the patient is <1 mSv depending on whether the patient is surrounded in the immediate vicinity by pregnant women or children. Those who will consciously provide care for the patient can exceed this limit. In this case, the limit is 5 mSv [81].

According to the Turkish Atomic Energy Agency (TAEK) criteria, the patient can be discharged when the dose rate measured 1 m away from the patient falls to <30 μSv/h. The corresponding radioactive substance dose is 600 MBq and the 185–555 MBq (5–15 mCi) radioactive iodine doses commonly administered in Graves patients do not exceed this limit. Therefore, treatment can be performed outpatient in Graves patients. In patients who are given higher doses such as 800 MBq in compulsory cases, the activity on them can be retained under observation until the dose rate measured from 600 MBq, that is 1 m <30 μSv/h, and can be discharged when this condition is met [82].

Abundant fluid consumption should be recommended, especially in the first 24 h after treatment.

5.16 Post-RAI Treatment Follow-Up Results

Thyrotoxic symptoms are expected to regress within 4–5 weeks. 40–80% of patients become euthyroid after 8–16 weeks [83]. Treatment success (providing euthyroidism or hypothyroidism) is associated with the given dose. For example, the success rate is 50% with a single dose in patients given 50μCi per gram of tissue, while this rate is 80% with 190μCi [40, 84, 85]. After RAI administration, any antithyroid medication may be started from Day 5 in order to reach euthyroidism more quickly. ß-blocker agents can also be used to reduce symptoms that may be caused by free hormones released from the gland by destruction. Since radiation thyroiditis can be painful, analgesics with peripheral anti-inflammatory properties can be used. Steroids are rarely needed.

It has been reported that the response to RAI treatment can only be understood by a reduction in the size of the gland with USG after 6 months; and if a minimal response is observed before that, it will not be appropriate to repeat iodine treatment immediately, and RAI can be repeated only if it is considered that the disease does not respond to treatment after 6 months. However, surgery is recommended instead of repeated doses in RAI-resistant disease [40].

5.17 Concluding Remarks

Radioactive iodine therapy in Graves patients is a cheap, effective, easy-to-apply, and reliable treatment method with a low side effect profile due to its selective and destructive effects on thyroid tissue. Although most patients require life-long thyroid hormone replacement, it is the preferred treatment method except in cases where treatment efficacy is reduced, such as severe ophthalmopathy or excessive hyperplasia of the thyroid gland, due to the more vital consequences of long-term uncontrolled hyperthyroidism-related complications compared to hypothyroidism in toxic diffuse goiter patients.

References

1. Brent GA. Clinical practice. Graves' disease. N Engl J Med. 2008;358:2594.
2. Davies TF. Graves' disease: pathogenesis. In: Braverman LE, Utiger RD, editors. Werner & Ingbar's the thyroid. 8th ed. Philadelphia: Lippincott Williams & Wilkins; 2000. p. 518.
3. McLachlan SM, Pegg CA, Atherton MC, et al. TSH receptor antibody synthesis by thyroid lymphocytes. Clin Endocrinol. 1986;24:223–30.
4. Eckstein AK, Plicht M, Lax H, et al. Thyrotropin receptor autoantibodies are independent risk factors for Graves' ophthalmopathy and help to predict severity and outcome of the disease. J Clin Endocrinol Metab. 2006;91:3464–70.
5. Nordyke RA, Gilbert FI Jr, Harada AS. Graves' disease. Influence of age on clinical findings. Arch Intern Med. 1988;148:626–31.
6. Trzepacz PT, Klein I, Roberts M, et al. Graves' disease: an analysis of thyroid hormone levels and hyperthyroid signs and symptoms. Am J Med. 1989;87:558–61.
7. Krassas GE, Pontikides N, Kaltsas T, et al. Menstrual disturbances in thyrotoxicosis. Clin Endocrinol (Oxf). 1994;40:641–4.
8. Kidd GS, Glass AR, Vigersky RA. The hypothalamic-pituitary-testicular axis in thyrotoxicosis. J Clin Endocrinol Metab. 1979;48:798–802.
9. Trivalle C, Doucet J, Chassagne P, et al. Differences in the signs and symptoms of hyperthyroidism in older and younger patients. J Am Geriatr Soc. 1996;44:50–3.
10. Woeber KA. Thyrotoxicosis and the heart. N Engl J Med. 1992;327:94–8.
11. Ayres J, Rees J, Clark TJ, et al. Thyrotoxicosis and dyspnoea. Clin Endocrinol. 1982;16:65–71.
12. Boelaert K, Torlinska B, Holder RL, et al. Older subjects with hyperthyroidism present with a paucity of symptoms and signs: a large cross-sectional study. J Clin Endocrinol Metab. 2010;95:2715–26.
13. Tanda ML, Piantanida E, Liparulo L, et al. Prevalence and natural history of Graves' orbitopathy in a large series of patients with newly diagnosed graves' hyperthyroidism seen at a single center. J Clin Endocrinol Metab. 2013;98:1443–9.
14. Vijayakumar A, Ashwath G, Thimmappa D. Thyrotoxic periodic paralysis: clinical challenges. J Thyroid Res. 2014;2014:649502.
15. Charkes ND. Graves' disease with functioning nodules (Marine-Lenhart syndrome). J Nucl Med. 1973;13(12):885–92.
16. Davey RX, Clarke MI, Webster AR. Thyroid function testing based on assay of thyroid- stimulating hormone: assessing an algorithm's reliability. Med J Aust. 1996;164:329–32.
17. Laurberg P, Vestergaard H, Nielsen S, et al. Sources of circulating 3,5,3'-triiodothyronine in hyperthyroidism estimated after blocking of type 1 and type 2

iodothyronine deiodinases. J Clin Endocrinol Metab. 2007;92:2149–56.
18. Intenzo C, dePapp A, Jabbour S, et al. Scintigraphic manifestations of thyrotoxicosis. Radiographics. 2003;23:857–69.
19. Intenzo C, Capuzzi D, Jabbour S, et al. Scinitigraphic features of autoimmune thyroiditis. Radiographics. 2001;21:957–64.
20. Castagnone D, Rivolta R, Rescalli S, et al. Color Doppler sonography in Graves' disease: value in assessing activity of disease and predicting outcome. AJR Am J Roentgenol. 1996;166(1):203–7.
21. Imseis RE, Vanmiddlesworth L, Massie JD, et al. Pretreatment with propylthiouracil but not methimazole reduces the therapeutic efficacy of iodine-131 in hyperthyroidism. J Clin Endocrinol Metab. 1998;83:685–7.
22. Santos RB, Romaldini JH, Ward LS. Propylthiouracil reduces the effectiveness of radioiodine treatment in hyperthyroid patients with Graves' disease. Thyroid. 2004;14:525–30.
23. Nakamura H, Noh JY, Itoh K, et al. Comparison of methimazole and propylthiouracil in patients with hyperthyroidism caused by Graves' disease. J Clin Endocrinol Metab. 2007;92:2157–62.
24. Watanabe N, Narimatsu H, Noh JY, et al. Antithyroid drug-induced hematopoietic damage: a retrospective cohort study of agranulocytosis and pancytopenia involving 50,385 patients with Graves' disease. J Clin Endocrinol Metab. 2012;97:E49–53.
25. Wang MT, Lee WJ, Huang TY, et al. Antithyroid drug-related hepatotoxicity in hyperthyroidism patients: a population-based cohort study. Br J Clin Pharmacol. 2014;78:619–29.
26. Elfenbein DM, Schneider DF, Havlena J, et al. Clinical and socioeconomic factors influence treatment decisions in Graves' disease. Ann Surg Oncol. 2015;22:1196–9.
27. Erbil Y, Ozluk Y, Giriş M, et al. Effect of lugol solution on thyroid gland blood flow and microvessel density in the patients with Graves' disease. J Clin Endocrinol Metab. 2007;92:2182–9.
28. Saha GB. Characteristics of specific radiopharmaceuticals. In: Fundamentals of nuclear pharmacy. 4th ed. New York: Springer Verlag; 1998. p. 112–47.
29. Saha GB. Diagnostic uses of radiopharmaceuticals in nuclear medicine. In: Fundamentals of nuclear pharmacy. 4th ed. New York: Springer Verlag; 1998. p. 238–319.
30. Kowalsky RJ, Perry JR. Radiopharmaceuticals in nuclear medicine practice. Norwalk, Conn: Appleton & Lange; 1987.
31. Swanson DP, Clinton HM, Thrall JH. Radiopharmaceuticals in medical imaging. New York: Macmillan; 1990.
32. Siegel JA. Guide for diagnostic nuclear medicine and radiopharmaceutical therapy. Reston, VA: Society of Nuclear Medicine; 2004.
33. Clinton HM, Witcofski RL. Nuclear pharmacy: an introduction to the clinical application of radiopharmaceuticals. Philadelphia: Lea & Febiger; 1986.
34. Kwee SA, Coel MN, Patrick DF. Iodine - 131 radiotherapy for benign thyroid disease. In: Eary JF, Brenner W, editors. Nuclear medicine therapy. New York: Informa Healthcare; 2007. p. 169–89.
35. Freitas EJ. Therapeutic options in the management of toxic and nontoxic nodular goiter. Semin Nucl Med. 2000;2:88–97.
36. Ross DS, Burch HB, Cooper DS, et al. 2016 American Thyroid Association Guidelines for Diagnosis and Management of Hyperthyroidism and other causes of Thyrotoxicosis. Thyroid. 2016;26(10):1343–421.
37. Bartalena L, Marcocci C, Bogazzi F, et al. Relation between therapy for hyperthyroidism and the course of Graves' ophthalmopathy. N Engl J Med. 1998;338:73–8.
38. Träisk F, Tallstedt L, Abraham-Nordling M, et al. Thyroid-associated ophthalmopathy after treatment for Graves' hyperthyroidism with antithyroid drugs or iodine-131. J Clin Endocrinol Metab. 2009;94:3700–7.
39. Kahaly GJ, Bartalena L, Hegedüs L. The American Thyroid Association/American Association of Clinical Endocrinologist Guidelines for hyperthyroidism and other causes of thyrotoxicosis: a European perspective. Thyroid. 2011;21(6):585–91.
40. Alexander EK, Larsen PR. High dose of (131) I therapy for the treatment of hyperthyroidism caused by Graves' disease. J Clin Endocrinol Metab. 2002;87:1073–7.
41. Royal College of Physicians of London. Radioiodine in thema- nagement of benignthyroid disease: clinical guidelines. London: RCP; 2007. http://www.rcplondon.ac.uk/pubs/contents/0621b67a-4880-4a1b-9942-57a666efee4a.pdf
42. Rivkees SA, Cornelius EA. Influence of iodine-131 dose on the outcome of hyperthyroidism in children. Pediatrics. 2003;111:745–9.
43. Stokkel MPM, Junak DH, Lassmann M, et al. EANM procedure guidelines for therapy of benign thyroid disease. Eur J Nucl Med Mol Imaging. 2010;37:2218–28.
44. Brunn J, Block U, Ruf G, et al. Volumetric analysis of thyroid lobes by real-time ultrasound. Dtsch Med Wschr. 1981;106:1338–40.
45. Moschetta M, Ianora AA, Testini M, et al. Multidetector computed tomography in the preoperative evaluation of retrosternal goiters: a useful procedure for patients for whom magnetic resonance imaging is contraindicated. Thyroid. 2010;20:181–7.
46. Cooper DS, Doherty GM, Haugen BR, et al. Revised American Thyroid Association management guidelines for patients with thyroid nodules and differentiated thyroid cancer. Thyroid. 2009;19:1167–214.
47. Fisher WD, Voorhess ML, Gardner LI. Congenital hypothyroidism in infant following maternal I-131 therapy with a review of hazards of environmental radioisotope contamination. J Pediatr. 1963;62:132–46.
48. Berg GE, Nystrom EH, Jacobsson L, et al. Radioiodine treatment of hyperthyroidism in a pregnant women. J Nucl Med. 1998;39:357–61.

49. Azizi F, Smyth P. Breastfeeding and maternal and infant iodine nutrition. Clin Endocrinol. 2009;70:803–9.
50. Bonnema SJ, Bennedbaek FN, Veje A, et al. Propylthiouracil before I-131 therapy of hyperthyroid diseases; effect on cure rate evaluated by a randomized clinical trial. J Clin Endocrinol Metab. 2004;89:4439–44.
51. Braga M, Walpert N, Burch HB, et al. The effect of methimazole on cure rates after radioiodine treatment for Graves' hyperthyroidism: a randomized clinical trial. Thyroid. 2002;12:135–9.
52. Kobe C, Weber I, Eschner W, et al. Graves' disease and radioiodine therapy: is success of ablation dependent on the choice of thyreostatic medication? Nuklearmedizin. 2008;47:153–66.
53. de Rooij A, Vandenbroucke JP, Smit JW, et al. Clinical outcomes after estimated versus calculated activity of radioiodine for the treatment of hyperthyroidism: systematic review and meta-analysis. Eur J Endocrinol. 2009;161:771–7.
54. Boelaert K, Maisonneuve P, Torlinska B, et al. Comparison of mortality in hyperthyroidism during periods of treatment with thionamides and after radio- iodine. J Clin Endocrinol Metab. 2013;98:1869–82.
55. Franklyn JA, Maisonneuve P, Sheppard MC, et al. Mortality after the treatment of hyperthyroidism with radioactive iodine. N Engl J Med. 1998;338:712–8.
56. Reiners C, Schneider P. Radioiodine therapy of thyroid autonomy. Eur J Nucl Med. 2002;29:471–8.
57. Marinelli LD, Quimby EH, Hine GJ. Dosage determination with radioactive isotopes; practical considerations in therapy and protection. Am J Roentgenol Radium Ther. 1948;59:260–81.
58. Peters H, Fischer C, Bogner U, et al. Treatment of Graves' hyperthyroidism with radio- iodine: results of a prospective randomized study. Thyroid. 1997;7:247–51.
59. Peters H, Fischer C, Bogner U, et al. Radioiodine therapy of Graves' hyperthyroidism: standard vs. calculated 131iodine activity. Results from a prospective, randomized, multicentre study. Eur J Clin Investig. 1995;25:186–93.
60. Peters H, Fischer C, Bogner U, et al. Reduction in thyroid volume after radioiodine therapy of Graves' hyperthyroidism: results of a prospective, randomized, multicentre study. Eur J Clin Investig. 1996;26:59–63.
61. Holst JP, Burman KD, Atkins F, et al. Radioiodine therapy for thyroid cancer and hyperthyroidism in patients with end-stage renal disease on hemodialysis. Thyroid. 2005;15:1321–31.
62. Nibhanupudy JR, Hamilton W, Sridhar R, et al. Iodine-131 treatment of hyperthyroidism in a patient on dialysis for chronic renal failure. Am J Nephrol. 1993;13:214–7.
63. Robertson JS, Gorman CA. Gonadal radiation dose and its genetic significance in radioiodine therapy of hyperthyroidism. J Nucl Med. 1976;17(9):826–35.
64. McDermott MT, Kidd GS, Dodson LE Jr, et al. Radioiodine-induced thyroid storm. Case report and literature review. Am J Med. 1983;75:353–9.
65. Walter MA, Briel M, Christ-Crain M, et al. Effects of antithyroid drugs on radioiodine treatment: systematic review and meta-analysis of randomised controlled trials. BMJ. 2007;334:514.
66. Klein I, Danzi S. Thyroid disease and the heart. Circulation. 2007;116:1725–35.
67. Klein I. Endocrine disorders and cardiovascular disease. In: Libby P, et al., editors. Braunwald's heart dis- ease: a textbook of cardiovascular medicine. 8th ed. Philadelphia, PA: Saunders/Elsevier; 2008. p. 2033–47.
68. Royal College of Physicians of London. Radioiodine in management of benign thyroid disease: clinical guidelines. Report of a working party. Sudbury, Suffolk, Great Britain: The Lavenham Press Ltd; 2007.
69. Tuttle RM, Becker DV, Hurley JR. Radioiodine treatment of thyroid disease. In: Sandler MP, Coleman RE, Patton JA, Wackers FJ, Gottsscalk A, editors. Diagnostic nuclear medicine. 4th ed. Philadelphia, PA: Lippincott Williams & Wilkins; 2003. p. 653–70.
70. Laurberg P, Wallin G, Tallstedt L, et al. TSH-receptor autoimmunity in Graves' disease after therapy with anti-thyroid drugs, surgery, or radioiodine: a 5-year prospective randomized study. Eur J Endocrinol. 2008;158:69–75.
71. Franklyn JA, Maisonneuve P, Sheppard M, et al. Cancer incidence and mortality after radioiodine treatment for hyperthyroidism: a population based cohort study. Lancet. 1999;353:2111–5.
72. Dobyns BM, Sheline GE, Workman JB, et al. Malignant and benign neoplasms of the thyroid in patients treated for hyperthyroidism: a report of the cooperative thyrotoxicosis therapy follow-up study. J Clin Endocrinol Metab. 1974;38:976–98.
73. Boice JD Jr. Radiation induced thyroid cancer – what's new? J Natl Cancer Inst. 2005;97:703–5.
74. Lucignani G. Long-term risks in hyperthyroid patients treated with radioiodine: is there anything new? Eur J Nucl Med Mol Imaging. 2007;34:1504–9.
75. Dickman PW, Holm LE, Lundell G Jr, et al. Thyroid cancer risk after thyroid examination with I-131: a population-based cohort study in Sweden. Int J Cancer. 2003;106:580–7.
76. Hieu TT, Russell AW, Cuneo R, et al. Cancer risk after medical exposure to ra- dioactive iodine in benign thyroid diseases: a meta- analysis. Endocr Relat Cancer. 2012;19:645–55.
77. Ceccarelli C, Canale D, Battisti P, et al. Testicular function after 131I therapy for hyperthyroidism. Clin Endocrinol. 2006;65:446–52.
78. Read CH Jr, Tansey MJ, Menda Y. A 36-year retrospective analysis of the efficacy and safety of radioactive iodine in treating young Graves' patients. J Clin Endocrinol Metab. 2004;89:4229–33.
79. American Thyroid Association Taskforce on Radioiodine Safety, Sisson JC, Freitas J, et al.

Radiation safety in the treatment of patients with thyroid diseases by radioiodine 131I : practice recommendations of the American Thyroid Association. Thyroid. 2011;21:335.
80. United States Nuclear Regulatory Commission (NRC). Consolidated Guidance About Materials Licenses: Program-Specific Guidance About Medical Use Licenses, 2008. http://www.nrc.gov/reading-rm/doc-collections/nuregs/staff/sr1556/v9/r2/sr1556v9r2-final.pdf#08-36.
81. Release of Patients After Radionuclide Therapy Safety Reports Series No. 63 Vienna, 2009 STI/PUB/1417; (ISBN:978-92-0-108909-0); 77 pp.
82. Radyasyon Güvenliği Yönetmeliği, Ek- 5 I-131 ile Tedavi Gören Hastaların Taburcu Edilme Koşulları, 2010.
83. Stan MN, Durski JM, Brito JP, et al. Cohort study on radioactive iodine-induced hypothyroidism: implications for Graves' ophthalmopathy and optimal timing for thyroid hormone assessment. Thyroid. 2013;23:620–5.
84. Goolden AW, Stewart JS. Long-term results from graded low dose radioactive iodine therapy for thyrotoxicosis. Clin Endocrinol. 1986;24:217–22.
85. Sridama V, McCormick M, Kaplan EL, et al. Long-term follow-up study of compensated low-dose 131I therapy for Graves' disease. N Engl J Med. 1984;311:426–32.

6 Radionuclide Therapy in Malignant Thyroid Diseases: Differentiated Thyroid Cancer

Gülin Uçmak

6.1 Epidemiology

According to "Turkey Cancer Statistics" published by the Public Health Directorate of the Ministry of Health in Turkey, thyroid cancers rank second in all age groups in women in Turkey after breast cancer, first in girls and women between the ages of 15 and 24 and fifth in boys [1]. The project, which was created to provide up-to-date estimates about the incidence, mortality, and prevalence of major cancer types at the national level in many countries of the world, ranks 4th in all age groups in women in the USA according to Globocan 2012 data [2]. According to the SEER (Surveillance, Epidemiology and End Results) data, the number of thyroid cancer cases per 100,000 people in 1992 was 5.8, while it was reported as 14.6 in 2015. With 53,990 new cases in 2018, it is estimated that it will constitute 3.1% of all cancers [3]. The reason for the increase in the incidence of thyroid cancer is an increase in actual disease formation due to ionized radiation, environmental factors, eating habits and obesity, as well as an improvement in diagnostic standards and medical experience [4–6]. Lim et al. reported in their study on the incidence of thyroid cancer and mortality rate in the USA between 1974 and 2013; it was found that with the real increase in papillary thyroid carcinoma (PTC), an increase in the mortality rate was observed in advanced PTC cases, despite all standard, adjuvant treatments and systemic treatments. The authors stated that clinical trials were needed to optimize new systemic therapies in advanced DTC, including iodine-resistant PTC [6].

Differentiated thyroid cancers (DTC) originate from thyroid follicular cells. The majority of DTC (>90%) is papillary and follicular type and approximately 80–85% are papillary thyroid cancers [7]. In DTC, long-term disease progression is generally good. Ten-year survival in the middle-aged group in DTC is 80–90%. However, 5–20% local-regional recurrence and 10–15% distant metastasis may occur. The disease-specific mortality rate in DTC is approximately 9% and >50% in the presence of distant metastasis [8–11].

The prognosis in DTC is related to the individual characteristics that should be determined for each patient such as age at diagnosis, histological type, degree of differentiation-tumor heterogeneity, molecular profile (such as $BRAF^{V600E}$, RAS, TERT), extrathyroidal spread, diffuse vascular invasion, presence of distant metastasis, radioactive iodine (RAI) treatment and uptake, adequacy and feasibility of surgery, application of adjuvant treatments at the right time and adequacy, correct selection of follow-up plan, and diagnostic tests. There have always been debates and disputes regarding the management of DTC in the world. The reason is that there are few

G. Uçmak (✉)
Department of Nuclear Medicine, University of Health Sciences, Dr. A.Y. Ankara Oncology Training and Research Hospital, Ankara, Turkey
e-mail: gulin.ucmak@sbu.edu.tr

R. Bekiş et al. (eds.), *Radionuclide Therapy*, https://doi.org/10.1007/978-3-030-97220-2_6

prospective randomized studies on this subject, the difference in data due to the diagnosis and treatment approaches that have changed over time since the past and the biological-molecular characteristics and individual behavior of DTC.

Guidelines review health outcomes and evidence-based medical data and provide recommendations. In the purpose section of the guidelines, it is stated that "they should be seen as complementary information for physicians rather than as a clinical provision."

In this chapter, the topic of DTC and Radionuclide therapy will be shared through current guidelines, literature, and my experience.

6.2 Histopathological Classification in Thyroid Cancers

Histopathology in DTCs is the most basic basis for clinical staging and determination of prognostic risk factors [11]. The World Health Organization (WHO) pathology classification for thyroid cancers is presented below as updated (Table 6.1) [12].

6.2.1 Papillary Thyroid Cancer

PTC, which contains approximately 80–85% of DTC, develops from thyroid follicle cells with microscopic nuclear properties and is the most common variant. It has been reported that approximately 67% can be seen in thyroid, 20–25% in thyroid and cervical lymph nodes, and 13% only in lymph nodes in some series at the time of diagnosis [13]. The frequency of micrometastasis, which is of less clinical importance than macrometastases, can reach 80–90% with molecular pathology methods [14–16]. Exposure to ionized radiation in childhood (medical, Chernobyl), Hashimoto thyroiditis, and familial adenomatous polyposis are risk factors for PTC. Although the classic PTC prognosis is good, tall cell, columnar cell, and hobnail variants exhibit aggressive behavior. Increased local recurrence, distant metastasis, decreased disease-free survival, and disease-related mortality rates are high in these variants. $BRAF^{V600E}$ mutation is common in these tumors [17–19].

Diffuse sclerosing variant constitutes 1–2% of PTC and is mostly seen in young women or children [12]. Lymph node and lung metastasis are

Table 6.1 WHO classification in thyroid cancers

Papillary cancer	Follicular cancer	Poorly differentiated	Others thyroid cancer
Classic type (most frequent)	Minimally invasive	Insular carcinoma	Anaplastic carcinoma
Microcarcinoma	Encapsulated angioinvasive		Medullary carcinoma
Encapsulated PTC	Diffuse invasive		Squamous cell carcinoma
Follicular variant			Others
Diffuse sclerosing variant	Rare variants		
Tall cell variant	Clear cell variant		
Columnar cell variant	Signet-ring cell follicular carcinoma		
Cribriform-morular variant			
Solid trabecular variant			
Oncocytic or oxyphilic variant	**Hurthle cell carcinoma (oncocytic)**[b]		
Spindle cell variant			
Clear cell variant			
Warthin-like variant			
Fibromatosis-fasciitis-like stromal PTC			
Hobnail variant[a]			

[a]Newly defined
[b]Separately defined in the new classification

common. Although it has been emphasized historically that it is more aggressive than classic PTC, 10-year survival is >90% similar.

The reasons are adequate surgical and adjuvant treatments (RAI, external beam radiation therapy –RT), and that it is mostly monitored in young and children [20].

Solid trabecular variant is rarely (3%) seen in adults, more frequently in children (post-Chernobyl) with RET/PTC3 rearrangement and has a higher risk of relapse [21]. In the oncocytic-Hurthle cell variant of PTC, the nucleus properties are papillary, but the cytoplasm is oncocytic. It is more common in women and is often associated with autoimmune thyroiditis. In general, the disease behaves like classic PTC. Warthin-like variant is very rare, similar to salivary gland tumors. In general, metastasis is not seen and tumor diameter is < 2 cm and its behavior is like classic PTC [12].

Although PTC microcarcinomas (<1 cm) are generally good prognosis, the treatment/follow-up approach is the most controversial group. Microcarcinomas are pathologies in which nodal involvement can be observed at the rate of 12–31%, capsular invasion and multifocality are frequently observed, and distant metastasis is rarely observed [22, 23]. In one of the recent studies, $BRAF^{V600E}$ mutation, subcapsular localization, peri-intratumoral fibrosis, and multifocality have been reported to be used in risk determination in microcarcinomas [24].

In encapsulated follicular variant PTC, the tumor shows a follicular pattern, while its characteristic nucleus properties are similar to papillary carcinoma. It does not show capsular/vascular invasion, RAS mutation is frequently observed, and the risk of recurrence is low. However, if the tumor does not encapsulate but shows an infiltrative pattern, $BRAF^{V600E}$ mutation is frequently observed in this group and should be treated like classic PTC [25, 26].

6.2.2 Follicular Thyroid Cancer (FTC)

FTC, which develops from thyroid follicle cells that make up approximately 10–12% of DTCs, is defined according to tumor capsular/vascular invasion characteristics, and no diagnostic nuclear properties are observed in PTC. It is distinguished from follicular adenoma by tumor capsule and/or vascular invasion, and mitotic activity is not used for malignant indicator. It develops in areas with epidemiological iodine deficiency and usually in the adult age group (>50) and is rare in children [10, 12].

Classic FTC has minimally invasive and widespread invasive forms. Minimally invasive encapsulated FTC shows only capsule invasion and has a good prognosis. If FTC is encapsulated and vascular invasion is limited (<4), it has a better prognosis than the widely invasive form and is evaluated separately in the WHO classification. In widely invasive FTC, widespread vascular invasion and extrathyroidal spread occur. Lymphatic metastasis is low (<5%) in FTCs, whereas distant metastasis (most commonly lung, bone) reaching 69% can be seen in widely invasive carcinoma. In the long term, mortality was observed as 50%. Molecular-cytogenetically, 49% NRAS-HRAS mutations and 36% PAX8/PPARγ rearrangements are observed. It has been shown that rearrangements in tumor trigger invasive behavior [27, 28]. The clear cell variant of FTC is rare, similar to classic FTC and distinguished by Tg staining from parathyroid adenoma/carcinoma and clear cell tumor metastasis of the kidney.

In the oncocytic variant-Hurthle cell carcinoma, follicular neoplasia was coated with oncocytic tumor cells at a rate of >75%. Capsule and/or vessel invasion is present in Hurthle cell carcinoma. Lymph metastasis (30%), extrathyroidal spread, local recurrence, and iodine refractory metastatic disease are more common and more aggressive than classic FTC [29].

6.2.3 Poorly Differentiated Thyroid Cancer (Insular Carcinoma)

In insular carcinoma, the microscopic growth pattern of the tumor is solid/trabecular/insular, its core properties are removed from papillary cancer, and the loss of partial differentiation is characteristic. Clinical outcome and prognosis are poor (10-year survival of approximately 50%). Studies have shown that tumor size, high mitotic rate and Ki-67 index (≥4%), tumor necrosis, and >45 years of age are indicators of poor prognosis. In the absence of these features other than insular/trabecular/solid pattern, the tumor should not be called poorly differentiated as it will not exhibit aggressive behavior [30, 31].

6.3 Diagnosis and Preoperative Staging in Thyroid Cancers

Thyroid nodules can be detected by palpation or randomly (<1 cm) by ultrasonography (USG) or other imaging methods. USG is the most sensitive method for thyroid nodules (especially PTC). It is important to evaluate the complete clinical history and thyroid gland and cervical lymph nodes with physical examination in the patient with thyroid nodules. In addition to the characteristics of the nodule in USG, the history of treatment with ionized radiation involving the neck region in childhood, familial thyroid cancer, or medullary thyroid cancer should also be considered in terms of malignancy. Thyroid function tests and thyroid scintigraphy (routinely with Tc-99m) are used in differential diagnosis. If the serum TSH level is below normal and the nodule is hyperfunctional-active in thyroid scintigraphy, the risk of malignancy is very low. However, high serum TSH levels may indicate an increased risk of malignancy in the presence of hypofunctional nodules on scintigraphy [32, 33].

Serum thyroglobulin (Tg), serum calcitonin measurements, and positron emission tomography (PET/CT) are not routinely recommended in the evaluation of thyroid nodules. However, in some patients, for example, in cases suspected of PTC as a result of cytology and considered for subtotal thyroidectomy, serum calcitonin levels may change the surgical approach. Fine-needle aspiration biopsy (FNAB) is recommended if focally increased F-18 fluorodeoxyglucose (FDG) uptake is observed accidentally on PET/CT examination and a nodule of >1 cm is confirmed in this area on USG. One recent meta-analysis found cancer in about 35% of FDG-positive thyroid nodules [34].

Characteristics associated with thyroid cancer in ultrasonography, especially those defined for PTC, include the presence of microcalcification, hypoechogenicity, irregular-infiltrative or lobulated borders, transverse images with a larger height than transverse, and extrathyroidal extension. Unlike these, FTC may have more hyperechogenic or isoechoic, rounded, smoothly bounded, and intranodular vascularity of the nodule. The follicular variant of thyroid papillary cancer may also show similar sonographic features. FNAB is recommended sonographically for nodules > 1cm and nodules > 1.5 cm with moderate- to high-risk features defined above in terms of malignancy. Bilateral cervical lymph nodes should be carefully examined in the presence of nodules and FNAB, and/or Tg washout test should be performed in the presence of suspicion (>8 mm) [35].

According to current guidelines, it was accepted that the risk of cytopathological category and malignancy should be performed according to the "Bethesda diagnosis classification" at the diagnosis stage [36, 37]. According to the guidelines, it is recommended to consider repeating biopsy for cytopathology with non-diagnostic/insufficient material, follow-up, or surgical excision taking into account the USG characteristics of the nodule and clinical risk factors if reported. In benign cytology, if the feature of the nodule on USG is in the risk group for malignancy, 6–12 months of USG follow-up and FNAB can be performed in the presence of suspicious findings. Surgery is inevitable in malignant cytopathology. The behavior pattern is slightly more complicated in cytopathology results with uncertain significance of atypia/follicular lesion (AUS/FLUS) (Tr3) and suspected malignancy. In this case, FNAB repetition or molecular tests (BRAF, RET/PTC, PAX8/PPARγ) can be performed by interviewing the patient, or surgical excision for follow-up or diagnostic purposes can be preferred considering the sonographic pattern, clinical risk factors, and patient preference. The type of surgery (lobectomy, total thyroidectomy) should also be determined according to the clinical-sonographic risk factors of the patient with a personalized approach [35, 38].

When thyroid nodules are detected in pregnant women, if the nodule is risky according to the sonographic risk assessment and if the patient is euthyroid or hypothyroid, FNAB should be performed. If TSH is suppressed, FNAB can be postponed after birth and breastfeeding [38].

The importance of evaluating cervical lymph nodes in the preoperative period (central and lateral compartment, Fig. 6.1) is indisputable in terms of correct staging, contributing to patient management with the appropriate surgical procedure and prognosis [39, 40]. Since the differentiation of benign and malignant lymph nodes cannot always be made clearly on neck USG, cytopathological diagnosis should be made by FNAB on suspicious lymph nodes before primary surgery if it will change the surgical procedure. As lymph node metastasis in DTC produces Tg, Tg washout test is a highly reliable method, and intracellular Tg does not interact with circulating anti-Tg antibodies (anti-Tg). However, it has also been reported that intact thyroid tissue (especially for central lymph nodes) may cause false positivity and may result in false negativity due to very high anti-Tg values in circulation [41]. In the literature, different threshold values such as 0.9–39 ng/ml have been given for Tg washout positivity value [35]. In the guideline published by the European Thyroid Community, it was suggested that lymph node Tg washout threshold values should be considered negative if Tg is <1 ng/ml, correlated with cytology if Tg is 1–10 ng/ml, and positive if Tg is >10 ng/ml [35]. Lee et al. reported lymph node metastasis with 100% sensitivity and specificity with positive cytology and positive Tg washout [42]. Studies have emphasized that preoperative neck mapping can predict lymphatic spread and can be a guide for effective surgical planning [40] (Fig. 6.2).

Although there are studies in the literature in terms of the place of preoperative serum Tg levels in patient management and indicator of disease progression, there is no clear data [43]. Therefore, preoperative serum Tg values have no place in thyroid cancer management.

In addition to neck USG evaluation in preoperative staging in patients with primary thyroid malignancy and clinical findings suspicious of advanced disease (such as neck palpated masses, primary tumor invasion), evaluation with IV

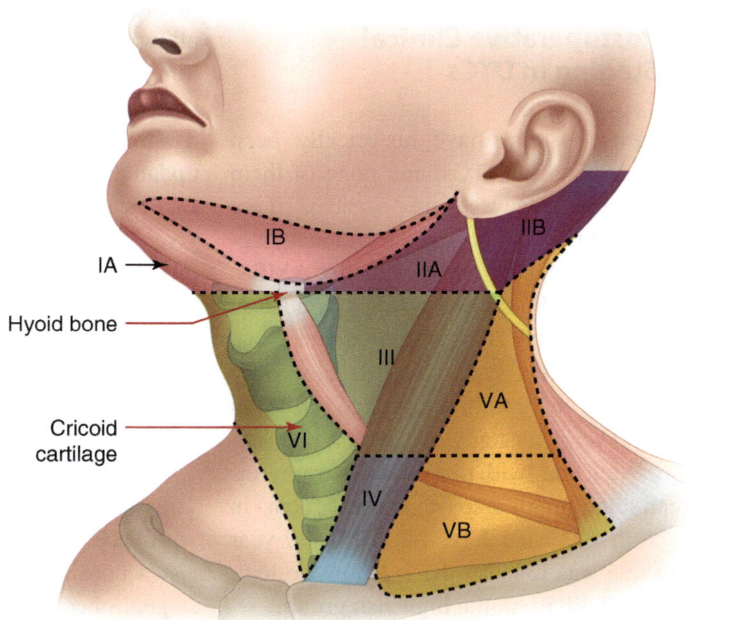

Fig. 6.1 Cervical lymph node levels (Levels I–VII). Level I, submental (IA) and submandibular (IB) lymph nodes. Level II, upper jugular lymph nodes. Level III, middle jugular lymph nodes. Level IV, lower jugular lymph nodes. Level V, posterior triangle. Level VI (central compartment), prelaryngeal, pretracheal, paratracheal lymph nodes, and upper mediastinal lymph nodes (also called Level VII) [39]

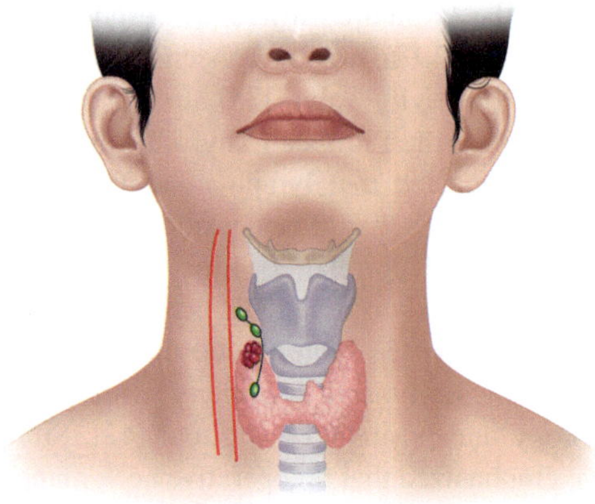

Fig. 6.2 In the preoperative neck mapping of a 39-year-old female patient, malignant (FNAB malignant) nodule in the upper pole of the right thyroid lobe and three right central millimetric lymph nodes were mapped. Postoperative pathology; 1.2 × 0.8 × 0.8 cm classic papillary thyroid Ca, surgical margin and lymphovascular invasion positive, right central 2 metastatic, 1 reactive lymph nodes

contrast CT and MRI especially in terms of tracheal and esophageal invasion and evaluation of mediastinal lymph nodes and distant metastases with PET/CT in poorly differentiated thyroid pathologies may be useful for patient management in preoperative staging.

6.4 Postoperative Clinical Staging in DTCs

Many staging systems have historically been used in the staging of DTCs, and none of them fully predict recurrence risk and prognosis. If we talk about the historical process of clinical staging and prognostic factors, we can list AMES, AGES, and MACIS scoring systems and more accepted, renewed 8th TNM staging system.

The AMES scoring system was developed by the Lahey clinic in 1988 based on age (40 years for males, 50 years for females), distant metastasis, tumor extension (with or without extrathyroidal spread), and tumor size (<5 cm or >5 cm) in patients with PTC and FTC [44]. The 20-year mortality rate was found to be 1.2% in the low-risk group and 39.5% in the high-risk group.

The AGES scoring system was developed by the Mayo Clinic in 1987 with a follow-up of 1938 PTC patients [45]. In the AGES system, the variables of age (40 years limit), grade, tumor extension spread (invasions-distant metastasis), and tumor size were used. The disease-related 20-year mortality rate was found to be 1% in the low-risk (86% patients, score <4) group and 36% in the high-risk (score ≥ 4) group.

In 1993, the MACIS scoring system was defined by the Mayo Clinic, which included 2284 PTC patients [46]. In the MACIS scoring, the variables of metastasis, age (40 years limit), adequate surgery, and tumor size were used. The 20-year disease-specific survival was found to be 99% in the low-risk group (83% of patients, score <6), and the disease-related mortality rate was found to be 32% in the high-risk group (17% of patients, score ≥ 6).

The 10-year recurrence rate was reported as 9% and 19% in the low- and high-risk groups, respectively.

The TNM (tumor, node, metastasis) staging system was first published by the UICC (Union for International Cancer Control) Committee in 1958 with clinical staging recommendations for breast and laryngeal cancers [47]. The TNM staging system, which has been updated over time, includes TNM staging and prognostic factors in all types of cancer, identifies and records the anatomical prevalence of the disease in the diagnosis (stages 0–4), and then remains unchanged in the dynamic process. In the 8th edition [11] of the updated TNM system in 2018, the age limit for DTC staging was changed from 45 years to 55 years of age (Table 6.2). In addition, prognostic factors were identified in DTCs (Table 6.3).

6.5 Treatment of DTC

6.5.1 Surgery

The standard treatment for a patient diagnosed with DTC is surgery. The surgical technique varies according to the preoperative evaluation stage. Lobectomy, near-total thyroidectomy, cen-

Table 6.2 TNM staging [11]

Primary tumor (T)	
TX	No primary tumor assessment
T0	No primary tumor
T1	Tumor <2 cm, intrathyroidal
T1a	Tumor <1 cm, intrathyroidal
T1b	Tumor 1–2 cm, intrathyroidal
T2	Tumor >2 cm - ≤4 cm, intrathyroidal
T3	Tumor >4 cm, gross extrathyroidal spread to intrathyroidal or only strap muscles (sternothyroid, sternothyroid, or omohyoid muscles)
T3a	Tumor >4 cm, intrathyroidal
T3b	Gross extrathyroidal spread of tumor to strap muscles of any size (sternothyroid, sternothyroid, or omohyoid muscles)
T4a	Tumor (any size) has crossed the thyroid capsule and spread to the subcutaneous soft tissues, larynx, trachea, esophagus, or recurrent laryngeal nerve (any)
T4b	Tumor invaded the prevertebral fascia, involving mediastinal vessels or carotid
Regional lymph node (N)	
NX	Regional lymph nodes not assessed
N0	No regional lymph node metastasis
N1	Regional lymph node metastasis
N1a	Level VI (metastasis in pretracheal, paratracheal, and prelaryngeal/Delphian lymph nodes or upper mediastinal lymph nodes)
N1b	Unilateral, bilateral other cervical lymph nodes (Levels I, II III, IV or V) or retropharyngeal metastasis
Distant metastasis (M)	
M0	No distant metastasis
M1	Distant metastasis
Clinical staging	
Papillary and follicular < 55 years	
Stage I	Any T any N and M0
Stage II	Any T any N M1
Papillary and follicular ≥ 55 years	
Stage I	T1a, T1b, T2 N0 M0
Stage II	T3 N0 M0 T1, T2, T3 N1 M0
Stage III	T4a any N M0
Stage IVA	T4b any N M0
Stage IVB	Any T any N M1

Table 6.3 Prognostic factors for survival in follicular cell-derived DTC [11]

Prognostic factors	Tumor-associated	Patient-associated	Other conditions
Key factors	Extrathyroidal spread (Category T) Category M Post-treatment Tg Values	Age	Residual disease: R0, R1, R2
Additional factors	Category N BRAF V600E mutation in metastatic sites	Sex	Adequacy of surgery RAI ablation Endemic goiter
New – promising	Molecular profile		

tral lymph node dissection (LND), lateral LND, and some cases are among the approaches of thyroid surgery. Correct preoperative staging and surgical procedure reduce the risk of recurrence of the disease and death.If we list the importance of the initial treatment approach:

1. At the beginning, the level of surgery and possible risks are determined and reduced.
2. Removal of the primary tumor, evaluation of extracapsular spread, and removal of metastatic lymph nodes affect disease progression (in terms of persistent-recurrent disease).
3. Adequacy of surgery is one of the most important prognosis determinants.
4. All normal thyroid tissue should be removed for RAI ablation/treatment efficacy.
5. Accurate staging allows initial determination of risk factors and follow-up decision.

6.5.2 Guidelines [38, 48] Recommend Surgical Approach in Patients Diagnosed with DTC

(a) Tumor diameter < 1 cm, no clinical lymph node metastasis (clinical N0) and extrathyroidal spread, lobectomy is recommended if there is no clear indication for removal of the opposite lobe. In small, unifocal, and intrathyroidal tumors, lobectomy alone is sufficient if there is no history of head and neck RT and family history (strong recommendation, moderate evidence).

(b) Although the first surgical approach may be bilateral total thyroidectomy (BTT) in cases with a tumor diameter of 1–4 cm, without clinical lymph node metastasis (clinical N0) and extrathyroidal spread, it is recommended that lobectomy can be performed in low-risk PTC and FTC; on the other hand, considering the feasibility of RAI, facilitation of follow-up, patient preference, and characteristics of the disease, BTT is preferred instead of lobectomy (strong recommendation, moderate evidence).

(c) BTT is recommended in case of tumor diameter > 4 cm, extrathyroidal spread (clinical T4), clinical lymph node metastasis (clinical N1), and any distant metastasis (strong recommendation, moderate evidence).

Considering the recommendations regarding the surgical approach in cases diagnosed with DTC, the personalized approach associated with patient and disease characteristics such as preferences, genetical-histopathological characteristics, and family and radiation history comes to the forefront in tumors <1 cm and especially those between 1 and 4 cm, and in this case, the choice of lobectomy or BTT is left to the patient and treatment team. Here, different socio-cultural and economic structures should be taken into consideration for each country.

6.5.3 For LND According to Current Guidelines [38, 48, 49]

(a) Prophylactic central LND is not recommended in noninvasive T1, T2 tumors, clinically N0, without aggressive pathology, PTC and FTC.

(b) Prophylactic central LND is recommended in PTC with clinical metastasis (cN1b) in the lateral compartment, even if it is clinically N0 in T3, T4 tumors,

(c) Therapeutic LND is recommended for lateral compartment lymph nodes with clinically central lymph node involvement and proven by biopsy.

6.6 Postoperative Nuclear Medicine Clinical Approach in DTC

The postoperative evaluation process begins with the admission or consultation of patients with operated DTC to the nuclear medicine clinic. Currently, there are no randomized controlled trials in the postoperative pathway, diagnostic strategy, and clear decisions on RAI ablation/

treatment in DTC patients. Postoperative evaluation is the most important step in the evaluation of the pathology report at the first stage followed by staging risk assessment in terms of RAI treatment requirement/dose, re-surgery requirement (complementary or metastasis surgery), RT decision, and follow-up plan.

"Postoperative Nuclear Medicine" Approach at 4–6 Weeks Postoperatively in Patients with DTC Who Underwent BTT or Subtotal Thyroidectomy-Lobectomy.

1. The pathology report should be carefully and thoroughly examined (tumor diameter, localization, lymph node metastasis, lymphovascular-capsule invasions, extrathyroidal spread, poor variants, presence of lymphocytic thyroiditis, immunohistochemistry staining and molecular profile, if any).
2. TSH, fT3, fT4, anti-Tg, and postoperative Tg level (preferably stimulated Tg value).
3. Ca, CBC, KCFT, and routine biochemistry.
4. Neck USG.
5. Tc-99 m thyroid scintigraphy (in terms of residual tissue, Tc-99 m whole-body scan, hormone replacement should be discontinued for 3–4 weeks in selected cases).
6. In some selected patients with known or suspected critical organ metastases, I-131 diagnostic whole-body scan-SPECT/CT with 2 mCi before RAI treatment (within 72 h).
7. FDG PET/CT before RAI treatment; in terms of additional treatment requirement (operation, RT) and follow-up in selected patients with high-risk or poorly differentiated histopathology, and/or unexplained with routine examinations or clinically incompatible postoperative high Tg levels (Fig. 6.3).
8. Initial selection and planning of patients requiring reoperation (complementary thyroidectomy, regional or distant metastasis surgery) or RT. *Complementary thyroidectomy* is recommended in our clinic in the patient group (lobectomy-subtotal thyroidectomy) who did not undergo adequate surgery initially (usually in the low-risk group before

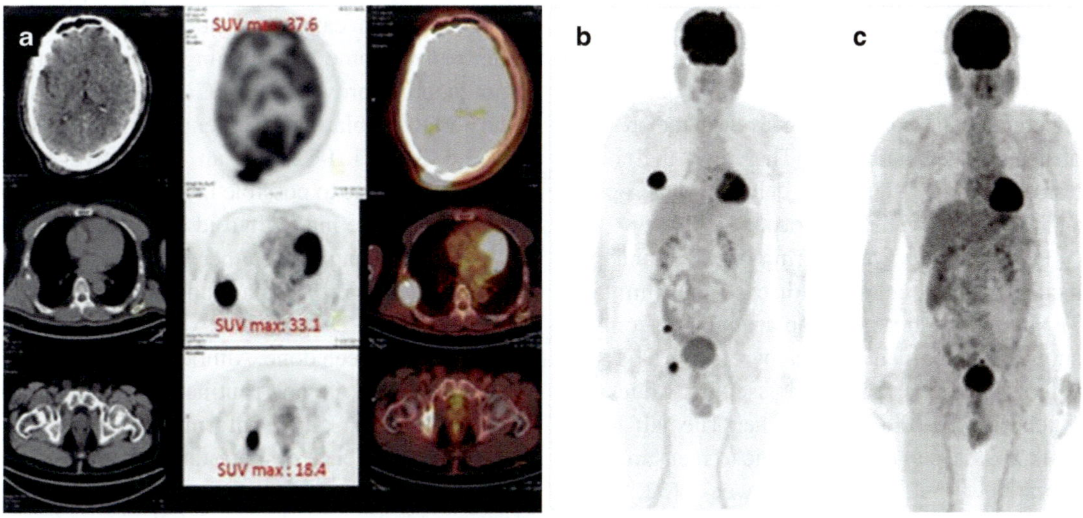

Fig. 6.3 A 52-year-old male patient; 3.6 cm PTC and thyroid capsule invasion as a result of right frontal mass resection and BTT, post-op stimulated Tg > 1000 ng/ml, TSH 60 mU/L, neck USG normal (high-risk patient). The patient followed up for 10 years who has received thoracic surgery and cranial RT, 200 mCi RAI treatment followed by 2 more doses of RAI treatment due to multiple bone metastases observed and residual tumor in cranium in FDG PET/CT imaging at post-op staging (**a**. transverse fusion sections, **b**. PET MIP image), Tg 2 ng/ml in suppression and no structural disease (**c**. PET MIP image, focal FDG uptake in the colon at bladder superior level, endoscopy and biopsy: villous adenoma)

surgery) in terms of recurrence risk and prognosis, taking into account clinical-pathological and social-cultural characteristics, or in order to facilitate follow-up. RT may be adjuvant or palliative in the postoperative period. Preferably RAI treatment should be planned earlier unless critical organ irradiation such as emergency airway is required, as post-RT iodine uptake may deteriorate (radiation effect-stunning). RAI treatment should be given after 2–3 months if RT has been given or is required to be given before [49].

6.7 Importance of Postoperative Tg

Thyroglobulin is a glycoprotein produced in normal thyroid and tumoral thyroid follicle cells in DTC. In DTC, suppressed or stimulated Tg levels in the postoperative process largely predict residual thyroid tissue, residual disease, additional treatment requirement, and disease progression. Anti-Tg are positive in 15–25% of patients with thyroid cancer [50] and reduce the reliability of Tg, leading to false-negative results. Therefore, Tg and anti-Tg should be examined together both postoperatively and during follow-up. Furthermore, false-negative or false-positive results can be obtained by affecting both Tg and anti-Tg levels in the presence of heterophilic antibodies. Therefore, the correct results can be obtained by detecting heterophilic antibodies in large laboratories [51].

Prognostically, in determining risk and predicting residue-recurrence disease, the stimulated Tg value (with hormone replacement discontinuation or recombinant human thyrotropin (rhTSH)) is more sensitive than suppressed Tg values and is generally 5–10 times or higher. The half-life of Tg is 1–3 days and the best time to measure postoperative stimulated Tg is 3–4 weeks [52, 53].

There is no optimum cutoff value for postoperative Tg (suppressed or stimulated). This is because Tg is released from normal thyroid tissue and thyroid cancer cells, and values vary due to the amount of diseased tissue and TSH level. Studies have shown that Tg with postoperative stimulation strongly predicts poor prognosis if it is >10–30 ng/ml and remission if it is <1–2 ng/ml [54, 55]. In current guidelines such as ATA [38] and NCCN [48], if the stimulated or suppressed Tg value is <1 ng/ml, it is predictable that no metastatic focus will be detected except thyroid bed in the imaging performed after RAI treatment. However, if postoperative Tg is >5–10 ng/ml, it was emphasized that the possibility of detecting metastatic focus showing iodine uptake after RAI treatment would increase and postoperative Tg was recommended to be used in the RAI ablation-treatment decision in the low-intermediate risk group. If the patient has unexpected and incompatible Tg elevation after evaluation, neck USG and other conventional imaging (CT, MR) should be investigated first in terms of possible regional residual disease-metastasis and with FDG PET/CT in selected cases.

6.8 Postoperative Diagnostic Scan

Current guidelines suggest that postoperative diagnostic scan can be "done if necessary." In order to overcome the stunning effect, it is recommended to provide 1–3 mCi I-131 diagnostic scan and RAI ablation/treatment within 72 h or to use 1.5–3 mCi I-123 as an alternative [38]. Furthermore, due to possible intense involvement in residual tissue in the thyroid bed (star artifact) or low dose, imaging of other areas can be prevented (e.g., micronodular lung metastases) in diagnostic scan. Diagnostic RAI scan is sensitive if ablation has been done. Although postoperative diagnostic scan is not routinely performed in every case in our clinic, information is obtained about the prevalence of metastatic disease with 2 mCi I-131 within 72 h before treatment and the degree of iodine uptake, especially in terms of unexpected very high Tg values or critical organ metastases (such as brain-cranial, diffuse lung, spinal involvement), and accordingly, measures to be taken during hospitalization with the RAI dose (steroid use/dose, consultation requirement, etc.) (Fig. 6.4).

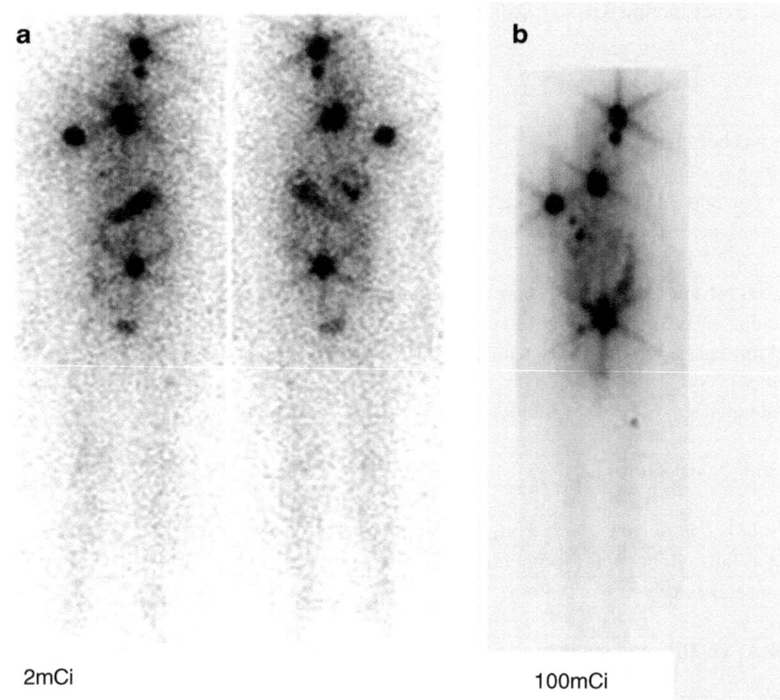

Fig. 6.4 A 45-year-old female patient, FTC (operated cranial metastasis), postoperative Tg > 1000 ng/ml. MRI: Bone defect on the left and cerebral parenchymal herniation in the subgaleal area. Tumor burden-RAI uptake intensity, RAI dose and possible complications in treatment – diagnostic I-131 scan (**a**: anterior and posterior) with 2 mCi in terms of measures to be taken for cerebral edema and scan after the RAI treatment dose given by planning premedication accordingly, intensive uptake in the neck (**b**: anterior and posterior) seen more prominently and in more foci, bone and lung metastases

6.9 Postoperative Risk Identification

Since staging systems (AJCC/TNM) were inadequate in predicting recurrence risk in DTCs, ATA identified low-, intermediate-, and high-risk groups in terms of structural recurrence risk in patients without macroscopic disease in 2009 [56] and made modifications with additional prognostic factors in 2015 (Table 6.4). In FTC, the prevalence of invasion, lymph node involvement prevalence, and mutation status are the parameters added. However, the importance of the effects of these modifications in risk determination is yet to be studied. What is noteworthy in the low- and moderate-risk group is the "involvement in the neck inside or outside thyroid bed if RAI treatment is given," because disease detection at the molecular level is possible by nuclear medicine imaging methods without anatomical change or without the lesion reaching the pathological dimension level. Therefore, the detection of micronodular-miliary (<1mm) lung metastases, the detection of metastatic lymph nodes not anatomically pathological in size, and some bone metastases can be performed by scan after RAI treatment at molecular level [57, 58]. As can be seen, although the current guidelines show a more conservative attitude toward RAI ablation/treatment indications, behavior is essential according to patient factors.

Determination of the postoperative-initial risk in DTC is the most important information that forms the basis for additional surgical intervention, additional imaging, RAI treatment decision, and the dose to be administered. In determining

Table 6.4 ATA 2015 structural recurrence modified risk classification

Low risk
PTC, provided that all of the following features are present
• No local or distant metastases
• The entire macroscopic tumor has been removed
• No tumor invasion to surrounding tissues and structures
• No aggressive tumor histology (such as tall cell, hobnail variant, columnar cell carcinoma)
• *If I131 has been given, there is no involvement outside the thyroid bed in the scan after treatment*
• No vascular invasion[a]
• Clinically N0 or ≤ 5 pathological N1 micrometastases (maximum diameter < 0.2 cm)[a]
Intrathyroidal, encapsulated follicular variant papillary thyroid cancer[a]
Intrathyroidal, well-differentiated follicular thyroid cancer, with capsular invasion and without vascular invasion or with minimal vascular invasion (<4 foci)[a]
Intrathyroidal papillary microcarcinoma, single focus or multifocal, *BRAF V600E* mutation (if known)[a]
Intermediate risk
Microscopic tumor invasion to perithyroidal soft tissues
PTC with vascular invasion
Neck involvement outside the thyroid bed in the first whole-body RAI scan after I131 treatment
Aggressive tumor histology (such as tall cell, hobnail variant, columnar cell carcinoma)[a]
Intrathyroidal papillary thyroid cancer, primary tumor 1–4 cm
BRAFV600E mutation (if known)[a]
Spread outside the thyroid and BRAF*V600E* mutation in multifocal papillary microcarcinoma (if known)[a]
High risk
Macroscopic tumor invasion to perithyroidal soft tissues (wide extrathyroidal spread)
Distant metastasis
Postoperative serum TG elevation suggestive of distant metastasis
Pathological N1 metastatic lymph node with largest diameter > 3 cm in any of them[a]

[a]Proposed modifications not included in ATA 2009
Clinically N1 or > 5 pathological N1 with the largest diameter < 3 cm
Incomplete tumor resection
Follicular thyroid cancer with diffuse vascular invasion (>4 foci)

the initial risks in the postoperative period, postoperative poor histopathological features, the size and prevalence of lymphatic metastasis, extrathyroidal spread, and postoperative Tg elevation predicting possible metastatic disease are observed as the most important risk factors for the correct planning of initial treatment in DTC.

6.10 RAI Ablation and Treatment

6.10.1 Iodine Metabolism and Radioactive Iodine in DTC

Although neoplastic cells in PTC and FTC are similar to normal thyroid cells, deterioration in iodine metabolism is the most characteristic feature and Tg production is ongoing. Peroxidase activity is the enzyme that converts iodine (I^-) to iodine (I^0) and is the beginning of organification. Iodine binds to tyrosine in Tg by iodinase and this is called organification. Since there is no iodine organification in the cancer cell, thyroid hormone synthesis is low (although rarely functional thyroid metastases can be seen with hyperthyroidism/thyrotoxicosis). The biological half-life of iodine is reduced in the tumor cell. TSH receptors are expressed in these tumors and increase radioactive iodine (RAI) uptake. As Tg production increases, tumor growth increases. Even if TSH receptor, NIS, and thyroid peroxidase (TPO) expression are reduced in the tumor, they are normally expressed. Therefore, suppression of TSH in DTCs (suppression treatment) is one of the most important steps of treatment. TSH stimulation is required to increase RAI uptake in the tumor cell. NIS expression is even lower in metastatic foci, and this may actually be an indicator of the onset of dedifferentiation with metastases. As cancer cells move away from differentiation, Tg production decreases or does not exist [59].

RAI, the ancestor of theranostic practices in which diagnosis and treatment were performed with the same agent, was first applied in 1946 by Seidlin et al., and since then RAI treatment has been the most common and successful of nuclear medicine radionuclide therapy applications [60]. I-131, a nuclear reactor product, is produced by nuclear fission of uranium. It has 53 protons and 78 neutrons and its atomic number is 131. In order for I-131 to transition to a stable state, the neutron is converted to proton and exits to negative electron (β particle). Meanwhile, the number of protons becomes 54, and Xe-131, which is stimulated, decays to stable Xe-131 and 364 keV photon (gamma) release occurs. As a result of β (−) decay, β particles (electrons) are ejected in different energies and cause apoptosis and cell death by progressing 1–2 mm in the concentrated tissue. Treatment with the highest β particle energy of 606 keV (90%) and an average of 192 keV and imaging with 364 keV gamma energy are provided. Its physical half-life is 8 days. Na-iodine has high specific activity and oral forms as a solution or capsule. High-dose I-131 is taken orally unless there is an obstacle. The capsule form is safer than the liquid form. While the effective half-life in normal thyroid tissue is 6–8 days, it is 1–3 days or less in cancerous tissue [61]. This shows us how the efficacy of RAI treatment in metastatic/tumoral tissue can be variable and lower than normal with tumor biology-NIS expression, i.e., differentiation-heterogeneity. In addition, it should not be overlooked that I-131 involvement will be different according to tissue size and mass, and the dose exposed will also differ. Therefore, for effective RAI treatment in DTCs, it is very important to provide RAI treatment after removal of normal thyroid tissue and surgical removal of large metastatic foci to reduce tumor burden, if appropriate.

6.11 RAI Dosimetry

RAI ablation refers to the elimination of residual thyroid tissue after the operation in thyroid cancer, and RAI treatment refers to the elimination of metastatic-recurrent tumor tissues with the effect of RAI. There are two main approaches known to determine the I-131 dose after thyroidectomy in thyroid cancer patients. These are empirical/fixed-dose approach and dosimetric approach. The empirical-fixed-dose approach is a fairly easy-to-apply method that is most commonly used in routine practice. However, in this application, differences in individual biological and physical characteristics (iodine uptake level and retention differences in tissue, elimination difference, heterogeneity, etc.) are ignored. In the personalized dosimetric approach, maximum treatment efficacy and radiation safety are aimed with a minimum effective dose to the target tissues. The most common formulation of medical radiation dose (Medical Internal Radiation Dosimetry, MIRD) is used for dosimetric examinations in nuclear medicine clinical applications [62]. The MIRD method is based on dose calculation on the human body and its organ models in standard measures. Since dosimetric whole-body imaging and blood samples are taken at successive times and calculations are made, it is difficult and cumbersome, but it is recommended to be performed in selected cases, especially in the metastatic-recurrent disease group requiring high levels of activity.

There are two basic concepts as bone marrow and lesion dosimetry in the dosimetric approach. In the bone marrow-based approach, it is aimed to calculate the maximum safe radiation dose for the bone marrow, and in the lesion-based approach, it is aimed to calculate the minimum dose required to damage the tumor.

Bone marrow dosimetry (AHASA: As High As Safely Administrable) was first studied in 1962 by Benue et al. in 59 patients with metastatic thyroid cancer and reported as a safe limit dose for <2 Gy bone marrow [63]. Later, Leeper et al. suggested that the blood dose should be below 2 Gy and the total body retention at 48 h should be below 120 mCi and below 80 mCi in the presence of diffuse lung metastases [64]. Finally, it was emphasized in ATA guidelines that caution should be exercised in >150 mCi activities, especially in elderly patients over 70 years of age and in cases of renal failure [38].

In the lesion-based dosimetric approach (ALARA: As Low As Reasonably Achievable), the aim is to determine the minimum radiation dose required for the destruction of residual thyroid tissue or metastatic foci. Maxon et al. conducted a study using planar scintigraphy in 1983 and obtained significant results in response to treatment when an average dose of 300 Gy was administered to successfully ablate the remaining thyroid tissue and over 80 Gy was administered to eliminate metastases [61]. The lesion-based dosimetric approach has been reported to be suitable for larger lesions due to difficulties in volume calculation in smaller lesions (e.g., disseminated lung metastases) [65].

In addition to I-131 gamma camera studies, dosimetric studies with I-124 (half-life 4.18 days) PET/CT come to the forefront because it enables more accurate uptake measurement due to the fact that spatial resolution is much better, there is adequate attenuation-scattering correction, and more accurate lesion volume can be detected [66, 67]. It has also been suggested that I-124 PET/CT lesion dosimetry can be used as a prognostic indicator predicting lesion-based I-131 response [68].

Although the importance of the dosimetric approach in the treatment of thyroid cancer in selected cases (such as large and inoperable lymph nodes, distant metastasis) is known in terms of its contribution and dose-response relationship, fixed-dose application is generally preferred in the world in routine practice due to application difficulties and some limitations (such as lesion size, shape, tumor heterogeneity, different biokinetics, and bioavailability of RAI in the target tissue).

6.12 RAI Ablation/Treatment Purpose

Definition: RAI ablation/treatment is the first of the theranostic practices, and it is a standard therapy with proven recurrence and survival effectiveness after BTT in DTC.

6.12.1 Purpose

1. **RAI ablation:** It means ablation of normal thyroid tissue after total thyroidectomy. After ablation, the level of Tg produced in normal thyroid tissue becomes undetectable and can be used as a specific tumor marker, and the sensitivity of diagnostic I-131 scan increases when normal thyroid tissue is ablated.
2. **RAI adjuvant therapy:** It reduces the disease-specific risk of death by the destruction of suspected but unproven tumor foci (intermediate-high risk group for relatively recurrent disease).
3. **RAI treatment:** Treatment of persistent and metastatic disease contributes to progression-free and overall survival.

6.13 RAI Indications

The recommendations of the current guidelines for RAI are given in Table 6.5. Considering the recommendations, as in the risk classification, it is emphasized that patient-specific clinicopathological features (tumor size, histological features, degree of lymphatic invasion, prevalence of lymphatic metastasis), postoperative Tg and anti-Tg, surgical competence, age, and preoperative and postoperative USG quality affect patient management and RAI decision. The age limit among the criteria is still 45 years, although it has been raised to 55 years, especially for the female sex in the new TNM classification [11]. There is not enough data yet available to guide the molecular profile to the RAI treatment decision [38].

RAI Ablation/Treatment Decision of Our Clinic:

1- RAI ablation is not routinely recommended in the low-risk group of patients who underwent lobectomy and are not candidates for complementary thyroidectomy; who underwent adequate surgery (BTT); who did not have significant residual tissue findings in favor of thyroid scintigraphy and USG; who had tumor <1 cm; who are <45 years; who did not have aggressive tumor histology, lymphovascular

Table 6.5 Recommendations for RAI in ATA 2015 [38] and NCCN 2018 [48] guidelines

	RAI not routinely recommended (provided that all are present	RAI may be recommended in selected patients (if any of the following is present)	RAI recommended (if any of the following is present)
ATA 2015	– Tumor <1 cm (single or <1 cm multifocal) – No poor histopathological features	– Tumor 1–4 cm, poor histopathological features – Tumor >4 cm – Microscopic extrathyroidal spread (T3) – Central lymph node metastasis (N1a, especially >45 years) – Lateral and mediastinal lymph node metastasis (N1b, especially >45 years)	– Macroscopic extrathyroidal spread (T4, tumor size does not matter) – Distant metastasis
NCCN 2018	– Tumor <2 cm classic PTC – Intrathyroidal – Single or ≤1 cm multifocal – Anti-Tg negative – Postoperative unstimulated Tg < 1 ng/ml	– Tumor 2–4 cm – High-risk histopathologies – Lymphatic-minor vascular invasion – Cervical lymph node metastasis – >1 cm multifocality – Postoperative unstimulated Tg < 5–10 ng/ml – Microscopic positive margin	– Extrathyroidal spread – Tumor >4 cm – Postoperative unstimulated Tg > 5–10 ng/ml – Distant metastasis

invasion, extrathyroidal spread, and lymph node metastasis-extracapsular spread; who were anti-Tg negative; who had Tg < 1 ng/ml in postoperative suppression; or whose stimulated Tg level was consistent with residual thyroid tissue.

2- RAI ablation/treatment is recommended in patients with tumor of any size but with histopathologically poor prognostic features (extrathyroidal spread, aggressive-malignant variants), tumor >4 cm, lymphatic-vascular invasion, lymph node metastasis-extracapsular spread, presence of distant metastasis, inadequate surgery-incomplete macroscopic tumor resection (also evaluated in terms of reoperation and/or RT), "postoperative high Tg" level incompatible with residual thyroid tissue and the initially determined disease status, unexplained high anti-Tg level and pathological findings in postoperative USG (also evaluated in terms of reoperation), age > 45 years and male sex, and in case of any of radiation exposure characteristics.

Table 6.6 RAI purpose and dose recommendations

RAI purpose	ATA 2015	NCCN 2018
Ablation	30–100 mCi	30–50 mCi
Adjuvant treatment	30–150 mCi	50–100 mCi
Treatment	100–200 mCi	100–200 mCi

6.14 RAI Dose

Since the dosimetric approach is not practical in routine use, fixed-dose administration is widely used except in selected cases (such as elderly patients, renal failure), and the guidelines also recommend the simpler fixed-dose approach (Table 6.6). The dose values given in Table 6.6 cover different risk groups according to the purpose in patients who have undergone BTT and RAI decision has been made [38, 48].

There are numerous studies in the literature on low-dose and high-dose RAI administration in low-risk patients. Some of the studies argue that 30 mCi and 100 mCi ablation have similar success and that low-dose administration may be preferred in the low-risk group considering that possible acute and long-term side effects of RAI can be reduced and do not require hospitalization [69, 70]. Schlumberger et al. emphasized in their randomized prospective study that the combination of low-dose RAI ablation with rhTSH also improves the quality of life [70]. However, a recent meta-analysis reported that 100 mCi administration was more successful than low-dose administration [71]. It has also been reported in studies that low-dose RAI administrations increase incomplete biochemical and structural responses in the moderate-risk group and repeated doses should be given [72]. The important thing about low-dose RAI ablation is that individual risk assessment should be done correctly.

Samuel et al. showed that effective half-life in target tissue was shortened compared to previous RAI at repeated RAI doses [73]. Patients with DTC may be exposed to repeated doses that are thought to alter iodine biokinetics and lead to dedifferentiation in the tumor cell due to inadequate initial RAI dose. In this case, especially in metastatic DTC, considering the heterogeneity of tumor cells with less differentiation and lower RAI involvement, it is concluded that inadequate dose administration at the beginning will adversely affect survival [74].

There is no standard dose of RAI in pediatric DTCs. In general, empirical dosing can be determined by the age, weight, and body surface area of the patient. The RAI dose can be 1–1.5 mCi/kg, or it can be planned by adapting the adult dose to the pediatric group for a similar disease condition, for example, 1/3 of the adult dose for 5 years of age, ½ for 10 years of age, and 5/6 for 15 years of age. Dosimetric approach is appropriate for repeated RAI therapies and diffuse lung metastases [75].

For RAI ablation and treatment in DTCs, correct selection of the initial RAI dose within safe limits – at maximum efficacy – is essential in RAI applications. If RAI ablation is to be performed in low-risk patients, it should be kept in mind that the general tendency is low-dose applications (30 mCi), low-dose decision should be made carefully in the moderate-risk group (preferably 100 mCi), and repeated RAI treatments may be required in the high-risk group, so the initial dose should be selected at the appropriate high dose (150–200 mCi) and should not be given below the previous dose at repeated doses.

6.15 Cumulative Dose

There is no clear limit on cumulative dose in the literature or guidelines. However, in patients with ongoing RAI uptake and response, if there is no problem in terms of the bone marrow and lungs, repeated doses (should be at least 9–12 months apart) can be given. Especially in children with diffuse lung metastasis, if complete remission is not observed after 3–4 cycles and the disease with low tumor load continues, it is recommended not to continue RAI treatment and to remain under follow-up in TSH suppression [74]. In addition, if the cumulative dose is above 600 mCi, it has been reported to increase the risk of secondary malignancy [76]. This dose limit has been used in subsequent studies in the literature, but it has also been shown in studies that this level should not be used as a limit and higher doses can be administered using the dosimetric approach [74].

6.16 Empirical Dosing in Scan-Negative, Tg-Positive Cases

In patients with increased serum Tg levels, negative I-131 whole-body scan, no obvious pathology detected on CT/MR and FDG PET/CT, and unsuitable for local treatments, it is generally a 150 mCi dose of RAI application. The contribution of empirical dose RAI treatment to survival is unclear and the degree of recommendation and level of evidence in guidelines are poor [38, 48]. It is also recommended to decide according to the personalized risk assessment in selected cases [49]. A meta-analysis published in the literature on empirical dose administration involving 16 studies, 438 patients (negative diagnostic scan, increased serum Tg) reported a 61% post-treatment iodine-positive foci and a 56% decrease in

Tg in this group during follow-up [77]. Kabasakal et al. reported that 79% of patients had involvement in scan-negative and Tg-positive cases, especially in micrometastatic disease after high-dose RAI treatment, and treatment effectiveness was observed [78]. In our current clinical practice, in cases with Tg-positive under suppression therapy and uptake in the previous RAI treatment dose scan (mostly micronodular lung metastases), re-treatment is planned without diagnostic scan.

6.17 RAI Treatment Contraindications

Pregnancy: RAI crosses the placenta freely and the fetal thyroid concentrates iodine after 12 weeks and causes severe hypothyroidism due to the thyroid gland damaged by the radiation effect. Furthermore, exposure to fetal radiation develops from the maternal bladder as a result of the excretion of RAI [79].

Breastfeeding: Since RAI is excreted in milk, breastfeeding should be discontinued at least 8 weeks.

before treatment and breastfeeding should not be continued afterward [38, 79].

Iodine intake: Since exogenous iodine intake will compete with RAI and if iodine-containing IV contrast agents have been used in both treatment and diagnostic procedures, RAI should be delayed for at least 8 weeks. RAI treatment should not be given if the patient is taking amiodarone, an iodine-containing medicine, or if they have used it within 12 months. Although there is no definitive data on low iodine diet before RAI treatment scan, a low iodine diet (≤50 μg/day) is recommended for 1–2 weeks before RAI [49].

6.18 TSH Stimulation

TSH stimulation should be >30 μIU/ml for effective RAI uptake. Optimum TSH stimulation level is unclear based on available data. TSH stimulation can be accomplished by discontinuation of hormone replacement or administration of rhTSH in low-risk patients.

Discontinuation of hormone replacement: If RAI ablation/treatment can be planned in 4–6 weeks after the operation, T3 preparation is given for 2 weeks (50–75 μg/day, the half-life of T3 in the blood is approximately 18–24 h), and it is discontinued for 2 weeks. Discontinuation of T4 preparation for 3–4 weeks on average is sufficient for TSH stimulation if the patient is receiving hormone replacement (half-life of T4 in blood is approximately 1 week) [10]. In case of hypothyroidism (high TSH levels), the renal clearance of RAI decreases, and its bioavailability increases in thyroid/cancer cells. However, radiation exposure throughout the whole body increases and intestinal motility decreases in the hypothyroid process.

rhTSH administration: Hypothyroidism (even in the short term) is an important symptom that affects quality of life. Guidelines recommend the use of FDA-approved rhTSH for TSH stimulation in RAI ablation/adjuvant therapy in patients with low-risk DTC or moderate-risk DTC without widespread lymph node metastasis [38, 48, 49]. Apart from the low-risk group, rhTSH may also be recommended in the group with psychiatric and cardiovascular diseases that cannot tolerate the symptoms of hypothyroidism, which may cause serious undesirable effects related to the disease, and in patients who do not have TSH elevation despite hormone replacement discontinuation (ATA 2015 low level of evidence). There are insufficient data for the use of rhTSH in the high-risk and recurrence-metastatic patient group, and it is not recommended.

rhTSH 0.9 mg IM is administered on two consecutive days, and serum Tg levels are measured on day 3 and day 5 (>2 ng/ml suggests the presence of thyroid tissue/metastatic cells) [38, 48]. Some studies have shown that the success of ablation is lower with rhTSH stimulation compared to endogenous TSH stimulation since the RAI bioavailability and iodine intake in the euthyroid patient will decrease, although it is not statistically significant [80]. There are also studies suggesting the discontinuation of T4 a few days before ablation with a low iodine diet for 2 weeks [81].

6.19 RAI Ablation/Post-treatment Scan

It has been reported that 10–50% more foci are detected with SPECT/CT imaging, which provides anatomical correlation with whole-body scan after RAI ablation/treatment, compared to low-dose diagnostic scan, and there is a 9–15% change in patient management [82]. Post-treatment scan can be performed between 3 and 10 days. Although there are studies showing higher target tissue uptake in the scan performed on the 7th post-treatment day, the optimum timing is unclear.

In our study comparing whole-body scan findings performed after RAI diagnostic scan and treatment (day 4) in 75 patients with DTC in 1999, 29% of the patients had iodine uptake in new or additional areas and more than half (64%) had residual thyroid tissue, lymph node, and bone metastasis, including lung metastasis [83]. In our clinic, scan/SPECT is routinely performed with treatment doses for more than 20 years, and diagnostic accuracy is increased with low-dose SPECT/CT imaging for anatomical correlation in cases required in recent years with developing technology (Fig. 6.5).

6.20 RAI Complications

6.20.1 Side Effects and Early Complications That May Occur During Hospitalization

Nausea (≈30%), edema-pain in the cervical-thyroid region (radiation thyroiditis, ≈10–20%), and salivary glands (sialadenitis, ≈30%) are the most common side effects during hospitalization. In the weeks following RAI treatment, complications are mostly transient when measures are taken (such as hydration, anti-inflammatory medicines, antiemetics, steroids) and can be more frequently observed in high-dose – short interval administrations (≥100–200 mCi) may develop such as salivary gland dysfunction-sialadenitis, taste disturbance, minimal bone marrow suppression, transient pancytopenia, gastritis, cystitis,

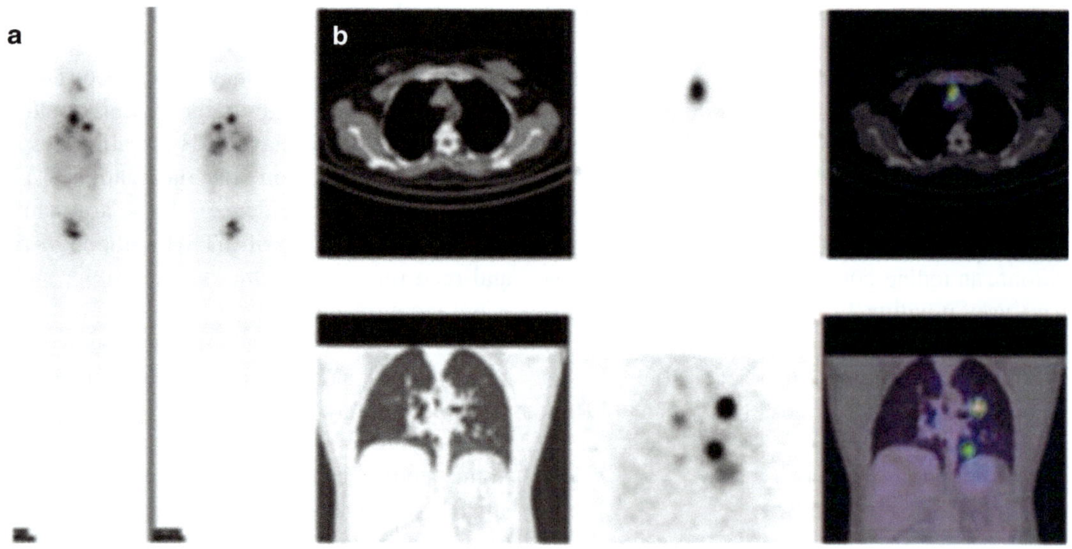

Fig. 6.5 Postoperative Tg 1.5 ng/ml, anti-Tg > 500 IU/ml in female patient diagnosed with PTC, lymph node metastasis, and lymphocytic thyroiditis. Intense focal and heterogeneous RAI uptake was observed in the anterior mediastinum (sternum?, LAP?) and both lungs in the whole-body scan of the patient who received 150 mCi RAI treatment (**a**). In the SPECT/CT (**b**) study, it was distinguished that the iodine uptake observed in the middle part of the anterior mediastinum belonged to the prevascular lymph node. Note: No distinctive anatomical lesion is observed in the correlation of heterogeneous and focal RAI uptakes observed in both lungs (detection of micrometastatic foci by molecular theranostic imaging)

and glossitis [65]. Bone marrow suppression is usually observed in patients with extensive bone metastases and cumulative dose >500–600 mCi and is transient. Bone marrow radiation exposure increases in patients with impaired renal function. Therefore, it is recommended to know kidney functions and to perform complete blood tests before RAI treatment [38].

Temporary impairment of testicular and ovarian functions may occur. It has been reported that temporary amenorrhea and fertility disorder may be due to impairment of pituitary-gonadal axis due to hypothyroidism rather than dose relationship [84]. It has been reported that testicular dysfunction is seen at a rate of 10–50% when the RAI treatment dose is >100 mCi, and this effect can be reduced by hydration and may be permanent as the cumulative dose increases, and sperm bank is recommended at doses of ≥400 mCi [38].

Radiation pneumonitis is a rare complication in lung metastases. Complications secondary to edema (such as cerebral edema, spinal cord compression) may be observed in critical organ metastases. However, such undesirable complications can be prevented by measures to be taken such as adequate hydration and steroid use during and after hospitalization.

After RAI treatment, the release of radioactive iodoproteins from the thyroid gland in patients with excessive residual thyroid tissue or, in rare cases, hormones released by RAI treatment during the thyrotoxic process in hyperfunctional metastatic cases may cause thyroid crisis. Patients with thyrotoxic metastatic DTC should be euthyroid before RAI treatment [85].

6.21 Late Complications

Xerostomy is the most common (2–4%) and dental problems can also be observed in these patients. Precautions should be taken to protect salivary glands, especially in high-dose activities. There are publications in the literature on the use of cholinergic agents, amifostine, and lemon candy other than hydration to prevent salivary gland injury. In a study, the recommended time for lemon candy use is 24 h after RAI treatment, and it has been reported that salivary gland damage will increase when used immediately after treatment [86]. However, there is no recommendation-level evidence in the guidelines for the prevention of salivary gland injury.

There is insufficient evidence of genetic abnormality and decreased fertility secondary to RAI treatment. 1.8% genetic defects were detected in patients receiving high-dose treatment activities, and this rate was not different from the normal population [87].

Although some studies on secondary malignancies indicate that the incidence will increase and some indicate that the risk is very low or does not exist, the relative risk for secondary malignancies (especially hematological malignancies) compared to the general population has been reported to be approximately 1.2–1.9/10,000 patients per year [87]. In a broad series, multicenter, and long-term meta-analysis, it was emphasized that the risk of secondary malignancy (such as breast, prostate, leukemia, salivary gland, colorectal) increased slightly in the first 10 years, especially in patients diagnosed with thyroid cancer in the 25–49 age group and that the risk of leukemia increased especially in the group receiving RAI treatment [76, 88]. The risk of leukemia may increase with high doses (>900 mCi) and short treatment intervals. Regardless of RAI treatment, the relatively increased risk of thyroid cancer and secondary malignancy (especially breast cancer) should be investigated taking into account molecular, genetic, and environmental factors. In a study by Marti et al. in terms of secondary malignancy risk, in 3850 pediatric and young adult (<25 years) thyroid cancer patients with an average follow-up of 15.5 years, they reported that patients who receive RAI for DTC experience an elevated risk of secondary malignancies mainly salivary cancer. It has also been reported that these risks appear to be only slightly higher than in adult patients and that salivary gland cancer is associated with a 1.7-fold increased risk per 10,000 people/year in pediatric DTC patients receiving RAI treatment [89].

Radiation-secondary pulmonary fibrosis is a rare complication in diffuse micronodular lung metastases with RAI uptake given at repeated doses and at short intervals as a result of radiation pneumonitis [90]. In case of clinical suspicion, chest disease consultation and pulmonary function tests should be performed; if there is a problem, RAI treatment should not be continued and the dose of RAI treatment should be determined with a dosimetric approach. Lung fibrosis was not observed during long-term follow-ups in the patient group with lung metastasis in our clinic, whose premedication was carefully planned and RAI treatment was given and intense diffuse RAI uptake was observed in the treatment dose scan [91].

6.22 RAI Treatment Hospitalization

RAI treatment practices, radiation safety rules, and discharge conditions vary in international regulations. RAI treatment in Turkey is provided in isolated bed services of nuclear medicine clinics, in rooms licensed by the national regulatory authority Nuclear Regulatory Agency (NDK). In terms of radiation safety, room designs, ventilation, wall thicknesses, shower baths and toilets, surrounding areas, and radioactive liquid-solid waste tanks must comply with the standards set by NDK (www.ndk.org.tr).

In the discharge guide of patients receiving radionuclide therapy published by NDK, the limit value of liquid radioactive wastes containing urine and feces of patients receiving I-131 inpatient treatment is 10 Bq/ml. It is also stated that if it exceeds 10 Bq/ml, liquid radioactive waste should be held in the tank system. Therefore, tank systems are installed in all high-dose RAI treatment services in the volumes determined according to the number of beds. The length of hospital stay is determined according to the dose rate determined by NDK and is as follows: "Patients given I-131 radioactive substance above 800 MBq can be discharged by providing other conditions and following the instructions after being kept in a separate isolated room approved by the NDK until the amount of radioactivity in the body falls below 600 MBq and the dose rate 1 meter away from the patient falls below 30 μSv/h." Since iodine will be retained in small amounts in thyroid in cancer patients with normal thyroid tissue removed or ablated, the activity passes into the urine in a short time. The amount excreted in urine usually varies according to the size of the remaining tissue and metastatic tissue. In most cases, 50–60% of the activity is eliminated from the body within the first 24 h and 85% within the 3–5 days of hospitalization [92].

Admission Procedure of Patients Who Will Receive High-Dose RAI Treatment due to DTC and Considerations

1. Patients who will undergo RAI treatment/ablation will present to the nuclear medicine clinic on the morning of their appointment. RAI treatment information and consent form is signed. It is confirmed again that hormone replacement is discontinued and there is no exogenous iodine intake.
2. ECOG performance level of the patients should be ≤2.
3. After the general physical examinations of the patients, pre-hospitalization blood tests are requested (TSH, Tg, anti-Tg, fT3, fT4, CBC, Ca, FBG, βHCG). Female patients of childbearing age should be asked for a pregnancy test. It should be confirmed that breastfeeding is discontinued in breastfeeding women (at least 8 weeks ago).
4. Renal and liver function tests, hepatitis markers, and necessary tests for cardiac problems, diabetes, and lung diseases should be requested during pre-hospitalization – RAI treatment planning and the patient's comorbid diseases and medications used during hospitalization should be known, precautions should be taken, and if necessary, relevant clinics should be consulted. Psychiatric consultation should be requested, especially for the presence of psychiatric illness or anxiety-depression disorders, and the necessary medication should be initiated or readjusted (hypothyroidism may trigger or increase these diseases).

5. Necessary precautions should be taken in terms of radiation safety in patients with catheters.
6. Otolaryngological examination should be absolutely performed in patients with cord vocal paralysis and respiratory distress.

6.23 Before RAI Treatment What to Do in Service and Premedication-Medication

The physician and nurse in charge of the service inform the patient about the side effects and measures to be taken during RAI treatment. The most important of these measures is adequate hydration (3–4 L/day), regular emptying of the bladder and showering every day, taking lemon candy after 24 h, and paying attention to hygiene when going to the toilet and flushing. It should be stated that the patient will not be able to go out of service during the RAI treatment hospitalization process and will be able to reach the responsible physician and nurse with their phone numbers when necessary.

6.23.1 List of Medications Ordered for Inpatient

1. Steroid: Preferably dexamethasone for short-term use is given to prevent possible local edema secondary to residual tissue, pressure secondary to edema in cranial-spinal region metastases, and possible peritumoral edema and dyspnea in lung metastases. Before steroids, diabetes, viral hepatitis, electrolyte balance, and gastrointestinal diseases should be carefully examined. In general, oral form steroids are preferred during hospitalization, IM and IV can be administered in necessary cases, and oral initiation is appropriate in critical organ metastases a few days before treatment. In rhTSH applications, steroids can also be started before injection. Patients on steroids take their doses during hospitalization and reduce them after discharge.
2. Antiemetics: Preferably selective serotonin 5-HT3 receptor blockers (antiemetic effect may be increased with dexamethasone).
3. Antiacid-gastroprotective agents: Proton pump inhibitors, such as H2 receptor blockers.
4. Anti-inflammatory analgesic: Acetaminophen can be preferred.
5. Laxative: In some cases, laxatives may be given for constipation due to hypothyroidism, thereby reducing the intestinal radiation dose.

After checking the information, premedication, and all desired test results, the patient is preferably given RAI in capsule form with sufficient water (does not take food for 2–3 h).

6.24 Discharge

Procedures performed in our clinic on the day of discharge after high-dose RAI treatment:

1. Epicrisis and prescription: It includes all the patient's history, examinations, and consultations, administered RAI dose, control time, and then treatment dose scan findings are added to the system. When preparing the prescription, hormone replacement (levothyroxine-LT4) is gradually increased (the targeted dose is increased by 25–50 μg every 3 days, in the morning on an empty stomach at once); preferably in hypocalcemic patients requiring calcium support, preparations combined with vitamin D are prescribed; if the steroid is started, it is gradually reduced and discontinued (should be taken on a full stomach) and care should be taken to add gastroprotective agents as long as the steroid is taken. On the day of discharge, the prescription content is explained, and the first follow-up visit time is notified to the patient (generally after 2.5–3 months).
2. Post-treatment scan: The generally recommended time is 3–10 days for scan time after RAI treatment. In our clinic, a treatment dose scan is generally performed after 4–7 days. After the treatment dose scan, SPECT/CT imaging is added to the required areas.

3. Measurement and recording of radiation dose rates: When the patients are discharged, dose rates are measured from a distance of 1 m. At the dose rate determined and permitted by NDK (<30 μSv/h, as per NDK radiation safety regulation annex 5), an information form containing the points to be considered (NDK radiation safety regulation annex 6) is given to the patient and archived. In the patient who is discharged according to the regulation and has a body radioactivity amount of <600 MBq or a dose rate of <30 μSv/h, the period to be considered in terms of radiation safety is 15 days on average, and it is carefully reminded again that there should be no close contact with pregnant and children.
4. Birth control should be provided for at least 6 months, preferably 1 year in women and at least 4 months in men after RAI treatment.
5. Due to hypothyroidism or radiation safety, working patients are given a medical report appropriate to the current situation.

6.25 TSH Suppression

Levothyroxine (L-T4) treatment is part of adjuvant therapy in DTC, other than hormone replacement. With TSH suppression, Tg production and growth of tumor cells are suppressed, reducing the risk of recurrence and disease-specific death. Caution should also be exercised with regard to age and cardiovascular diseases on a patient-by-patient basis while considering the risk of disease in the treatment of suppression. Tachycardia, arrhythmia, and their effects on bone metabolism (demineralization), especially in the postmenopausal period, are important. Although its effect on bone metabolism has not been proven alone, since the loss of mineralization will increase in the postmenopausal period, it increases the risk of osteoporosis, and bone density measurements should be made. There is no adverse effect on bone maturation in children [10].

Although the purity of commercial forms of L-T4 is close to 100%, bioavailability varies for each patient. In order to ensure that dose adjustment is reliable in the general approach, it is recommended that the patient continues with whatever preparation they are taking. Since the L-T4 half-life in blood is 6–8 days, it is appropriate to take it as a single dose per day. After L-T4 oral intake, approximately 80% is absorbed from the intestine, although it varies individually. Since L-T4 absorption will be affected after eating, it should be taken at once 20–30 min before breakfast on an empty stomach in the morning. Even small dose changes can cause significant clinical effects in susceptible cases. Therefore, age, sex, body weight, clinical status, and metabolism are important in dose adjustment [93]. The L-T4 suppression dose is generally 2–2.5 ug/kg. However, suppression may occur at higher doses in children and young adults and at lower doses in >40 years of age [10, 48].

Hormone replacement monitoring should be performed more frequently during pregnancy. Since the need for L-T4 will increase, thyroid function tests should be performed at intervals of 1.5–2 months and L-T4 dose should be adjusted. The L-T4 dose should also be re-adjusted for appropriate TSH level after birth.

TSH is suppressed according to the initially recurrence risk in DTC patients. However, suppression levels can be changed by dynamic risk stratification according to treatment response during follow-up. In the presence of persistent disease, if there is no contraindication, TSH must be <0.1 mU/L.

If the high-risk patient is biochemical and clinically disease-free at baseline, TSH should be retained at 0.1–0.5 mU/L for 5–10 years and then re-evaluated [38, 49]. TSH should be retained at normal levels in low-risk DTC undergoing lobectomy.

6.26 Renal Failure and RAI Ablation/Treatment

There are no guidelines for renal failure and RAI treatment. Although there is not much information in the current guidelines on this subject, it is stated that the whole body and bone marrow dose will increase in renal failure due to the fact that the main elimination of I-131 is from the kidneys, so it would be appropriate to apply dosimetry or reduce the standard dose [38, 81, 94].

In healthy individuals, 50–60% of the RAI dose given is excreted within the first 24 h and 80–85% within 48 h [92]. In some studies, in chronic kidney disease and renal failure, the total body concentration of RAI increases approximately 1.5–3-fold and 9–fold, respectively [95]. Therefore, the radiation dose and side effects also increase. Although there are some differences in RAI dose and hemodialysis timing in RAI ablation/treatment planning in DTC patients with renal failure in the literature, a fixed dose with reduced RAI dose (25% on average) is generally preferred. The aim is maximum treatment efficacy, minimum extrathyroidal concentration, and side effect. Accordingly, hemodialysis is performed before treatment and after RAI treatment, and hemodialysis is generally initiated after 1 or 2 days and continued for 3–5 days considering the maximum uptake time of RAI in thyroid tissue (up to 48 h) [96].

6.27 Follow-Up in DTCs

Low-risk cases undergoing BTT and not being given RAI can be monitored periodically at 6–12 month intervals for neck USG, thyroid function tests, and Tg and anti-Tg levels in terms of hormone replacement regulation. Although ATA suggested Tg follow-up in this group in 2015, it is thought that Tg will not provide much information in the presence of residual tissue since its sensitivity decreases. TSH levels can be retained within the normal reference range.

Initial control of patients receiving RAI ablation and treatment is 2.5–3 months later (treatment efficacy and blood tests before 1.5–2 months may not be reliable). Physical examination is performed by reviewing the patient's history, clinicopathological characteristics, initial risk, and treatment dose scan result. TFT, Tg, anti-Tg, Ca, CBC, neck USG, I-131 diagnostic scan, and CT/MRI follow-up or PET/CT examination are requested in necessary cases. Dynamic risk assessment is performed in response and follow-up after the first treatment.

6.28 Determining "Dynamic Risk" and Clinical Approach in Follow-Up

The initial risk may change after the treatments applied during the follow-up process, which is called "dynamic risk determination system." Similar to the repeated risk assessment and clinical approach-follow-up plan according to the results of Tg, anti-Tg, USG, and diagnostic scan routinely applied in our clinic after the first treatment, a new risk classification has been created with the proposed modifications along with the treatment response in the last published ATA guidelines [38]. For treatment response:**Excellent response**: No evidence of clinical, biochemical, or structural disease.

Biochemical incomplete response: Abnormal Tg or increased anti-Tg antibody levels without localizable disease.**Structural incomplete response**: Persistent or newly defined regional or distant metastasis.

Unclear response: Nonspecific biochemical or structural findings that cannot be classified as benign or malignant. Suppressed Tg < 1 ng/ml or stimulated Tg < 10 ng/ml. This includes patients with stable or decreased anti-Tg antibody levels without definite structural disease evidence.

Management approach based on dynamic risk analyses in DTC ensures that initial risk markers are used to manage follow-up and treatment decisions. Thus, the initial decisions are then modified, taking into account the patient's response to treatment. This system determines the intensity and extent of treatment and follow-up processes using risk estimates that vary over time for each individual patient.

The table published in ATA 2015 in terms of treatment response evaluation and clinical approach in patients with DTC who underwent BTT and received RAI treatment and is basically consistent with our clinical experience is presented below (Table 6.7).

Table 6.7 Treatment response evaluation and clinical approach in patients with DTC who underwent BTT and received RAI treatment (ATA 2015)

Treatment response	Definition	Clinical course	Effects on approach
Excellent response	Negative imaging, supressed $Tg < 0.2$ ng/ml, or stimulated $Tg < 1$ ng/ml	– 1–4% recurrence – < 1% disease-specific death	Follow-up time and TSH suppression time will decrease in a short while
Biochemical incomplete response	Negative imaging, supressed $Tg \geq 1$ ng/ml or stimulated ≥ 10 ng/ml, or increasing anti-Tg levels	– 30% resolve spontaneously during follow-up and become disease-free – 20% become disease-free with additional treatment – 20% structural recurrence – < 1% disease-specific mortality	-If decreasing or stable Tg values are observed, follow-up with TSH suppression is suitable - Increasing Tg or anti-Tg levels require additional evaluation (in terms of foci) and additional treatment
Structural incomplete response	Structural or functional disease finding – At any Tg level – Independent of anti-Tg	– 50–85% persistent disease despite additional treatment – Disease-specific mortality rate reaches 11% in regional metastasis and 50% in distant metastasis	– Additional treatments may be required Or – Follow-up may be performed depending on multiple clinical-pathological factors such as size, localization, growth rate, RAI uptake, F18-FDG uptake of lesion(s), and specific pathology of the structural lesion
Unclear response	– Nonspecific findings on imaging – Slight uptake in thyroid bed on RAI scan – Non-stimulated Tg at detectable levels but $Tg < 1$ ng/ml – Stimulated Tg at detectable levels but $Tg < 10$ ng/ml or – Stable or decreasing anti-Tg levels in the absence of structural or functional disease	– 15–20% structural disease during follow-up – In the remaining, nonspecific changes resolve spontaneously or remain stable – < 1% disease-specific mortality	– May be followed up with appropriate serial imaging and serum Tg levels – Nonspecific clinical findings becoming suspicious over time should be evaluated with further additional imaging or biopsy

6.29 Treatment Response and Clinical Approach by Baseline Risks

6.29.1 Low Risk

If the patient, who was initially in the "low risk" group, had the expected excellent response as a result of the biochemical complete response and negative I-131 diagnostic scan (once after treatment), periodic USG, Tg, anti-Tg, TSH (in the range of 0.5–1 mU/L), and Ca controls are performed every 9–12 months. Thereafter, routine diagnostic scan and stimulated Tg control are not required. If there is a very low biochemical or structural incomplete response or uncertain response, the frequency of follow-ups is increased.

6.29.2 Intermediate–High Risk

After the initial treatment that should be performed in the "intermediate-risk" and "high-risk" groups according to the initial risk assessment, if the treatment response meets the criteria of "excellent response," we should keep TSH in the range of 0.1–0.5 mU/L for at least 5–10 years in the intermediate- to high-risk patients with whom we initially target TSH <0.1 mU/L suppression. Periodic checks should be continued every 6–12 months. Routine diagnostic I-131 scan should also be performed 1–2 times at 9–12 month intervals, as it will also allow stimulated Tg control.

Patients with a "biochemical incomplete response" whose Tg is stable or tends to decrease in suppression should be closely monitored for TSH suppression and neck USG checks should be performed every 6 months. If there is no contraindication in patients with diffuse lung metastasis or other metastatic patients who are not considered for operation, RAI treatment should be planned again in a safe range. If suppressed/stimulated Tg or anti-Tg levels tends to increase gradually and there are no pathological findings in neck US during follow-up, CT, MRI (especially brain metastasis at rapidly increasing Tg levels should be considered), or FDG PET/CT imaging should be performed and the focus/foci of the disease should be sought. If structural pathology is detected on imaging, operability and/or RT indication should be questioned.

Patients with a "structural incomplete response" (detected by USG, CT, FDG PET/CT, or MRI) require a multidisciplinary approach. The size of the structural disease should be monitored and the operability or RT requirement should be determined first. If additional treatments cannot be performed or combined, RAI treatment should be planned again, if there is a response to previous RAI treatment and the patient is eligible. In structural disease without RAI uptake (iodine refractory) and inoperable, first local treatments (such as RT, ablative treatments), then systemic treatments should be considered and suppression treatment should be continued as long as Tg production continues. When additional lesions are observed in DTC with structural disease, possible secondary malignancies should be excluded and histopathological diagnosis should be made if clinically necessary.

Periodic follow-ups (TSH, Tg, anti-Tg, USG) and annual diagnostic I-131 scan (SPECT, SPECT/CT) and stimulated Tg follow-up should be performed routinely at 6–12 months in patients with *uncertain treatment response*. Nonspecific findings may remain stable or reach normal limits during follow-up. In some cases, the findings may become more specific clinical findings. In this case, focus is detected by additional diagnostic imaging and biopsy if necessary. As mentioned in the subsequent biochemical or structural incomplete treatment response, additional treatments such as RAI treatment and/or operation, RT, and other local or systemic treatments may be required.

6.30 Microcarcinomas

Carcinomas with a tumor diameter of <1 cm are defined as microcarcinomas. It accounts for approximately 30% of DTCs and management of microcarcinomas has been one of the most controversial issues over the years [97]. Almost all of them are papillary microcarcinomas (PMCs), very rarely there may be follicular and medullary microcarcinomas. In general, the guidelines report that only lobectomy is sufficient without RAI ablation in unifocal PMC without local invasion, lymph node metastasis, and other poor prognostic-histopathological features, since their prognosis is excellent. TSH can be maintained within normal limits. In a meta-analysis, PMC distant metastasis was reported to be 0.4% and local-regional recurrences were reported to be 12–50% [49]. It has been reported that lymph node micrometastases are observed more as tumor diameter increases and the rate increases up to 57% with SPECT and SPECT/CT studies [98]. While 5-year recurrence-free survival was 78.6% in PMCs without RAI ablation, it was shown to be 95% in those undergoing RAI ablation [99]. The mortality rate was reported to be 0.34% in a meta-analysis involving 9379 PMK patients [100].

If we list the risk factors in terms of recurrence in PMCs, multifocal-bilateral, infiltrative pattern, desmoplastic fibrosis, extrathyroidal spread, relatively larger tumor size (6–10 mm), histopathologically poor variants/less differentiated component, incidental FDG PET-positive nodule, disproportionate Tg elevation in patients undergoing BTT, anti-Tg elevation in patients without thyroiditis pathology, nodular lesion in residual tissue in patients undergoing lobectomy or subtotal thyroidectomy, $BRAF^{V600E}$ mutation, and history of neck RT [49, 101]. According to all mentioned risk factors, active follow-up, complementary thyroidectomy, and/or RAI ablation should be decided with a patient-specific individual approach in PMCs. Dynamic risk criteria, treatment response, and follow-up of PMC patients undergoing BTT and RAI ablation are similar to other DTCs.

6.31 F-18 FDG PET/CT During Follow-Up

The use of PET/CT in follow-up is usually for the high-risk DTC patient group with Tg>10 ng/ml, normal neck USG, and RAI negative. Monitoring FDG-positive metastatic lesions in PET/CT provides prognostic information and shows aggressive behavior. In addition, FDG PET/CT allows patient selection for surgical, local, or systemic treatments, and post-treatment response is evaluated [38]. In a prospective study conducted by Uçmak et al. in our clinic, the contribution of PET/CT to patient management was investigated in 105 patients with recurrent-metastatic disease suspected to have negative iodine uptake, high Tg values, negative anti-Tg antibodies, and no pathological findings on neck USG, and follow-up data were reported [102]. When the relationship between Tg values and PET positivity was evaluated in our study, a correlation was observed between PET positivity and stimulated and suppressed Tg values (p: 0.0001) and the threshold values determined by ROC analysis in terms of PET positivity were 38.2 ng/ml (77% area under the curve) for stimulated Tg and 1.9 ng/ml (80% area under the curve) for suppressed Tg. Sensitivity, specificity, and accuracy values of PET/CT were 94%, 100%, and 93%, respectively, for Tg> 38.2 ng/ml. After PET/CT, the treatment plan was changed in 39% of patients (operation, RT, or other local treatments). Of the 75 PET-positive cases, 69 were correctly positive and 6 (6/69, 9%) of these patients had disease-specific mortality at 5-year follow-up, while all PET-negative patients (30/105) survived during follow-up. However, recurrences were observed during follow-up in the patient group with negative PET, high stimulated Tg values (97.3 ± 139.4 ng/ml), and suppressed Tg value >1 ng/ml (3.9 ng/ml average) (Fig. 6.6). Although PET was negative and stimulated Tg values were high (mean 28 ± 29.8 ng/ml), no recurrence was observed during approximately 5-year follow-up in the suppressed (<1 ng/ml) patient group under T4. It has been argued that this can predict good prognosis-disease-free survival if PET is negative and Tg is "suppressible," even if stimulated Tg values are high. In another retrospective study conducted by Akkaş et al., prognostic factors affecting disease-specific survival were investigated in 77 patients with PET-positive recurrent and/or metastatic DTC. Accordingly, in the multivariate analysis, the absence of vascular inva-

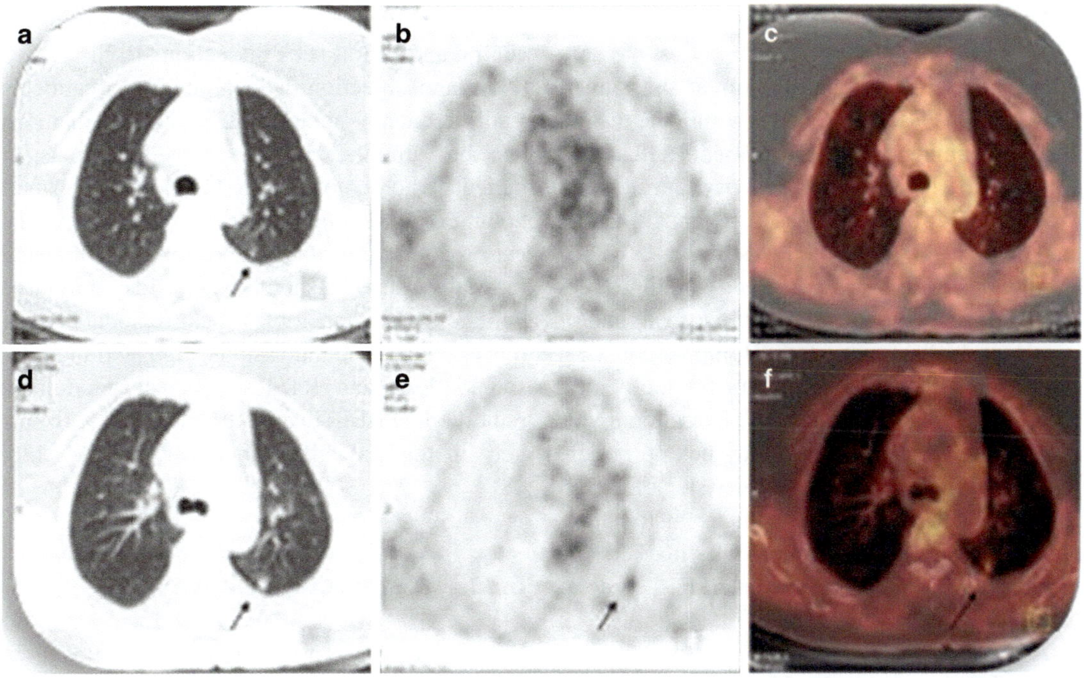

Fig. 6.6 In the PET/CT examination (**a**–**c**) performed while Tg was 4 ng/ml under suppression in the patient with Hurthle cell thyroid cancer, millimetric nodule was observed in the upper lobe of the left lung, and pathological FDG uptake was not observed. After 7 months, Tg increased to 7 ng/ml under suppression. It is noteworthy that nodule size increases and pathological FDG involvement is observed in follow-up PET/CT examination (**d**–**f**)

sion (*p*: 0.04) and the surgical feasibility of recurrence or metastasis (*p*: 0.0001) and the suppression of Tg (*p*: 0.01) were found to be significant, while TNM staging, the number-localization of FDG-positive lesions, and SUV max values did not affect the clinical course [103].

We have previously stated that increased levels of *anti-Tg* after surgery and RAI require a personal approach and follow-up in terms of possible recurrent disease. In these cases, first neck USG and then RAI diagnostic scan can be considered. However, the neck USG may show local-regional recurrence, and RAI scan is usually insufficient, given the low spatial resolution and the fact that the lesion may be iodine-negative. FDG PET/CT imaging was investigated in RAI negative and anti-Tg positive cases. The first study was conducted by Chung et al. in 2002 in 26 DTCs which were Tg negative with anti-Tg increase, and recurrence was detected with PET in 50% of patients. Sensitivity, specificity, and accuracy of FDG PET/CT were 84.6%, 92.3%, and 88.4%, respectively [104]. In another study, Özkan et al. found the sensitivity, specificity, and accuracy of FDG PET/CT to be 75%, 76%, and 80%, respectively, in 31 DTCs which were Tg negative, RAI negative, and USG and thorax CT negative with no initial diagnosis of thyroiditis and increased anti-Tg levels [105]. In conclusion, current studies at persistent or increased anti-Tg levels with Tg negativity during follow-up indicate that FDG PET/CT should be used as an additional test to demonstrate persistent-recurrent disease, especially in RAI-negative patients. If PET is negative, it is argued that there is no persistent-recurrent disease, and anti-Tg levels will tend to decrease during follow-up, but if PET is positive, it will be accompanied by a malignant-aggressive disease [106].

6.32 Local-Regional Recurrence

Local-regional recurrences occur at the rate of 5–30% in DTC, and 66% occur within the first 10 years after diagnosis and treatment, and in my clinical experience, many of them occur at 6 and 7 years [10, 48]. In most cases, diagnosis can be made with detailed and high-resolution USG, Tg washout test, and biopsy. Current guidelines recommend therapeutic central compartment and/or lateral neck dissection if the lymph node with evidence of metastasis is >8mm for the central compartment and >1 cm for the lateral compartment. However, observation may be appropriate in low-volume disease. As in every step of DTCs, individual characteristics (such as histopathology, RAI or FDG uptake, molecular markers, Tg increase rate) should be considered in the operation decision [38, 48, 49].

After the operation, 60–90% of the patients' serum Tg values decrease, 30–50% of them have undetectable levels of Tg (<0.2 ng/ml), and approximately 80% of the patients have a treatment response in terms of structural disease [38].

Recurrence surgery in the neck is very difficult due to previous operations and therapies (such as RT and fibrosis), surgical complications increase, and success decreases. In recent years, although few in the literature, preoperative metastatic lesions are labeled with radio-guided occult lesion localization (ROLL) technique in local-regional recurrences in DTCs, and surgery is performed under the guidance of a gamma probe. In a study conducted in our clinic in conjunction with nuclear medicine and general surgery, preoperative neck mapping and labeling with the ROLL (radioactive labeling with Tc-99m MAA) technique was performed for lymph node metastases proven by biopsy and Tg washout test in 20 patients with BTT and/or central/lateral neck dissection. Patients were operated under the guidance of gamma probe. Thirty-four lesions (85%) of the 40 lesions removed by ROLL technique in 20 patients, and 64% of the other 60 lesions found to be suspicious during the operation were found to be metastatic. In the study, it was concluded that ROLL technique and preoperative neck mapping were quite safe and successful in local-regional recurrent DTCs planned for central and lateral neck dissection [107].

Ethanol injection or local ablative treatments (radiofrequency ablation-RFA or laser ablation) can be administered in repeated sessions in patients who do not want to be operated on small volume lymph node metastases or in whom surgery is contraindicated. The results are promising in small series. RT should be considered in large volume and inoperable local-regional recurrences, soft tissue invasions, and extranodular spread. RAI and RT/dose intensity-modulated radiotherapy (IMRT) are recommended with surgery in tracheal and esophageal invasions [38, 48].

6.33 Metastatic Disease

Distant metastases are the main cause of death in DTCs, and approximately 50% are seen at diagnosis. 35% of Hurthle cell carcinomas (>40 years of age) have distant metastases at diagnosis. In a meta-analysis involving 13 studies and 1231 patients, 49% of distant metastases were in the lung, 25% were in the bone, 15% were in the lung and bone, and the rest were in other organs (brain, soft tissue, skin, and liver) [48, 108]. The main factors affecting disease progression in metastatic DTC are the age of diagnosis, metastasis region-prevalence, RAI uptake, and operability. Ten-year overall survival in distant metastases is between 25% and 40% [109]. There is no specified limit on the cumulative RAI dose in distant metastases with ongoing RAI uptake, but repeated doses above 600 mCi have been reported to not contribute much to complete remission [110].

6.34 Lung Metastases

It can be of micronodular and macronodular type. Metastases may be <1cm, even <2mm in size, and may not be viewed on both diagnostic scan and X-ray and CT (Fig. 6.5). Micronodular-diffuse lung metastases are common in young and children, while macronodular metastases are more common in older patients and have a worse course. In young patients, survival in diffuse RAI-positive, radiology-negative micronodular lung metastases is much longer, and 10-year survival is >50% and the chance of cure is quite high if nodule size is <2 mm [111]. Stimulated Tg values are >10 ng/ml in almost all of them. Tg values under suppression may not be detected in micronodular lung metastases (radiology negative) [108, 111]. The standard RAI treatment dose in lung metastases is 200 mCi, but a dosimetric approach can also be used for dose selection.

In general, selecting the first dose of RAI in metastatic disease in DTCs at the maximum safe dose is important for disease progression. Routine diagnostic I-131 scan during follow-up in metastatic DTC with RAI uptake and high Tg levels under suppression will not change the treatment strategy, and it is generally not necessary due to its hypothyroidism effects and its reducing RAI uptake in subsequent treatments (stunning).

Surgery may be considered in selected cases in lung metastases. Although the contribution of lung metastasectomy surgery to overall survival is unclear, Moneke et al. investigated the contribution of metastasectomy to disease progression in 43 patients with iodine refractory lung metastasis in their retrospective study [112]. In the patient group followed up for an average of 77 months, 72% of the patients who underwent R0 resection had a 10-year survival rate of 100% and 77%, and the survival rate was 62% and 22% in the incomplete resection group, respectively (*P*: 0.01). As a result, it was emphasized that tumor burden was reduced and Tg values decreased significantly and contributed to survival, especially in those who underwent R0 resection with lung metastasectomy.

Local treatments such as RFA or "stereotactic body radiation therapy" (SBRT) may be an alternative to surgery for lung metastases. Due to the repeatability of RFA, it can be applied especially in <3 cm cases without soft tissue-vessel or mediastinal invasion. Otherwise, recurrences are seen in a short time [38].

Recurrent treatments should be considered on a patient-based basis and possible complications should not be underestimated. The contribution of repeated treatments to long-term disease progression in patients with low RAI uptake and negative diagnostic scan is unclear [78, 113]. Sabra et al. reported that 44% remained stable and 56% progressed even though a decrease in Tg was observed in these cases [113]. In a study by our clinic, prognostic factors were investigated in 80 patients with lung metastasis who received BTT and RAI treatment and had an average follow-up of 5 years. At the end of the study, >45 years of age, postoperatively stimulated Tg>100ng/ml, non-PTC histology, and extrapulmonary metastasis were found to be statistically significant in terms of poor prognostic factors affecting clinical course [91].

6.35 Bone Metastases

Since bone metastases in DTCs are generally lytic in nature, bone scintigraphy may not be successful in showing the disease. Bone metastases are better visualized anatomically by CT, MRI, and molecular PET/CT imaging. However, whole-body scan/SPECT after RAI therapy dose or SPECT/CT for anatomical correlation has the highest accuracy in diagnosis, especially in terms of structurally small micrometastasis detection. Tg values are higher than in lung metastases and prognosis is worse. The prognosis in bone metastases is associated with RAI uptake, the prevalence of metastasis, and the presence of accompanying non-bone metastases. Bone metastases of DTC have almost no chance of cure with RAI therapy alone. Although the rate of cure is quite low, survival increases with metastasis surgery, RT, other local treatments, and RAI therapy (multidisciplinary approach – combined treatments) and there may be a chance of cure (Fig. 6.7). Local tumor control with SBRT was reported to be 88–100% in cases undergoing surgery. In incomplete resection, complementary RT to surgery or palliative RT should be considered in terms of pain palliation, spinal cord compression, and pathological fracture risk. However, the repeatability of RT in vertebral metastases is limited to the cumulative spinal cord dose. RFA and

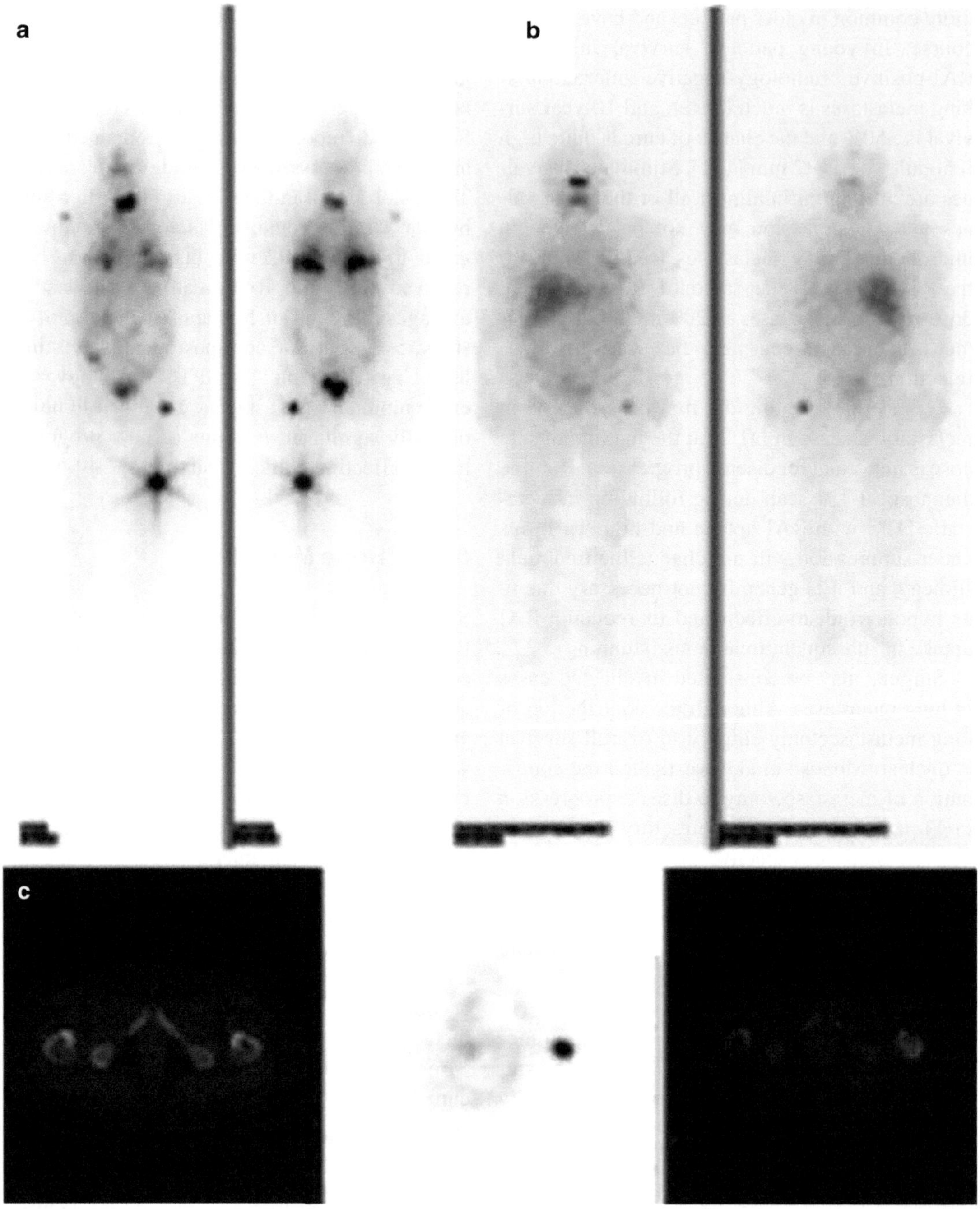

Fig. 6.7 A 53-year-old female patient with FTC (5.5 cm, thyroid capsule invasion). Stimulated Tg 2149 ng/ml, RAI uptake in neck thyroid site, and multiple bone-pulmonary metastases on scan (**a**) on the first treatment dose (250 mCi). On the fourth treatment dose (300 mCi) scan and SPECT/CT study (**b**, **c**), no significant RAI uptake is observed except proximal to the left femur and stimulated Tg is 74 ng/ml. Suppressed Tg is 7.9 ng/ml during follow-up. Combined additional local treatments for left femoral lesion may be considered in the patient with significant treatment response in RAI treatment

cryoablation are promising especially in local control, pain control, and lesion stabilization with cementoplasty [38, 49].

Bone-targeted agents such as "bisphosphonates and denosumab" are recommended in current guidelines in extensive and RAI refractory bone metastases [38, 49]. The effect of kinase inhibitors on bone metastases is low compared to other metastases (such as lung, lymph node and other soft tissue metastases). Denosumab is a human monoclonal (IgG2) antibody against "Receptor activator of nuclear factor kappa-B ligand (RANKL)." In bone microarchitecture, it reduces the risk of fracture by reducing the differentiation of precursor cells to mature osteoclasts, osteoclast function, and life span of osteoclasts. In DTC bone metastases, bone-targeted agents improve symptoms and quality of life by reducing fracture risk, delaying pain and neurological complications. Adequate renal functions, serum Ca level, and dental evaluation are important before treatment. Hypocalcemia and mandibular osteonecrosis are the possible risks of these agents. Ca and vitamin D supplementation and oral and dental health controls can reduce risks. Denosumab has been reported to have less risk than zoledronic acid [38].

6.36 Brain Metastasis

Brain metastases are rare in DTCs at about 1% [114]. It is usually associated with advanced age patients and advanced disease. In progressive Tg increases during follow-up, brain metastases should be kept in mind and brain MRI should be performed. Surgery and SBRT are the primary treatments for brain metastases. There are little data demonstrating the effectiveness of RAI treatment in brain metastases with RAI uptake. Starting high-dose corticosteroids before RT and RAI treatment is important to prevent possible cerebral edema. Local control can be achieved if the number of metastatic foci is low, but since patients generally have poor prognostic characteristics, they are mostly lost due to extracerebral progressive disease [115, 116].

6.37 Iodine-Refractory Disease

Surgery, adjuvant RAI ablation/ treatment, and TSH suppression in DTCs lead to a 10-year survival rate of approximately 90%. However, about 20% local recurrence and 10% distant metastasis may develop, and surgery, EBRT, and other local treatments are applied with RAI treatment. All these multidisciplinary approaches provide a complete treatment response in only one-third of the cases, while the remaining two-thirds develop RAI refractory DTC and have a poor prognosis [117]. Reduction of NIS expression in RAI refractory DTC pathogenesis is associated with decreased Tg, TSH, and thyroperoxidase (TPO) receptors. Thus, DTC cells lose the ability to concentrate RAI. In addition, the MAPK (mitogen-activated protein kinase) pathway is also responsible for dedifferentiation and progression. The most known activators of the MAPK pathway are BRAF mutations [118].

Definition of RAI refractory DTC includes (**a**) the absence of RAI uptake in metastatic tissue other than thyroid bed in the first treatment, (**b**) reduction and loss of uptake in structurally existing tumoral tissue with previous RAI uptake (false negativity should be ruled out, e.g., non-radioactive iodine intake), (**c**) RAI uptake is observed in some lesions, while in some lesions there is no uptake, and (**d**) structural progression in metastatic disease despite RAI uptake [119]. In addition, it is reported that DTC cases with no RAI cumulative treatment dose >600 mCi effective treatment response are also in the RAI refractory group [38, 120].

Neck USG and FDG PET/CT (stimulated Tg > 10 ng/ml) should be considered primarily for the diagnosis of RAI refractory disease. Somatostatin receptor imaging plays a complementary role in PET/CT [121], diagnostic CT, and MRI. In the treatment, personal factors such as the localization, prevalence of structural disease, and the time of Tg duplication should be taken into consideration. Depending on the current situation, active monitoring, local therapies, and systemic therapies should be administered, respectively.

6.38 Systemic (Targeted) Therapies

Targeted chemotherapies mainly have two mechanisms of action with inhibition of angiogenesis and cell proliferation. In recent years, multikinase inhibitors (MKIs) have been used in RAI refractory DTCs with their antiangiogenic properties. Sorafenib and lenvatinib are FDA-approved for RAI refractory DTCs. Phase III clinical trials of both drugs have been published, and they have been shown to improve progression-free survival in progressive DTC [122, 123]. In the randomized placebo-controlled clinical phase III studies DECISION (sorafenib) [122] and SELECT (lenvatinib) [123], progression-free survival (PFS) was investigated in RAI refractory DTC patients, and treatment response assessment was performed according to RECIST criteria. The median PFS was 10.8 months versus 5.8 months ($p < 0.0001$) in 417 patients with refractory DTC in the sorafenib (800 mg/day) group compared to the placebo group, respectively. In the lenvatinib (24 mg/day) group, median PFS was 18.3 months versus 3.6 months ($p < 0.001$) in 392 patients with progressive DTC. In both studies, the contribution to overall survival was not statistically significant. Regarding the side effects of both drugs, hypertension, bleeding, intestinal symptoms (diarrhea), impaired liver and kidney function, weight loss, skin lesions (hand-foot skin reactions), and mucositis are side effects that may impair the quality of life or even cause death. Furthermore, an increase in TSH levels can be observed, so it should be checked frequently and the suppression level should be adjusted [119, 124]. In addition to the side effects of the drugs, timing and patient selection are very important for systemic treatment. Systemic therapies may be considered in rapidly growing (<12 months), progressive, symptomatic patients with large tumor burden and no response to local therapies or in whom local therapies cannot be applied. Increased serum Tg alone does not create indications in terms of systemic treatment; there should be symptomatic-structural disease progression [125].

Lin et al. used FDG PET/CT SUV max values and serum Tg levels in terms of biochemical response at 4 and 8 weeks after treatment to assess the early molecular treatment response together with RECIST in evaluating the treatment response after apatinib (750 mg/day) in 10 DTC patients with progressive-RAI refractory. In addition to RECIST 1.1, they suggested that serum Tg and FDG PET/CT SUV max values could be used to evaluate early treatment response [126]. Since molecular imaging with PET/CT is also used in addition to anatomical imaging in routine patient selection for MKI, morphological (USG, CT, MR) imaging, biochemical (serum Tg), and molecular imaging (PET/CT) play a complementary and integrative role in terms of RECIST criteria in the treatment response and follow-up process.

Today, the extension studies of sorafenib and lenvatinib are still ongoing and initial clinical studies on different MKIs (such as pazopanib, axitinib, selumetinib, everolimus, gefitinib) are also ongoing in progressive RAI refractory DTCs, and the results are promising [127, 128].

6.39 Redifferentiation Therapy

Studies limited to retinoic acid, PPARγ agonists (such as rosiglitazone, piaglitazone), and histone deacetylase inhibitors (such as HDI-valproic acid, panobinostat), which are older for regulating impaired or decreased NIS function in dedifferentiated thyroid cancers, have shown that RAI uptake can be increased, but no clear results have been obtained due to the few number of patients and prospective studies and differences in administration [129–131]. Recently, clinical studies to improve NIS restoration and RAI uptake with BRAF (dabrafenib), mitogen-activated and extracellular signal regulated kinase-MEK inhibitors (selumetinib), and MKIs (sorafenib) have been ongoing [132, 133].

6.40 Other Theranostic Approaches

In recent years, peptide receptor radionuclide therapy (PRRT) with imaging and theranostic approach with somatostatin receptors (especially SSTR-2 and SSTR-5) is promising in iodine-refractory or iodine-negative DTCs. Budiawan et al. treated 16 patients with thyroid cancer (8 medullary, 4 FTC, 3 Hurthle cell cancer, and 1 mixed) with Y-90 and Lu-177 DOTATATE and reported a promising treatment response and survival benefit (mean survival 4.2 years and mean progression-free survival 25 months after the first PRRT) with minimal toxicity [134].

Czepczynski et al. administered Y-90 DOTATOC (100 mCi) treatment with a 12-week interval in 11 iodine-negative DTC patients. They were able to complete four doses in six patients and reported an average survival of 21 months [135]. Although PRRT appears promising in iodine-negative DTCs, randomized prospective studies are needed in larger series on this subject.

Tumor-associated neovascularization and PSMA (prostate-specific membrane antigen) expression in poorly differentiated and anaplastic thyroid cancers has recently been one of the research topics. It is emphasized that it can open a new window in terms of PSMA-targeted anti-neovascular or radioligand treatments in the future in dedifferentiated thyroid cancers and should be investigated [136]. Verma et al. found that metastatic foci were 81.8% and 93.7% positive in FDG PET/CT and Ga-68 PSMA PET/CT imaging in ten patients with metastatic DTC, respectively. They localized metastatic lesions in two iodine-negative and Tg-positive patients with Ga-68 PSMA PET/CT and argued that PSMA imaging could be used in the selection of patients with iodine-negative-refractory DTC who have no other treatment option and can benefit from PSMA-targeted radionuclide therapies [137].

6.41 Concluding Remarks

In this section, in which diagnosis, treatment, and follow-up plans in DTCs have been reviewed with current data, guidelines, and clinical experience, the importance of dynamic risk factors in the postoperative process and post-treatment follow-up, the limit of thyroid surgery with an approach based on risk analysis, the need and limit for central-cervical lymph node dissection, the need for adjuvant RAI ablation/treatment, the need and level of TSH suppression, the determination of follow-up intensity and duration, external irradiation, and other local and systemic treatments have been discussed.

Each DTC patient has unique clinical-histopathological risks and needs a personalized treatment and follow-up plan. In addition, the fact that national and international regulations may differ and socio-cultural and economic characteristics may affect the treatment and follow-up plan in this disease requiring long-term follow-up should be taken into consideration.

In RAI ablation/treatment applications, which are the first of the theranostic practices and reduce the risk of recurrence and disease-specific death based on evidence in DTCs throughout the decades, the indication should be determined correctly, the necessary dose and frequency of treatment should be applied, a dosimetric approach should be considered in selected cases, precautions should be taken in terms of possible short- and long-term complications, and unnecessary treatments should be avoided.

References

1. TCSB HalkSağlığıGenelMüdürlüğü, Türkiye-Kanserİstatistikleri 2015. https://hsgm.saglik.gov.tr/tr/kanser-istatistikleri.
2. Ferlay J, Soerjomataram I, Ervik M, et al. GLOBOCAN 2012 v1.0, Cancer Incidence and Mortality Worldwide: IARC CancerBase No. 11 [Internet]. Lyon, France: International Agency for

Research on Cancer; 2013. ErişimAdresi: http://globocan.iarc.fr
3. Noone AM, Howlader N, Krapcho M, et al. SEER Cancer Statistics Review, 1975–2015. Bethesda, MD., https://seer.cancer.gov/csr/1975_2015/, based on November 2017 SEER data submission, posted to the SEER web site: National Cancer Institute; 2018.
4. Dal Maso L, Bosetti C, VecchiaC L, et al. Risk factors for thyroid cancer. Cancer Causes Control. 2009;20(1):75–86.
5. Aschebrook-Kilfoy B, Schechter RB, Shih YC, Kaplan EL, Chiu BC, Angelos P, et al. The clinical and economic burden of a sustained increase in thyroid cancer incidence. Cancer Epidemiol Biomark Prev. 2013;22(7):1252–9.
6. Lim H, Devesa SS, Sosa JA, et al. Trends in thyroid cancer incidence and mortality in the United States, 1974–2013. JAMA. 2017;317(13):1338–48.
7. Sherman SI. Thyroid carcinoma. Lancet. 2003;361:501–11.
8. Durante C, Haddy N, Baudin E, et al. Long-term outcome of 444 patients with distant metastases from papillary andfollicular thyroid carcinoma: benefits and limits of radioiodine therapy. J Clin Endocrinol Metab. 2006;91:2892–9.
9. Schlumberger M, Pacini F. Thyroid tumors. 2nd ed. Nucleon, 2003, pp. 193–207.
10. Amin MB, Edge SB, Greene FL, et al., editors. AJCC cancer staging manual. 8th ed. New York: Springer; 2017.
11. Andrey Bychkov. Thyroid cancer World Health Organization (WHO) classification. Revised: 9 January 2018, last major update September 2017 Copyright: (c) 2002–2018, PathologyOutlines.com, Inc. PubMed Search: WHO classification of thyroid cancer.
12. Islam S. Papillary carcinoma—general. Pathology Outlines.com website. http://www.pathologyoutlines.com/topic/thyroidpapillary.html. Accessed December 2nd, 2018.
13. Maceri DR, Babyak J, Ossakow SJ. Lateral neck mass. Sole presenting sign of metastatic thyroid cancer. Arch Otolaryngol Head Neck Surg. 1986;112(1):47–9.
14. Ahn JE, Lee JH, Yi JS, et al. Diagnostic accuracy of CT and ultrasonography for evaluating metastatic cervical lymph nodes in patients with thyroid cancer. World J Surg. 2008;32(7):1552–8.
15. Arturi F, Russo D, Giuffrida D, et al. Early diagnosis by genetic analysis of differentiated thyroid cancer metastases in small lymph nodes. J Clin Endocrinol Metab. 1997;82(5):1638–41.
16. Xing M. BRAF mutation in thyroid cancer. Endocr Relat Cancer. 2005;12:245–62.
17. Chen JH, Faquin WC, Lloyd RV, et al. Clinicopathological and molecular characterization of nine cases of columnar cell variant of papillary thyroid carcinoma. Mod Pathol. 2011;24:739–49.
18. Asioli S, Erickson LA, Sebo TJ, et al. Papillary thyroid carcinoma with prominent hobnail features: a new aggressive variant of moderately differentiated papillary carcinoma. A clinicopathologic, immunohistochemical, and molecular study of eight cases. Am J Surg Pathol. 2010;34:44–52.
19. Lam AK, Lo CY. Diffusesclerosing variant of papillary carcinoma of the thyroid: a 35-year comparative study at a single institution. Ann Surg Oncol. 2006;13(2):176–81.
20. Thomas GA, Bunnell H, Cook HA, et al. High prevalence of RET/PTC rearrangements in Ukrainian and Belarussian post-Chernobyl thyroid papillary carcinomas: a strong correlation between RET/PTC3 and the solid- follicular variant. J Clin Endocrinol Metab. 1999;84(11):4232–8.
21. Lim YC, Choi EC, Yoon YH, et al. Central lymph node metastases in unilateral papillary thyroid microcarcinoma. Br J Surg. 2009;96(3):253–7.
22. Hay ID, Hutchinson ME, Gonzalez-Losada T, et al. Papillary thyroid microcarcinoma: a study of 900 cases observed in a 60-year period. Surgery. 2008;144(6):980–79.
23. Niemeier LA, KuffnerAkatsu H, et al. A combined molecular-pathologic score improves risk stratification of thyroid papillary microcarcinoma. Cancer. 2012;118(8):2069–77.
24. Rivera M, Ricarte-Filho J, Knauf J, et al. Molecular genotyping of papillary thyroid carcinoma follicular variant according to its histological subtypes (encapsulated vs infiltrative) reveals distinct BRAF and RAS mutation patterns. Mod Pathol. 2010;23:1191–200.
25. Howitt BE, Jia Y, Sholl LM, et al. Molecular alterations in partially-encapsulated or well-circumscribed follicular variant of papillary thyroid carcinoma. Thyroid. 2013;23:1256–62.
26. Nikiforova MN, Lynch RA, Biddinger PW, et al. RAS point mutations and PAX8-PPAR gamma rearrangement in thyroid tumors: evidence for distinct molecular pathways in thyroid follicular carcinoma. J Clin Endocrinol Metab. 2003;88(5):2318–26.
27. Nikiforova MN, Biddinger PW, Caudill CM, et al. PAX8-PPAR gamma rearrangement in thyroid tumors: RT- PCR and immunohistochemical analyses. Am J Surg Pathol. 2002;26(8):1016–23.
28. Nikiforov YE, Ohori NP. Follicular carcinoma. In: Nikiforov YE, Biddinger PW, Thompson LDR, editors. Diagnostic pathology and molecular genetics of the thyroid. 2nd ed. Philadelphia, PA: Lippincott Williams and Wilkins; 2012. p. 152–82.
29. Hiltzik D, Carlson DL, Tuttle RM, et al. Poorly differentiated thyroid carcinomas defined on the basis of mitosis and necrosis: a clinicopathologic study of 58 patients. Cancer. 2006;106:1286–95.
30. Gnemmi V, Renaud F, Do Cao C, et al. Poorly differentiated thyroid carcinomas: application of the Turin proposal provides prognostic results similar to those from the assessment of high-grade features. Histopathology. 2014;64:263–73.
31. Boelaert K, Horacek J, Holder RL, et al. Serum thyrotropin concentration as a novel predictor of

malignancy in thyroid nodules investigated by fine-needle aspiration. J Clin Endocrinol Metab. 2006;91(11):4253–5.
32. Haymart MR, Repplinger DJ, Leverson GE, et al. Higher serum thyroid stimulating hormone level in thyroid nodule patients is associated with greater risks of differentiated thyroid cancer and advanced tumor stage. J Clin Endocrinol Metab. 2008;93(3):809–14.
33. Soelberg KK, Bonnema SJ, Brix TH, et al. Risk of malignancy in thyroid incidentalomas detected by 18F- fluorodeoxyglucose positron emission tomography: a systematic review. Thyroid. 2012;22:918–25.
34. Leenhardt L, Erdogan MF, Hegedus L, et al. European Thyroid Association Guidelines for cervical ultrasound scan and ultrasound-guided techniques in the postoperative management of patients with thyroid cancer. Eur Thyroid J. 2013;2013(2):147–59.
35. Cibas ES, Ali SZ. The Bethesda system for reporting thyroid cytopathology. Am J ClinPathol. 2009;132:658–65.
36. Bongiovanni M, Spitale A, Faquin WC, et al. The Bethesda system for reporting thyroid cytopathology: a meta-analysis. Acta Cytol. 2012;56:333–9.
37. Haugen BR, Alexander EK, Bible KC, et al. 2015 American Thyroid Association management guidelines for adult patients with thyroid nodules and differentiated thyroid cancer: the American Thyroid Association guidelines task force on thyroid nodules and differentiated thyroid cancer. Thyroid. 2016;26:1–133.
38. Harish K. Neck dissections: radical to conservative. World J Surg Oncol. 2005;3:21. https://doi.org/10.1186/1477-7819-3-21.
39. Kocharyan D, Schwenter F, Bélair M. The relevance of preoperative ultrasound cervical mapping in patients with thyroid cancer. Can J Surg. 2016;59(2):113–7.
40. Jeon MJ, Park JW, Han JM, et al. Serum antithyroglobulin antibodies interfere with thyroglobulin detection in fine-needle aspirates of metastatic neck nodes in papillary thyroid carcinoma. J Clin Endocrinol Metab. 2013;98:153–60.
41. Lee MJ, Ross DS, Mueller PR, et al. Fine-needle biopsy cervical lymph nodes in patients with thyroid cancer: a prospective comparison of cytopathologic and tissue marker analysis. Radiology. 1993;187(3):851–4.
42. McLeod DS, Cooper DS, Ladenson PW, For the National Thyroid Cancer Treatment Cooperative Study Group, et al. Prognosis of differentiated thyroid cancer in relation to serum thyrotropin and thyroglobulin antibody status at time of diagnosis. Thyroid. 2014;24:35–42.
43. Cady B, Rossi R. An expanded view on risk group definition in differentiated thyroid carcinoma. Surgery. 1988;104:947–53.
44. Hay I, Grant CS, Taylor W, et al. Ipsilateral lobectomy versus bilateral lobar dissection in papillary thyroid carcinoma: a retrospective analysis of surgical outcome using a novel prognostic system. Surgery. 1987;102:1088–95.
45. Hay ID, Bergstralh EJ, Goellner JR, et al. Predicting outcome in papillary thyroid carcinoma: Development of a reliable prognostic scoring system in a cohort of 1779 patients surgically treated at one institution during 1940 through 1989. Surgery. 1993;114:1050–8.
46. International Union Against Cancer (UICC) Committee on Clinical Stage Classification and Applied Statistics. Clinical Stage Classification and Presentation of Results, Malignant Tumours of the Breast and Larynx. Paris, 1958. www.iarc.fr.
47. NCCN Clinical Practice Guidelines in ONCOLOGY: Thyroid Carcinoma V2 2018. www.nccn.org.
48. Perros P, Colley S, Boelaert K, et al. British Thyroid Association Guidelines for the management of thyroid cancer. Clin Endocrinol. 2014;81(suppl. 1):1–122.
49. Spencer CA, LoPresti JS, Fatemi S, et al. Detection of residual and recurrent differentiated thyroid carcinoma by serum thyroglobulin measurement. Thyroid. 1999;9:435–41.
50. Giovanella L, Keller F, Ceriani L, et al. Heterophile antibodies may falsely increase or decrease thyroglobulin measurement in patients with differentiated thyroid carcinoma. Clin Chem Lab Med. 2009;47:952–4.
51. Rosario PW, Filho AFCM, Prates BS, et al. Postoperative stimulated thyroglobulin of less than 1 ng/ml as a criterion to spare low-risk patients with papillary thyroid cancer from radioactive iodine ablation. Thyroid. 2012;22(11):1140–3.
52. Yang X, Liang J, Jun Li T, et al. Postoperative stimulated thyroglobulin level and recurrence risk stratification in differentiated thyroid cancer. Chin Med J. 2015;128(8):1058–64.
53. Kim TY, Kim WB, Kim ES, et al. Serum thyroglobulin levels at the time of 131I remnant ablation just after thyroidectomy are useful for early prediction of clinical recurrence in low-risk patients with differentiated thyroid carcinoma. J Clin Endocrinol Metab. 2005;90:1440–5.
54. Piccardo A, Arecco F, Puntoni M, et al. Focus on high-risk DTC patients: high postoperative serum thyroglobulin level is a strong predictor of disease persistence and is associated to progression-free survival and overall survival. ClinNucl Med. 2013;38:18–24.
55. Cooper DS, Doherty GM, Haugen BR, et al. Revised American thyroid association management guidelines for patients with thyroid nodules and differentiated thyroid cancer. Thyroid. 2009;19(11):1167–214.
56. Sisson JC, Jamadar DA, Kazerooni EA, et al. Treatment of micronodular lung métastases of papillary thyroid cancer: are the tumors too small for effective irradiation from radioiodine? Thyroid. 1998;8(3):215–21.

57. Muresan MM, Olivier P, Lecle're J, et al. Bone metastases from differentiated thyroid carcinoma. Endocr Relat Cancer. 2008;15:37–49.
58. Filetti S, Bidart JM, Arturi F, et al. Sodium/iodide symporter: a key transport system in thyroid cancer cell metabolism. Eur J Endocrinol. 1999;141:443–57.
59. Seidlin SM, Marinelli LD, Oshry E. Radioactive iodine therapy: effect on functioning metastases of adenocarcinoma of thyroid. JAMA. 1946;132:838–47.
60. Maxon HR, Thomas SR, Hertzberg VS, et al. Relation between effective radiation dose and outcome of radioiodine therapy for thyroid cancer. N Engl J Med. 1983;309:937–41.
61. Zanzonico PB. Internal radionuclide radiation dosimetry: a review of basic concepts and recent developments. J Nucl Med. 2000;41:297–308.
62. Benua RS, Cicale NR, Sonenberg M, et al. The relation of radioiodine dosimetry to results and complications in the treatment of metastatic thyroid cancer. Am J Roentgenol Radium Ther Nucl Med. 1962;87:171–82.
63. Leeper RD, Shimaoka K. Treatment of metastatic thyroid cancer. Clin Endocrinol Metab. 1980;9:383–404.
64. Hong CM, Ahn B-C. Factors associated with dose determination of radioactive iodine therapy for differentiated thyroid cancer. Nucl Med Mol Imag. 2018;52(4):247–53.
65. Freudenberg LS, Jentzen W, Stahl A, et al. Clinical applications of 124I-PET/CT in patients with differentiated thyroid cancer. Eur J Nucl Med Mol Imaging. 2011;38(Suppl. 1):S48–56.
66. Chen MK, Cheng DW. What is the role of dosimetry in patients with advanced thyroid cancer? Curr Opin Oncol. 2015;27:33–7.
67. Wierts R, Brans B, Havekes B, et al. Dose–response relationship in differentiated thyroid cancer patients undergoing radioiodine treatment assessed by means of 124I PET/CT. J Nucl Med. 2016; https://doi.org/10.2967/jnumed.115.168799.
68. Mallick U, Harmer C, Yap B, et al. Ablation with low-dose radioiodine and thyrotropin alfa in thyroid cancer. N Engl J Med. 2012;366:1674–85.
69. Schlumberger M, Catargi B, Borget I, et al. Strategies of radioiodine ablation in patients with low-risk thyroid cancer. N Engl J Med. 2012;366:1663–73.
70. Song X, Meng Z, Jia Q, et al. Different radioiodine dose for remnant thyroid ablation in patients with differentiated thyroid cancer: a meta-analysis. Clin Nucl Med. 2015;40:774–9.
71. Jeong JH, Kong EJ, Jeong SY, et al. Clinical outcomes of low-dose and high-dose postoperative radioiodine therapy in patients with intermediate-risk differentiated thyroid cancer. Nucl Med Commun. 2017;38:228–33.
72. Samuel AM, Rajashekharrao B, Shah DH. Pulmonary metastases in children and adolescents with well-differentiated thyroid cancer. J Nucl Med. 1998;39:1531–6.
73. Verburg FA, Hänscheid H, Luster M. Radioactive iodine (RAI) therapy for metastatic differentiated thyroid cancer. Best Pract Res Clin Endocrinol Metab. 2017;31:279–90.
74. Francis GL, Waguespack SG, Bauer AJ. Management guidelines for children with thyroid nodules and differentiated thyroid cancer. Thyroid. 2015;25(7):716–59.
75. Rubino C, de Vathaire F, Dottorini ME, et al. Second primary malignancies in thyroid cancer patients. Br J Cancer. 2003;89:1638–44.
76. Chao M. Management of differentiated thyroid cancer with rising thyroglobulin and negative diagnostic radioiodine whole body scan. Clin Oncol. 2010;22:438–47.
77. Kabasakal L, Selcuk NA, Shafipour H, et al. Treatment of iodine-negative thyroglobulin positive thyroid cancer: differences in outcome in patients with macrometastases and patients with micrometastases. Eur J Nucl Med Mol Imaging. 2004;31:1500–4.
78. Gorman CA. Radioiodine and pregnancy. Thyroid. 1999;9(7):721–6.
79. Benbassat CA, Mechlis-Frish S, Hirsch D. Clinicopathological characteristics and long-term outcome in patientswith distant metastases from differentiated thyroid cancer. World J Surg. 2006;30:1088–95.
80. Hänscheid H, Lassmann M, Luster M, et al. Iodine biokinetics and dosimetry in radioiodine therapy of thyroid cancer: procedures and results of a prospective international controlled study of ablation after rhTSH or hormone withdrawal. J Nucl Med. 2006;47(4):648–54.
81. Silberstein EB, Alavi A, Balon HR, et al. The SNM Practice Guideline for therapy of thyroid disease with 131I. J Nucl Med. 2012;53(10):1633–51.
82. Ciappuccini R, Heutte N, Trzepla G, et al. Postablation (131)I scintigraphy with neck and thorax SPECT-CT and stimulated serum thyroglobulin level predict the outcome of patients with differentiated thyroid cancer. Eur J Endocrinol. 2011;164:961–9.
83. Vural G, Erçakmak N, Aslan S, et al. Diagnostic and post-therapy I-131 whole body scans in patients with well-differentiated thyroid carcinoma. J Nucl Med. 1999;40(5):235.
84. Garsi JP, Schlumberger M, Rubino C, et al. Therapeutic administration of 131I for differentiated thyroid cancer: radiation dose to ovaries and outcome of pregnancies. J Nucl Med. 2008;49(5):845–52.
85. Özülker T, Adaş M, Günay S. Thyroid and parathyroid diseases: a case-based guide. In: Uçmak G, Akkaş BE, editors. Thyrotoxicosis caused by functioning metastases of differentiated thyroid cancer. Springer; 2019. p. 193–200. https://doi.org/10.1007/978-3-319-78476-2-51.
86. Nakada K, Ishibashi T, Takei T, et al. Does lemon candy decrease salivary gland damage after radio-

iodine therapy for thyroid cancer? J Nucl Med. 2005;46:261–6.
87. Petrich T, Widjaja A, Musholt TJ, et al. Outcome after radioiodine therapy in 107 patients with differentiated thyroid carcinoma and initial bone metastases: side-effects and influence of age. Eur J Nucl Med. 2001;28(2):203–8.
88. Brown AP, Chen J, Hitchcock YJ, et al. The risk of second primary malignancies up to three decades after the treatment of differentiated thyroid cancer. J Clin Endocrinol Metab. 2008;93:504–15.
89. Marti JL, Jain KS, Morris LGT. Increased risk of second primary malignancy in pediatric and young adult patients treated with radioactive iodine for differentiated thyroid cancer. Thyroid. 2015;25(6):681–7.
90. Chen L, Shen Y, Luo Q, et al. Pulmonary fibrosis following radioiodine therapy of pulmonary metastases from differentiated thyroid carcinoma. Thyroid. 2010;20:337–40.
91. Vural GU, Tazeler Z, Demirel BB, et al. Treatment and long term follow up results of differentiated thyroid carcinoma patients with lung metastasis. Eur J Nucl Med. 2011;38(suppl 2):346–7.
92. Hays MT, Wegner LH. A mathematical and physiological model for early distribution of radioiodine in man. J Appl Physiol. 1965;20:1319–28.
93. Jonklaas J, Bianco AC, Bauer AJ, et al. Guidelines for the treatment of hypothyroidism: prepared by the american thyroid association task force on thyroid hormone replacement. Thyroid. 2014;24(12):1670–751.
94. Luster M, Clarke SE, Dietlein M, et al. Guidelines for radioiodine therapy of differentiated thyroid cancer. Eur J Nucl Med Mol Imaging. 2008;35(10):1941–59.
95. Saracyn M, Bilski M, Kaminski G, et al. Can radioiodine be administered effectively and safely to a patient with severe chronic kidney disease? Clin Endocrinol. 2014;81:169–74.
96. Bhat M, Mozzor M, Chugh S, et al. Dosing of radioactive iodine in end-stage renal disease patient with thyroid cancer. Endocrinol Diab Metab. 2017:17-0111, 1–6. https://doi.org/10.1530/EDM-17-0111.
97. Hughes DT, Haymart MR, Miller BS, et al. The most commonly occurring papillary thyroid cancer in the United States is now a microcarcinoma in a patient older than 45 years. Thyroid. 2011;21:231–6.
98. Gallicchio R, Giacomobono S, Capacchione D, et al. Should patients with remnants from thyroid microcarcinoma really not be treated with iodine-131 ablation? Endocrine. 2013;44:426–33.
99. Creach KM, Siegel BA, Nussenbaum B, et al. Radioactive iodine therapy decreases recurrence in thyroid papillary microcarcinoma. ISRN Endocrinol. 2012;2012:816386.
100. Roti E, degli Uberti EC, Bondanelli M, et al. Thyroid papillary microcarcinoma: a descriptive and meta-analysis study. Eur J Endocrinol. 2008;159:659–73.
101. Dietlein M, Eschner W, Grünwald F, Lassmann M, Verburg FA, Luster M. Procedure guidelines for radioiodine therapy of differentiated thyroid cancer. Version 4. Nuklearmedizin. 2016;55:77–89.
102. UçmakVural G, Akkaş BE, Erçakmak N, et al. Prognostic significance of FDG-PET/CT on the follow up of patients of differentiated thyroid carcinoma with negative I-131 whole body scan and elevated thyroglobulin levels: correlation with clinical and histhopathological characteristics and long-term follow-up data. Clin Nucl Med. 2012;37(10):953–9.
103. Akkaş BE, Demirel BB, Vural G, U. Prognostic factors effecting disease specific survival in patients with recurrent and/or metastatic differentiated thyroid carcinoma detected by PET/CT. Thyroid. 2013;24(2):287–95.
104. Chung JK, Park YJ, Kim TY, et al. Clinical significance of elevated level of serum antithyroglobulin antibody in patients with differentiated thyroid cancer after thyroid ablation. Clin Endocrinol. 2002;57:215–21.
105. Ozkan E, Aras G, Kucuk NO. Correlation of F18-FDG PET/CT findings with histopathological results in differentiated thyroid cancer patients who have increased thyroglobulin or antithyroglobulin antibody levels and negative I-131 whole-body scan results. Clin Nucl Med. 2013;38:326–31.
106. Bogsrud TV, Hay ID, Karantanis D, et al. Prognostic value of F18-FDG-PET in patients with differentiated thyroid carcinoma and circulating antithyroglobulin autoantibodies. Nucl Med Commun. 2011;32:245–51.
107. Gulcelik MA, Karaman N, Dogan L, et al. Radioguided occult lesion localization for locally recurrent thyroid carcinoma. Eur Arch Otorhinolaryngol. 2017;274(7):2915–9.
108. Pacini F, Cetani F, Miccoli P, et al. Outcome of 309 patients with metastatic differentiated thyroid carcinoma treated with radioiodine. World J Surg. 1994;18(4):600–4.
109. Mazzaferri EL, KloosR T. Current approaches to primary therapy for papillary and follicular thyroid cancer. J Clin Endocrinol Metab. 2001;86(4):1447–63.
110. Thies ED, Tanase K, Maeder U, et al. The number of 131I therapy courses needed to achieve complete remission is an indicator of prognosis in patients with differentiated thyroid carcinoma. Eur J Nucl Med Mol Imaging. 2014;41:2281–90.
111. Ilgan S, Karacalioglu AO, Pabuscu Y, et al. Iodine-131 treatment and high-resolution CT: results in patients with lung metastases from differentiated thyroid carcinoma. Eur J Nucl Med Mol Imaging. 2004;31:825–30.
112. Moneke I, Kaifia JT, Kloesera R, et al. Pulmonary metastasectomy for thyroid cancer as salvage therapy for radioactive iodine-refractory metastases. Eur J Cardiothorac Surg. 2018;53(3):625–30.
113. Sabra MM, Grewal RK, Tala H, et al. Clinical outcomes following empiric radioiodine therapy in patients with structurally identifiable metastatic follicular cell-derived thyroid carcinoma with negative

diagnostic but positive post-therapy 131 I whole-body scans. Thyroid. 2012;22:877–83.
114. Henriques de Figueiredo B, Godbert Y, Soubeyran I, et al. Brain metastases from thyroid carcinoma : A retrospective study of 21 patients. Thyroid. 2014;24:270–7.
115. Choi J, Kim JW, Keum YS, et al. The Largest Known Survival Analysis of Patients with Brain Metastasis from Thyroid Cancer Based on Prognostic Groups. PLoS One. 2016;29(11):e0154739. https://doi.org/10.1371/journal.pone.0154739.
116. Özülker T, Adaş M, Günay S. Thyroid and parathyroid diseases: a case-based guide. In: Uçmak G, Akkaş BE, editors. . Differentiated thyroid cancer with brain metastasis, Springer; 2019. p. 323–30. https://doi.org/10.1007/978-3-319-78476-2-51.
117. Durante C, Haddy N, Baudin E, et al. Long-term outcome of 444 patients with distant metastases from papillary and follicular thyroid carcinoma: benefits and limits of radioiodine therapy. J Clin Endocrinol Metab. 2006;91:2892–9.
118. Phay JE, Ringel MD. Metastatic mechanisms in follicular cell-derived thyroid cancer. Endocr Relat Cancer. 2013;20:R307–19. https://doi.org/10.1530/ERC-13-0187.
119. Cabanillas ME, McFadden DG, Durante C. Thyroid cancer. Lancet. 2016;388:2783–95.
120. Schlumberger M, Brose M, Elisei R, et al. Definition and management of radioactive iodine-refractory differentiated thyroid cancer. Lancet Diabetes Endocrinol. 2014;2:356–8.
121. Binse I, Poeppel TD, Ruhlmann M, et al. 68Ga-DOTATOC PET/CT in patients with iodine- and 18F-FDG– negative differentiated thyroid carcinoma and elevated serum thyroglobulin. J Nucl Med. 2016;57:1512–7.
122. Brose MS, Nutting CM, Jarzab B, et al. Sorafenib in radioactive iodine-refractory, locally advanced or metastatic differentiated thyroid cancer: a randomised, double-blind, phase 3 trial. Lancet. 2014;384:319–28.
123. Schlumberger M, Tahara M, Wirth LJ, et al. Lenvatinib versus placebo in radioiodine-refractory thyroid cancer. N Engl J Med. 2015;372:621–30.
124. Jin Y, Van Nostrand D, Cheng L, Liu M, Chen L. Radioiodine refractory differentiated thyroid cancer. Crit Rev Oncol Hematol. 2018;125:111–20.
125. Schmidt A, Iglesias L, Klain M, et al. Radioactive iodine-refractory differentiated thyroid cancer: an uncommon but challenging situation. Arch Endocrinol Metab. 2017;61(1):81–9.
126. Li J, Qin S, Xu J, et al. Randomized, double-blind, placebo-controlled phase III trial of Apatinib in patients with chemotherapy-refractory advanced or metastatic adenocarcinoma of the stomach or gastroesophageal junction. J Clin Oncol. 2016;34(13):1448–54.
127. Lim SM, Chang H, Yoon MJ, et al. A multicenter, phase II trial of everolimus in locally advanced or metastatic thyroid cancer of all histologic subtypes. Ann Oncol. 2013;24:3089–93.
128. Hayes DN, Lucas AS, Tanvetyanon T, et al. Phase II efficacy and pharmacogenomic study of selumetinib (AZD6244; ARRY-142886) in iodine-131 refractory papillary thyroid carcinoma with or without follicular elements. Clin Cancer Res. 2012;18:2056–65.
129. Philips JC, Petite C, Willi JP, et al. Effect of peroxisome proliferator-activated receptor gamma agonist, rosiglitazone, on dedifferentiated thyroid cancers. Nucl Med Commun. 2004;25:1183–6.
130. Nilubol N, Merkel R, Yang L, et al. A phase II trial of valproic acid in patients with advanced, radioiodine-resistant thyroid cancers of follicular cell origin. Clin Endocrinol. 2016;86:128–33.
131. Özülker T, Adaş M, Günay S. Thyroid and parathyroid diseases: a case-based guide. In: Uçmak G, Akkaş BE, editors. Rosiglitazone effect on radioiodine uptake in a case of dedifferentiated thyroid carcinoma. Springer; 2019. p. 297–303. https://doi.org/10.1007/978-3-319-78476-2-51.
132. Rothenberg SM, McFadden DG, Palmer EL, et al. Redifferentiation of iodine-refractory BRAF V600E-mutant metastatic papillary thyroid cancer with dabrafenib. Clin Cancer Res. 2015;21(5):1028–35.
133. Ruan M, Liu M, Dong Q, et al. Iodide- and glucose-handling gene expression regulated by sorafenib or cabozantinib in papillary thyroid cancer. J Clin Endocrinol Metab. 2015;100:1771–9.
134. Budiawan H, Salavati A, Kulkarni HR, et al. Peptide receptor radionuclide therapy of treatment-refractory metastatic thyroid cancer using (90)Yttrium and (177) Lutetium labeled somatostatin analogs: toxicity, response and survival analysis. Am J Nucl Med Mol Imaging. 2013;4(1):39–52.
135. Czepczyński R, Matysiak-Grześ M, Gryczyńska M, et al. Peptide receptor radionuclide therapy of differentiated thyroid cancer: efficacy and toxicity. Arch Immunol Ther Exp (Warsz). 2015;63(2):147–54.
136. Heitkötter B, Ko S, Trautmann M, et al. Neovascular PSMA expression is a common feature in malignant neoplasms of the thyroid. Oncotarget. 2018;9(11):9867–74.
137. Verma P, Malhotra G, Agrawal R, et al. Evidence of prostate-specific membrane antigen expression in metastatic differentiated thyroid cancer using 68Ga-PSMA-HBED-CC PET/CT. Clin Nucl Med. 2018;43(8):e265–8. https://doi.org/10.1097/RLU.0000000000002161.

7 Radionuclide Therapy in Malignant Thyroid Diseases: Medullary Thyroid Cancer

Evrim Sürer Budak and Funda Aydın

Medullary thyroid cancer (MTC) is a rare neuroendocrine tumor originating from parafollicular C cells that produce calcitonin (Ct). It constitutes 2–5% of all thyroid malignancies. It can be seen in sporadic form or hereditary form as a component of multiple neuroendocrine neoplasia (MEN) type 2. Its prognosis is poor compared to differentiated thyroid cancers. At the time of diagnosis, 35–50% of MTC patients are diagnosed with regional metastasis; 13–15% are diagnosed with distant metastasis to organs such as lungs, bones, and liver [1, 2]. According to SEER data, 10-year survival in gland-limited MTCs is approximately 95.6%, and overall survival in patients with regional disease is 75.5% [1]. The 10-year survival rate of those with distant metastasis at the time of diagnosis is approximately 20% [1, 2].

7.1 Preoperative Diagnosis

Staging and re-staging is very important as surgery is the only curative treatment option and also the diagnosis of advanced disease or recurrences is also critical for the evaluation of other treatment options.

E. S. Budak
Department of Nuclear Medicine, University of Health Sciences, Antalya Training and Research Hospital, Antalya, Turkey
e-mail: evrimsurer@hotmail.com

F. Aydın (✉)
Faculty of Medicine, Department of Nuclear Medicine, Akdeniz University, Antalya, Turkey
e-mail: afunda@akdeniz.edu.tr

7.2 Laboratory

Serum Ct and carcinoembryonic antigen (CEA) measurements are routinely performed in preoperative evaluation. Basal serum Ct concentration is correlated with tumor burden; it also gives an idea about tumor differentiation. Machens et al. showed that there was a correlation between Ct level and prognosis; distant metastasis and extrathyroidal extension were high in both familial and sporadic cases at Ct levels above 150 pg/mL [3]. Ct level above 500 pg/mL, nodal metastasis, and re-operative status are the best indicators that correlate with unsuccessful biochemical course [3].

Since pheochromocytoma or primary hyperparathyroidism or both can be seen together in patients with MEN type 2, RET (rearranged during transfection) protoonkogen mutation should be investigated in these patients.

7.3 Imaging

7.3.1 Conventional Morphological Methods

In preoperative diagnosis, all patients undergo detailed neck ultrasonography (USG) examination. Conventional morphological imaging methods

R. Bekiş et al. (eds.), *Radionuclide Therapy*, https://doi.org/10.1007/978-3-030-97220-2_7

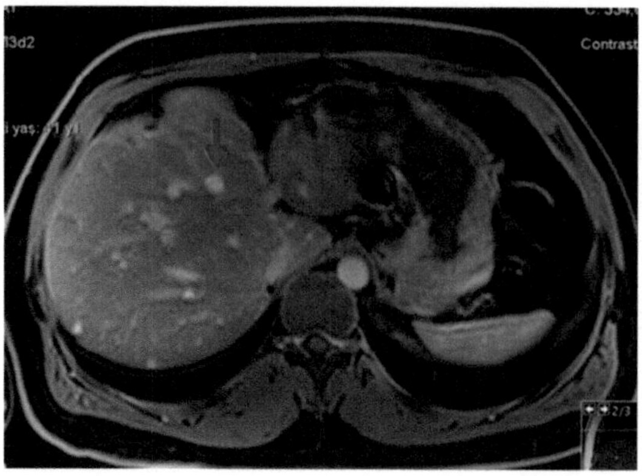

Fig. 7.1 A 44-year-old male patient with medullary thyroid Ca; calcitonin 1196 pg/mL. Metastatic lesion (arrow) in liver segment 4B on MRI. The patient also has multiple bone metastases

such as computed tomography (CT) and magnetic resonance imaging (MRI) are also used to detect distant metastasis (Fig. 7.1). Local or distant recurrence/metastases may be misdiagnosed by morphological imaging methods. In these cases, functional imaging methods should be preferred. Evaluation of whole body by just one method is another advantage of functional imaging.

7.3.2 Conventional Nuclear Medicine Methods

Commonly used radiopharmaceuticals in nuclear medicine functional imaging of metastatic medullary thyroid cancer are technetium-99m-(V)-dimercaptosuccinic acid (Tc-99m-V-DMSA), thallium-201 chloride (Tl-201), Tc-99m-sestamibi, iodine-131/iodine-123-metaiodobenzylguanidine (I-123/I-131-MIBG), and indium-111 (In-111) or technetium-99m (Tc-99m) labeled somatostatin receptor radiopharmaceuticals [4–7].

Tc-99m-V-DMSA: It can be used in primary tumor evaluation and detection of recurrences. Its sensitivity varies between 19 and 88%. Using Tc-99m as radionuclide for labeling is an advantage. The distribution pattern is similar to phosphate ion, and this is the basic principle of its use in MTCs. Today, it is not commonly used in the practice by the invention of more effective methods with higher sensitivity.

MIBG: It is an analog of guanethidine and has a similar structure to norepinephrine. It can be labeled with iodine-123 or 131. I-123 MIBG is more preferable for imaging while I-131 MIBG for treatment option. I-123 MIBG is not recommended because of its low sensitivity (25–30%) in MTC% [7] (Fig. 7.2a, b). I-131 MIBG can be preferred especially if MIBG treatment is planned. It enables also retention measurements and shows the distribution pattern of tumor. Thyroid blockade should be performed before MIBG administration in non-thyroidectomized patients. In addition, medications interacting with MIBG should also be discontinued.

Somatostatin receptor imaging: MTC cells express somatostatin receptor (SSR) which allows scanning and treatment by this mechanism. Somatostatin (SS) is a cyclic peptide hormone with 2 bioactive forms. It is responsible for endocrine system regulation, neurotransmission modulation, and membrane G protein-mediated cell proliferation. Five subtypes have been identified in humans (SSTR1–5; SSTR2 has two subgroups, SSTR2A-2B). Papotti et al. showed that MTCs expressed 57% SSTR5, 47% SSTR3, 43% SSTR1, 33% SSTR2, and 4% SSTR4 [8]. The native form has a quite short half-life; by the development of synthetic SS analogs, its half-life has been considerably extended.

The most commonly used radiopharmaceuticals in scintigraphic imaging are In-pentetreotide (OctreoScan), which is the In-111-DTPA-D-Phe111 conjugate of octreotide. Other Tc-99m-labeled somatostatin analogs are Tc-99m-HYNIC-TATE octreotide, Tc-99m-EDDA/HYNIC-TOC, and Tc-99m-demotate. These show high affinity for SSTR2 which is lesser for SSTR5. In vitro studies have shown that when TATE chelates with DTPA or DOTA, SSTR2 affinity increases 14–17 times compared to octreotide and 8–10 times compared to TOC [9]. In studies, the sensitivity of these radiopharmaceuticals in tumor detection varies between 50% and 70%. It is stated that the degree of retention is directly related to high Ct and CEA levels [10].

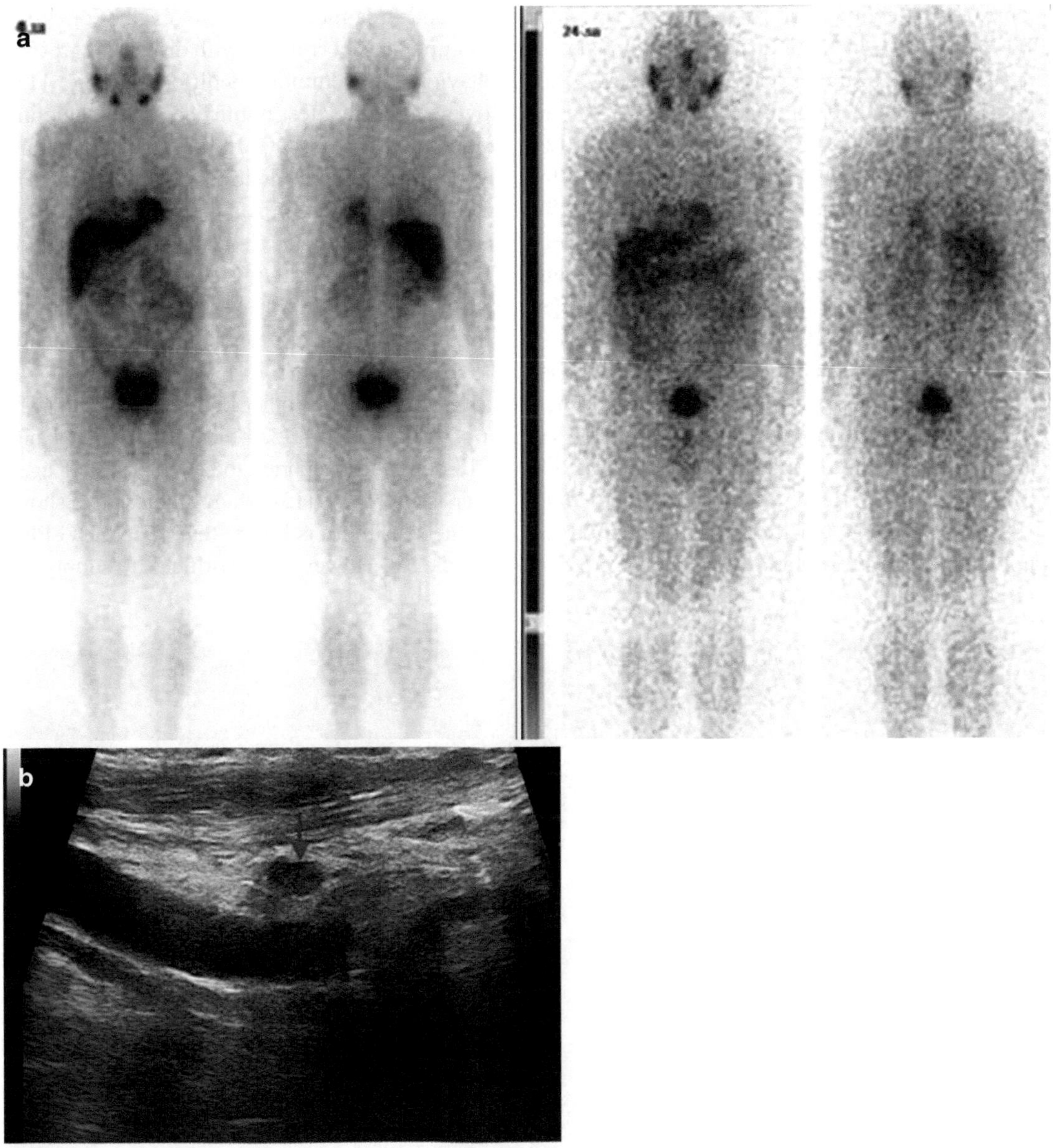

Fig. 7.2 (**a**) A 73-year-old male with operated medullary Ca, elevated calcitonin during follow-up; I-123 MIBG whole-body imaging showed no pathological findings. (**b**) A 73-year-old male with operated medullary Ca, elevated calcitonin during follow-up; left inferior cervical pathological LAP (arrow) on USG examination

7.3.3 PET/CT and Radiopharmaceuticals

Fluorodeoxyglucose (FDG): It is the main PET agent used in oncology and the mechanism of involvement is through the glycolytic pathway. It is labeled with Flourine-18 (F-18). Its involvement in neoplastic cells correlates with poor differentiation and high proliferative activity. As tumors become dedifferentiated, more aggressive, and cell proliferation increases, FDG uptake also increases. F-18-FDG PET/CT is an important imaging tool in patients with biochemical recurrence in MTC. Treglia et al. evaluated the recurrence detection performance of F-18-FDG PET or PET/CT in MTC in their meta-analysis consisting of 24 studies [11]. Accordingly, the overall recurrence detection rate was 75% in cases with a Ct level above 1000 ng/mL and 40% in cases with a Ct level below 150 ng/mL. In addition, the recurrence detection rate was 69% in cases which CEA was above 5 ng/mL and 45% in cases which CEA was equal to or below 5 ng/mL. Recurrence detection rate was 26% in cases with Ct doubling time above 24 months and 67% in cases where it was below 24 months. The recurrence detection rate was 33% in cases with a CEA doubling time above 24 months and 91% in cases with a CEA duplication time below 24 months [11, 12]. Recent studies indicate that F-18-FDG PET/CT will be a useful method in targeted treatment evaluation, prognosis prediction, and treatment response evaluation since FDG uptake is correlated with disease aggressive behavior and tumor dedifferentiation [13]. However, in the latest published MTC guideline, preoperative F-18-FDG PET/CT is not recommended in routine evaluation and follow-up. The main recommendation for the use of F-18-FDG PET/CT is persistent Ct levels (150 pg/mL or CEA level above 30 ng/mL at the 3rd month after thyroidectomy) and in cases where conventional imaging methods are negative or inconclusive [14, 15] (Figs. 7.3 and 7.4).

F-18-DOPA: The other PET agent used in MTC is 6-[F-18]-L-fluoro-L-3, 4-dihydroxyphenylalanine (F-18-dopa). It is reported to be the best PET agent in persistent MTCs [15]. Many studies have shown that the sensitivity is higher than F-18-FDG PET/CT [15, 16]. However, it is difficult to supply and

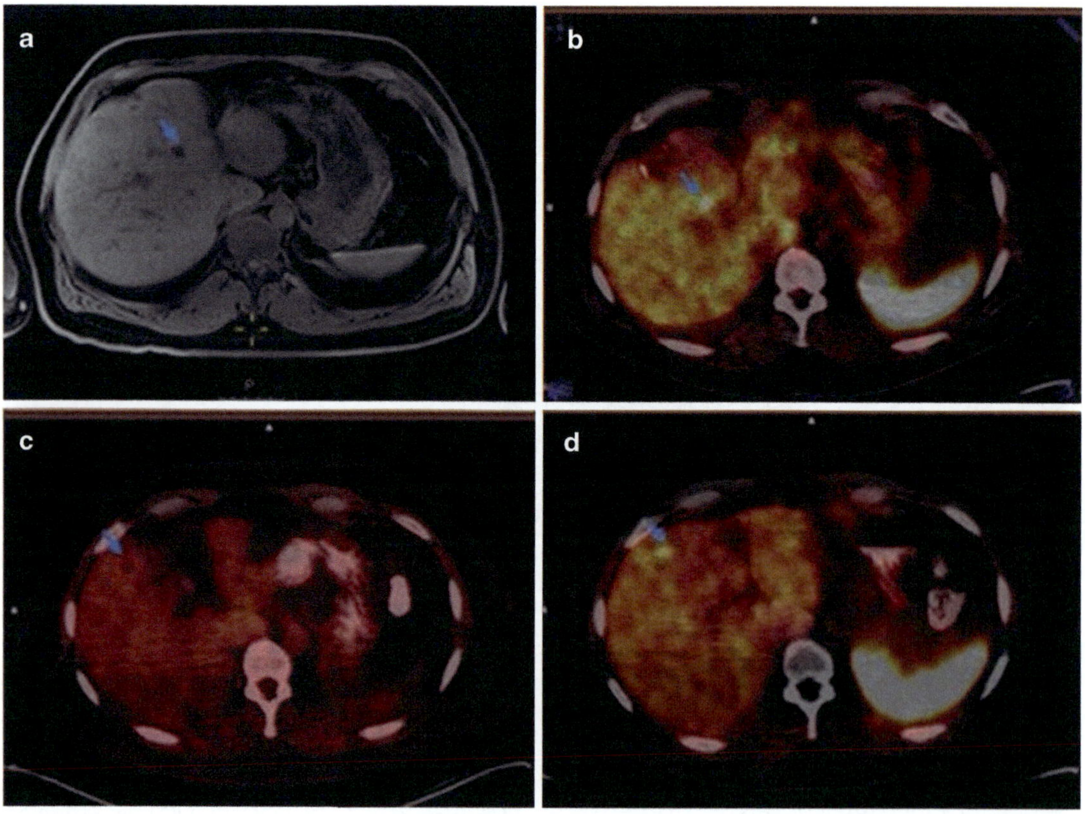

Fig. 7.3 A 44-year-old male with calcitonin elevation (1196 pg/mL). (**a**) Metastatic lesion (arrow) in liver segment 4A on MRI. (**b**) The same lesion is SSR positive (arrow) on Ga-68-PEPTIDE PET imaging. (**c**) F-18-FDG PET imaging shows another hypometabolic lesion in segment 8/4A (arrow). (**d**) The same lesion is SSR positive on Ga-68-PEPTIDE PET imaging (arrow)

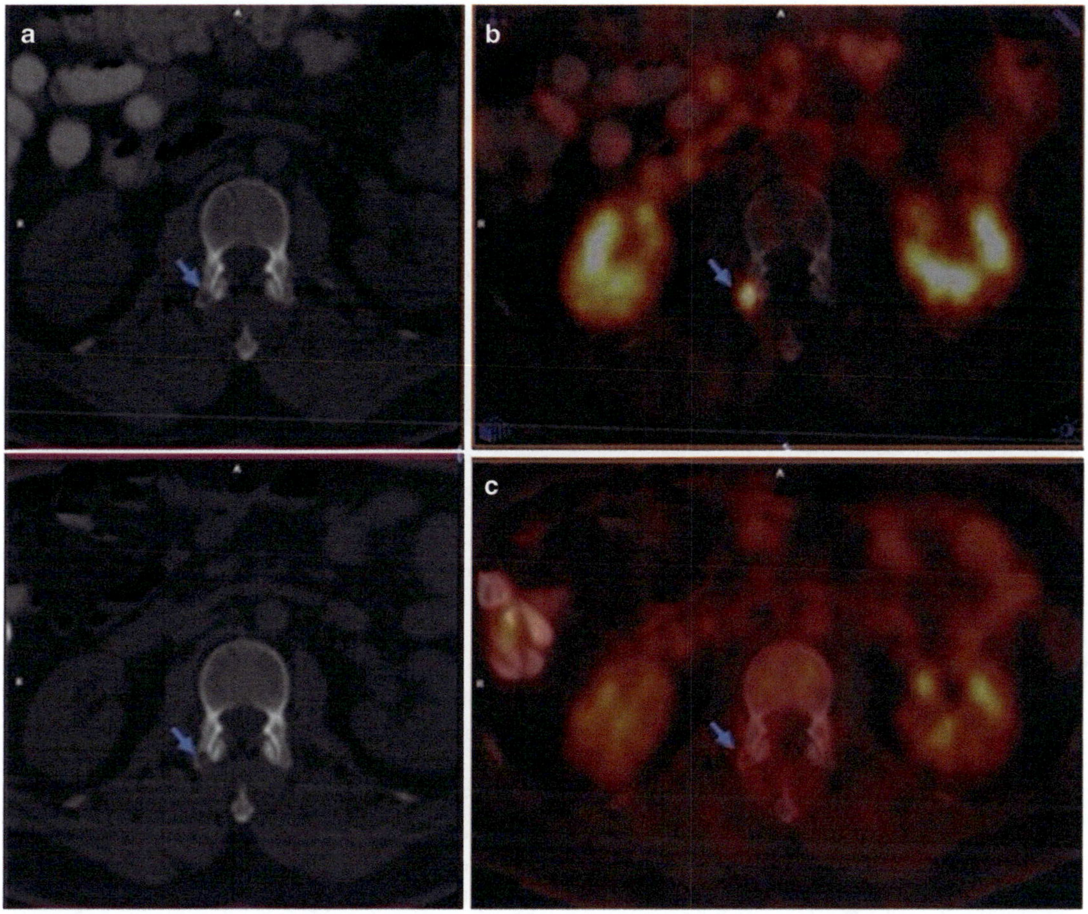

Fig. 7.4 A 44-year-old male with calcitonin elevation (1196 pg/mL). (**a**) Lytic lesion (arrow) in right posterior of L2 vertebra on CT. (**b**) SSR positive (arrow) on Ga-68-PEPTIDE PET imaging. (**c**) F-18-FDG PET imaging shows no FDG avidity (hypometabolic) (arrow)

since tumor detection rate can decrease by 40% in early and late time images, the optimal imaging time needs to be modified according to the patient.

Ga-68 labeled agents: Similar to SS analogs labeled with In-111 and Tc-99m, in PET imaging Ga-68 labeled agents are also used. The most known of these are DOTA labeled Tyr3-octreotate (DOTATATE) and DOTA-D-Phe1-Tyr3-octreotide (DOTATOC). Many studies have shown that they are effective imaging method in MTCs with elevated Ct and CEA levels, for localization of recurrent or metastatic disease, as well as staging and re-staging [17] (Fig. 7.5a, b). An important limitation is metastatic liver lesions especially showing equal uptake with liver activity can be missed out [18]. In a retrospective study involving 18 patients with residual or recurrent disease, the diagnostic performance of F-18-DOPA PET/CT, F-18-FDG PET/CT, and Ga-68-DOTATATE PET/CT were compared. F-18-DOPA PET/CT was found superior and more sensitive than others in detecting lesions. However, F-18-FDG PET/CT provided more valuable information in prognosis evaluation, and Ga-68-DOTATATE PET/CT was found to be more advantageous in radionuclide therapy selection [16, 19–21].

New and promising agents: Ga-68 and copper-64 (Cu-64) labeled cholecystokinin-2 (CCK-2) peptide, Ga-68 labeled anti-CEA, anti-HSG

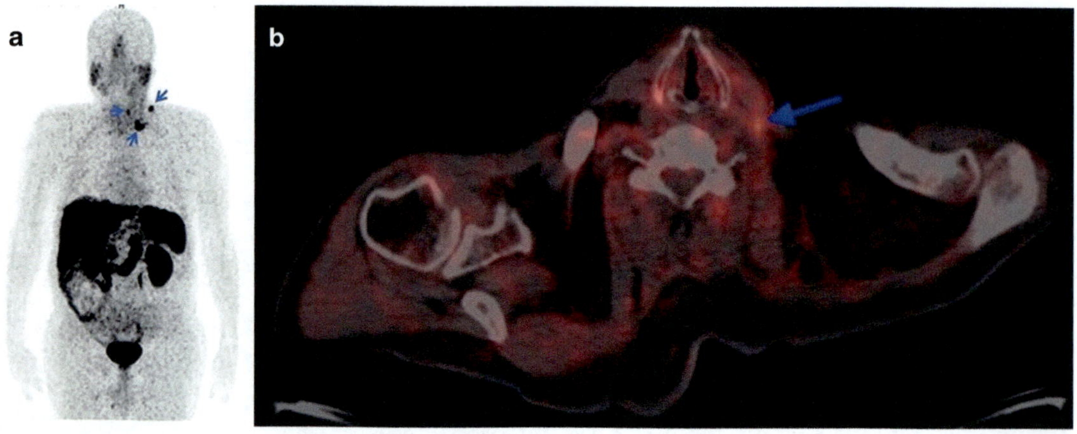

Fig. 7.5 (**a**) A 73-year-old male with elevated calcitonin levels; recurrence in left thyroid bed shown by USG and left inferior cervical pathological LAP; MIP image of Ga-68-PEPTIDE PET/CT imaging; SSR-positive lesions (arrow). (**b**) A 73-year-old male with elevated calcitonin levels. Neck USG was suspicious for recurrence in left thyroid bed and inferior cervical level pathological LAP was detected on the left side Ga-68-PEPTIDE PET/CT revealed receptor-positive lymph node (arrow) at left cervical level 3. Lymph node was dissected, and pathological examination is consistent with medullary thyroid Ca metastasis

trivalent humanized BsMAb TF2 and Ga-68 labeled histamine peptide, 3-O-methyl-6-Fluoro--18-dopa (F-18-OMFD), carbon-11 (C-11)-hydroxyl-tryptophan, In-111-CP04, and C-11-DOPA. Studies on these agents are ongoing and clinical data are still being collected.

7.4 Treatment Approaches in Medullary Thyroid Carcinoma

7.4.1 Primary Treatment: Surgery

The standard treatment procedure of MTC in neck limited disease and with no cervical lymph node and distant metastasis on preoperative imaging is total thyroidectomy and central LN dissection [21]. Prophylactic central LN dissection is not recommended in thyroid limited small MTCs with a Ct level <20 pg/mL because LN metastasis is not an expected finding in cases where preoperative Ct level is <20 pg/mL (normal reference value <10 pg/mL). An important issue is whether lateral LN dissection should be added to primary surgery or not in cases with no suspicious LN metastases clinically either on USG examination. As a grade 1 recommendation in the revised ATA guideline, it is said that lateral compartment LN dissection (levels 2–5) decision can be made depending on serum Ct levels in cases with no suspicious cervical LN metastasis on USG and distant metastasis [22]. In preoperative evaluation, contralateral neck dissection should also be planned if the basal serum Ct level is higher than 200 pg/mL in patients with positive ipsilateral and negative contralateral neck compartment.

At the onset of accompanying pheochromocytoma, adrenalectomy should be planned before thyroidectomy [23].

7.4.1.1 Treatment in Local Advanced or Metastatic MTCs

In patients with locally advanced or metastatic disease at the time of initial diagnosis, the purpose of treatment is more palliative and total thyroidectomy and dissection of involved LN compartments are recommended. In most cases, aggressive surgery in the central and lateral neck region is avoided in terms of protecting speech, swallowing, parathyroid functions, and shoulder mobility. Non-surgical methods such as external beam radiotherapy (EBRT), systemic medical treatment or radiofrequency ablation (RFA), cryoablation, and embolization are used to provide local tumor control. If surgery is performed for eradication, operation decision should be based on patient's expectations, quality of life, and other medical comorbidities. The first treatment option in cervical recurrences is reoperation, and RT can be added according to the extensiveness of the disease.

In cases with distant metastasis, the purpose of treatment is to reduce symptoms and improve quality of life. The most common distant metastasis side for MTC is the liver. Patients usually have symptoms such as pain and diarrhea. Surgical resection of lesions is recommended for symptom-free survival [24]. In case of multiple and unresectable metastases, RFA is an effective treatment method due to its low morbidity. Transarterial chemoembolization of the liver in diffuse lesions provides symptom control and partial response (PR) in one-third of patients with stable liver and kidney functions and organ involvement below 30% [25].

Lung metastases associated with mediastinal nodal disease should be considered surgically if symptomatic and resectable [24]. Alternatively, RFA can be tried.

Bone metastases are commonly seen in the vertebra, pelvis, costa, femur, skull, and humerus. If possible, for long-term symptomatic cure, resection and postoperative RT are recommended [26]. The use of biphosphates in combination with RFA, vertebroplasty, or kyphoplasty is also beneficial for palliation [27–29].

If possible, single brain metastases should be resected for palliation and survival [30]. EBRT can be considered in multiple brain metastases unsuitable for surgery [22, 30].

Although soft tissue metastases such as breast [31], testicle [32], and skin [33] are mostly suitable for excision or RT, these patients usually pass on in less than 1 year as these are a sign of widespread disease.

Consequently, small and isolated metastases can be followed up if Ct level is stable [34]. Systemic treatment should be preferred in symptomatic progressive metastases that cannot be resected and in cases where symptomatic improvement cannot be achieved with a single method [35].

7.4.1.2 Treatment in Persistent or Recurrent MTCs

Serum Ct and CEA levels should be measured at the postoperative 3rd month in terms of detection of residual disease. Patients with normal CEA levels and undetectable Ct values are considered biochemically cured and have a very good prognosis [36–38]. Postoperative biochemical remission is the best predictive factor for recurrence-free survival [39]. Further research in patients with persistent hypercalcitoninemia depends on serum Ct levels (150 pg/mL). In addition, the doubling time of Ct and CEA is a useful tumor marker and helps to predict prognosis and aggressive tumor behavior [40].

Treatment approaches in the case of recurrent or residual disease are follow-up/active follow-up, surgical resection, EBRT, RFA, cryoablation, embolization, and systemic treatments such as chemotherapy (CT), molecular targeted therapy (MTT), and immunotherapy. The treatment approach depends on many variables such as the nature of the disease (localized/systemic), tumor burden, distance of metastatic foci to vital organs, and the presence of disease-related additional symptoms [23]. Patients with detectable Ct and/or abnormal CEA values but no structural foci can be followed up. In these patients, postoperative adjuvant EBRT is not recommended.

External radiotherapy should be used in selected conditions as it will affect the success of probable surgery and the patient's quality of life by inducing fibrosis. Postoperative head and neck adjuvant EBRT is applied to patients with a high risk of local recurrence (microscopic or macroscopic residual MTC, extrathyroidal spread, or wide LN metastasis) or airway obstruction [22]. Active follow-up is the best option in recurrent MTCs with asymptomatic subcentimetric LN metastasis. However, EBRT can be applied to patients with unresectable gross tumor or cervical soft tissue lesion in the thyroid bed to provide locoregional control. EBRT is used in the treatment of multiple brain or mediastinal metastases (while surgery is preferable for solitary gross lung, liver, and brain metastases), palliation of painful bone lesions, and reduction of fracture risk [22].

7.4.2 Systemic Therapy

7.4.2.1 Clinical Indications for Systemic Therapy

Targeted systemic treatments should be preferred when well tolerated and more accessible local treatments are depleted. Molecular markers such as Ct and CEA levels and clinical and radiological findings also guide the decision to start treatment. MTCs with progressive or symptomatic metastasis cannot be treated with surgery, local treatments, or RT, and these are candidates for systemic treatment.

7.4.2.2 Molecular Principles

MTC has a detectable relationship with RET proto-oncogene mutation, whether hereditary (MEN2 and FMTC) or sporadic. MTC is hereditary by 25% and occurs as a component of an inherited syndrome; 75% is sporadic [41]. RET is mutated in almost all familial cases and roughly 50% of sporadic cases [42]. RET activation stimulates mitogenic and vital mechanisms through RAS and phosphoinositide-3-kinase 2 (PI3K/AKT/mTOR) pathways [43–45].

The tyrosine kinase (TK) receptor activates germline mutations of RET proto-oncogene and is found in almost all patients with MEN2A and MEN2B. Somatic RET mutation was reported in 50–60% of sporadic MTC cases. In addition, somatic RAS mutations can be detected in MTC patients without somatic RET mutation [44, 46]. In addition, vascular endothelial growth factor receptors (VEGF-1 and VEGF-2) are frequently overexpressed from MTC tumor cells and vascular endothelium [47]. Since angiogenesis plays a critical role in tumor development and metastasis, increased VGEF expression increases thyroid cancer cell growth, LN metastasis, local invasion, and distant metastasis development [48]. Therefore, the most successful agents in treatment are those targeting VEGF and TK.

7.4.2.3 Agents Used in Systemic Therapy

Cold SS analogs (octreotide): When administered in the short or long term, symptomatic MTC patients improve neuroendocrine symptoms, especially diarrhea and flushing, and biochemical markers; however, data on objective tumor response are anecdotal [49]. No significant antiproliferative effect has been achieved with cold octreotide treatment in advanced MTC, and the results are not very encouraging.

Tyrosine kinase-multikinase inhibitors (TKIs): Cabozantinib and vandetanib are first-generation TKIs developed for use in MTC. Sorafenib, sunitinib, pazopanib, and lenvatinib are second-generation TKIs used in MTC. They are used when cabozantinib and vandetanib are inappropriate [35]. Motesanib, axitinib, imatinib, gefitinib, and ponatinib are also targeted monokinase inhibitors (MSIs), and promising results are obtained in preclinical or phase 1–2 studies, but there are not enough data in terms of clinical use in MTC. Other agents being developed are other MSIs such as nintedanib, anlotinib, regorafenib, and farnesyl transferase inhibitors (FTI or tipifarnib). In addition, statins such as lovastatin have been found to have antitumor effects in K-Ras-dependent thyroid tumors [50].

Monotherapy agents and epigenetic therapy: These include mTOR inhibitors such as nelfinavir (NFV) and everolimus.

Conventional cytotoxic chemotherapy: The chemotherapy results reported in MTC are uncertain. Traditional cytotoxic agents such as dacarbazine and capecitabine are not preferred in these patients due to their limited benefits and common side effects in first-line treatment [51].

I-131 MIBG: Patients with documented pathological uptake by I-123 MIBG imaging are adequate for I-131 MIBG therapy. The administered MIBG treatment dose varies according to tumor burden and ranges between 100 and 300 mCi. During treatment, dose-related side effects such as tachycardia, pallor, nausea, vomiting, and abdominal pain may occur. Treatments can be evaluated personally and repeated periodically. Limitations in treatment include myelosuppression, renal dysfunction, and lack of response to treatment.

7.5 Peptide Receptor Radionuclide Therapy

7.5.1 General Information

Although the choice of appropriate treatment in metastatic or inoperable MTCs is still controversial, it requires a multidisciplinary approach. The first nuclear medicine treatment method used in MTC is MIBG. After the low treatment rates detected with MIBG, new treatment options were investigated. By considering the SSR overexpression in tumors and symptom control detected with somatostatin analogs, the option "Peptide Receptor Radionuclide Therapy (PRRT)" in which radionuclide-labeled somatostatin analogs are used in the treatment has been developed. Thus, not only diagnosis but also targeted treatment has been achieved. The antitumor mechanism of PRRT is based on receptor-mediated internalization and intracellular retention of radiopeptide. As a result, radiation reaches the intracellular compartments of the cancer cell, resulting in tumor shrinkage and even depletion [52]. Another potential goal of PRRT is to create an antiangiogenic response by inducing upregulation of SSTR2 in peritumoral vessels. Another advantage is the small size of peptides than the antibodies because their pharmacokinetics are better and their antigenic properties are lower, making them almost ideal ligands for receptor-based radionuclide imaging and treatment. The most important advantage of PRRT over systemic treatment is its selectivity (due to its high affinity to SSR2) and relatively low toxicity. In addition, hospitalization periods are shorter. Depending on the characteristics of the radionuclide used, the patient can be discharged even on the same day. The first radiolabeled somatostatin analog used in the treatment was In-111-DTPA-octreotide in the early 1990s, and very good results were obtained in symptom control. However, partial remission rates were found to be very low.

7.5.2 Peptide Receptor Radionuclide Therapy Agents

The synthetic SS analog consists of a peptide (a cyclic octapeptide such as octreotide or Tyr-3-octreotate/octreotide), a radioactive component (yttrium-Y or lutetium-Lu), and a chelator (such as DTPA or DOTA). Y and Lu achieve tumor ablation directly or by anti-angiogenic pathway. The most commonly used radionuclide-labeled peptides are yttrium-90 (Y-90) or lutetium-177 (Lu-177) DOTA-Tyr3-octreotide (DOTATOC), DOTA-LANREOTIDE (DOTALAN), DOTA-1-NAL3-octreotide (DOTANOC), and DOTA-Tyr-3-octreotate (DOTATATE). The difference between Tyr-3-octreotate and Tyr-3-octreotide is the displacement of treoninol in the terminal treonin part, which is associated with higher receptor binding, better internalization, and greater tumor radiation. DOTATATE's SSTR2 affinity is 6–9 times higher than DOTATOC, but its affinity for other receptors is lower (low for SSTR5 and SSTR3 and very low for SSTR1 and SSTR4). In addition to SSTR2, DOTANOC has a very high affinity for SSTR3 and SSTR5. This broad receptor affinity leads to a high in vivo uptake in the whole body and normal tissue, resulting in a higher risk of bone marrow toxicity. The side effects are known to be directly associated with the ligand type used.

Radionuclide selection: Y-90 is a pure beta emitter. Its half-life is 64 h and its maximum tissue penetration is 12 mm. High tissue penetration causes a "cross-fire" effect on adjacent tumor cells. The high energy of the radioisotope (935 keV) is directly responsible for the tumor effect.

The half-life of Lu-177 is 6.7 days. It has 497 and 133 keV beta emissions and its maximum tissue penetration is 2 mm. It also emits 208 (11%) and 113 (7%) keV gamma (which allows post-therapeutic dosimetry) [52]. Lu-177 is more effective in lesions below 2 cm (Fig. 7.6a, b). Phase 1 and 2 studies have shown that Y-90 will be more effective in larger lesions with low vascularization and Lu-177-labeled SS analogs in smaller lesions and that com-

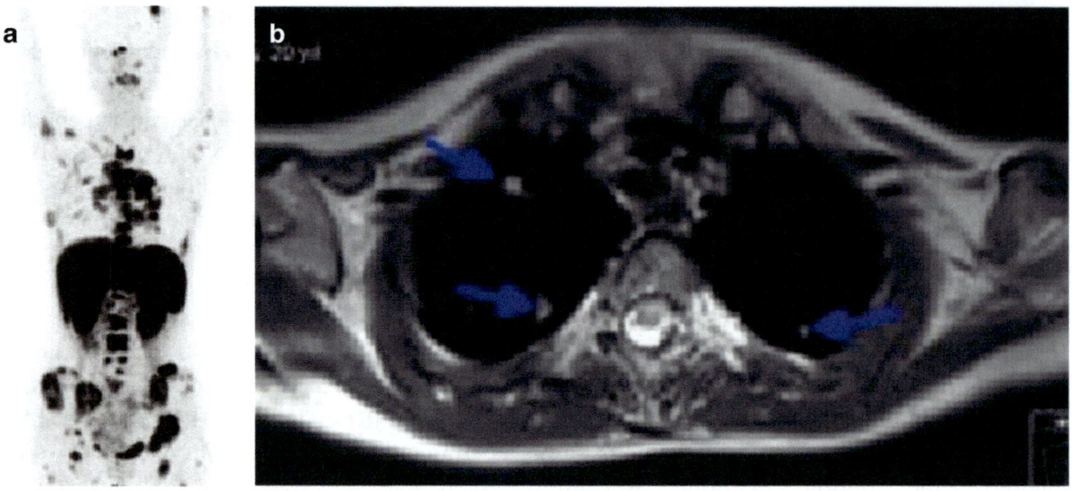

Fig. 7.6 (**a**) A 20-year-old, female, operated medullary thyroid Ca, had chemotherapy and radiotherapy to neck region and systemic Lu-177 peptide receptor therapy; Ga-68 peptide PET/CT MIP image; diffuse SSR-positive metastatic lesions in the lungs and bones. (**b**) A 20-year-old female, operated medullary thyroid Ca, had chemotherapy and longitudinal radiotherapy as well as Lu-177 peptide receptor therapy; millimetric metastatic nodules (arrow) in the lung on thoracic MRI scan

bined treatments may be the best treatment approach [53]. Intra-arterial administration of radiolabeled SS analogs also provides a better tumor/normal tissue uptake rate and the results are promising.

7.5.3 Combination of Chemotherapy and PRRT

Clinical trial results suggest that combined treatments increase the effectiveness of PRRT by increasing the antitumoral effect. The first successful study with proven reliability is the combination of 5-fluorouracil and PRRT. Subsequently, a randomized study using the combination of capecitabine and Lu-177 PRRT in gastroenteropancreatic tumors was performed, and 94% of 33 patients achieved tumor control and stabilization. Although three patients could not complete chemotherapy due to capecitabine-induced angina, all completed PRRT cycles. These and similar studies are promising in terms of obtaining similar results in MTCs.

7.5.4 Peptide Receptor Radionuclide Therapy Indication

The indication is inoperable, recurrence-metastatic and symptomatic MTC patients whose SSTR expression is demonstrated by peptide receptor imaging [54].

7.5.5 Contraindication

Definitive contraindication: Pregnancy, concomitant severe acute disease, severe psychiatric disorder

Relative contraindication: Breastfeeding (if cannot be discontinued)

Severe renal impairment: While normal renal function is essential in the treatment with Y-90, mild to moderate renal failure (creatine <1.7 mg/dL) can be tolerated for Lu-177 treatment. Glomerular filtration rate (GFR) and tubular extraction rate (SWEAT) must be at least 60% of the age-adjusted value.

Severe hematological impairment: Bone marrow (BM) reserve should be sufficient before PRRT.

Recommended values are WBC < 3000/μL, neutrophil < 1000/μL, PLT < 75,000/μL (for Lu-177-DoTATATE); PLT < 90,000/μL (for Y-90-DOTATOC), and RBC < 3,000,000/μL [54].

7.5.6 Warnings

Dose-limiting organs are the kidneys. Renal and BM side effects are mild if necessary precautions are taken. Renal function tests (BUN, creatine, renal clearance) should be performed in all patients. All pediatric patients, as well as patients at risk for renal toxicity and failure, should undergo specific tests such as 24-h urinary GFR measurement, MAG3 scintigraphy/SWEAT measurement, and Tc-99m-DTPA GFR measurement before treatment. Renal obstructions leading to potential hydronephrosis and sudden onset failure conditions should be excluded or corrected before treatment. Patients with a history of EBRT in areas such as pelvis/spine or history of pre-PRRT cytotoxic chemotherapy are at high risk of developing post-treatment BM toxicity. BM biopsy may be performed in suspicious cases. Platelet monitoring depending on the treatment type and doses may be guiding in terms of treatment cycle planning and dose decision. Caution should also be taken in terms of suspected liver failure [54].

7.5.7 Pretreatment Assessment

Prior to treatment, the patient must have a histopathologically documented diagnosis of MTC and SSTR expression indicated by one of the SSTR imaging methods in the existing lesions. The patient's performance score is also one of the factors affecting the treatment decision (Karnofsky performance >60% or ECOG <2) [54].

7.5.8 Patient Preparation

SS analogs labeled with Y-90 and Lu-177 are secreted into glomeruli and then reabsorbed from proximal tubules, which is the most important cause of renal toxicity. Risk factors such as underlying hypertension or diabetes may aggregate renal toxicity. Positively charged amino acids (aa) such as L-lysine or L-arginine are used to reduce renal retention by competitively inhibiting reabsorption of radiopeptides from proximal tubules. Concomitant amino acid administration causes a 9–53% reduction in renal dose absorption [55]. Large volumes should be preferred for hydration when preparing amino acid solution (such as 2 L); however, caution should be exercised in cases of cardiac insufficiency. Optimal dilution is 25 g lysine/arginine in 1 L isotonic. Hyperosmolar solutions should be avoided due to electrolyte imbalance. Antiemetic and/or steroid is started to prevent nausea and vomiting before aa infusion and antiemetic and saline infusion is repeated as necessary. Aa infusion is started 30–60 min before radiopeptide administration and maintained for 4 h. Care should be taken in this process for electrolyte imbalance (hyperkalemia and hypernatremia) and metabolic acidosis. Mild nausea and vomiting due to metabolic acidosis may be observed. Hydration with saline and repeated corticosteroids and antiemetics can be applied for these side effects [54].

Amino Acid Infusion Protocols

- **One-day 50 g protocol:** 25 g lysine + 25 g arginine in 2 L saline/4 h.
- **3-day 25 g protocol:** 25 g lysine-1 L volume on the first day/4 h; posttherapy 2nd and 3rd days 12.5 g lysine-500 mL volume/3 h; maximum protection and minimum side effects are aimed.
- **3-day 50 g protocol:** 25 g lysine + 25 g arginine-2 L volume/4 h, 2nd and 3rd day 12.5 g lysine- 500 mL volume/twice a day for 3 h.
- **One-day 50 g + gelofusine protocol:** 25 g lysine + 25 g arginine/4 h; bolus gelofusine infusion from 1 mL/kg 10 min before radio-

peptide injection and 0.02 mL/kg/min gelofusine infusion 3 h after radiopeptide injection in 2 L saline. Vital follow-up is recommended during infusion for immunogenic side effects [54].

7.5.9 Discontinuation of Somatostatin Analogs

Short-acting analogs should be discontinued at least 24 h before treatment and long-acting analogs 4–6 weeks before treatment as SS analogs used in treatment will create competition in receptor binding [54].

7.5.10 Treatment (Dose, Form, Duration)

Vascular access is ensured and aa infusion is started 30 min before radiopharmaceutical injection. Then, according to the infusion system to be used, the final volume is diluted with radiopharmaceutical saline to be 10–100 mL and radiopharmaceutical infusion is continued with aa infusion for approximately 30 min. Amino acid infusion is maintained for a total of 4 h. Vital signs (blood pressure, pulse) should be monitored for possible symptoms. Caution should be paid to contamination due to urinary excretion during the first 48 h. Contraception is recommended for at least 6 months in female patients in the reproductive period. Temporary infertility due to Sertoli cell damage may also occur in male patients [54].

7.6 For Y-90-Dotatate/ Y-90-Dotatoc

- 3.7 GBq (100 mCi)/m^2 body surface; 2 times at 6–12 week intervals
- 2.78–4.44 GBq (75–120 mCi); 2–4 times at 6–12 week intervals

7.7 For Lu-177-Dotatate/ Lu-177-Dotatoc

- 5.55-7.4 GBq (150–200 mCi)/m^2; 3–5 times at 6–12 week intervals

7.7.1 Combined Administration

Co-administration of Y-90 and Lu-177 peptides may have additional therapeutic contributions. However, these treatments should be performed by centers with sufficient equipment and experience. The given activities should be calculated personally for each patient.

7.7.2 Consecutive Administration

- Y-90: 2.5–5.0 GBq (68–135 mCi)
- Lu-177: 5.55–7.4 GBq (150–200 mCi)
- 2–3 times at 6–16 week intervals

Combined administrations of Lu-177 and Y-90 are also tried.

7.7.3 Complications and Precautions

The dose is reduced in patients with impaired renal and/or hematological functions, and treatment is planned according to clinical/laboratory and dosimetric parameters. After nephrology consultation, intensive hydration (2–3 L) and diuretic administration (in cases of dilated renal pelvis or delayed output) are recommended in patients with impaired renal function if there is no clinical contraindication such as heart failure. Lu-177 treatment should be preferred in these patients if possible.

In patients with impaired hematological functions, hematology consultation, blood support following treatment if necessary, or granulocyte stimulating factor (GSF)/erythropoietin applications starting at least 10 days after the treatment can be planned; autologous peripheral stem cell transplantation can also be performed in cases of very severe failure [54].

7.7.4 Side Effects

7.7.4.1 Acute Side Effects

Acute side effects develop secondary to amino acid and radiopeptide administration and are generally mild. Metabolic acidosis induced by amino acid infusion causes nausea and headache in the majority of patients, rarely causes vomiting [56]. Care should also be taken against possible electrolyte imbalance (hyperkalemia and hypernatremia). These side effects can be corrected with appropriate hydration and repeated antiemetic/corticosteroids. Symptoms may exacerbate in the early period with PRRT in hormone-secreting functional tumors; follow-up of vital signs and treatment for symptoms are recommended in these patients. Hepatic toxicity is not an expected finding in patients without or low hepatic metastasis. However, toxicity may occur in patients with massive liver metastases or impaired liver functions. Therefore, appropriate radioisotope and dose selection is essential; Lu-177-labeled peptides should be preferred and dose should be reduced properly. Temporary hair loss may occur after Lu-177-DOTATATE treatment, and this resolves spontaneously within 3–6 months [54].

7.7.4.2 Delayed Side Effects

Renal toxicity: Since kidneys are dose-limiting organs, aa infusion is essential before treatment. However, after PRRT with Lu-177-DOTATATE and Y-90-DOTATOC, annual renal clearance loss of 3.8% and 7.3% can develop, respectively [57]. Delayed renal toxicity after treatment with Y-90-DOTATOC is more common in patients with long-term and uncontrolled hypertension and diabetes [58].

Bone marrow toxicity: Severe (grades 3 and 4), mostly reversible acute bone marrow toxicity can develop in a rate of 10–13% with Y-90-DOTATOC and 2–3% with Lu-177-DOTATATE therapy. It usually occurs 4–6 weeks after treatment. A transient decrease in platelets, leukocytes, and hemoglobin may be detected in 15% of the cases. However, sporadic cases of myelodysplastic syndrome or acute myeloid leukemia have also been reported at a total dose of 2.7 Ci (100 GBq) [59].

Endocrine toxicity: Despite SSR expression detected in the majority of endocrine organs, no toxicity/loss of endocrine function has been reported in these organs after treatment [58].

7.7.5 Follow-Up and Patient Management

Follow-up is necessary for side effects. Serum creatinine levels and creatinine clearance should be examined. More detailed tests such as GFR measurement with Tc-99m-DTPA or Tc-99m-MAG3 clearance calculation can also be performed in high-risk patients [54].

7.7.5.1 Inter-Cycle Follow-Up

A complete blood cell count should be performed every 2–4 weeks or more frequently in high risk patients. Renal and liver functions are checked before each cycle and if blood values are lower than the initial pre-PRRT values, dose reduction or extension of the cycle intervals may be possible. PRRT may also be discontinued in severe cases [54].

7.7.5.2 Intermediate and Long-Term Follow-Up

Complete blood cell count and liver and kidney function tests should be performed at 8–12 week intervals in the first 12 months and then two times a year if clinically required. Treatment response is assessed based on clinical, biochemical, morphological, and PET/CT results and the patient's clinical well-being/symptomatic response. Preferably contrast-enhanced CT or MRI is used to evaluate the morphological response. In some cases, the combination of both may be complementary. Follow-up should always be performed using the same imaging method; examinations can be repeated every 3–6 months, depending on the disease duration and tumor biology. However, this period may be extended up to 12 months in patients with durable response. World Health Organization (WHO), SWOG, and RECIST criteria are used to evaluate the objective response [60–62]. Functional imaging is also very valuable in follow-up and better reflects tumor behavior combined with morphological imaging [54].

7.7.5.3 Re-treatment Decision

It can be applied as salvage treatment in cases where there is no more appropriate treatment option [63]. In a progressive disease previously responded to PRRT, a re-treatment decision may be made considering the total radiation doses taken to the kidney and bone marrow in the previous treatment. Treatment eligibility criteria are the same as the first treatment, and treatment can be continued with the same or a different radionuclide. In this case, the use of Lu-177-labeled peptides is safer in terms of protecting kidney functions. If Lu-177-labeled peptides are used, whole-body scan should be performed after each cycle in order to evaluate the distribution pattern of radiopharmaceutical and functional response.

7.7.5.4 Quality of Life After Peptide Receptor Radionuclide Therapy

Vaisman et al. evaluated the quality of life in MTC in a small group of patients; they reported an improvement in general health quality and pain after PRRT with Lu-177-octreotate [21].

7.7.6 Prognosis

Although the results of PRRT are encouraging, complete remission is rare and recurrences may eventually be detected. Bodei et al. published a series of 21 MTC patients with non-resectable locoregional disease or distant metastasis. All patients were treated with Y-90-DOTATOC. The overall antitumor response (objective response + stable disease) was 67% in the patients, while only 2 patients had a complete response (10%). Partial or minor response was not detected in any patient. Seven patients (33%) did not respond to treatment and progressed. The overall response time (complete remission + stable disease) was between 3 and 40 months. In one patient (5%), serum Ct and CEA levels returned to normal levels after treatment; in the other five patients (24%), biochemically partial remission was detected. On the basis of serum markers, stabilization was observed in 3 patients (13%) and an increase was observed in 12 patients (57%). None of the patients developed toxicity. Since a better treatment response is observed in smaller tumors, it is recommended to start PRRT in the early stages of the disease [64].

Iten et al. investigated the response, survival, and long-term safety profile in 31 metastatic MTC patients treated with Y-90-DOTATOC in their phase 2 study [65]. Median survival was 91 months from the time of initial diagnosis and 15.7 months after the first treatment. Survival rates of patients who responded to treatment were significantly higher than those who did not (108.8 vs. 80.4 months).

In the current literature, data on median progression-free (PFS) and median overall survival after PRRT are inadequate and further studies are required.

7.8 Conclusion

The inoperable, recurrent-metastatic and symptomatic MTC patients with documented pathological SSTR expression on I-123 MIBG or peptide receptor imaging can be treated by radionuclide therapy methods. Treatments can be managed individually and repeated periodically. The most important advantage of PRRT over systemic treatment is its relatively low toxicity and SSR selectivity. Theranostic radionuclide therapy methods that can demonstrate the functional extent of the disease and enables to evaluate therapy response will be preferred in the early stages of the disease in combination with chemotherapy and other radionuclide therapies in the future.

References

1. Roman S, Lin R, Sosa JA. Prognosis of medullary thyroid carcinoma. Demographic, clinical and pathologic predictors of survival in 1252 cases. Cancer.

2006;107(9):2134–42. https://doi.org/10.1002/cncr.22244.
2. Leboulleux S, Baudin E, Travagli JP, et al. Medullary thyroid carcinoma. Clin Endocrinol. 2004;61(3):299–310. https://doi.org/10.1111/j.1365-2265.
3. Machens A, Schneyer U, Holzhausen HJ, et al. Prospects of remission in medullary thyroid carcinoma according to basal calcitonin level. J Clin Endocrinol Metab. 2005;90(4):2029–34. https://doi.org/10.1210/jc.2004-1836.
4. Ozkan ZG, Kuyumcu S, Uzum AK, et al. Comparison of Ga-DOTATATE PET-CT, 1F-FDG PET-CT and 99mTc- (V)DMSA scintigraphy in the detection of recurrent or metastatic medullary thyroid carcinoma. Nucl Med Commun. 2015;36:242–50.
5. Krishnamurthy A, Kumar RK, Ravishankaran P, et al. Exploring the role of technitium-99m dimercaptosuccinyl acid (V) scan in medullary carcinoma thyroid patients with postoperative persistent hypercalcitoninemia in the era of positron emission tomography-computerized tomography. Indian J Nucl Med. 2014;29:146–50.
6. Roosenburg S, Laverman P, Joosten L, et al. PET and SPECT imaging of a radiolabeled minigastrin analogue conjugated with DOTA, NOTA, and NODAGA and labeled with (64)Cu, (68)Ga, and (111)In. Mol Pharm. 2014;11:3930–7.
7. Castellani MR, Seregni E, Maccauro M, et al. MIBG for diagnosis and therapy of medullary thyroid carcinoma: is there still a role? Q J Nucl Med Mol Imaging. 2008;52:430–40.
8. Papotti M, Kumar U, Volante M. Immunohistochemical detection of somatostatin receptor types 1–5 in medullary carcinoma of the thyroid. Clin Endocrinol (Oxf). 2001;54:641–9.
9. http://www.eanm.org/publications/guidelines/gl_onco_fv.pdf.
10. Kwekkeboom DJ, Reubi JC, Lamberts SW, Bruining HA, Mulder AH, et al. In vivo somatostatin receptor imaging in medullary thyroid carcinoma. J Clin Endocrinol Metab. 1993;76:1413–7.
11. Treglia G, Muoio B, Giovanella L, et al. The role of positron emission tomography and positron emission tomography/computed tomography in thyroid tumours: an overview. Eur Arch Otorhinolaryngol. 2013;270:1783–7.
12. Rufini V, Castaldi P, Treglia G, et al. Nuclear medicine procedures in the diagnosis and therapy of medullary thyroid carcinoma. Biomed Pharmacother. 2008;62:139–46.
13. Salaun PY, Campion L, Ansquer C, et al. Â1â¸F-FDG PET predicts survival after pretargeted radioimmunotherapy in patients with progressive metastatic medullary thyroid carcinoma. Eur J Nucl Med Mol Imaging. 2014;41:1501–10.
14. Treglia G, Cocciolillo F, Di Nardo F, et al. Detection rate of recurrent medullary thyroid carcinoma using fluorine-18 dihydroxyphenylalanine positron emission tomography: a meta- analysis. Acad Radiol. 2012;19:1290–9.
15. Santhanam P, Taïeb D. Role of (18) F-FDOPA PET/CT imaging in endocrinology. Clin Endocrinol (Oxf). 2014;81:789–98.
16. Treglia G, Castaldi P, Villani MF, et al. Comparison of 18F-DOPA, 18F-FDG and 68Ga-somatostatin analogue PET/CT in patients with recurrent medullary thyroid carcinoma. Eur J Nucl Med Mol Imaging. 2012;39:569–80.
17. Lapa C, Werner RA, Schmid JS, et al. Prognostic value of positron emission tomography-assessed tumor heterogeneity in patients with thyroid cancer undergoing treatment with radiopeptide therapy. Nucl Med Biol. 2015;42:349–54.
18. von Guggenberg E, Dietrich H, Skvortsova I, et al. 99mTc-labelled HYNIC-minigastrin with reduced kidney uptake for targeting of CCK-2 receptor-positive tumours. Eur J Nucl Med Mol Imaging. 2007;34:1209–18.
19. Palaniswamy SS, Subramanyam P. Diagnostic utility of PETCT in thyroid malignancies: an update. Ann Nucl Med. 2013;27:681–93.
20. Verbeek HH, Plukker JT, Koopmans KP, et al. Clinical relevance of 18F-FDG PET and 18F-DOPA PET in recurrent medullary thyroid carcinoma. J Nucl Med. 2012;53:1863–71.
21. Vaisman F, de Castro PH, Lopes FP, et al. Is there a role for peptide receptor radionuclide therapy in medullary thyroid cancer? Clin Nucl Med. 2015;40:123–7.
22. Wells SA Jr, Asa SL, Dralle H, et al. Revised American Thyroid Association guidelines for the management of medullary thyroid carcinoma. Thyroid. 2015;25:567–610.
23. Cabanillas ME, McFadden DG, Durante C. Thyroid cancer. Lancet. 2016. May 27 [Epub]; https://doi.org/10.1016/S0140-6736(16)30172-6.
24. Chen H, Roberts JR, Ball DW, et al. Effective long-term palliation of symptomatic, incurable metastatic medullary thyroid cancer by operative resection. Ann Surg. 1998;227(6):887. https://doi.org/10.1097/00000658-199806000-00012.
25. Fromigué J, De Baere T, Baudin E, et al. Chemoembolization for Liver metastases from medullary thyroid carcinoma. J Clin Endocrinol Metab. 2006;91(7):2496–9. https://doi.org/10.1210/jc.2005-2401.
26. Munoz-Bendix C, Santacroce A, Gierga K, et al. Recurrent spinal metastasis of a sporadic medullary carcinoma of the thyroid after radiation therapy: a case report and review of the literature. Clin Case Rep. 2016;4(1):9–18. https://doi.org/10.1002/ccr3.409.
27. Wexler JA. Approach to the thyroid cancer patient with bone metastases. J Clin Endocrinol Metab. 2011;96:2296–307. https://doi.org/10.1210/jc.2010-1996.
28. Quan GM, Pointillart V, Palussiere J, et al. Multidisciplinary treatment and survival of patients with vertebral metastases from thyroid carcinoma. Thyroid. 2012;22:125–30. https://doi.org/10.1089/thy.2010.0248.

29. Frassica DA. General principles of external beam radiation therapy for skeletal metastases. Clin Orthop Relat Res. 2003;145:S158–64. https://doi.org/10.1097/01.blo.0000093057.96273.fb.
30. McWilliams RR, Giannini C, Hay ID, et al. Management of brain metastases from thyroid carcinoma. Cancer. 2003;98:356–62. https://doi.org/10.1002/cncr.11488.
31. Mandanas S, Margaritidou E, Christoforidou V, et al. Breast metastasis from medullary thyroid carcinoma in a male patient: case report and review of the literature. Rare Tumors. 2015;7(2):5765. https://doi.org/10.4081/rt.2015.5765.
32. Appetecchia M, Barnabei A, Pompeo V, et al. Testicular and inguinal lymph node metastases of medullary thyroid cancer: a case report and review of the literature. BMC Endocr Disord. 2014;14(1):84. https://doi.org/10.1186/1472-6823-14-84.
33. Nashed C, Sakpal SV, Cherneykin S, et al. Medullary thyroid carcinoma metastatic to skin. J Cutan Pathol. 2010;37:1237–40. https://doi.org/10.1111/j.1600-0560.2009.01365.x.
34. Schlumberger M, Bastholt L, Dralle H, et al. European thyroid association guidelines for metastatic medullary thyroid cancer. Eur Thyroid J. 2012;1(1):5–14. https://doi.org/10.1159/000336977.
35. National Comprehensive Cancer Network. Clinical Practice Guidelines in Oncology (NCCN Guidelines). Thyroid carcinoma. Version 1.2016. Fort Washington, PA: NCCN; 2016.
36. Lindsey SC, Ganly I, Palmer F, et al. Response to initial therapy predicts clinical outcomes in medullary thyroid cancer. Thyroid. 2015;25:242–9.
37. Tuttle RM, Ganly I. Risk stratification in medullary thyroid cancer: moving beyond static anatomic staging. Oral Oncol. 2013;49:695–701.
38. Yang JH, Lindsey SC, Camacho CP, et al. Integration of a postoperative calcitonin measurement into an anatomical staging system improves initial risk stratification in medullary thyroid cancer. Clin Endocrinol (Oxf). 2015;83:938–42.
39. Jung KY, Kim SM, Yoo WS, et al. Postoperative biochemical remission of serum calcitonin is the best predictive factor for recurrence-free survival of medullary thyroid cancer: a large-scale retrospective analysis over 30 years. Clin Endocrinol (Oxf). 2016;84:587–97.
40. Meijer JA, le Cessie S, van den Hout WB, et al. Calcitonin and carcinoembryonic antigen doubling times as prognostic factors in medullary thyroid carcinoma: a structured meta- analysis. Clin Endocrinol (Oxf). 2010;72:534–42.
41. Cakir M, Grossman AB. Medullary thyroid cancer: molecular biology and novel molecular therapies. Neuroendocrinology. 2009;90(4):323–48. https://doi.org/10.1159/000220827.
42. de Groot JW, Links TP, Plukker JT, et al. RET as a diagnostic and therapeutic target in sporadic and hereditary endocrine tumor. Endocr Rev. 2006;27:535–60. https://doi.org/10.1210/er.2006-0017.
43. Schubbert S, Shannon K, Bollag G. Hyperactive Ras in developmental disorders and cancer. Nat Rev Cancer. 2007;7:295–308. https://doi.org/10.1038/nrc2175.
44. Moura MM, Cavaco BM, Pinto AE, et al. High prevalence of RAS mutations in RET-negative sporadic medullary thyroid carcinomas. J Clin Endocrinol Metab. 2011;96:E863–8. https://doi.org/10.1210/jc.2010-1921.
45. Hay N, Sonenberg N. Upstream and downstream of mTOR. Genes Dev. 2004;18:1926–45. https://doi.org/10.1101/gad.1212704.
46. Moura MM, Cavaco BM, Pinto AE, et al. Correlation of RET somatic mutations with clinicopathological features in sporadic medullary thyroid carcinomas. Br J Cancer. 2009;100:1777–83.
47. Lin JD, Chao TC. Vascular endothelial growth factor in thyroid cancers. Cancer Biother Radiopharm. 2005;20:648–61.
48. Kim BH, Kim IJ, Kim SS, et al. Relationship between biological marker expression and fluorine-18 fluorodeoxyglucose uptake in incidentally detected thyroid cancer. Cancer Biother Radiopharm. 2010;25:309–15.
49. Frank-Raue K, Ziegler R, Raue F. The use of octreotide in the treatment of medullary thyroid carcinoma. Horm Metab Res Suppl. 1993;27:44–7.
50. Wang CY, Zhong WB, Chang TC, et al. Lovastatin, a 3-hydroxy-3-methylglutaryl coenzyme A reductase inhibitor, induces apoptosis and differentiation in human anaplastic thyroid carcinoma cells. J Clin Endocrinol Metab. 2003;88:3021–6. https://doi.org/10.1210/jc.2002-021834.
51. Bajetta E, Rimassa L, Carnaghi C, et al. 5-Fluorouracil, dacarbazine, and epirubicin in the treatment of patients with neuroendocrine tumors. Cancer. 1998;83:372–8.
52. Baum RP, Kulkarni HR. THERANOSTICS: From molecular imaging using Ga-68 labeled tracers and PET/CT to personalized radio-nuclide therapy—the Bad Berka experience. Theranostics. 2012;2:437–47.
53. Traub-Weidinger T, Von Guggenberg E, Dobrozemsky G, et al. Preliminary experience with (68)Ga-DOTA-lanreotide positron emission tomography. Q J Nucl Med Mol Imaging. 2010;54:52–60.
54. Zaknun JJ, Bodei L, Mueller-Brand J, et al. The joint IAEA, EANM, and SNMMI practical guidance on peptide receptor radionuclide therapy (PRRNT) in neuroendocrine tumours. Eur J Nucl Med Mol Imaging. 2013;40(5):800–16. Published online 2013 Feb 7. https://doi.org/10.1007/s00259-012-2330-6.
55. de Jong M, Krenning EP. New advances in peptide receptor radio-nuclide therapy. J Nucl Med. 2002;43:617–20.
56. Jamar F, Barone R, Mathieu I, et al. (86YDOTA0)-DPhe1-Tyr3-octreotide (SMT487)—a phase 1 clinical study: pharmacokinetics, biodistribution and renal protective effect of different regimens of amino acid co-infusion. Eur J Nucl Med Mol Imaging. 2003;30:510–8.
57. Valkema R, Pauwels SA, Kvols LK, et al. Long-term follow-up of renal function after peptide receptor

radiation therapy with 90Y-DOTA0, Tyr3-octreotide and 177Lu-DOTA0,Tyr3- octreotate. J Nucl Med. 2005;46:83S–91S.
58. Teunissen JJ, Kwekkeboom DJ, Kooij PP, et al. Peptide receptor radionuclide therapy for non-radioiodine-avid differentiated thyroid carcinoma. J Nucl Med. 2005;46(Suppl. 1):107S–14S.
59. Imhof A, Brunner P, Marincek N, et al. Response, survival, and long-term toxicity after therapy with the radiolabeled somatostatin analogue [90Y-DOTA]-TOC in metastasized neuroendocrine cancers. J Clin Oncol. 2011;29:2416–23.
60. World Health Organization. WHO handbook for reporting results of cancer treatment. Geneva: World Health Organization; 1979. Available from: http://whqlibdoc.who.int/offset/WHO_OFFSET_48.pdf
61. Green S, Weiss G. Southwest Oncology Group standard response criteria, endpoint, definitions and toxicity criteria. Invest New Drugs. 1992;10:239–53.
62. Van Persijn Van Meerten EL, Gelderblom H, Bloem J. RECIST revised: implications for the radiologist. A review article on the modified RECIST guideline. Eur Radiol. 2010;20:1456–67.
63. Sowa-Staszczak A, Pach D, Kunikowska J, et al. Efficacy and safety of 90Y-DOTATATE therapy in neuroendocrine tumours. Endokrynol Pol. 2011;62:392–400.
64. Bodei L, Handkiewicz-Junak D, Grana C, et al. Receptor radionuclide therapy with 90Y-DOTATOC in patients with medullary thyroid carcinomas. Cancer Biother Radiopharm. 2004;19:65–71.
65. Iten F, Muller B, Schindler C, et al. Responseto [90Yttrium-DOTA]-TOC treatment is associated with long-term survival benefit in metastasized medullary thyroid cancer: a phase II clinical trial. Clin Cancer Res. 2007;13:6696–702.

8 Systemic Treatments and Related Side Effects in Thyroid Cancer

Seher Nazlı Kazaz and İlhan Öztop

Thyroid cancers are the most common cancers of the endocrine system. Especially in recent years, its incidence has been increasing in women and developed countries [1]. Most thyroid cancers are caused by follicular epithelium. These are papillary, follicular, Hurthle cell, and anaplastic thyroid cancers, respectively. More rarely medullary thyroid cancer (MTC) and lymphomas are observed. The first two of these, papillary and follicular type thyroid cancers, are called differentiated thyroid cancers (DTCs). The prognosis is better in differentiated thyroid cancers, with 10-year survival rates exceeding 90%. The basic treatment approach in differentiated thyroid cancer consists of surgical and radioactive iodine (RAI) treatment and approaches that suppress thyroid-stimulating hormone (TSH) [1–5]. Although these approaches provide long-term disease control even in metastatic disease, the disease may become resistant to RAI treatment after a while. In this case, the available treatment options are follow-up, anti-angiogenic kinase inhibitors, and chemotherapy. The place of radiotherapy is quite limited. On the other hand, anaplastic thyroid cancer is a highly aggressive tumor and its prognosis is poor in general and its main treatment is systemic chemotherapy.

S. N. Kazaz (✉)
Faculty of Medicine, Department of Medical Oncology, Karadeniz Technical University, Trabzon, Turkey
e-mail: nazlikazaz@ktu.edu.tr

İ. Öztop
Dokuz Eylül University, Institute of Oncology, Izmir, Turkey
e-mail: ilhan.oztop@deu.edu.tr

8.1 Therapy in Differentiated Thyroid Cancers

The basic treatment approach in early-stage DTC is surgery. However, total thyroidectomy±therapeutic neck dissection is recommended in the presence of any of the risk factors such as known distant metastasis, extrathyroidal spread, tumor diameter greater than 4 cm, cervical lymph node involvement, poor differentiation, bilateral nodularity, and known radiation exposure; otherwise, subtotal thyroidectomy + isthmusectomy may also be performed. Adjuvant radioactive iodine (RAI) ablation treatment and TSH suppression treatment are applied according to postoperative risk factors [3].

Recurrences may occur in approximately one-third of differentiated thyroid cancers in the following period. Local recurrences occur mostly in cervical lymph nodes, while the most common distant metastasis is the lung. Repeat surgery is recommended in local recurrence, if possible. If imaging is positive in local recurrences that cannot be resected, firstly RAI and radiotherapy are recommended [3]. The basic treatment approach in metastatic DTC is RAI treatment with TSH suppression. However, some patients become

R. Bekiş et al. (eds.), *Radionuclide Therapy*, https://doi.org/10.1007/978-3-030-97220-2_8

resistant to RAI treatment during the course of the disease. Resistance to RAI treatment is mentioned in the absence of RAI uptake in any of the metastatic lesions, in the absence of uptake in one or more of the lesions, or in the case of RAI uptake but progression with treatment. Other treatment options in this group of patients include chemotherapy, radiotherapy, metastasectomy in appropriate cases, and molecular targeted treatments. In this sense, anti-angiogenic multiple kinase inhibitors constitute the most commonly used and most up-to-date treatment approach today. In particular, kinase inhibitors targeting the vascular endothelial growth factor receptor (VEGFR) pathway are the most commonly used agents. These drugs provide tumor stabilization and can provide long-term disease control. But today there is not enough data to suggest that it increases overall survival. With the introduction of this group of drugs, the role of chemotherapy in the treatment of DTC is quite limited [3–7].

The treatment recommendation of the American Thyroid Association (ATA) guidelines [4] in differentiated thyroid cancer is as follows: Multiple kinase inhibitors are recommended in patients with RAI resistant DTC, tumor >1–2 cm and growth rate at least 20% per year, or symptomatic metastatic disease. Among these, lenvatinib and sorafenib are the primary drugs. Other multiple kinase inhibitors and BRAF inhibitors are recommended in patients who are progressing or intolerant to multiple kinase inhibitors. Cytotoxic chemotherapy remains in the background. In addition, supportive therapies such as radiotherapy and bisphosphonate therapies are recommended for bone metastasis while continuing treatment suppressing TSH [3, 6].

8.2 Multiple Kinase Inhibitors

VEGF expression and peritumoral angiogenesis are increased in thyroid cancer cells [8, 9]. In addition, studies have found genetic alterations in MAPK (mitogen-activated protein kinase) and PI3K-AKT/mTOR pathway, PTEN mutation in Cowden syndrome, BRAF-V600E mutation in papillary thyroid cancer, and activating mutations in RAS (KRAS, HRAS, NRAS) oncogen. RAS mutation and increased VEGF expression are associated with poor prognosis. Other important signal transmission pathways are fibroblast growth factor receptor (FGFR) and platelet-derived growth factor receptor (PDGFR) [10–12]. Among these, most frequently, increased VEGF expression and activation in the MAPK pathway are retained responsible. Kinase inhibitors developed for these goals have found an important place in the treatment of DTC as in many tumors. Some kinase inhibitors selectively block one of these targets, while others block multiple targets (multiple kinase inhibitors). The main ones with clinical trials in thyroid cancers are sorafenib, lenvatinib, sunitinib, pazopanib, vandetanib, and cabozantinib, and their clinical activities will be briefly discussed.

Sorafenib is a multiple kinase inhibitor that blocks VEGFR 1, 2, and 3, platelet-derived growth factor receptor (PDGFR), common RET subtypes, c-kit, and to a lesser extent BRAF [13]. The efficacy of sorafenib in RAI-resistant DTC has been investigated in a randomized phase 3 study. In the study of a total of 417 patients, patients were randomized to sorafenib or placebo arms. In conclusion, sorafenib was superior to placebo in median progression-free survival (10.8 months vs. 5.8 months). Overall survival was longer in the sorafenib arm than in the placebo arm, but no statistical significance was achieved (HR 0.8; $P = 0.14$). Similarly, the 12% response rate obtained with sorafenib was not found to be significant. Generally, grade 1 and 2 side effects were observed. Hand-foot syndrome, diarrhea, alopecia, and rash were reported at a frequency of 76%, 68%, 67%, and 50% in the sorafenib arm. Toxicity rates leading to dose reduction and treatment discontinuation were reported as 78% and 14%, respectively [14] (Table 8.1). Sorafenib received FDA approval in 2013 for the treatment of RAI-resistant, recurrent, or metastatic progressive DTC [15].

Lenvatinib is a multiple kinase inhibitor that inhibits VEGFR, RET, and fibroblast growth factor receptor kinases 1–4 [16]. The efficacy of lenvatinib in RAI-resistant DTC has been investigated in a randomized phase 3 study. In the

Table 8.1 Phase 3 studies in local advanced or metastatic radioiodine-resistant thyroid cancers

Study	Drug	Phase	Histology	Previous treatment	Number of patients	Response rate	PFS (months)	*p*	OS (HR)	*p*
Decision [14]	Sorafenib Placebo	3	DTC	None	207 210	12% 0.5%	10.8 5.8	<0.001	0.80	0.14
Select [17]	Lenvatinib Placebo	3	DTC	Yes	261 131	64% 1.5%	18.3 3.6	<0.001	0.73	0.10
Zeta [29]	Vandetanib Placebo	3	MTC	Yes	231 100	45% 13%	30.5 19.3	<0.001	0.89	NS
Exam [30]	Cabozantinib Placebo	3	MTC	Yes	219 111	28% 0%	11.2 4.0	<0.001 <0.001	0.89 0.98	NS NS

SELECT study of a total of 392 patients, patients were randomized to lenvatinib or placebo arms. In conclusion, lenvatinib was superior to placebo in median progression-free survival (18.3 months vs. 3.6 months) and response rate (64.8% vs. 1.5%). The most common adverse reactions of grade 3 and above were reported as hypertension (42%), proteinuria (10%), fatigue (9%), diarrhea (8%), and venous and arterial thrombosis (3.8% and 2.7%).

Severe adverse reactions such as gastrointestinal perforation/fistula were reported as 2% in the lenvatinib arm and 0.8% in the placebo arm. 14% (37 patients) discontinued due to adverse events [17] (Table 8.1). This benefit with lenvatinib was observed in both the age group below 65 years and the age group above 65 years [18]. Lenvatinib received FDA approval in 2015 for the treatment of RAI-resistant, recurrent, or metastatic progressive DTC [19].

Sunitinib is a multiple kinase inhibitor that blocks VEGFR 1, 2, and 3 and RET subtypes 1 and 3 [20]. Partial response and stable disease were found to be 13% and 68%, respectively, in a phase 2 study in patients with DTC who progressed under RAI treatment and used sunitinib at a dose of 50 mg/day (28 days treatment and 14 days off) [21]. In another phase 2 study using sunitinib at a dose of 37.5 mg/day (continuous use) (35 patients with DTC and 7 patients with medullary thyroid cancer), 3% had a complete response, 28% had a partial response, and 46% achieved a stable disease response [22].

Pazopanib is an anti-angiogenic kinase inhibitor that blocks all VEGFRs [23]. It does not distinctively inhibit RET. The efficacy of pazopanib (800 mg/d) was investigated in a phase 2 study in 37 patients with RAI-resistant DTC. As a result, 49% partial response and 47% 1-year progression-free survival were found [24].

Vandetanib is a multiple kinase inhibitor that blocks VEGFR, RET, and epidermal growth factor receptor (EGFR) [25]. The efficacy of vandetanib in RAI-resistant DTC was investigated in a randomized study. In the study of a total of 145 patients, patients were randomized to vandetanib or placebo arms. In conclusion, median progression-free survival was longer in the vandetanib arm (11.1 months vs 5.9 months), with no significant difference in response rate (8% vs. 5%). The efficacy was reported to be higher in the papillary Ca subtype. Toxicities of grade 3 and above in the vandetanib arm were reported as QTc prolongation 14%, diarrhea 10%, and asthenia 7% [26]. Vandetanib is also highly effective in medullary thyroid cancer and is a kinase inhibitor recommended by treatment guidelines [3] (Table 8.1).

Cabozantinib is a multiple kinase inhibitor that blocks VEGFR, RET, and c-MET [27]. The efficacy of cabozantinib was investigated in a phase 2 study in 25 patients with RAI-resistant DTC who had previously used 1 or 2 lines of other kinase inhibitors. As a result, 40% partial response and 52% stable disease response were achieved. Median progression-free survival was 12.7 months [28]. Cabozantinib is also highly effective in medullary thyroid cancer like vandetanib and is a kinase inhibitor recommended by treatment guidelines [3] (Table 8.1).

Although multiple kinase inhibitors generally do not provide cure for the disease, they show significant clinical efficacy and delay progression. These drugs have their own class side effects. Optimal treatment management is very important when using multiple kinase inhibitors due to the unique clinical behavior pattern of DTCs. In this sense, both optimal dose use and good side effect management are necessary in order not to decrease efficacy [3, 5].

8.3 Side Effects of Multiple Kinase Inhibitors Targeting Vascular Endothelial Growth Factor Receptor

Major side effects include fatigue, diarrhea, hypertension, hand-foot syndrome, myelosuppression, bleeding, thyroid dysfunction, arterial thromboembolism, and Q-T prolongation [13, 16, 20, 23, 25, 27, 29–38].

8.4 BRAF Inhibitors

Another oncogenic abnormality that plays a role in the development and invasion of differentiated thyroid cancers is the presence of BRAF mutation. BRAF V600E mutation reaches 80% in papillary thyroid cancers. In this respect, phase 2 studies were conducted with BRAF inhibitors vemurafenib and dabrafenib. Fifty-one patients with papillary thyroid cancer with BRAF V-600 mutation resistant to RAI were treated with vemurafenib in a study. As a result of this study with approximately half of the patients having previously received anti-angiogenic kinase inhibitors, the response rate in the group that had not previously received anti-angiogenic kinase inhibitors was 38.5%, and median progression-free survival was 18.2 months, while these rates remained 27.3% and 8.9 months in the anti-angiogenic kinase inhibitor group, respectively [39]. In a phase 2 study with dabrafenib, another BRAF inhibitor, the efficacy of dabrafenib was investigated in 14 patients with BRAF (V600E)-mutant metastatic thyroid cancer, achieving a partial response of 29% and median progression-free survival of 11.3 months [40]. It is also stated that BRAF inhibitors can stimulate re-differentiation and thus RAI uptake in RAI-resistant patients [41, 42]. Studies on BRAF inhibitors and MEK inhibitors are ongoing.

8.5 Side Effects of BRAF Inhibitors

Major side effects include rash, fatigue, weight loss, alopecia, squamous cell carcinoma, and skin tumors in the form of non-squamous cell carcinoma [23, 43–45].

8.6 Cytotoxic Chemotherapy

Due to the introduction of kinase inhibitors in differentiated thyroid cancers and the long-term disease stabilization effects they provide, the role of cytotoxic chemotherapy is quite limited. However, it is stated that it can be considered as salvage treatment in the selected patient group with high performance status. Today, it is recommended as an alternative option in patients progressing or intolerant to kinase inhibitor treatments in DTC [46]. Doxorubicin is the most investigated and widely used agent among chemotherapeutic drugs. Doxorubicin, the main treatment agent for anaplastic thyroid cancer, is the only chemotherapeutic agent approved by the FDA in DTCs with a partial response rate of 30–40% in phase 2 studies in RAI-resistant cases [46–50]. Studies on the use of doxorubicin in DTC have reported that it is more effective every 3 weeks than weekly use and is more useful especially in patients with lung metastasis and patients with good performance status [46, 51]. It is stated that combination treatments do not significantly increase efficacy [49].

Main side effects of doxorubicin include cardiotoxicity, myelosuppression, alopecia, secondary malignancy, amenorrhea, infertility, mucositis, abdominal pain, anorexia, and urinary discoloration. Rare but serious side effects affecting treatment with doxorubicin are dose-dependent cardiotoxicity and are generally irreversible, and patients should be monitored by echocardiography at the beginning of and during treatment [52, 53].

8.7 Therapy in Medullary Thyroid Cancers

Medullary thyroid carcinoma is one of the rare thyroid malignancies and is also a member of the group of neuroendocrine tumors. It is the third most common thyroid malignancy and constitutes 3% of thyroid cancers. It develops from parafollicular C cells of the thyroid that produce calcitonin. It is divided into three groups as sporadic, hereditary, and familial. Calcitonin is a very important biomarker in diagnosing and determining recurrences and distant organ metastases. Carcinoembryonic antigen (CEA) is also used as a biomarker in MTC follow-up and evaluation of treatment response, although it is not specific. Its prognosis is worse than other subtypes because it causes distant organ metastases more frequently than papillary and follicular thyroid carcinomas. Approximately 13% of patients have distant organ metastases at the time of diagnosis. The mean overall survival in patients with metastatic MTC is 3 years [54–57].

The standard treatment for MTC is surgery. Thyroidectomy and prophylactic central lymph node dissection are performed surgically. Radiotherapy can be applied in incomplete surgery or surgical margin positivity. Cytotoxic chemotherapy has a limited role in recurrent and metastatic disease. With advances in molecular oncology, tyrosine kinase inhibitors (TKIs) come to the forefront in treatment. RET mutation is seen in sporadic MTC (30%–50%) as in hereditary MTC (95%) accompanying multiple endocrine neoplasia (MEN) syndromes [58]. RAS mutations occur in a group of patients (10%) without somatic RET mutations. MTC tumor cells and vascular endothelial cells overexpress VEGF receptors (VEGFR-1–VEGFR-2) [59]. In recent years, tyrosine kinase inhibitors (cabozantinib, vandetanib, sorafenib, sunitinib) targeting RET and VEGFR kinases have been used in many studies in patients with advanced MTC. Two TKIs (Vandetanib-2011, Cabozantinib-2012), whose phase 3 studies have been completed and demonstrated to prolong progression-free survival, have been approved by the FDA for use in patients with advanced MTC.

8.8 Multiple Kinase Inhibitors

There are two phase 2 studies and several retrospective studies involving a small number of MTC patients with sorafenib [60]. A meta-analysis of sorafenib studies evaluated 219 patients (159 patients with DTC, 52 patients with MTC, 8 patients with anaplastic thyroid carcinoma) and found partial response in 22% and progressive disease in only 6.5% of MTC patients. Hand-foot syndrome and diarrhea were observed in 70% of patients receiving sorafenib; fatigue, weight loss, and skin rash in 50%; hypertension in 36%; acute myocardial infarction in 3.8%; and severe hypokalemia in 2.5% (grades 3–4). Caution should be exercised with hypoparathyroidism after thyroidectomy in terms of secondary hypokalemia and other electrolyte imbalance. Cutaneous squamous cell carcinoma was observed in 6.8% of patients (6 patients in total, 4 patients with keratoacanthoma).

In the study, it was reported that 16% of the patients could not tolerate the drug due to toxicity and 56% had a dose reduction [61].

Thirty-five patients with advanced MTC were included in a phase 2 study with pazopanib in MTC. 35% of patients had a partial response lasting 29 weeks, 23% had a stable response, and 14% had progression, while 63% of the patients died during treatment. Tumor response rate was 14.3% and median PFS was 9.4 months. The most common side effects reported were fatigue, impaired liver function tests, hand-foot syndrome, diverticulitis, diarrhea, hypertension, and mood changes. Dose reduction is recommended for grade 3 and above side effects in patients using pazopanib. It should be retained in mind that there may be side effects such as proteinuria, gastrointestinal perforation, grade 3–4 hemorrhage, and severe thrombosis due to the use of pazopanib [62].

Fifty-nine patients with surgically unresectable progressive MTC were treated with lenvatinib in a phase 2 study. While the best response rate was 35% in all partial response patients, stable disease was detected in the other 44%. Similar response rates were observed in patients with or without prior VEGFR-targeted therapy. Median progression-free survival and overall survival were reported as 9.0 months and 16.6 months, respectively. Side effects such as diarrhea, hypertension, and decreased appetite were observed [63].

The efficacy of vandetanib in MTC has been investigated in phase 2 and phase 3 studies. In the phase 3 prospective, multicenter ZETA study, 331 locally advanced MTC patients with metastatic or progression were included, and patients were randomized 2:1 to vandetanib or placebo arms. In conclusion, vandetanib demonstrated superiority over placebo in PFS (30.5 vs. 19.3 months), with no overall difference in survival. However, patients with CEA doubling times greater than 24 months were unlikely to benefit from treatment, while the presence of somatic RET M918T mutation was predicted to increase progression-free survival [29] (Table 8.1). With this study, vandetanib received FDA approval in MTC. Diarrhea, fatigue, skin rash, folliculitis, photosensitivity, hypertension, and QT prolongation at grade 1–2 level have been reported as the side effect profile of vandetanib. 12% of patients in the vandetanib arm were unable to continue treatment due to toxicity, and the dose was reduced in 35% [29]. In planning treatment with vandetanib, dose adjustment according to renal function and routine blood tests, especially ECG, sodium, potassium, calcium, and magnesium monitoring, are recommended at 2, 4, 8, and 12 weeks after initiation of treatment. This interval can be extended if there is no problem. In addition, close monitoring of diarrhea is recommended [37].

Another multiple kinase inhibitor investigated in MTC is cabozantinib. In the phase 3, randomized, prospective, multicenter EXAM study with which cabozantinib received FDA approval, 330 advanced stage MTC patients were randomized 2:1 to cabozantinib or placebo arms. In conclusion, cabozantinib demonstrated superiority over placebo in PFS (11.2 vs. 4.0 months) (Table 8.1). Diarrhea, malaise, palmoplantar erythrodysesthesia, and gastrointestinal fistula were observed in the side effect profile. It was reported that 16% of patients could not continue treatment due to toxicities and 79% had a dose reduction [30]. In the subgroup analyses of this study, PFS was found to be significantly superior to placebo, especially in patients with M918T mutation (61 vs. 17 weeks) and RET mutation (47 vs. 8 weeks). Electrolyte, calcium, and TSH monitoring is also required at certain intervals in cabozantinib use [38].

8.9 Cytotoxic Chemotherapy

With the widespread use of targeted therapies in MTC, the use of cytotoxic drugs has been seriously reduced. Among chemotherapeutic drugs, single-agent doxorubicin, platinum-doxorubicin combination, 5-FU-dacarbazine, and cyclophosphamide-vincristine-dacarbazine combinations are the most commonly studied ones. Doxorubicin is FDA approved for all histological types of thyroid cancers, including MTC. However, less than 30% of patients achieved an objective response and the response time was very short. There are positive results with the use of capecitabine at the case level in resistant metastatic MTC cases [64]. After positive results in a prospective phase 2 CAPTEM study with the concomitant use of temozolomide and capecitabine in well-differentiated neuroendocrine tumors, there are cases in which partial response is achieved with the use of these two agents in metastatic MTC patients [65].

Studies with radioimmunotherapy and bispecific monoclonal antibody and iodine-labeled bivalent hapten use in patients with advanced MTC have shown promising results. However, there are no prospective, randomized clinical trials with other treatments or with comparison to placebo. Time is needed for the use of these treatments [66, 67].

8.10 Side Effect Management in Drugs Used in the Treatment of Thyroid Cancer

The severity of toxicities observed during treatment is usually graded according to assessment methods such as the National Cancer Institute Common Terminology Criteria for Adverse Events (NCI-CCTCAE) [68]. Approaches such as discontinuation, postponement, dose reduction, as well as specific approaches specific to toxicity are made depending on the type and degree of toxicity observed.

8.11 Management of Common Side Effects in Chemotherapeutics

Although the role of cytotoxic chemotherapy gradually decreases with longer-term responses with kinase inhibitors in differentiated thyroid cancers, it is stated that it can be considered as salvage treatment in patients with good performance status. Doxorubicin, the only chemotherapeutic agent approved by the FDA with a partial response rate of 30–40% in phase 2 studies, is used in this group of patients [46–50].

The main side effects of doxorubicin include cardiotoxicity, myelosuppression, alopecia, secondary malignancy, amenorrhea, infertility, mucositis, abdominal pain, anorexia, and urinary discoloration. Rare but severe side effects affecting treatment with doxorubicin are dose-dependent cardiotoxicity and are generally irreversible (type 1 cardiotoxicity). Although the guidelines do not yet recommend routine basal echocardiography (ECHO) at the beginning of the treatment, most experts believe that basal ECHO should be performed in order to facilitate the detection of newly developing adverse events during the treatment process. In addition, echocardiography should be monitored at regular intervals during treatment [52, 53]. Anthracyclines should be avoided in patients with low ejection fraction (EF) along with heart failure or left ventricular EF (LVEF) ≤40% on the basal ECHO. In asymptomatic patients with 40–50% basal LVEF and without heart failure, it is recommended that the treatment decision be made according to the profit/loss ratio. If anthracycline is to be used, it is recommended to provide blood pressure control in patients with hypertension; to initiate β blockers (recommended carvedilol, nebivolol) with ACE inhibitors/ARB before starting anthracyclines, for close ECHO monitoring; and to discontinue anthracycline if there is a 10% decrease compared to basal LVEF. Blood pressure control and ECHO monitoring are sufficient in patients with LVEF ≥50% and without heart failure [69]. For patients on doxorubicin, it is generally recommended to limit the lifetime dose to 450–550 mg/m^2. Some experts start dexrazoxane when lifetime anthracycline doses exceed 300 mg/m^2. Dexrazoxane is the only drug approved by the FDA to prevent anthracycline-mediated cardiotoxicity.

Another important and frequent side effect of doxorubicin is myelosuppression. It may be accompanied by leukopenia (≤75%; often develops within 10–14 days; recovery: on day 21), neutropenia (≤75%; often develops within 10–14 days; recovery: on day 21), anemia, and thrombocytopenia. Close monitoring is required. Acceleration of the exit time from neutropenia with granulocyte colony-stimulating agents (G-CSF) such as filgrastim according to the degree of neutropenia, close follow-up in terms of neutropenic fever, hospitalization if necessary, antibiotherapy, and platelet and erythrocyte transfusion replacements should be performed as needed. G-CSF prophylaxis should be performed, and dose modification should be performed according to the degree of toxicity in recurrent courses (Table 8.2) [52, 53, 68].

Doxorubicin may cause discoloration in the urine. Patients should be informed about this in order to prevent unnecessary fears. Another point to be considered in doxorubicin use is extravasation because it is a vesicant agent. It may result in severe local tissue damage and necrosis, which may require extensive excision of the affected area and skin graft. If extravasa-

Table 8.2 Hematological toxicity NCI-CTCAE v5.0 [68]

Blood element	Grade 1	Grade 2	Grade 3	Grade 4	Grade 5
Neutrophils	Between LLN and 1500/ microL	1000–1500/ microL	500–1000/microL	<500/microL	
Platelets	Between LLN and 75,000/ microL	50,000–75,000/ microL	25,000–50,000/microL	<25,000/microL	
Hemoglobin	Between LLN and 10.0 g/dL	8.0–10.0 g/dL	<8.0 g/dL	Life-threatening consequences; requiring urgent intervention	Death
Febrile neutropenia			Absolute number of neutrophils <1000 microL and presence of body temperature > 38.30 °C at a single measurement or ≥ 38.00 °C lasting longer than 1 h	Life-threatening consequences; requiring urgent intervention	Death

NCI CTCAE, National Cancer Institute Common Terminology Criteria for Adverse Events; LLN, lower limit of normal; Cell/microL, cell/mm^3 or cell × 10^9/L

tion is suspected, the infusion should be terminated immediately and ice applied to the affected area. It is very important to ensure and control the placement of appropriate needles or catheters before and during infusion to avoid extravasation [52, 53].

8.12 Management of Common Side Effects in Tyrosine Kinase Inhibitors

Thyroid kinase inhibitors, which are more commonly used today in metastatic differentiated thyroid cancers, have group side effects and agent-specific side effects. First of all, comorbidities and risk profile should be well evaluated with detailed anamnesis before treatment. Stabilization of comorbidities, evaluation of the drugs to be taken concurrently in terms of interaction, and patient education on the side effects of the disease and the treatment agent are very important. The severity of toxicities is usually graded according to assessment methods such as the National Cancer Institute Common Terminology Criteria for Adverse Events (NCI-CTC) [3, 5, 70–72].

8.13 Skin Toxicity Management

Several skin side effects have been reported with sorafenib, vandetanib, and lenvatinib. Hand-foot syndrome (HFSR) (37% with sorafenib, 6% with pazopanib) and rash (41% with vandetanib) are most common, followed by squamoproliferative lesions. More rarely, seborrheic dermatitis, subungual splinter hemorrhages, erythema multiforme, and eruptive melanocytic lesions are observed [73, 74].

There is no evidence yet in randomized studies that determine the best management strategy for HFSR [75]. However, expert opinions are available from an international consensus group [76]. The most important of these recommendations is the removal of existing hyperkeratotic areas and calluses using appropriately sterilized tools, avoiding exposure of hands and feet to hot water, and avoiding excessive friction on the skin in daily activities. It should be emphasized that severe exercises that exert excessive stress especially on the palms and/or soles of the feet should be avoided, especially during the first treatment period.

It should be recommended to wear padded soles throughout treatment to reduce foot pres-

Table 8.3 Grading in hand-foot syndrome [5, 68, 76, 77]

Grade	Symptoms
Grade 1	Numbness, dysesthesia, paresthesia, tingling, painless edema, erythema, and restlessness in hands and feet, not affecting daily activity
Grade 2	Painful erythema, edema, and restlessness in hands and feet, affecting daily activity
Grade 3	Peeling, cracking, erosion, severe pain, and restlessness in hands and feet, unable to perform daily activities

sure. Patients should be warned to wear thick cotton gloves or socks to prevent injury and to keep palms and soles dry [76, 77].

For patients who develop HFSR while taking sorafenib, the following management strategies are recommended by this group [70, 76] (Table 8.3):

- No dose adjustment is required for mild (grade 1) symptoms. Hot water should be avoided and the use of topical softeners should be encouraged. Keratolytics such as topical urea (20–40%) or salicylic acid (6–10%) may be recommended.
- Treatment for grade 2 HFSR should continue as in grade 1 HFSR, but with topical corticosteroids (clobetasol 0.05% ointment) added to erythematous areas twice daily. Topical analgesics such as 2% lidocaine may be sufficient. If necessary, the dose of sorafenib may be temporarily reduced by up to 50% for at least 7 days until HFSR grade 0 or 1 is reached, and then the full dose is resumed.
- For grade 3 HFSR, treatment according to grade 1 or 2 HFSR should be provided upon temporary discontinuation of the drug for at least 7 days until grade 1 or 2. Treatment should continue up to 50% of the dose. Dose increase can be attempted if the side effect is not repeated [76, 77].

Sorafenib is also associated with cutaneous squamoproliferative lesions, including keratoacanthomas (KA) and squamous cell carcinomas (SCC) [78]. Twenty-two squamoproliferative lesions were seen in 13 patients within nine months of initiation in a series after starting sorafenib. One was reported as classic invasive SCC, 5 as KA-like SCC, and 16 as classic KA [78]. In a retrospective study of 131 patients receiving sorafenib for metastatic renal cell carcinoma, 7 were diagnosed with SCC and 2 were diagnosed with KA [79]. Squamoproliferative lesions that develop during treatment with sorafenib should be treated in a similar manner to lesions that develop in patients who have not taken any drug (usually with complete surgical excision). There is no definite evidence to continue against discontinuation of sorafenib in patients who develop SCC or KA during treatment. Close clinical follow-up is required during treatment [70].

In clinical trials, skin reactions with vemurafenib were also common in metastatic/unresectable thyroid cancer, and the incidence of serious adverse effects was reported to be 26.9% for squamous cell carcinoma and 7.6% for keratoacanthoma [39]. Vemurafenib-related phototoxic reactions are thought to be associated with UVA radiation and can be prevented by the use of broad-spectrum sunscreens [80].

Stevens-Johnson syndrome (SJS) and toxic epidermal necrolysis (TEN) have been reported in patients receiving vemurafenib [81–83].

Among patients receiving dabrafenib, verrucal keratotic lesions with low to moderate epidermal dysplasia were reported up to 66%, and keratoacanthomas or well-differentiated cutaneous SCC were reported between 6% and 26% in melanoma use [84–86]. These side effects have not been reported with dabrafenib in thyroid cancer (in combination with trametinib). The risk of developing skin SCC with BRAF inhibitors increases up to 30 percent in patients older than 60 years of age [87]. Most lesions develop during the first 3 months of treatment and may occur in sun-protected areas. Cutaneous SCC developing in patients treated with these agents is treated with surgical excision, and patients can generally continue treatment without dose adjustment [88]. Trametinib and cobimetinib are mitogen-activated protein kinase (MAPK) kinase enzyme (MEK1 and MEK2) inhibitors [89, 90] approved for the treatment of metastatic melanoma, a BRAF V600E or V600K mutation, in combination with dabrafenib and vemurafenib. Trametinib was also approved in combination with dabrafenib in unresectable-metastatic BRAF mutant anaplastic thyroid cancer [91]. Data from combination therapy studies with dabrafenib+trametinib for advanced melanoma indicate that combination therapy is associated with a marked cutaneous toxicity reduction compared to vemurafenib or dabrafenib alone [86, 92]. Patients should be managed with close dermatological follow-up during these treatments [70].

8.14 Thyroid Dysfunction Management

Thyroid dysfunction is seen more frequently in patients receiving sunitinib for metastatic RCC but also in patients treated with sorafenib [71, 93]. In the analysis of thyroid function in RCC data, hypothyroidism was observed in 7 (18%) of 39 patients and hyperthyroidism in 1 patient [94]. Two of the hypothyroidism patients (5% of the total) were symptomatic and required thyroid replacement therapy [95].

Hypothyroidism has also been reported among pazopanib-treated patients and therefore appears to be a class effect of these agents [95–97]. Regular monitoring of TSH levels at baseline and during treatment is recommended in patients treated with antiangiogenic TKIs due to the high frequency of hypothyroidism, initial evaluation of thyroid function tests, and subsequent and every 4–12 weeks monitoring in symptomatic patients. Symptomatic patients with hypothyroidism should receive thyroid hormone support. No discontinuation of the agent causing toxicity and no dose modification is usually necessary [3, 5, 71].

8.15 Gastrointestinal Toxicities Side Effect Management

Diarrhea, nausea, and vomiting have been observed in all antiangiogenic TKIs and are generally mild. In clinical trials, diarrhea was reported in 30–79% (highest with vandetanib) of all grades and severe diarrhea (grade 3/4) in 3–17% [26, 98–104]. In addition to being a VEGFR inhibitor, vandetanib is also an epidermal growth factor receptor (EGFR) inhibitor. Therefore, the higher incidence of diarrhea associated with this agent is attributed to this [26, 101].

Nausea (all grades) was reported in 23–58% of patients treated with antiangiogenic TKIs in clinical trials. Sunitinib-, lenvatinib-, and cabozantinib-treated patients had the highest rates. Vomiting of any grade was reported in 10–48% of patients treated with pazopanib and sorafenib with the lowest and highest rates with sunitinib, lenvatinib, and cabozantinib [17, 105–107].

Nausea and vomiting are rarely severe and are usually controlled with oral antiemetics. However, caution should be exercised in combining vandetanib, lenvatinib, sunitinib, and sorafenib with serotonin antagonists such as granisetron and ondansetron due to QTc interval prolongation and torsades de pointes potential (especially with BRAF inhibitors) [71].

Infectious agents should be treated in accordance with their degree after being excluded in addition to performing fluid-electrolyte replacement in case of diarrhea. It is generally sufficient to prevent food and supplements that increase symptomatic management and gastrointestinal motility with an oral antidiarrheal agent such as loperamide in the treatment of grade 1 or 2 diarrhea. Treatment should be discontinued for grade 3 or 4 diarrhea, and dose modifications may be required to control diarrhea if the drug is continued (Table 8.4) [68, 71, 108].

8.16 Hepatotoxicity Management

Serious and occasionally fatal hepatotoxicity has been observed in clinical studies with all VEGFR TKIs. The risk of elevated serum alanine transaminase (ALT), aspartate transaminase (AST), alkaline phosphatase (ALP), and bilirubin during treatment with VEGFR TKIs was discussed in a meta-analysis of 18,282 patients from 52 randomized controlled trials [109]. The incidence of hepatic failure in VEGFR TKIs was found to be

Table 8.4 Diarrhea NCI-CTCAE v5.0 [68]

Adverse event	Grade 1	Grade 2	Grade 3	Grade 4	Grade 5
Diarrhea	<4 increase in daily defecation relative to baseline	4–6 increase in daily defecation relative to baseline	≥7 increase in daily defecation relative to baseline; requiring hospitalization	Life-threatening results; requiring urgent intervention	Death
	Moderate increase in stool coming from ostomy relative to baseline	Moderate increase in stool coming from ostomy relative to baseline	Severe increase in stool coming from ostomy relative to baseline; limitation of self-care		

NCI CTCAE, National Cancer Institute Common Terminology Criteria for Adverse Events

0.8% in general. Relative risks (RRs) for elevations in all grades in ALT, AST, ALP, and bilirubin in patients receiving VEGFR TKI were 1.57 ($p < 0.001$), 1.57 ($p < 0.001$), 1.20 ($p < 0.001$), and 1.55 ($p < 0.001$), respectively, compared to patients not treated with VEGFR TKI. While there was a statistically significant increase in the relative risk of ALT and AST for high-grade elevations, the risk increase in ALP and bilirubin elevation was not statistically significant [109].

Sorafenib-induced hepatitis can be accompanied by hepatocellular hepatic injury, which is a significant increase in transaminases that can result in hepatic failure and death. There may also be increases in bilirubin and INR. It is recommended to exclude the causes such as viral hepatitis or progressive malignancy first and to discontinue the drug considering drug-related hepatotoxicity in case of a significant increase in transaminases (Table 8.5) [5, 68, 71, 109].

Polymorphisms in the enzyme diphosphoglucuronosyltransferase 1A1 (UGT 1A1), which causes Gilbert syndrome (UGT1A1 * 28 alleles), are thought to be associated with pazopanib- and sorafenib-induced hyperbilirubinemia. Isolated hyperbilirubinemia in these patients may represent a benign manifestation of Gilbert syndrome, in which case continuation of treatment is recommended [110–112].

In general, liver function tests (LFTs) should be periodically evaluated at baseline and during treatment in patients treated with any of these agents. Evaluation of liver function tests is recommended, especially for patients treated with pazopanib, at baseline and at weeks 3, 5, 7, 9, 12, and 16 and periodically thereafter, and interruption or complete discontinuation of treatment is recommended in patients with bilirubin levels 3 times and above [71, 113, 114].

8.17 Management of Cardiovascular Side Effects

The main cardiovascular side effects are hypertension, arteriovenous thromboembolisms, LV dysfunction, and QT prolongation, which are seen as group side effects in this group of drugs [72].

Hypertension: Among VEGF receptor tyrosine kinase inhibitors, it is not clear whether any agent causes hypertension more frequently. In a meta-analysis, pazopanib was reported to cause hypertension in all grades at a higher rate than sorafenib and sunitinib (36%, 23%, and 22%, respectively), while high-grade hypertension rates were reported to be similar (6.5%, 5.7%, and 6.8%, respectively) [36]. On the other hand, both all-grade (68%) and severe (42%) hypertension rates were found to be higher with lenvatinib [17]. It has been reported in some studies that there is a relationship between antiangiogenic TKIs and antitumor efficacy during treatment and the development of systolic or diastolic hypertension [115–117].

Active control of hypertension in the use of these agents allows patients to tolerate effective treatment doses for a long time [118]. Recommendations in this regard include risk assessment for potential cardiovascular complications, identification and treatment of existing

Table 8.5 Hepatobiliary toxicity NCI-CTCAE v5.0 [68]

Adverse event	Grade 1	Grade 2	Grade 3	Grade 4	Grade 5
ALP increase	If baseline is normal, ULN to 2.5 × ULN	If baseline is normal, 2.5–5 × ULN	If baseline is normal, 5–20 × ULN	If baseline is normal, >20 × ULN	
	If baseline is abnormal, 2–2.5 × baseline	If baseline is abnormal, 2.5–5 × baseline	If baseline is abnormal, 5–20 × baseline	If baseline is abnormal, >20 × baseline	
ALT increase	If baseline is normal, ULN to 3 × ULN If baseline is abnormal, 1.5–3 × baseline	If baseline is normal, 3–5 x ULN If baseline is abnormal, 3–5 × baseline	If baseline is normal, 5–20 × ULN If baseline is abnormal, 5–20 × baseline	If baseline is normal, >20 × ULN If baseline is abnormal, >20 × baseline	
AST increase	If baseline is normal, ULN to 3 × ULN; if baseline is abnormal, 1.5–3 × baseline	If baseline is normal, 3–5 × ULN; if baseline is abnormal, 3–5 × baseline	If baseline is normal, 5–20 × ULN; if baseline is abnormal, 5–20 × baseline	If baseline is normal, >20 × ULN; if baseline is abnormal, >20 × baseline	
Serum bilirubin increase	If baseline is normal, ULN to 1.5 × ULN	If baseline is normal, 1.5–3 × ULN	If baseline is normal, 3–10 × ULN	If baseline is normal, >10 × ULN	
	If baseline is abnormal, 1–1.5 × baseline	If baseline is abnormal, 1.5–3 × baseline	If baseline is abnormal, 3–10 × baseline	If baseline is abnormal, >10 × baseline	
GGT increase	If baseline is normal, ULN to 2.5 × ULN	If baseline is normal, 2.5–5 × ULN	If baseline is normal, 5–20 × ULN	If baseline is normal, >20 × ULN	
	If baseline is abnormal, 2–2.5 × baseline	If baseline is abnormal, 2.5–5 × baseline	If baseline is abnormal, 5–20 × baseline	If baseline is abnormal, >20 × baseline	
Liver failure			Asterixis, moderate encephalopathy, liver injury due to the drug, limitation of self-care	Life-threatening outcomes, moderate-severe encephalopathy, coma	Death
Portal hypertension		Decrease in portal vein flow	Reverse/retrograde portal vein flow with varicose and/or acid	Life-threatening outcomes, requiring urgent intervention	Death

NCI CTCAE, National Cancer Institute Common Terminology Criteria for Adverse Events; ULN, upper limit of normal; ALP, alkaline phosphatase; ALT, alanine aminotransferase; AST, aspartate aminotransferase; GGT, gamma-glutamyl transpeptidase

hypertension before using these agents, active monitoring of blood pressure during treatment, more frequent measurements in the first few weeks of treatment, and lower blood pressure in those with pre-existing cardiovascular risk factors such as diabetes or chronic kidney disease [5, 72].

Patients who develop hypertension during treatment (defined as hypertension; blood pressure ≥ 140/90 mmHg, or 20 mmHg increase in diastolic blood pressure compared to basal) should be treated with antihypertensives. Agent selection should be based on the severity of hypertension and the urgency of blood pressure control. It is very important to avoid drugs with verapamil or diltiazem that inhibit it with agents that undergo partial metabolism with cytochrome p450 such as sunitinib/sorafenib even though it is not an optimal antihypertensive agent recommendation [72, 119].

Arterial/Venous Thromboembolism: Venous thromboembolism (VTE) is more common in anti-VEGF monoclonal antibodies and less common in anti-VEGF TKIs. In a systematic meta-analysis of 10 studies involving 10,255 patients (87% diagnosed with RCC) treated with sunitinib or sorafenib, the risk of arterial embolism was 1.4%, with a threefold increase in RR compared to controls [120]. Similarly, arterial thromboembolisms (ATE) were observed in 3% of pazopanib-treated patients in the placebo-controlled randomized pazopanib study in advanced RCC [121]. In a placebo-controlled lenvatinib study, ATEs occurred in 5% of the treated group and 2% of the placebo-treated group [122].

There is no adequate information to recommend the use of routine anticoagulation to prevent VTE in patients receiving or starting treatment with antiangiogenic TKIs. The NCCN Oncology Clinical Practice Guidelines recommend aspirin or anticoagulant prophylaxis based on the presence or absence of risk factors for VTE. NCCN has not defined the use of angiogenesis inhibitors for VTE in cancer patients as a risk factor, but expert opinions support prophylaxis with ponatinib, which is used in chronic myeloid leukemia due to the high risk of arterial and venous thromboembolism [3, 5, 72].

Both prevention and rapid management of arterial thromboembolic events are important. Cardiovascular risk factors (hypertension, hyperlipidemia, and diabetes) should be predetermined and aggressively managed prior to initiating treatment with antiangiogenic TKIs. Baseline blood pressure should be monitored, and the drug should preferably not be administered within 6 to 12 months in patients with severe cardiovascular events. Low-dose aspirin prophylaxis is appropriate in patients with ATE or other high-risk patients [123, 124]. Antiangiogenic treatment should be discontinued and ATE should be managed in other patients who develop ATE while receiving antiangiogenic TKI.

Left Ventricular Dysfunction/Myocardial Ischemia: Left ventricular (LV) function may decrease in patients treated with any of the VEGF-targeted treatments. A meta-analysis of 21 randomized studies using various VEGFR TKIs evaluated 10,647 patients. In the group without TKI, 37 of 4895 patients and 138 of 5752 patients receiving VEGFR TKI developed heart failure of any grade (0.75% versus 2.39%). In the group without TKI versus TKI, the RR of high-grade heart failure in all grades was 2.69 ($p < 0.001$; 95% CI 1.86–3.87) and 1.65 ($p = 0.227$, 95% CI 0.73–3.70), respectively [125]. In a placebo-controlled study in patients with advanced thyroid cancer, 7% cardiac dysfunction was reported in the lenvatinib arm versus 2% in the placebo arm. In most of the cases, ejection fraction was found to decrease on echocardiography [122].

It is recommended that LVEF of the patients be screened with ECHO or MUGA and basic evaluation with ECG [72]. Some sources have suggested that patients receiving these drugs should be treated as "stage A" heart failure patients (but without structural heart disease or symptoms, i.e., at risk of heart failure) [126]. The American Heart Association guideline states that it may be reasonable to consider those who receive potentially cardiotoxic agents for LV dysfunction as stage A heart failure in 2013 [127]. Monitoring of LVEF is generally recommended in patients treated with VEGFR TKI. US prescribing information for sunitinib recommends dose reduction or discontinuation in patients with clinical signs of cardiac failure and no clinical evidence of cardiac failure, but with an ejection fraction <50% and/or > 20% below baseline [128].

QT Prolongation/Cardiac Arrhythmia: Many drugs delay cardiac repolarization. This is an effect reflected on ECG in the QTc interval. Although a long QTc interval is not immediately harmful, it can be associated with potentially fatal cardiac arrhythmias. Triggered ventricular tachyarrhythmia (VT) is the most typical and most common, also known as torsades de pointes. It is often transient but can be fatal if it persists, causing impaired cerebral circulatory symptoms or ventricular fibrillation. The risk of other VEGFR TKIs, including sorafenib and pazopanib, is lower while vandetanib and sunitinib, inhibitors of VEGFR tyrosine kinase, are more

Table 8.6 NCI CTCAE v5.0 ECG QTc interval prolongation grading [5, 68, 72]

Adverse effect	Grade 1	Grade 2	Grade 3	Grade 4	Grade 5
Prolonged	QTc 450–480	QTc 481–500	QTc ≥501 ms;	Torsades de	Death
QTc interval on ECG	ms	ms	>60 ms change relative to baseline	pointes; polymorphic VT; serious arrhythmia symptoms	

NCI CTCAE, National Cancer Institute Common Terminology Criteria for Adverse Events; QTc, corrected QT interval

associated with QTc prolongation [129, 130]. In addition, QTc prolongation and cardiomyopathy can also be seen in BRAF inhibitors [5, 72].

Specific guidelines for the evaluation and monitoring of the QTc interval and recommendations for managing the drug by toxicity grade are available, especially for vandetanib and lenvatinib (Table 8.6). Guidelines for other antiangiogenic TKIs are not yet available. Concomitant drugs should be carefully reviewed, especially drugs that increase QTc should be evaluated for any patient receiving treatment with antiangiogenic TKI. Those with a history of QT interval prolongation, a history of arrhythmia, and pre-existing heart disease, bradycardia, or electrolyte disorder may be more prone to develop QTc prolongation. Dose reduction for TKI may be required if antiangiogenic TKIs are to be taken concomitantly with strong CYP3A4 inhibitors that may increase plasma concentrations.

Patients who develop arrhythmia should be evaluated and treated separately with cardiological consultation according to the definition of arrhythmia [5, 16, 25, 72].

References

1. Siegel RL, Miller KD, Jemal A. Cancer statistics, 2017. CA Cancer J Clin. 2017;67(1):7–30.
2. Yu GP, Li JC, Branovan D, et al. Thyroid Cancer incidence and survival in the national cancer institute surveillance, epidemiology, and end results race/ethnicity groups. Thyroid. 2010;20(5):465–73.
3. National Comprehensive Cancer Network (NCCN) Website. NCCN Clinical practice guidelines in oncology. Available at: https://www.nccn.org/professionals/physician_gls/pdf/thyroid.pdf. Accessed on 30 January, 2019.
4. Haugen BR, Alexander EK, Bible KC, et al. 2015 American Thyroid Association Management Guidelines for adult patients with thyroid nodules and differentiated thyroid cancer: The American Thyroid Association Guidelines Task Force on thyroid nodules and differentiated thyroid cancer. Thyroid. 2016;26(1):1–133.
5. UpToDate website. Available at: https://www.uptodate.com/contents/differentiated-thyroid-cancer-overview-of-management.
6. Haugen BR, Sherman SI. Evolving approaches to patients with advanced differentiated thyroid cancer. Endocr Rev. 2013;34(3):439–55.
7. Schlumberger M, Sherman SI. Clinical trials for progressive differentiated thyroid cancer: patient selection, study design, and recent advances. Thyroid. 2009;19(12):1393–400.
8. Ishiwata T, Iino Y, Takei H, et al. Tumor angiogenesis as an independent prognostic indicator in human papillary thyroid carcinoma. Oncol Rep. 1998;5:1343–8.
9. Lennard CM, Patel A, Wilson J, et al. Intensity of vascular endothelial growth factor expression is associated with increased risk of recurrence and decreased disease-free survival in papillary thyroid cancer. Surgery. 2001;129:552–8.
10. Fagin JA, Mitsiades N. Molecular pathology of thyroid cancer: diagnostic and clinical implications. Best Pract Res Clin Endocrinol Metab. 2008;22(6):955–69.
11. Nikiforova MN, Nikiforov YE. Molecular diagnostics and predictors in thyroid cancer. Thyroid. 2009;19(12):1351–61.
12. Narayanan S, Colevas AD. Current standards in treatment of radioiodine refractory thyroid cancer. Curr Treat Options in Oncol. 2016;17(6):30. https://doi.org/10.1007/s11864-016-0404-6.
13. Nexavar (sorafenib) [product monograph]. Toronto, ON: Bayer Inc.; May 2013.
14. Brose MS, Nutting CM, Jarzab B, et al. Sorafenib in radioactive iodine-refractory, locally advanced or metastatic differentiated thyroid cancer: a ran-

domised, double-blind, phase 3 trial. Lancet. 2014;384(9940):319–28.
15. http://www.fda.gov/NewsEvents/Newsroom/PressAnnouncements/ucm376443.htm (Accessed on December 02, 2013).
16. Lenvima (lenvatinib) [product monograph]. Mississauga, ON: Eisai Limited; December 2018.
17. Schlumberger M, Tahara M, Wirth LJ, et al. Lenvatinib versus placebo in radioiodine-refractory thyroid cancer. N Engl J Med. 2015;372(7):621–30.
18. Brose MS, Worden FP, Newbold KL, et al. Effect of age on the efficacy and safety of lenvatinib in radioiodine-refractory differentiated thyroid cancer in the phase III SELECT trial. J Clin Oncol. 2017;35:2692–9.
19. http://www.fda.gov/NewsEvents/Newsroom/PressAnnouncements/ucm434288.htm. Accessed on February 13, 2015.
20. Sutent (sunitinib) [product monograph]. Kirkland, QC: Pfizer Canada Inc; October 2018.
21. Cohen EE, Needles BM, Cullen KJ, et al. Phase 2 study of sunitinib in refractory thyroid cancer. J Clin Oncol (Meeting Abstracts). 2008;26
22. Carr LL, Mankoff DA, Goulart BH, et al. Phase II study of daily sunitinib in FDG-PET-positive, iodine- refractory differentiated thyroid cancer and metastatic medullary carcinoma of the thyroid with functional imaging correlation. Clin Cancer Res. 2010;16(21):5260–8.
23. Votrient (pazopanib) [product monograph]. Dorval, QC: Novartis Pharmaceuticals Canada Inc; January 2018.
24. Bible KC, Suman VJ, Molina JR, et al. Efficacy of pazopanib in progressive, radioiodine-refractory, metastatic differentiated thyroid cancers: results of a phase 2 consortium study. Lancet Oncol. 2010;11(10):962–72.
25. Caprelsa (vandetanib) [product monograph] Mississauga, ON: Genzyme Canada; May 2017.
26. Leboulleux S, Bastholt L, Krause T, et al. Vandetanib in locally advanced or metastatic differentiated thyroid cancer: a randomised, double-blind, phase 2 trial. Lancet Oncol. 2012;13(9):897–905.
27. Cabometyx (cabozantinib) [product monograph]. Mississauga, ON: Ipsen Biopharmaceuticals Canada Inc.; September 2018.
28. Cabanillas ME, de Souza JA, Geyer S, et al. Cabozantinib as salvage therapy for patients with tyrosine kinase inhibitor-refractory differentiated thyroid cancer: results of a multicenter phase II international thyroid oncology group trial. J Clin Oncol. 2017;35(29):3315–21.
29. Wells SA Jr, Robinson BG, Gagel RF, et al. Vandetanib in patients with locally advanced or metastatic medullary thyroid cancer: a randomized, double-blind phase III trial. J Clin Oncol. 2012;30:134–41.
30. Elisei R, Schlumberger MJ, Muller SP, et al. Cabozantinib in progressive medullary thyroid cancer. J Clin Oncol. 2013;31:3639–46.
31. Qi WX, Min DL, Shen Z, et al. Risk of venous thromboembolic events associated with VEGFR-TKIs: a systematic review and meta-analysis. Int J Cancer. 2013;132(12):2967–74.
32. http://www.bccancer.bc.ca/drug-database-site/Drug%20Index/Sorafenib_monograph.pdf
33. http://www.bccancer.bc.ca/drug-database-site/Drug%20Index/Lenvatinib_monograph.pdf
34. http://www.bccancer.bc.ca/drug-database-site/Drug%20Index/Sunitinib_monograph.pdf
35. http://www.bccancer.bc.ca/drug-database-site/Drug%20Index/Pazopanib_monograph.pdf
36. Qi WX, Lin F, Sun YJ, et al. Incidence and risk of hypertension with pazopanib in patients with cancer: a meta-analysis. Cancer Chemother Pharmacol. 2013;71(2):431–9.
37. http://www.bccancer.bc.ca/drug-database-site/Drug%20Index/Vandetanib_monograph.pdf
38. http://www.bccancer.bc.ca/drug-database-site/Drug%20Index/Cabozantinib_monograph.pdf
39. Brose MS, Cabanillas ME, Cohen EE, et al. Vemurafenib in patients with BRAF(V600E)-positive metastatic or unresectable papillary thyroid cancer refractory to radioactive iodine: a non-randomised, multicentre, open-label, phase 2 trial. Lancet Oncol. 2016;17(9):1272–82.
40. Falchook GS, Millward M, Hong D, et al. BRAF inhibitor dabrafenib in patients with metastatic BRAF-mutant thyroid cancer. Thyroid. 2015;25(1):71–7.
41. Huillard O, Tenenbaum F, Clerc J, Goldwasser F, Groussin L. Restoring radioiodine uptake in BRAF V600E-mutated papillary thyroid cancer. J Endocr Soc. 2017;1(4):285–7.
42. Dunn LA, Sherman EJ, Baxi SS, et al. Vemurafenib redifferentiation of BRAF mutant, RAİ-refractory thyroid cancers. J Clin Endocrinol Metab. 2018; https://doi.org/10.1210/jc.2018-01478.
43. Zelboraf (vemurafenib) [product monograph]. Mississauga, ON: Hoffman-La Roche Limited; February 2018.
44. http://www.bccancer.bc.ca/drug-database-site/Drug%20Index/Vemurafenib_monograph.pdf
45. http://www.bccancer.bc.ca/drug-database-site/Drug%20Index/Dabrafenib_monograph.pdf
46. Sherman SI. Cytotoxic chemotherapy for differentiated thyroid carcinoma. Clin Oncol (R Coll Radiol). 2010;22(6):464–8.
47. Bonadonna G, Monfardini S, De Lena M, et al. Phase I and preliminary phase II evaluation of Adriamycin (NSC 123127). Cancer Res. 1970;30:2572–82.
48. Gottlieb JA, Hill CS Jr. Chemotherapy of thyroid cancer with Adriamycin: experience with 30 patients. N Engl J Med. 1974;290:193–7.
49. Ahuja S, Ernst H. Chemotherapy of thyroid carcinoma. J Endocrinol Investig. 1987;10:303–10.
50. Matuszczyk A, Petersenn S, Bockisch A, et al. Chemotherapy with doxorubicin in progressive medullary and thyroid carcinoma of the follicular epithelium. Horm Metab Res. 2008;40:210–3.

51. Carter SK, Blum RH. New chemotherapeutic agents--bleomycin and adriamycin. CA Cancer J Clin. 1974;24(6):322–31.
52. Doxorubicin [product monograph]. Caledon, ON: Panda Pharmaceuticals, Inc; August 2017.
53. http://www.bccancer.bc.ca/drug-database-site/Drug%20Index/Doxorubicine_monograph.pdf
54. Pacini F, De Groot LJ. Thyroid cancer. In: De Groot LJ, et al., editors. Endotext. South Dartmouth, MA: MDText.com, Inc; 2000.
55. Schlumberger M, Bastholt L, Dralle H, et al. 2012 European thyroid association guidelines for metastatic medullary thyroid cancer. Eur Thyroid J. 2012;1(1):5–14.
56. Wells SA Jr, Asa SL, Dralle H, et al. Revised American Thyroid Association guidelines for the management of medullary thyroid carcinoma. Thyroid. 2015;25(6):567–610.
57. Chen H, Sippel RS, O'Dorisio MS, et al. The North American Neuroendocrine Tumor Society consensus guideline for the diagnosis and management of neuroendocrine tumors: pheochromocytoma, paraganglioma, and medullary thyroid cancer. Pancreas. 2010;39(6):775–83.
58. Dvorakova S, Vaclavikova E, Sykorova V, et al. Somatic mutations in the RET proto-oncogene in sporadic medullary thyroid carcinomas. Mol Cell Endocrinol. 2008;12(1–2):21–7.
59. Capp C, Wajner SM, Siqueira DR, et al. Increased expression of vascular endothelial growth factor and its receptors, VEGFR-1 and VEGFR-2, in medullary thyroid carcinoma. Thyroid. 2010;20(8):863–71.
60. de Castroneves LA, Negrão MV, de Freitas RM, et al. Sorafenib for the treatment of progressive metastatic medullary thyroid cancer: efficacy and safety analysis. Thyroid. 2016;26(3):414–9.
61. Thomas L, Lai SY, Dong W, et al. Sorafenib in metastatic thyroid cancer: a systematic review. Oncologist. 2014;19(3):251–8.
62. Bible KC, Suman VJ, Molina JR, et al. A multicenter phase 2 trial of pazopanib in metastatic and progressive medullary thyroid carcinoma: MC057H. J Clin Endocrinol Metab. 2014;99(5):1687–93.
63. Schlumberger M, Jarzab B, Cabanillas ME, et al. A Phase II trial of the multitargeted tyrosine kinase inhibitor lenvatinib (E7080) in advanced medullary thyroid cancer. Clin Cancer Res. 2016;22(1):44.
64. Paiva CE, Michelin OC. Use of capecitabine in refractory metastatic medullary thyroid carcinoma. Thyroid. 2008;18(5):587. https://doi.org/10.1089/thy.2007.0220.
65. Lacin S, Esin E, Karakas Y, Yalcin S. Metastatic medullary thyroid cancer: a dramatic response to a systemic chemotherapy (temozolomide and capecitabine) regimen. Onco Targets Ther. 2015;8:1039–42.
66. Kraeber-Bodere F, et al. Targeting, toxicity, and efficacy of 2-step, pretargeted radioimmunotherapy using a chimeric bispecific anti-body and 131I-labeled bivalent hapten in a phase I optimization clinical trial. J Nucl Med. 2006;47(2):247–55.
67. Salaun PY, et al. Phase II trial of anticarcinoembryonic antigen pretargeted radioimmunotherapy in progressive metastatic medullary thyroid carcinoma: biomarker response and survival improvement. J Nucl Med. 2012;53(8):1185–92.
68. https://ctep.cancer.gov/protocoldevelopment/electronic_applications/docs/CTCAE_v5_Quick_Reference_8.5x11.pdf. Accessed on March 09, 2018.
69. Schwartz RG, McKenzie WB, Alexander J, et al. Congestive heart failure and left ventricular dysfunction complicating doxorubicin therapy. seven-year experience using serial radionuclide angiocardiography. Am J Med. 1987;82(6):1109–18.
70. UpToDate website. Available at: https://www.uptodate.com/contents/cutaneous-side-effects-of-molecularly-targeted-therapy-and-other-biologic-agents-used-for-cancer-therapy
71. UpToDate website. Available at: https://www.uptodate.com/contents/toxicity-of-molecularly-targeted-antiangiogenic-agents-non-cardiovascular-effects
72. UpToDate website. Available at: https://www.uptodate.com/contents/toxicity-of-molecularly-targeted-antiangiogenic-agents-cardiovascular-effects
73. Massey PR, Okman JS, Wilkerson J, et al. Tyrosine kinase inhibitors directed against the vascular endothelial growth factor receptor (VEGFR) have distinct cutaneous toxicity profiles: a meta-analysis and review of the literature. Support Care Cancer. 2015 Jun;23(6):1827–35.
74. http://www.accessdata.fda.gov/drugsatfda_docs/label/2010/022465s002lbl.pdf. Accessed on September 22, 2010.
75. Anderson R, Jatoi A, Robert C, et al. Search for evidence-based approaches for the prevention and palliation of hand-foot skin reaction (HFSR) caused by the multikinase inhibitors (MKIs). Oncologist. 2009 Mar;14(3):291–302.
76. Lacouture ME, Wu S, Robert C, et al. Evolving strategies for the management of hand-foot skin reaction associated with the multitargeted kinase inhibitors sorafenib and sunitinib. Oncologist. 2008;13(9):1001–11.
77. Boone SL, Jameson G, Von Hoff D, et al. Blackberry-induced hand-foot skin reaction to sunitinib. Investig New Drugs. 2009;27(4):389–90.
78. Arnault JP, Wechsler J, Escudier B, et al. Keratoacanthomas and squamous cell carcinomas in patients receiving sorafenib. J Clin Oncol. 2009;27(23):e59. Epub 2009 Jul 13
79. Dubauskas Z, Kunishige J, Prieto VG, et al. Cutaneous squamous cell carcinoma and inflammation of actinic keratoses associated with sorafenib. Clin Genitourin Cancer. 2009;7(1):20–3.
80. Dummer R, Rinderknecht J, Goldinger SM. Ultraviolet A and photosensitivity during vemurafenib therapy. N Engl J Med. 2012;366(5):480–1.
81. Bellón T, Lerma V, González-Valle O, et al. Vemurafenib-induced toxic epidermal necrolysis:

possible cross-reactivity with other sulfonamide compounds. Br J Dermatol. 2016;174(3):621–4.
82. Jeudy G, Dalac-Rat S, Bonniaud B, et al. Successful switch to dabrafenib after vemurafenib-induced toxic epidermal necrolysis. Br J Dermatol. 2015;172(5):1454–5.
83. Sinha R, Lecamwasam K, Purshouse K, et al. Toxic epidermal necrolysis in a patient receiving vemurafenib for treatment of metastatic malignant melanoma. Br J Dermatol. 2014;170(4):997–9.
84. Ascierto PA, Minor D, Ribas A, et al. Phase II trial (BREAK-2) of the BRAF inhibitor dabrafenib (GSK2118436) in patients with metastatic melanoma. J Clin Oncol. 2013;31(26):3205–11.
85. Anforth R, Fernandez-Peñas P, Long GV. Cutaneous toxicities of RAF inhibitors. Lancet Oncol. 2013;14(1):e11–8.
86. Carlos G, Anforth R, Clements A, et al. Cutaneous toxic effects of BRAF inhibitors alone and in combination with MEK inhibitors for metastatic melanoma. JAMA Dermatol. 2015;151(10):1103–9.
87. Anforth R, Menzies A, Byth K, et al. Factors influencing the development of cutaneous squamous cell carcinoma in patients on BRAF inhibitor therapy. J Am Acad Dermatol. 2015;72(5):809–15.
88. Zelboraf (vemurafenib) prescribing information, www.accessdata.fda.gov/drugsatfda_docs/label/2011/202429s000lbl.pdf. Accessed on October 11, 2011.
89. http://www.accessdata.fda.gov/drugsatfda_docs/label/2013/204114s000lbl.pdf. Accessed on August 13, 2013.
90. http://www.accessdata.fda.gov/drugsatfda_docs/label/2015/206192s000lbl.pdf (Accessed on November 24, 2015).
91. https://www.accessdata.fda.gov/drugsatfda_docs/label/2018/202806s010lbl.pdf. Revised on May, 2018.
92. Robert C, Karaszewska B, Schachter J, et al. Improved overall survival in melanoma with combined dabrafenib and trametinib. N Engl J Med. 2015;372(1):30–9.
93. Feldt S, Schüssel K, Quinzler R, et al. Incidence of thyroid hormone therapy in patients treated with sunitinib or sorafenib: a cohort study. Eur J Cancer. 2012;48(7):974–81.
94. Tamaskar I, Bukowski R, Elson P, et al. Thyroid function test abnormalities in patients with metastatic renal cell carcinoma treated with sorafenib. Ann Oncol. 2008;19(2):265–8.
95. Fujiwara Y, Kiyota N, Chayahara N, et al. Management of axitinib (AG-013736)-induced fatigue and thyroid dysfunction, and predictive biomarkers of axitinib exposure: results from phase I studies in Japanese patients. Investig New Drugs. 2012;30(3):1055–64.
96. Figlin RA, de Souza P, McDermott D, et al. Analysis of PTEN and HIF-1alpha and correlation with efficacy in patients with advanced renal cell carcinoma treated with temsirolimus versus interferon-alpha. Cancer. 2009;115(16):3651–60.
97. Sternberg CN, Davis ID, Mardiak J, et al. Pazopanib in locally advanced or metastatic renal cell carcinoma: results of a randomized phase III trial. J Clin Oncol. 2010;28(6):1061–8.
98. Grothey A, Van Cutsem E, Sobrero A, et al. Regorafenib monotherapy for previously treated metastatic colorectal cancer (CORRECT): an international, multicentre, randomised, placebo-controlled, phase 3 trial. Lancet. 2013;381:303–12.
99. Wells SA Jr, Gosnell JE, Gagel RF, et al. Vandetanib for the treatment of patients with locally advanced or metastatic hereditary medullary thyroid cancer. J Clin Oncol. 2010;28:767–72.
100. Rini BI, Escudier B, Tomczak P, et al. Comparative effectiveness of axitinib versus sorafenib in advanced renal cell carcinoma (AXIS): a randomised phase 3 trial. Lancet. 2011;378:1931–9.
101. Lee JS, Hirsh V, Park K, et al. Vandetanib Versus placebo in patients with advanced non-small-cell lung cancer after prior therapy with an epidermal growth factor receptor tyrosine kinase inhibitor: a randomized, double-blind phase III trial (ZEPHYR). J Clin Oncol. 2012;30:1114–21.
102. Motzer RJ, Hutson TE, Tomczak P, et al. Sunitinib versus interferon alfa in metastatic renal-cell carcinoma. N Engl J Med. 2007;356:115–24.
103. Demetri GD, van Oosterom AT, Garrett CR, et al. Efficacy and safety of sunitinib in patients with advanced gastrointestinal stromal tumour after failure of imatinib: a randomised controlled trial. Lancet. 2006;368:1329–38.
104. Natale RB, Thongprasert S, Greco FA, et al. Phase III trial of vandetanib compared with erlotinib in patients with previously treated advanced non-small-cell lung cancer. J Clin Oncol. 2011;29:1059–66.
105. Smith DC, Smith MR, Sweeney C, et al. Cabozantinib in patients with advanced prostate cancer: results of a phase II randomized discontinuation trial. J Clin Oncol. 2013;31:412–9.
106. Raymond E, Dahan L, Raoul JL, et al. Sunitinib malate for the treatment of pancreatic neuroendocrine tumors. N Engl J Med. 2011;364:501.
107. Motzer RJ, Hutson TE, Tomczak P, et al. Overall survival and updated results for sunitinib compared with interferon alfa in patients with metastatic renal cell carcinoma. J Clin Oncol. 2009;27:3584–90.
108. Eisen T, Sternberg CN, Robert C, et al. Targeted therapies for renal cell carcinoma: review of adverse event management strategies. J Natl Cancer Inst. 2012;104:93–113.
109. Ghatalia P, Je Y, Mouallem NE, et al. Hepatotoxicity with vascular endothelial growth factor receptor tyrosine kinase inhibitors: a meta-analysis of randomized clinical trials. Crit Rev Oncol Hematol. 2015;93:257–76.
110. Xu CF, Reck BH, Xue Z, et al. Pazopanib-induced hyperbilirubinemia is associated with Gilbert's syndrome UGT1A1 polymorphism. Br J Cancer. 2010;102:1371–7.

111. Motzer RJ, Johnson T, Choueiri TK, et al. Hyperbilirubinemia in pazopanib- or sunitinib-treated patients in COMPARZ is associated with UGT1A1 polymorphisms. Ann Oncol. 2013;24:2927–8.
112. Peer CJ, Sissung TM, Kim A, et al. Sorafenib is an inhibitor of UGT1A1 but is metabolized by UGT1A9: implications of genetic variants on pharmacokinetics and hyperbilirubinemia. Clin Cancer Res. 2012;18:2099–107.
113. Shibata SI, Chung V, Synold TW, et al. Phase I study of pazopanib in patients with advanced solid tumors and hepatic dysfunction: a National Cancer Institute Organ Dysfunction Working Group study. Clin Cancer Res. 2013;19:3631–9.
114. Shibata S, Longmate J, Chung VM, et al. A phase I and pharmacokinetic single agent study of pazopanib in patients with advanced malignancies and varying degrees of liver dysfunction (Abstract 2571). J Clin Oncol 2010; 28:221s. Abstract available online at http://www.asco.org/ASCOv2/Meetings/Abstracts?&vmview=abst_detail_view&confID=74&abstractID=44621. Accessed on January 06, 2012.
115. Rini BI, Cohen DP, Lu DR, et al. Hypertension as a biomarker of efficacy in patients with metastatic renal cell carcinoma treated with sunitinib. J Natl Cancer Inst. 2011;103:763–73.
116. Estfan B, Byrne M, Kim R. Sorafenib in advanced hepatocellular carcinoma: hypertension as a potential surrogate marker for efficacy. Am J Clin Oncol. 2013;36:319.
117. Donskov F, Michaelson MD, Puzanov I, et al. Sunitinib-associated hypertension and neutropenia as efficacy biomarkers in metastatic renal cell carcinoma patients. Br J Cancer. 2015;113:1571–80.
118. Maitland ML, Bakris GL, Black HR, et al. Initial assessment, surveillance, and management of blood pressure in patients receiving vascular endothelial growth factor signaling pathway inhibitors. J Natl Cancer Inst. 2010;102:596–604.
119. Sica DA. Angiogenesis inhibitors and hypertension: an emerging issue. J Clin Oncol. 2006;24:1329–31.
120. Choueiri TK, Schutz FA, Je Y, et al. Risk of arterial thromboembolic events with sunitinib and sorafenib: a systematic review and meta-analysis of clinical trials. J Clin Oncol. 2010;28:2280–5.
121. Sternberg CN, Szczylik C, Lee ES, et al. A randomized, double-blind phase III study of pazopanib in treatment-naive and cytokine-pretreated patients with advanced renal cell carcinoma (RCC) (abstract #5021). J Clin Oncol. 2009;27:240s.
122. http://www.accessdata.fda.gov/drugsatfda_docs/label/2015/206947s000lbl.pdf?et_cid=35470087&et_rid=907466112&linkid=http%3a%2f%2fwww.accessdata.fda.gov%2fdrugsatfda_docs%2flabel%2f2015%2f206947s000lbl.pdf. Accessed on February 20, 2015.
123. Patrono C, Coller B, FitzGerald GA, et al. Platelet-active drugs: the relationships among dose, effectiveness, and side effects: the Seventh ACCP Conference on Antithrombotic and Thrombolytic Therapy. Chest. 2004;126:234S.
124. Tran H, Anand SS. Oral antiplatelet therapy in cerebrovascular disease, coronary artery disease, and peripheral arterial disease. JAMA. 2004;292:1867–74.
125. Ghatalia P, Morgan CJ, Je Y, et al. Congestive heart failure with vascular endothelial growth factor receptor tyrosine kinase inhibitors. Crit Rev Oncol Hematol. 2015;94:228–37.
126. Chintalgattu V, Patel SS, Khakoo AY. Cardiovascular effects of tyrosine kinase inhibitors used for gastrointestinal stromal tumors. Hematol Oncol Clin North Am. 2009;23:97–107.
127. Yancy CW, Jessup M, Bozkurt B, et al. 2013 ACCF/AHA guideline for the management of heart failure: a report of the American College of Cardiology Foundation/American Heart Association Task Force on Practice Guidelines. J Am Coll Cardiol. 2013;62:e147–239.
128. FDA-approved manufacturer's package insert for sunitinib available at http://dailymed.nlm.nih.gov/dailymed/lookup.cfm?setid=43a4d7f8-48ae-4a63-9108-2fa8e3ea9d9c. Accessed on December 18, 2012.
129. Shah RR, Morganroth J, Shah DR. Cardiovascular safety of tyrosine kinase inhibitors: with a special focus on cardiac repolarisation (QT interval). Drug Saf. 2013;36:295–316.
130. Ghatalia P, Je Y, Kaymakcalan MD, et al. QTc interval prolongation with vascular endothelial growth factor receptor tyrosine kinase inhibitors. Br J Cancer. 2015;112:296–305.

Part III

Clinical Information: Neuroendocrine Tumors

Radionuclide Therapy in Neuroendocrine Tumors

9

Levent Kabasakal, Emre Demirci, and Nalan Alan Selçuk

9.1 Epidemiology of Neuroendocrine Tumors

Neuroendocrine tumors (NET) are considered rare malignancies and their incidence is reported as 2–5/100,000 in various sources [1, 2]. In a comprehensive epidemiology study conducted by Yao et al. in 2004 by examining the US Surveillance, Epidemiology and End Results records (SEER database), the NET incidence was found to be 5.25/100,000. However, in this study, the rate of increase in the NET incidence was found to be higher than the rate of increase in general malignancy and the incidence was found to have increased from 1.9 to 5.25 out of 100,000 in the last 30 years. More importantly, its prevalence at publication date (2004) was found to be 103,312 (35/100,000) for the United States due to its relatively longer survival [3]. According to these results, the prevalence of NET, which is considered to be rare, is higher than the total prevalence of gastric and pancreatic cancers for 2004 with the effect of relatively long survival times [3]. Increased awareness of NET among clinicians is thought to have an effect on the increase in the incidence of NET overtime in addition to the recently used advanced imaging methods and diagnostic examinations [1, 4].

9.2 Diagnosis and Staging

For histopathological classification, guidelines first published by the World Health Organization (WHO) in 1980, undergoing significant changes in 2010 and last updated in 2017, are frequently preferred [5, 6]. In this classification, the NETs were categorized as low, moderate, and high grade according to the Ki-67 proliferation (MIB) and mitotic indices. Those with Ki-67 index below 3 are classified as grade 1, those between 3 and 20 are classified as grade 2, and those greater than 20 are classified as grade 3. According to WHO 2017 criteria, grade 3 NETs were divided into two groups as well-differentiated neuroendocrine tumors and less differentiated neuroendocrine carcinomas. Well-differentiated NETs in the grade 3 group are also classified as "Well-differentiated neuroendocrine tumors" with grade I and II NETs and distinguished from G3 neuroendocrine carcinomas with their clinical behavior [5–7]. The histopathological grades largely determine the behaviors of NETs. Well-differentiated NETs show somatostatin expression and longer survival is expected from this patient group [3, 8]. In addition, the histological grade is as impor-

L. Kabasakal (✉)
Cerrahpasa Medical Faculty, Department of Nuclear Medicine, Istanbul University-Cerrahpasa, İstanbul, Turkey
e-mail: lkabasakal@tsnm.org

E. Demirci · N. A. Selçuk
Faculty of Medicine, Department of Nuclear Medicine, Yeditepe University, İstanbul, Turkey
e-mail: emre.demirci@yeditepe.edu.tr; nalanselcuk@yeditepe.edu.tr

R. Bekiş et al. (eds.), *Radionuclide Therapy*, https://doi.org/10.1007/978-3-030-97220-2_9

tant as the TNM stage in the selection of imaging and treatment methods [9].

NETs can originate from different parts of the body. Although the histological grade is prioritized, the organ from which it originates is also of great importance in the course of the disease and also affects the treatment choice [3]. Therefore, it is important to determine the localization of the primary tumor in common metastatic patient groups.

9.3 Standard of Care

The only method that provides a full cure in the current treatment of NETs is early surgery [3, 10, 11]. However, up to 50% of patients can be diagnosed in the localized stage, especially due to the clinically silent onset of nonfunctional NET and late onset of symptoms. In addition, the early diagnosis rate in pancreatic, ileum-jejunum, and cecum-derived NETs decreases to 14–18% [1, 3]. Distant metastasis is observed in patients at the time of diagnosis at rates ranging from 21% to 50% according to the histological stages of NETs. [3]. Long-acting octreotide analogs in grade I and II NETs are among the standard treatments and used for disease stabilization or symptom control [12]. In the metastatic group, systemic treatment alternatives such as streptozocin, capecitabine, gemcitabine, topotecan, paclitaxel, oxaliplatin, and temozolomide can be used in different combinations. Among the targeted agents, sunitinib, a tyrosine kinase inhibitor, and everolimus, an mTOR inhibitor, can be preferred in well-differentiated NETs [13–16]. Interferon treatment has also been shown to be useful symptomatically in selected patients [17].

The European Society for Medical Oncology (ESMO) guidelines recommend the use of somatostatin analogs alone or in combination with another systemic antineoplastic (such as alpha interferon, everolimus, or bevacizumab) in SRS-positive WHO grade I NETs. It is also recommended for symptom control in WHO grade 2 and 3 NETs [18]. The biological half-life of natural somatostatin is less than 3 min and its clinical use is therefore not possible. Therefore, longer half-life synthetic somatostatin analogs have been developed. Octreotide (sandostatin-LAR®) and lanreotide (Somatuline®) administered by intramuscular injection every 4 weeks are preferred for long-term use [19].

Radiotherapy has a limited area of use in the treatment of NETs, and it is stated that it can be used in selected cases for the control of brain metastases but there is no complete consensus in the guidelines. It is stated that peptide receptor radionuclide therapy (PRRT) should be prioritized instead of radiotherapy, especially in the presence of brain metastasis and other organ metastases [20].

PRRT, one of the nuclear medicine methods, has been used as a standard method for many years [21, 22].

9.4 Peptide Receptor Radionuclide Therapy

9.4.1 Key Information

NETs express somatostatin receptors at different rates, and this is one of the most important factors in the selection of treatment and imaging methods [23]. Somatostatin shows its effects through its receptors located in the plasma membrane, and five subtypes (sstr 1-5) have been identified [24]. Various rates of expression of these five subreceptor types are observed in different tissues and benign or malignant neoplasms in the body. Ssrt-2 is much denser than other tissues, especially in neuroendocrine tumors, and thanks to this feature, it is the target for radionuclide therapies. Somatostatin analogs (e.g., octreotide), which are synthetic molecules formed by keeping the receptor-binding portion of the somatostatin molecule, are stable in vivo and also bind to certain receptor subtypes with higher affinity. They can be used for imaging by labeling with radioisotopes such as Tc-99m, In-111, Ga-68, or for treatment by labeling with radionuclides emitting beta and alpha particles (Fig. 9.1) [23, 25].

In all radionuclide therapies, the basic principle is to deliver the therapeutic dose of radiation locally or systemically to the target tissue. In neuroendocrine tumors, treatment is performed with the principle that octreotide analogs carry radio-

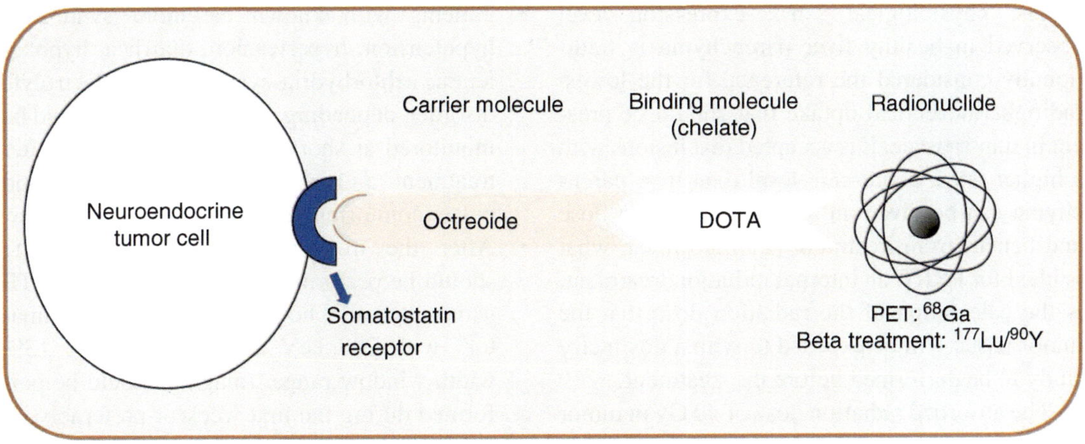

Fig. 9.1 General diagram of Ga-68-DOTATATE (PET radiopharmaceutical), Lu-177-DOTATATE, and Y-90-DOTATATE (treatment radiopharmaceuticals) used for theranostic applications in neuroendocrine tumors

nuclides such as Y-90 and Lu-177 into the cell and is called PRRT due to the peptide structure of octreotide analogs. PRRT first started with In-111 isotope. Afterward, Y-90, which has high energy beta particles reaching 11 mm in tissue, has become preferred for PRRT, and much higher treatment efficacy has been achieved compared to In-111. However, Lu-177 isotope, which has more appropriate physical properties, has begun to be preferred especially because of the prominent kidney toxicity of Y-90. The main spread of PRRT has been with Lu-177-labeled sst analogs [26]. Although many radionuclides are used for PRRT today, there are only phase 3 studies completed for Lu-177-DOTATATE among current radiopharmaceuticals [22].

9.4.2 Indications

PRRT is indicated for the treatment of the patients with adequate somatostatin receptor type 2 expression and metastatic or inoperable NETs [27, 28]. The indications and contraindications for PRRT according to the joint guidelines of the European Neuroendocrine Tumor Society (ENETS) and the International Atomic Energy Agency, the European Association of Nuclear Medicine, and the North American Society of Nuclear Medicine and Molecular Imaging (IAEA-EENM-SNMMI) are given in Table 9.1 [27–29].

Table 9.1 Indications for PRRT according to ENETS and IAEA-EENM-SNMMI guidelines [27–29]

• Histopathologically defined diagnosis:
– (Grade I–II NET and well-differentiated grade III NET) [21, 27]
– Pheochromocytoma and paraganglioma
– Neuroblastoma
– Medullary thyroid cancer
• Tumor uptake equal to or higher than liver uptake in SRS
• Presence of advanced stage (inoperable) disease
• Life expectancy at least 3–6 months
• Karnofsky performance scoring greater than 50%
• Informed patient consent
Contraindications for PRRT
• Continuation of pregnancy or breastfeeding
• Decreased renal function (creatinine clearance < 40 mL/min)
• Impairment of hematological functions (hemoglobin < 8 g/dL, platelet < 75 × 10^9/L, leukocyte < 2 × 10^9/L)
• Decrease in liver function (total bilirubin value > 3 times normal, albumin < 30 g/L, prothrombin time > 1.5 times longer)
• Cardiac failure

Although healthy kidney function is essential for the administration of Y-90-labeled peptides, a decrease in renal function for Lu-177-labeled peptides is a relative contraindication, and treatment can be applied if at least 70% of the GFR values expected for age can be achieved [27].

The physiological sstr-2 expression level observed in healthy liver parenchyma is traditionally considered the reference for the lowest radiopharmaceutical uptake that should be present in tumor tissue. It is accepted that lesions with a higher sstr-2 expression level than liver parenchyma can be given an adequate radiation dose and benefit from treatment [27]. However, what is ideal for PRRT, an internal radiation treatment, is the calculation of the radiation dose that the tumor tissue will be exposed to with a dosimetry study to be performed before the treatment.

The absorbed radiation dose of 40 Gy in tumor tissue generally provides the best responses, but more than 10 Gy responses can be obtained [30]. However, there are no controlled randomized trials to verify these data yet.

In cases with response to previous PRRT, Lu-177-DOTATATE treatment may be given again for salvage after progression monitoring. In these cases, the patient's hematological parameters, general condition and performance, tumor burden, toxicity in previous administrations, and side effects should be considered. Also, individual dose adjustments should be made according to the absorbed radiation doses to the organs in previous treatments [31].

9.4.3 PRRT: Administration

PRRT should be administered in healthcare centers with equipment and units that comply with the relevant legislation on radiation protection in the country where it is applied. The recommended administration protocol is as follows [27, 32, 33]:

- The volume of the radiopharmaceutical is recommended to be between 10 and 100 mL and should be administered intravenously by an infusion of 10–30 min. Administration also can be done using an automatic syringe pump. Another technique is to transfer the radiopharmaceutical to the patient's vascular access with the help of the pressure created by a 250 mL 0.9% NaCl isotonic solution connected to the vial with a short needle.
- Patients with known carcinoid syndrome, hypotension, hypertension, diarrhea, hypokalemia, achlorhydria syndrome, or electrolyte disorder, depending on the function, should be monitored at short intervals during and after treatment and routine blood pressure and pulse monitoring should be performed.
- After the treatment, whole-body imaging should be performed for Lu-177-DOTATATE using a "parallel hole medium energy collimator" with 208 keV energy peaks and 15% width window range. Imaging should be performed during the first week or preferably on day 4. If dosimetry is to be administered, the reference source containing 200 μCi Lu-177 in a 20 mL volume vial should be prepared daily and placed at the patient's head level and image should be taken. In addition, imaging should preferably be performed 3 times, ideally 4 times, on days 1, 4, and 7 for dosimetry administration. SPECT or SPECT/CT devices can be used according to the preferred method for dosimetry.
- Serotonin5-HT_3 receptor antagonists (e.g., ondansetron) are administered intravenously before the radiopeptide for antiemetic purposes.
- Low doses of dexamethasone are administered as IV shortly before the administration of the radiopeptide.
- PRRT is administered in radionuclide therapy rooms in accordance with national standards. Since there is a high probability of radioactive transmission in cases with incontinence, hospitalization is recommended. It is recommended that the patient should not have close contact with children and pregnant women for the first 3 days after treatment [33].

In order to reduce renal toxicity in PRRT administrations, arginine and lysine-containing amino acid solutions should be used according to the administration protocols specified in Table 9.2 [27]. This administration reduces the amount of radiation exposure to the kidney by 27% (9–53%) on average [9, 29]. Positively charged amino acids undergo megalin- and cubilin-mediated reabsorption in the proximal tubule after being

Table 9.2 Recommended amino acid protocols in the IAEA-EENM-SNMMI Guidelines [27]

One-day 50 g protocol	50 g solution containing arginine and lysine (25:25 g) is diluted in 2 L 0.9% NaCl solution and started 30 min before treatment and maintained for 4 h.
3-day 25 g protocol	25 g lysine is diluted in 1 L 0.9% NaCl solution on the first day of treatment and started 30-60 min before treatment and maintained for 4 h.
	After the end of this solution, 500 mL 0.9% NaCl solution with 12.5 g lysine is administered as infusions for at least 3 h twice a day on the second and third days of treatment. This protocol ensures renal protection while minimizing the side effects of amino acid administration.
3- day 50 g. amino acid protocol	In addition to the one-day protocol, 500 mL 0.9% NaCl solution containing 12.5 g lysine is administered as infusions for at least 3 h twice a day on the second and third days.
One-day 50 g amino acid and 0.02 succinyl gelatin (Gelofusine®) mL/kg combination protocol:	Gelofusine are administered intravenously 10 min before treatment in addition to the one-day protocol

filtered from glomeruli, and, if administered in combination with PRRT, they reduce the accumulation of radioactive agent in the kidneys by competing with radiopeptide during tubular reabsorption [34]. In addition, it has been shown that renal doses can be reduced with amifostine, a radioprotective agent, or diuretics that block renin-aldosterone-angiotensin system, although they are not yet included in the current guidelines [35]. It has also been reported that administration of amino acids reduces renal uptake but probably does not cause a significant change in tumor uptake due to differences in uptake mechanism [36]. If renal function is within normal limits, PRRT can be safely administered in patients with single kidney function. However, in patients with a single kidney, renal functions are known to be more affected in the long term (2–30% reduction in effective renal plasma flow) [37].

Treatment can be administered by using a fixed dose in PRRT or by making personalized dose selection according to the patient. It is stated that 22–30 GBq (600–800 mCi) doses can be administered in Lu-177-DOTATATE treatment applications without reaching the limits determined at the absorbed renal doses [27]. In dose selection according to the patient, the body surface, hematological and renal factors, and the patient's clinical status can be considered. Additionally, a personalized dose can be determined together with a dosimetry study. In the IAEA-EENM-SNMMI joint guidelines, it is recommended that the activity in Lu-177-DOTATATE treatment be administered at doses of 5.5–7.4 GBq (150–200 mCi) and at 10–12 week intervals in 2–6 cycles [27].

In another study conducted by Sansovini et al., antitumoral effect was observed in the group with low cumulative activity (18.5 GBq), but a more prominent antitumoral response was observed with 27.8 GBq activity. Therefore, it was stated that 27.8 GBq activity should be the target dose in PRRT [38].

In the Bad Berka Treatment Protocol, which is one of the most experienced centers in PRRT, long-term low dose treatment is also recommended [39]. In the phase 2 study with Lu-177-DOTATATE, the results of the treatments administered at 3.7 GBq (100 mCi) and 5.5 GBq (~150 mCi) doses were compared, and it was stated that the treatment responses were not lower in the low-dose group than in the high-dose group [22, 40]. The 4 × 7.4 GBq protocol was used in the phase 3 study (NETTER), which was completed in midgut NETs [22]. However, in cases where the administration is extended up to the maximum safe dose, median survival times up to two times can be reached compared to standard four cycles of administration [41].

Salvage treatment can be applied when progression develops again in the future follow-ups of the patients who received a response in the first four courses of Lu-177-DOTATATE treatment series. Since NETs can remain stable for a long time at this stage, it is generally recommended to wait for progression to start the second series. Unlike initial administrations, salvage treatments are recommended to be administered in two-cycle series and not exceeding 15 GBq dose in each series [31, 42].

PRRT can be administered neoadjuvant in selected patients, especially in locally advanced NET cases [43]. While fractionated protocols are recommended at longer intervals in metastatic patients and palliative applications, higher doses are recommended at shorter intervals in cases requiring neoadjuvant or regression [43].

The intraarterial administration of Lu-177-DOTATATE in liver metastases can be tried in selected cases. According to the very limited experience, a much higher treatment rate can be achieved compared to systemic administration (partial response rate of 75%), but it should be kept in mind that hematological side effects are also more pronounced than systemic administration [44]. Although agonists are typically used for targeting SST receptors, recent preclinical and limited clinical studies have shown that SST antagonists have much higher receptor affinity and retention times, and it has been reported that they may be more successful than analogs for treatment and imaging [45].

9.5 Combined Applications with Other Systemic Therapies

The combined administration of external radiotherapy and chemotherapy has been successfully applied in many tumors for many years, and the use of Lu-177-DOTATATE in combination with other systemic treatments has been investigated recently. Objective response rates in the combination of capecitabine-temozolomide and Lu-177-DOTATATE in NETs of pancreatic origin reach 80%, and progression-free survival duration reaches up to 4 years. In this protocol, it is recommended that oral capecitabine treatment should start 5 days before PRRT and continue for 14 days at a dose of 1500 mg/m^2 and 200 mg/m^2 oral temozolomide should be used in the last 5 days of the protocol [46]. If capecitabine is used alone during PRRT, a dose of 1650 mg/m^2 is recommended for 14 days. Although more prominent thrombocytopenia was observed in the protocol combined with temozolomide, limited hematological toxicities were generally observed. In another GEP-NET-based CT-PRRT combination, progression-free survival was 31 months, complete response was 16%, partial response was 41%, and stable response was 37% [47]. Administration of olaparib, a PAPR-1 inhibitor, in combination with Lu-177-DOTATATE treatment increases DNA damage and genomic instability in tumor cells compared to Lu-177-DOTATATE administration alone. However, there are no completed clinical trials yet [48, 49]. It has also been shown in preclinical studies that GMX1778, a NAMPT inhibitor, increases the cytotoxic effect of Lu-177-DOTATATE treatment [50].

9.5.1 Side Effects

Nausea and vomiting during PRRT are generally related to metabolic acidosis caused by positively charged amino acids administered to reduce nephrotoxicity [51]. Pre-PRRT administration of serotonin 5-HT$_3$ antagonists with corticosteroids to reduce this effect (e.g., ondansetron with dexamethasone 4–8 mg) is recommended [51, 52].

Although it is recommended to discontinue long-acting amino somatostatin analogs 3–4 weeks before treatment and to discontinue short-acting ones 24 h before treatment, there is no clear consensus on this issue. Many centers usually perform the application within the 4th week without changing the administration schedule of long-acting sst analogs [52]. Carcinoid crisis may occur due to sudden hormone release after PRRT in functional tumors, especially in cases with liver metastases. These symptoms can usually be controlled by the administration of short-acting sst analogs. Also serotonin agonists (cyproheptadine) can be used for supportive purposes 1–2 days before treatment in cases considered to be risky [51].

After Lu-177-DOTATATE administration, radiopharmaceutical was observed to accumulate in the proximal tubules of the kidney. Radiolabeled peptides are eliminated by glomerular filtration due to their small size and undergo tubular reabsorption by the megalin/cubilin system. In addition, sstr-2-mediated peritubular uptake has been reported to play a role in the accumulation of radiopeptides in the kidney [34]. The kidneys are dose-limiting organs, especially in treatments with Y-90-DOTATOC [53, 54]. Although there are no consensus dose limits for renal absorption doses in PRRT, the 23–28 gray (Gy) dose limit used in external radiotherapy applications is controversial and has been accepted as a reference [53]. It is known that age, hypertension, and diabetes are among the possible parameters that are effective in reducing creatinine clearance as a result of PRRT [53, 55]. Therefore, the 28 Gy limit specified for the kidney dose should be observed when treating patients with risk factors, while renal doses may increase up to 40 Gy in patients without risk factors [55]. The application of these limit values of external radiotherapy origin to Lu-177 is controversial. There are significant differences between treatment with internal beta radiation and radiobiological effects of external radiotherapy [4]. In addition, the low-energy beta radiation of Lu-177 accumulated in renal tubule cells can reach radiosensitive glomeruli in a more limited manner than the beta radiation of Y-90 due to the average penetration distance of less than 2 mm in tissue [4]. A long-term follow-up study by Bersma et al. examining the kidney functions of 323 patients receiving PRRT supports these hypotheses. According to this study (side effects within the framework of a common terminology criteria-CTCAE version 4.03), no grade 3 or 4 toxicity was observed after Lu-177-DOTATATE treatment and no annual loss of renal function was detected above 20% [56]. Sabet et al. found a decrease of 2–10 mL/min/m^2 in GFR values by 21% and a decrease of >10 mL/min/m^2 by 15% in patients treated with Lu-177-DOTATATE and grade 3 nephrotoxicity by 1.3% [57]. It is known that tubular extraction rate (TER) calculated by MAG3 has no role in predicting long-term nephrotoxicity [58].

Temporary leukopenia and thrombocytopenia usually occur according to the activity administered after PRRT. Severe (grade 3 or 4) hematotoxicity occurs in 4–5% of patients after 2–8 weeks. These include leukopenia, thrombocytopenia, and rarely severe anemia requiring transfusion [56]. The most important risk factors for hemotoxicity are initial cytopenia and decreased renal function (low GFR) [56, 59]. Although the presence of common bone metastases and previous cytotoxic treatments are accepted to increase hemotoxicity, some detailed analyses have shown that previous chemotherapy did not increase hematological side effects after PRRT [59, 60]. Advanced age (>70) and high tumor burden increase the likelihood of post-treatment anemia; the presence of diffuse bone metastasis increases the likelihood of thrombocytopenia after treatment [60]. The presence of a history of splenectomy appears to be a protective factor for hematotoxicity [59]. Due to the presence of intense sst-2 receptor in the spleen during PRRT, a patient receiving 7.4 GBq treatment is exposed to radiation at a median dose of 4.5 Gy. Accordingly, an average of 75% reduction in spleen sizes occurs, and this decrease in size is correlated with a decrease in hemoglobin levels in patients [37].

Due to the relatively high rate of somatostatin receptors in the pituitary gland, thyroid gland, adrenal glands, and pancreatic islet cells are exposed to higher radiation absorbed doses during PRRT (e.g., 5.8 ± 1.1/GBq for pituitary gland) [4]. However, transient and limited hormonal side effects are observed. Hypothyroidism was reported in 3% after PRRT. An 8% increase in HbA1c values was observed. Female patients have a decrease in gonadotropin levels in the postmenopausal period and male patients have a temporary effect on spermatogenesis [61].

9.5.2 Treatment Responses

In the meta-analysis of the retrospective series of Lu-177-DOTATATE treatment, the disease control rate (stable, partial response, and full response cases) was 83%, median progression-free survival was 25–34 months, and median overall survival was 42–71 months in pancreatic

SST (+) NETs [62]. In the phase 3 study of gastroenteropancreatic neuroendocrine tumors other than pancreas (NETTER study), progression-free survival was >30 months in the treatment arm and 8.4 months in the high-dose sst-analog arm. However, as of the date of publication of this book, the follow-up period required for the overall survival analysis has not been completed. In the largest published series in the literature ($n = 610$), complete response, partial response, stable disease, and progression rates were 2%, 39%, 46%, and 13%, respectively; progression-free and overall survival were 29 and 63 months [63]. Figure 9.2 shows Ga-68-DOTATATE PET MIP images of a sample patient with a complete response to Lu-177-DOTATATE treatment. In functional NETs, the success rate of treatment has been shown to reach up to 82% [64]. The treatment responses and survival durations obtained with selected prospective studies and case series with Lu-177-DOTATATE in the literature are shown in Table 9.3. While similar treatment responses are obtained in cases diagnosed with metastatic pheochromocytoma and paraganglioma, sympathetic discharge and symptom control, which are very important for this group of patients, are also contributed [64].

In patients who underwent Lu-177-DOTATATE again for *salvage* treatment with previous 3–4 courses of PRRT, complete response was 1%, partial response 18.2%, stable disease 45.4%, and progression 33.3%. The median progression-free survival in these cases was 13 months [31]. In another study conducted by Zwan V. et al., partial response was 15.5%, stable disease was 59.5%, median progression-free survival was 14.6 months, and overall survival of all Lu-177-DOTATATE administrations was 80 months in 181 patients receiving rescue treatment [42]. Recurrent PRRT administrations in

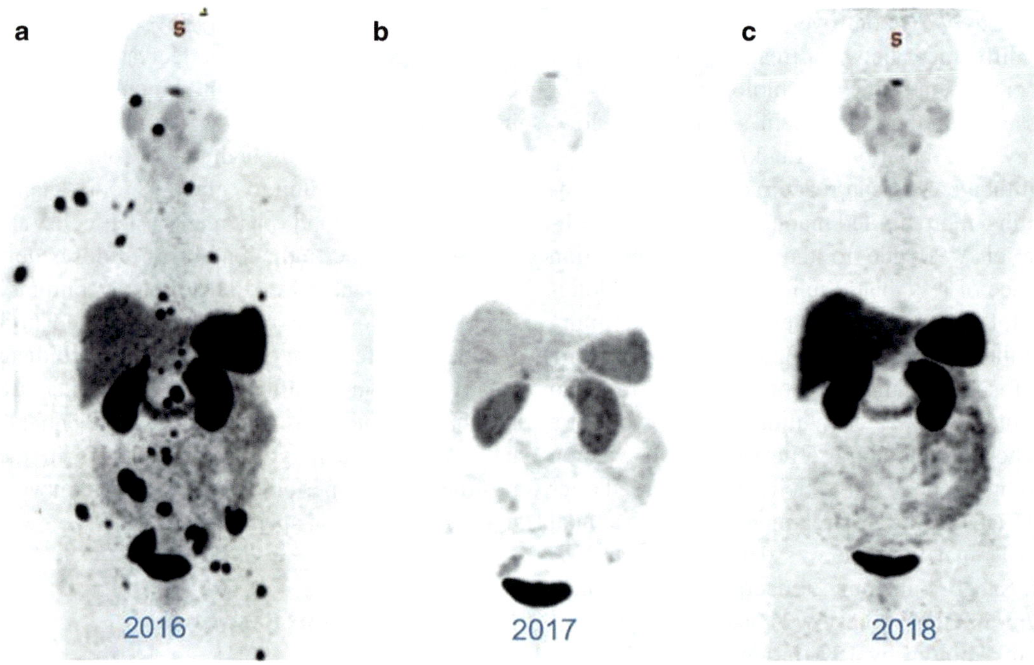

Fig. 9.2 Lu-177-DOTATATE treatment was applied at 3-month intervals (4 × 7.4 GBq) in the case referred for PRRT with NET diagnosis of WHO grade 2 and progressed bone metastases in 2016. After the standard protocol, a complete response was obtained after 2 × 3.6 GBq Lu-177-DOTATATE treatment. Diarrhea and gastrointestinal symptoms, which could not be controlled by sst analogs before treatment, decreased significantly from the first course and disappeared following the third course application. (**a**) Pre-treatment 68Ga-DOTATATE PET MIP image; (**b**) PET MIP image showing partial response obtained after 4 × 7.4 GBq Lu-177-DOTATATE; (**c**) PET MIP image showing complete response after 2 × 3.6 GBq Lu-177-DOTATATE administered additionally

Table 9.3 Selected studies with Lu-177-DOTATATE

Site	Primary area	Type of study	Progression before PRRT	*n*	CR	PR	SD	PD	PFS	OS
Rotterdam (Kwekkeboom 2008) [65]	GEPNET	Retrospective	43% (31% unknown)	310	2% (5)	28% (86)	35% (107)	20% (61)	40	46
Phase 2 (Paganelli 2014) [40]	GEPNET	Prospective		43	–	–	77% (33)	16% (7)	36	–
Phase 3 (Strosberg 2015) [66]	Non-pancreatic GEPNET	Prospective		221 (PRRT arm: 111)	1% (1)	18% (18)	66% (77)	4% (5)	40	Not yet reached
Istanbul (Demirci 2018) [21]	NET	Retrospective	81%	186 (160 cases according to RECIST)	3.1% (5)	46.9% (75)	21.9% (35)	28.1% (45)	36.4	55 (avg.)
Milan (Mariniello 2015) [67]	Lung NET	Retrospective	81.2%	48	–	29.2% (14)	45.8% (22)	25% (12)	28	58.8
Sweden (Garske-Román 2018) [41]	NET	Prospective observational	80.5%	200	0.5%	24.7%	71%	3.7%	29 (35[a] vs 17[b])	43 (54[a] vs 25[b])
Rotterdam (Brabander 2017) [63]	GEP-NET and lung NET	Retrospective	77.5%	610 (419 cases according to RECIST)	2% (9)	39% (165)	46% (192)	13% (53)	29	63
Italy, Switzerland, Netherlands, Germany, USA (Kim 2015) [68]	NET	Meta-analysis 3 prospective, 3 retrospective		473	Disease control rate: 81%			19%	–	–

CR, complete response; PR, partial response; SD, stable disease; P, progression; PFS, progression-free survival; OS, overall survival
[a]Dosimetry guided administration
[b]Standard dosing

the later stages should be initially considered as one of the treatment options in all cases benefiting from PRRT according to these results. Maximum tolerated dose limits should be considered in these retreatments and should be administrated in two cycles [31, 42].

PRRT has a significant palliative effect with the advantage of being a systemic radiation therapy. The time to a 10% decrease in the quality of life index in the follow-up of patients' symptoms was 6.1 months in the control group and 28.8 months in the PRRT group during the phase 3 study (NETTER) [69].

Renal and bone marrow absorbed dose values were reported to be 24–29 Gy and 1.2–2 Gy on average in patients who received 4 cycles of PRRT (30 GBq) as standard. It should be kept in mind that this radiation exposure occurs at very low dose rates and for long periods such as approximately 6–9 months and that its radiobiological effects are much lower compared to external radiotherapy [70].

9.6 Evaluation and Follow-Up of Treatment Response

Evaluating the treatment response in the NETs is a complex decision stage that requires examining the clinical status of the patient, biochemistry tests, and morphological and functional status of tumors [27]. The standard method for post-PRRT treatment follow-up is to perform 3–6 month intervals of serial ultrasound, contrast-enhanced CT, and MRI tests to investigate the morphological effects of treatment on tumors and to evaluate them according to the RECIST (Response Evaluation Criteria in Solid Tumors) criteria [18, 71].

However, it is stated that the imaging method, which is accepted as the "gold standard" in the determination of tumor burden in patients with well-differentiated NET diagnosis according to ENETS guidelines, is SRS performed with Ga-68-DOTA-sst analogs, and it is recommended to be repeated for follow-up 3 months after the operations or treatments administered [71]. Ga-68-DOTATOC PET/CT did not provide additional information compared to conventional CT, but it was stated that it could detect progressive disease earlier in the evaluation of the response after PRRT in metastatic NET according to the study conducted by Gabriel et al. in a small group of 29 patients [72]. EANM guidelines state that a somatostatin PET/CT scan should be performed 3 months after the last treatment and the planned 3 or 4 cycles of PRRT treatment in well-differentiated NET. However, octreotide PET or radiological methods can be used when there is a suspicion of progression [27]. ENETS guidelines suggest that the initial aggression of the disease should be taken into consideration in determining the timing of follow-up imaging. In addition, follow-up imaging is recommended at 3-month intervals in the presence of NET with high FDG affinity [28].

Interim evaluation can be performed after the second cycle, especially in cases at risk of rapid progression (FDG positive NET or cases known to show rapid progression in follow-ups). Treatment is continued in cases other than progression in the interim evaluation [33]. Post-treatment imaging with SPECT/CT can also be used to monitor treatment responses, but it should be considered that it may miss up to 10% of new lesions according to Ga-68-DOTATATE [73].

A complete blood count should be performed at 2, 4, and 6 weeks after treatment, and measurement is recommended at 1 week if combined with chemotherapy according to ENETS guidelines. Weekly follow-ups should be started and necessary supportive treatments should be performed if grade 3–4 toxicity is detected at any stage [28]. The most important parameter in post-PRRT follow-up is the follow-up of renal functions according to the IAEA-EENM-SNMMI joint guideline. Serum creatinine level should be monitored routinely and glomerular filtration rate (GFR) measurement or scintigraphic evaluation is recommended in patients with pre-treatment risk factors for renal toxicity. It is recommended that PRRT administrations should be delayed for a while or treatment is completely discontinued in patients with impaired renal and hematological functions in intermediate follow-ups according to the patient's clinic and degree of exposure [27]. Treatment should be discontinued if grade 3–4 hematotoxicity is observed that does not improve over 2–3 months after treatment and progressive disease is observed in interim evaluations [28].

9.7 Prognostic Factors

Karnofsky performance status score less than 70, weight loss, high chromogranin A values (>600), high neural-specific enolase values, NET presence of pancreatic origin, histologically NET grade 3 presence, high Ki-67 values, lack of total resection of the primary tumor, and presence of diffuse liver metastases lead to shorter survival times and lower disease control rates [21, 61, 74, 75]. There are controversial results regarding the application of the neutrophil/lymphocyte ratio (NLR), which is useful in predicting treatment responses and prognosis in many solid tumors, in the PRRT-administered NETs. However, lower progression-free survival was detected in high NLR values [61]. High somatostatin receptor expression and low FDG affinity in lesions also indicate that long survival times can be achieved with PRRT. The rate of progression after PRRT in FDG negative grade 2 NETs remains limited to 9%, while this rate increases to 32% in FDG-avid patients in the series published by Severi et al. [76]. FDG positivity was reported to be one of the most important prognostic factors, and median progression-free survival was 20 months in the FDG positive case group and 32 months in the FDG negative group in retrospective analyses of the Milan Group [76].

NET gene transcript analysis (NETest®) from peripheral blood samples is the most accurate method to predict PRRT response among the factors reported so far. Measurements made at the beginning of PRRT and during consecutive treatments can predict the PRRT result with high accuracy before the completion of the treatment protocol (area under the curve for prediction accuracy 0.90 ± 0.07) [74, 75].

9.8 Concluding Remarks

PRRT is a radionuclide therapy method that has been successfully used in well-differentiated neuroendocrine tumors for many years, and its effectiveness has been proven by many retrospective series and prospective studies. It is the therapy method that reaches the longest survival times in metastatic NETs. There are many aspects of research that are predicted to increase its effectiveness such as fractionation, combination with systemic treatments, application with alpha-emitting radionuclides, use of new carrier peptides, and intraarterial administrations.

References

1. Modlin IM, Lye KD, Kidd M. A 5-decade analysis of 13,715 carcinoid tumors. Cancer. 2003;97:934–59.
2. Hemminki K, Li X. Incidence trends and risk factors of carcinoid tumors: a nationwide epidemiologic study from Sweden. Cancer. 2001;92:2204–10.
3. Yao JC, Hassan M, Phan A, et al. One hundred years after "carcinoid": epidemiology of and prognostic factors for neuroendocrine tumors in 35,825 cases in the United States. J Clin Oncol. 2008;26:3063–72.
4. Niederle MB, Hackl M, Kaserer K, Niederle B. Gastroenteropancreatic neuroendocrine tumours: the current incidence and staging based on the WHO and European Neuroendocrine Tumour Society classification: an analysis based on prospectively collected parameters. Endocr Relat Cancer. 2010;17:909–18.
5. Lloyd RV, Osamura YR, Kloppel G, Rosai J. WHO classification of tumours of endocrine organs. WHO Press; 2017.
6. Klimstra DS, Modlin IR, Coppola D, Lloyd RV, Suster S. The pathologic classification of neuroendocrine tumors: a review of nomenclature, grading, and staging systems. Pancreas. 2010;39:707–12.
7. Klöppel G, Solcia E, Capella C, Heitz PU. Classification of neuroendocrine tumours. Ital J Gastroenterol Hepatol. 1999;31(Suppl. 2):S111–6.
8. Oberg K, Castellano D. Current knowledge on diagnosis and staging of neuroendocrine tumors. Cancer Metastasis Rev. 2011;30(Suppl. 1):3–7.
9. Plöckinger U, Rindi G, Arnold R, et al. Guidelines for the diagnosis and treatment of neuroendocrine gastrointestinal tumours. A consensus statement on behalf of the European Neuroendocrine Tumour Society (ENETS). Neuroendocrinology. 2004;80:394–424.
10. Norton JA, Warren RS, Kelly MG, Zuraek MB, Jensen RT. Aggressive surgery for metastatic liver neuroendocrine tumors. Surgery. 2003;134:1057–63. discussion 1063–5
11. Schnirer II, Yao JC, Ajani J, a. Carcinoid a comprehensive review. Acta Oncol (Madr). 2003;42:672–92.
12. Rinke A, Müller H-H, Schade-Brittinger C, et al. Placebo-controlled, double-blind, prospective, randomized study on the effect of octreotide LAR in the control of tumor growth in patients with metastatic neuroendocrine midgut tumors: a report

from the PROMID Study Group. J Clin Oncol. 2009;27:4656–63.
13. Moertel CG, Kvols LK, O'Connell MJ, Rubin J. Treatment of neuroendocrine carcinomas with combined etoposide and cisplatin. Evidence of major therapeutic activity in the anaplastic variants of these neoplasms. Cancer. 1991;68:227–32.
14. Raymond E, Dahan L, Raoul J-L, et al. Sunitinib malate for the treatment of pancreatic neuroendocrine tumors. N Engl J Med. 2011;364:501–13.
15. Yao JC, Shah MH, Ito T, et al. Everolimus for advanced pancreatic neuroendocrine tumors. N Engl J Med. 2011;364:514–23.
16. Kulke MH, Bergsland E, Emerson L, Fanta P, Goldner WS, Kunz PL, Saltz L. Neuroendocrine Tumors, version 1.2015. J Natl Compr Cancer Netw. 2014;
17. Faiss S, Pape U-F, Böhmig M, Dörffel Y, Mansmann U, Golder W, Riecken EO, Wiedenmann B. Prospective, randomized, multicenter trial on the antiproliferative effect of lanreotide, interferon alfa, and their combination for therapy of metastatic neuroendocrine gastroenteropancreatic tumors--the International Lanreotide and Interferon Alfa Study. J Clin Oncol. 2003;21:2689–96.
18. Oberg K, Akerström G, Rindi G, Jelic S. Neuroendocrine gastroenteropancreatic tumours: ESMO Clinical Practice Guidelines for diagnosis, treatment and follow-up. Ann Oncol. 2010;21(Suppl. 5):v223–7.
19. Oberg K. Consensus report on the use of somatostatin analogs for the management of neuroendocrine tumors of the gastroenteropancreatic system. Ann Oncol. 2004;15:966–73.
20. Pavel M, Grossman A, Arnold R, et al. ENETS consensus guidelines for the management of brain, cardiac and ovarian metastases from neuroendocrine tumors. Neuroendocrinology. 2010;91:326–32.
21. Demirci E, Kabasakal L, Toklu T, Ocak M, Şahin OE, Alan-Selcuk N, Araman A. 177Lu- DOTATATE therapy in patients with neuroendocrine tumours including high-grade (WHO G3) neuroendocrine tumours: response to treatment and long-term survival update. Nucl Med Commun. 2018;39:789–96.
22. Strosberg J, El-Haddad G, Wolin E, et al. Phase 3 trial of 177Lu-dotatate for midgut neuroendocrine tumors. N Engl J Med. 2017;376:125–35.
23. Reubi JC, Schär JC, Waser B, Wenger S, Heppeler A, Schmitt JS, Mäcke HR. Affinity profiles for human somatostatin receptor subtypes SST1-SST5 of somatostatin radiotracers selected for scintigraphic and radiotherapeutic use. Eur J Nucl Med. 2000;27:273–82.
24. Hoyer D, Bell GI, Berelowitz M, Epelbaum J, Feniuk W, Humphrey PP, O'Carroll AM, Patel YC, Schonbrunn A, Taylor JE. Classification and nomenclature of somatostatin receptors. Trends Pharmacol Sci. 1995;16:86–8.
25. Krenning EP, Kwekkeboom DJ, Bakker WH, Breeman WA, Kooij PP, Oei HY, van Hagen M, Postema PT, de Jong M, Reubi JC. Somatostatin receptor scintigraphy with [111In- DTPA-D-Phe1]- and [123I-Tyr3]-octreotide: the Rotterdam experience with more than 1000 patients. Eur J Nucl Med. 1993;20:716–31.
26. Bozkurt MF. Neuroendocrine tumours. Neuroendocr Tumours. 2015; https://doi.org/10.1007/978-3-662-45215-8.
27. Zaknun JJ, Bodei L, Mueller-Brand J, et al. The joint IAEA, EANM, and SNMMI practical guidance on peptide receptor radionuclide therapy (PRRNT) in neuroendocrine tumours. Eur J Nucl Med Mol Imaging. 2013;40:800–16.
28. Grozinsky-glasberg S, Arnold R, Cwikla J, Toumpanakis C, Davies P, Tiensuu E, Hicks RJ. ENETS Consensus Guidelines for the Standards of Care in Neuroendocrine Neoplasms: peptide receptor radionuclide therapy with radiolabelled somatostatin analogues. Neuroendocrinology. 2017;3000:295–309.
29. Kwekkeboom DJ, Krenning EP, Lebtahi R, Komminoth P, Kos-Kudła B, de Herder WW, Plöckinger U. ENETS Consensus Guidelines for the Standards of Care in Neuroendocrine Tumors: peptide receptor radionuclide therapy with radiolabeled somatostatin analogs. Neuroendocrinology. 2009;90:220–6.
30. Ilan E, Sandström M, Wassberg C, Sundin A, Garske-Román U, Eriksson B, Granberg D, Lubberink M. Dose response of pancreatic neuroendocrine tumors treated with peptide receptor radionuclide therapy using 177Lu-DOTATATE. J Nucl Med. 2015;56:177–82.
31. Sabet A, Haslerud T, Pape UF, Sabet A, Ahmadzadehfar H, Grünwald F, Guhlke S, Biersack HJ, Ezziddin S. Outcome and toxicity of salvage therapy with 177Lu-octreotate in patients with metastatic gastroenteropancreatic neuroendocrine tumours. Eur J Nucl Med Mol Imaging. 2014;41:205–10.
32. Cwikla JB, Sankowski A, Seklecka N, Buscombe JR, Nasierowska-Guttmejer A, Jeziorski KG, Mikolajczak R, Pawlak D, Stepien K, Walecki J. Efficacy of radionuclide therapy DOTATATE Y-90 in patients with progressive metastatic gastroenteropancreatic neuroendocrine carcinomas (GEP-NETs): a phase II study. Ann Oncol. 2010;21:787–94.
33. Mittra ES. Neuroendocrine tumor therapy: 177Lu-DOTATATE. AJR Am J Roentgenol. 2018;211(2):278–85.
34. Rolleman EJ, Melis M, Valkema R, Boerman OC, Krenning EP, de Jong M. Kidney protection during peptide receptor radionuclide therapy with somatostatin analogues. Eur J Nucl Med Mol Imaging. 2010;37:1018–31.
35. Melis M, Valkema R, Krenning EP, de Jong M. Reduction of renal uptake of radiolabeled octreotate by amifostine coadministration. J Nucl Med. 2012;53:749–53.
36. Jamar F, Barone R, Mathieu I, et al. 86Y-DOTA0-D-Phe1-Tyr3-octreotide (SMT487)--a phase 1 clinical study: pharmacokinetics, biodistribution and renal protective effect of different regimens of amino

acid co-infusion. Eur J Nucl Med Mol Imaging. 2003;30:510–8.
37. Svensson J, Hagmarker L, Magnander T, Wängberg B, Bernhardt P. Radiation exposure of the spleen during 177Lu-DOTATATE treatment and its correlation with haematological toxicity and spleen volume. EJNMMI Phys. 2016; https://doi.org/10.1186/s40658-016-0153-4.
38. Sansovini M, Severi S, Ambrosetti A, Monti M, Nanni O, Sarnelli A, Bodei L, Garaboldi L, Bartolomei M, Paganelli G. Treatment with the radiolabelled somatostatin analog Lu- DOTATATE for advanced pancreatic neuroendocrine tumors. Neuroendocrinology. 2013;97:347–54.
39. Baum RP, Kulkarni HR, Carreras C. Peptides and receptors in image-guided therapy: theranostics for neuroendocrine neoplasms. Semin Nucl Med. 2012;42:190–207.
40. Paganelli G, Sansovini M, Ambrosetti A, Severi S, Monti M, Scarpi E, Donati C, Ianniello A, Matteucci F, Amadori D. 177 Lu-Dota-octreotate radionuclide therapy of advanced gastrointestinal neuroendocrine tumors: results from a phase II study. Eur J Nucl Med Mol Imaging. 2014; https://doi.org/10.1007/s00259-014-2735-5.
41. Garske-Román U, Sandström M, Fröss Baron K, et al. Prospective observational study of 177Lu-DOTA-octreotate therapy in 200 patients with advanced metastasized neuroendocrine tumours (NETs): feasibility and impact of a dosimetry-guided study protocol on outcome and toxicity. Eur J Nucl Med Mol Imaging. 2018;45:970–88.
42. van der Zwan WA, Brabander T, BLR K, Teunissen JJM, Feelders RA, Hofland J, Krenning EP. Salvage peptide receptor radionuclide therapy with [177 Lu-DOTA , Tyr 3] octreotate in patients with bronchial and gastroenteropancreatic neuroendocrine tumours. Eur J Nucl Med Mol Imaging. 2019;46(3):704–17.
43. Sowa-Staszczak A, Pach D, Chrzan R, Trofimiuk M, Stefanska A, Tomaszuk M, Kołodziej M, Mikołajczak R, Pawlak D, Hubalewska-Dydejczyk A. Peptide receptor radionuclide therapy as a potential tool for neoadjuvant therapy in patients with inoperable neuroendocrine tumours (NETs). Eur J Nucl Med Mol Imaging. 2011;38:1669–74.
44. Limouris GS, Karfis I, Chatzioannou A, et al. Superselective hepatic arterial infusions as established technique ("ARETAIEION" Protocol) of [177Lu] DOTA-TATE in inoperable neuroendocrine liver metastases of gastro-entero-pancreatic (GEP) tumors. Q J Nucl Med Mol Imaging. 2012;56:551–8.
45. Wild D, Fani M, Behe M, Brink I, Rivier JEF, Reubi JC, Maecke HR, Weber WA. First clinical evidence that imaging with somatostatin receptor antagonists is feasible. J Nucl Med. 2011;52:1412–7.
46. Claringbold PG, Turner JH. Pancreatic neuroendocrine tumor control: durable objective response to combination 177Lu-Octreotate-capecitabine-temozolomide radiopeptide chemotherapy. Neuroendocrinology. 2016;103:432–9.
47. Kesavan M, Claringbold PG, Turner JH. Hematological toxicity of combined 177lu-octreotate radiopeptide chemotherapy of gastroenteropancreatic neuroendocrine tumors in long-term follow-up. Neuroendocrinology. 2014;99:108–17.
48. Soydal Ç, Akkuş P, Küçük NÖ. Nöroendokrin Neoplazilerde Peptid Reseptörlerle radyonüklit Tedavi ve İzlemi. In: Nükleer Onkol. Istanbul: Teranostik Uygulamalar; 2018. p. 49–52.
49. Nonnekens J, van Kranenburg M, Beerens CEMT, Suker M, Doukas M, van Eijck CHJ, de Jong M, van Gent DC. Potentiation of peptide receptor radionuclide therapy by the PARP inhibitor olaparib. Theranostics. 2016;6:1821–32.
50. Elf A-K, Bernhardt P, Hofving T, Arvidsson Y, Forssell-Aronsson E, Wängberg B, Nilsson O, Johanson V. NAMPT inhibitor GMX1778 enhances the efficacy of ^{177} Lu-DOTATATE treatment of neuroendocrine tumors. J Nucl Med. 2017;58:288–92.
51. Basu S, Ostwal V, Ranade R, Panda D. Supportive measures and finer practice points in 177Lu-DOTATATE PRRT for NET: aiming for optimal disease management. J Nucl Med. 2014;55:1916–7.
52. Guidance P, Tumours N (2013) Practical Guidance on Peptide Receptor Radionuclide Therapy (PRRNT) for neuroendocrine tumours.
53. Valkema R, Pauwels SA, Kvols LK, et al. Long-term follow-up of renal function after peptide receptor radiation therapy with (90)Y-DOTA(0),Tyr(3)-octreotide and (177)Lu- DOTA(0), Tyr(3)-octreotate. J Nucl Med. 2005;46(Suppl 1):83S–91S.
54. Vegt E, de Jong M, Wetzels JFM, Masereeuw R, Melis M, Oyen WJG, Gotthardt M, Boerman OC. Renal toxicity of radiolabeled peptides and antibody fragments: mechanisms, impact on radionuclide therapy, and strategies for prevention. J Nucl Med. 2010;51:1049–58.
55. Bodei L, Cremonesi M, Ferrari M, Pacifici M, Grana CM, Bartolomei M, Baio SM, Sansovini M, Paganelli G. Long-term evaluation of renal toxicity after peptide receptor radionuclide therapy with 90Y-DOTATOC and 177Lu-DOTATATE: the role of associated risk factors. Eur J Nucl Med Mol Imaging. 2008;35:1847–56.
56. Bergsma H, Konijnenberg MW, van der Zwan WA, Kam BLR, Teunissen JJM, Kooij PP, Mauff KAL, Krenning EP, Kwekkeboom DJ. Nephrotoxicity after PRRT with (177)Lu-DOTA- octreotate. Eur J Nucl Med Mol Imaging. 2016;43:1802–11.
57. Sabet A, Ezziddin K, Pape UF, Reichman K, Haslerud T, Ahmadzadehfar H, Biersack HJ, Nagarajah J, Ezziddin S. Accurate assessment of long-term nephrotoxicity after peptide receptor radionuclide therapy with 177Lu-octreotate. Eur J Nucl Med Mol Imaging. 2014;41:505–10.

58. Werner RA, Beykan S, Higuchi T, et al. The impact of 177Lu-octreotide therapy on 99mTc-MAG3 clearance is not predictive for late nephropathy. Oncotarget. 2016;7:41233–41.
59. Sabet A, Ezziddin K, Pape U-F, Ahmadzadehfar H, Mayer K, Poppel T, Guhlke S, Biersack H-J, Ezziddin S. Long-term hematotoxicity after peptide receptor radionuclide therapy with 177Lu-Octreotate. J Nucl Med. 2013;54:1857–61.
60. Bergsma H, Konijnenberg MW, Kam BLR, Teunissen JJM, Kooij PP, de Herder WW, Franssen GJH. Subacute haematotoxicity after PRRT with 177 Lu-DOTA-octreotate: prognostic factors , incidence and course. Eur J Nucl Med Mol Imaging. 2016;43(3):453–63.
61. Barriuso J, Custodio A, Afonso R, et al. Prognostic and predictive biomarkers for somatostatin analogs , peptide receptor radionuclide therapy and serotonin pathway targets in neuroendocrine tumours. Cancer Treat Rev. 2018;70:209–22.
62. Ramage J, Naraev BG, Halfdanarson TR. Peptide receptor radionuclide therapy for patients with advanced pancreatic neuroendocrine tumors. Semin Oncol. 2018; https://doi.org/10.1053/j.seminoncol.2018.08.004.
63. Brabander T, Van Der Zwan WA, Teunissen JJM, Kam BLR, Feelders RA, De Herder WW, Van Eijck CHJ, Franssen GJH, Krenning EP, Kwekkeboom DJ. Long-term efficacy, survival, and safety of [177Lu-DOTA0,Tyr3]octreotate in patients with gastroenteropancreatic and bronchial neuroendocrine tumors. Clin Cancer Res. 2017;23:4617–24.
64. Kong G, Grozinsky-glasberg S, Hofman MS, Callahan J, Meirovitz A, Maimon O, Pattison DA, Gross DJ, Hicks RJ. Efficacy of peptide receptor radionuclide therapy for functional metastatic paraganglioma and pheochromocytoma. J Clin Endocrinol Metab. 2017;102:3278–87.
65. Kwekkeboom DJ, de Herder WW, Kam BL, van Eijck CH, van Essen M, Kooij PP, Feelders RA, van Aken MO, Krenning EP (2008) Treatment with the radiolabeled somatostatin analog [177 Lu-DOTA 0,Tyr3] octreotate: toxicity, efficacy, and survival. J Clin Oncol 26:2124–2130.
66. Jonathan Strosberg, Edward Wolin, Beth Chasen, Matthew Kulke, David Bushnell, Martyn Caplin, Richard P. Baum, Erik Mittra, Timothy Hobday, Andrew Hendifar, Kjell Oberg, Maribel Lopera Sierra, Philippe Ruszniewski DK (2015) 177Lu-Dotatate Significantly Improves Progression-Free Survival in Patients with Midgut Neuroendocrine Tumours: Results of the Phase III NETTER-1 Trial. Pres. Sess. II 18th ECCO – 40th ESMO.
67. Mariniello A, Bodei L, Tinelli C, et al. Long-term results of PRRT in advanced bronchopulmonary carcinoid. Eur J Nucl Med Mol Imaging. 2016;43:441–52.
68. Kim SJ, Pak K, Koo PJ, Kwak JJ, Chang S. The efficacy of 177Lu-labelled peptide receptor radionuclide therapy in patients with neuroendocrine tumours: a meta-analysis. Eur J Nucl Med Mol Imaging. 2015;42:1964–70.
69. Strosberg J, Wolin E, Chasen B, et al. Health-related quality of life in patients with progressive midgut neuroendocrine tumors treated with 177 Lu-Dotatate in the Phase III NETTER-1 Trial. J Clin Oncol. 2018;36:2578–84.
70. Eberlein U, Cremonesi M, Lassmann M. Individualized dosimetry for theranostics: necessary, nice to have, or counterproductive? J Nucl Med. 2017;58:97S–103S.
71. Arnold R, Chen Y-J, Costa F, Falconi M, Gross D, Grossman AB, Hyrdel R, Kos-Kudła B, Salazar R, Plöckinger U. ENETS Consensus Guidelines for the standards of care in neuroendocrine tumors: follow-up and documentation. Neuroendocrinology. 2009;90:227–33.
72. Gabriel M, Oberauer A, Dobrozemsky G, Decristoforo C, Putzer D, Kendler D, Uprimny C, Kovacs P, Bale R, Virgolini IJ. 68Ga-DOTA-Tyr3-octreotide PET for assessing response to somatostatin-receptor-mediated radionuclide therapy. J Nucl Med. 2009;50:1427–34.
73. Sainz-Esteban A, Prasad V, Schuchardt C, Zachert C, Carril JM, Baum RP. Comparison of sequential planar 177Lu-DOTA-TATE dosimetry scans with 68Ga-DOTA-TATE PET/CT images in patients with metastasized neuroendocrine tumours undergoing peptide receptor radionuclide therapy. Eur J Nucl Med Mol Imaging. 2012;39:501–11.
74. Bodei L, Kidd M, Modlin IM, Severi S, Drozdov I, Nicolini S, Kwekkeboom DJ, Krenning EP, Baum RP, Paganelli G. Measurement of circulating transcripts and gene cluster analysis predicts and defines therapeutic efficacy of peptide receptor radionuclide therapy (PRRT) in neuroendocrine tumors. Eur J Nucl Med Mol Imaging. 2016;43:839–51.
75. Bodei L, Kidd MS, Singh A, Zwan WA Van Der, Severi S, Drozdov IA, Cwikla J, Baum RP, Kwekkeboom DJ (2018) PRRT genomic signature in blood for prediction of (177)Lu-octreotate efficacy. Eur J Nucl Med Mol Imaging 45(7): 1155–1169.
76. Severi S, Nanni O, Bodei L, Sansovini M, Ianniello A, Nicoletti S, Scarpi E, Matteucci F, Gilardi L, Paganelli G. Role of 18FDG PET/CT in patients treated with 177Lu-DOTATATE for advanced differentiated neuroendocrine tumours. Eur J Nucl Med Mol Imaging. 2013;40:881–8.

10 Systemic Treatments and Related Side Effects in Neuroendocrine Tumors

Seher Nazlı Kazaz and İlhan Öztop

Neuroendocrine tumors (NETs) are a heterogeneous group of tumors originating from neuroendocrine cells commonly found in the body. NETs of many organs, especially gastroenteropancreatic and lung NETs, can be monitored. It may cause local symptoms as well as various clinical conditions based on the hormones it secretes depending on the location [1–3]. Ki-67 index and mitotic index are classified as well-differentiated low grade (grade 1), well-differentiated intermediate grade (grade 2) NET, and poorly differentiated high grade (grade 3) neuroendocrine carcinoma (NEC) in the World Health Organization (WHO) gastroenteropancreatic NET classification [4].

The treatment approach in NET varies according to the degree of the tumor, location, local or metastatic status, the presence of only liver metastases or non-liver metastases in metastatic disease, whether it is symptomatic or not, and whether the tumor is somatostatin receptor-2 positive (SSTR-2) [5]. Surgical treatment can be applied for both the elimination of local pressure symptoms and cytoreductive therapy in metastatic disease while it is the basic treatment approach in localized disease in well-differentiated (grades 1–2). The main treatment of metastatic disease is systemic treatment and somatostatin analogs and molecular-based target treatments are commonly used for this purpose in well-differentiated NET. In addition, radionuclide therapies and local ablative approaches to the liver are also the main elements of treatment [1–3].

Somatostatin analogs are the leading drugs used in systemic treatment in well-differentiated NET. Today, octreotide and lanreotide are the drugs in this group. These drugs are used both for symptom control and for tumor stabilization effects. Antiangiogenic drugs and mammalian target of rapamycin (mTOR) pathway inhibitors are the most commonly used agents as molecular-based treatments. Capecitabine/temozolomide combination can be preferred more primarily in patients with high tumor burden or rapidly progressing disease in pancreatic NET. On the other hand, the platinum/etoposide combination is widely used in poorly differentiated NECs [1, 3, 6].

10.1 Somatostatin Analogs

Thulin et al. first demonstrated the effectiveness of somatostatin in carcinoid syndrome in 1978 [7]. However, the short half-life of somatostatin (2–3 min) limited its clinical use. Then, Bauer et al. synthesized octreotide in 1982 [8]. Octreotide was then used as 150 mcg/three times a day for symptom control in 25 patients with

S. N. Kazaz (✉)
Faculty of Medicine, Department of Medical Oncology, Karadeniz Technical University, Trabzon, Turkey
e-mail: nazlikazaz@ktu.edu.tr

İ. Öztop
Dokuz Eylül University, Institute of Oncology, Izmir, Turkey
e-mail: ilhan.oztop@deu.edu.tr

R. Bekiş et al. (eds.), *Radionuclide Therapy*, https://doi.org/10.1007/978-3-030-97220-2_10

metastatic carcinoid tumors with carcinoid syndrome and was shown to provide significant symptom control (22 out of 25) and a decrease in 5-hydroxyindoleacetic acid levels (18 out of 25) [9]. Subsequently, similar studies have shown this usefulness and have taken its place as a standard in the initial treatment of well-moderately differentiated GI-NETS [10–14]. Treatment in symptomatic well-differentiated NETs is initiated with short-acting octreotide and monthly intramuscular treatment is initiated in 20–30 mg forms generally [1, 3].

A PROMID study was then conducted to demonstrate the effect of octreotide on tumor stabilization. Octreotide LAR was compared with placebo at a dose of 30 mg and was found to be superior in terms of both median progression-free (PFS) (14.3 months vs. 6.0 months) and tumor stabilization (66.7% vs. 37.2%) in this study, which evaluated 85 patients with metastatic well-differentiated middle intestinal carcinoid tumors (functional and non-functional) without previous treatment. This usefulness was reported to be independent of functional status [15]. Similarly, a CLARINET study was conducted with lanreotide. Lanreotide was shown to provide a significant increase in progression-free survival compared to placebo (PFS: 65% vs. 33% at 2 years) in this study, which evaluated 204 patients with well-moderately differentiated GEP-NET and non-functional [16]. Lanreotide is used monthly at a dose of 120 mg. A meta-analysis evaluating 17 studies with octreotide and 11 studies with lanreotide in addition to these two studies showed that both drugs provide both symptom control and tumor stabilization [17].

Side effects related to some systems, especially the gastrointestinal tract, are observed even though somatostatin analogs are generally well tolerated. Gastrointestinal side effects include swelling, nausea, gas, and malabsorption in about one-third of patients. It can also cause moderate glucose intolerance, causing gallbladder sludge and gallstones to form due to a decrease in postprandial gallbladder contractility in approximately one-quarter of patients. Less sinus bradycardia, edema, hypertension, upper respiratory tract infection, nephrolithiasis, fever, and pain at the administration site can be observed. These side effects may vary depending on the dose and route of administration [18–20].

10.2 Molecular-Based Target Treatments

Drugs targeting the pathway of angiogenesis have been the focus of attention in treatment since neuroendocrine tumors are highly vascular tumors. In this sense, both bevacizumab, a monoclonal antibody developed against the vascular endothelial growth factor (VEGF) receptor, and VEGF receptor tyrosine kinase inhibitors (VEGFR-TKI) are used in treatment. On the other hand, everolimus, which inhibits the mTOR pathway, is another important target drug used in treatment. mTOR pathway both plays a role in the NET development and regulates angiogenesis by controlling the hypoxia-inducible factor (HIF). Therefore, inhibition of this pathway constitutes an important therapeutic goal in the NET treatment.

10.3 Vascular Endothelial Growth Factor Receptor Tyrosine Kinase Inhibitors

Sunitinib, sorafenib, and pazopanib are more prominent in pancreatic NET, while GI-NET is not at the same rate. Studies in patients with well-moderately differentiated pNET who progressed under therapy with somatostatin analog have shown that sunitinib provides an advantage in terms of PFS [21]. On the other hand, the results are generally unsatisfactory even though it has been shown that these drugs provide PFS advantage in some phase 2 studies investigating their effectiveness in GI-NET treatment. Overall, these studies have reported response rates ranging from 0% to 9% and progression-free survival rates ranging from 7.8 to 12.7 months [22–24].

The main side effects of VEGFR-TKIs are described as hypertension, edema, bleeding, weakness, anemia, leukopenia, proteinuria, serum uric acid increase, skin and hair color change, serum AST, and ALT increase, thyroid dysfunction, diarrhea, and QT prolongation [25–30].

10.3.1 Bevacizumab

Bevacizumab, a monoclonal antibody against VEGF, has also been investigated as a potential treatment option since neuroendocrine tumors are highly vascular tumors. Combination therapy was found to be superior in terms of both response rate (31% vs. 12%) and progression-free survival (16.7 months vs. 14.0 months) in a phase 2 study comparing bevacizumab in combination with everolimus alone in patients with metastatic pancreatic NET [31]. On the other hand, the effectiveness of bevacizumab in advanced carcinoid tumors was investigated in study SWOG S0518. Patients were randomized to Depot Octreotide Plus Interferon Alfa-2b versus Depot Octreotide Plus Bevacizumab groups in this randomized phase 3 study. No significant difference was found in terms of progression-free survival (16.6 months vs. 15.4 months) even though bevacizumab interferon was found to be superior to alpha-2b in terms of response rate (12% vs. 4%) [32].

The main side effects of bevacizumab include hypertension, bleeding, venous thromboembolism, delayed wound healing, peripheral edema, malaise, headache, nausea, vomiting, and an increase in serum creatinine [33–37].

10.3.2 mTOR Inhibitors

The effectiveness of everolimus, an mTOR pathway inhibitor, has been investigated in various well-moderately differentiated NET patient groups with a series of studies called RADIANT studies. Octreotide LAR (30 mg) + everolimus and octreotide LAR (30 mg) were compared in 429 patients with well-moderately differentiated GI-NETs (with carcinoid syndrome) in RADIANT-2 study. The addition of everolimus to octreotide has been reported to significantly prolong PFS (16.4 months vs. 11.3 months) as a result [38, 39]. Everolimus and placebo were compared in 302 patients with well-differentiated, non-functional lung, and GI-NET who progressed under octreotide treatment in RADIANT-4 study. Everolimus has been reported to be superior to placebo in terms of PFS (14.0 months vs. 5.5 months) as a result. The usefulness was found to be similar in both lung and GI-NET [40]. RADIANT-3 study was conducted on patients with pancreatic NET, and this study compared everolimus and placebo in 410 patients with grade 1–2 pancreatic NETs who progressed under octreotide treatment. Everolimus has been reported to be superior to placebo in terms of PFS (11.4 months vs. 5.4 months) [41] as a result. Everolimus has taken its place in the well-moderately differentiated NET treatment of progression under somatostatin analog in line with all these studies.

The main side effects of everolimus (>10% frequency) include edema, mucositis, hypercholesterolemia, hyperglycemia, malaise, rash, anemia, leukopenia, increased risk of infection, increased serum alkaline phosphatase, increased serum alanine transferase, and increased serum creatinine. On the other hand, pneumonitis is also an important side effect even though it is a rare side effect [42, 43].

10.4 Systemic Chemotherapy

10.4.1 Capecitabine/Temozolomide Chemotherapy

The combination of temozolomide, an alkylating agent, and capecitabine, an antimetabolite, has been investigated in retrospective studies and a prospective study. Combination therapy has been shown to be superior to temozolomide therapy alone and thus this combination has taken its place in unresectable/metastatic pancreatic NET treatment as a result [44, 45]. Capecitabine/temozolomide combination can be preferred more primarily in patients with high tumor burden or rapidly progressing disease with pancreatic NET.

The main side effects of temozolomide are described as malaise, headache, alopecia, nausea, vomiting, lymphocytopenia, neutropenia, thrombocytopenia, hepatic failure, peripheral edema, and fever [46, 47].

The main side effects of capecitabine include mucositis, diarrhea, palmar-plantar erythrodysesthesia (hand-foot syndrome), malaise, nausea, hematological toxicity, peripheral edema, hyperbilirubinemia, and fever. In addition, its interaction with warfarin is also emphasized [48, 49].

10.4.2 Platinum/Etoposide Chemotherapy

The main treatment in poorly differentiated NECs is systemic treatment and platinum/etoposide combination is commonly used for this purpose. As a platinum preference, cisplatin or carboplatin is used considering the patient's organ functions and hypersensitivity; platinum is used in combination with etoposide [50].

Side effects of cisplatin include major nausea, vomiting, nephrotoxicity, autotoxicity, and peripheral neuropathy. In addition, arterial spasms can lead to electrolyte abnormalities and cardiac rhythm disorders. Hematological toxicity and hypersensitivity are more prominent side effects in carboplatin. Anemia, thrombocytopenia, leukopenia, neutropenia, and neutropenic fever may be observed due to hematological toxicity [51].

Main side effects of etoposide include hematological toxicity and hypersensitivity, and hematological toxicity may lead to anemia, thrombocytopenia, leukopenia, neutropenia, and neutropenic fever. Apart from these, it also carries a lower risk of alopecia, weakness, loss of appetite, nausea, vomiting, cardiac, hepatic, renal toxicity, and secondary leukemia [52].

10.5 Side Effects and Management

Somatostatin analogs, molecular-based targeted agents, and systemic chemotherapies constitute systemic treatment options in well-differentiated neuroendocrine tumors. All of these treatments have different mechanisms of action and very different side effect profiles. It is important to evaluate the comorbid diseases, concomitant drugs of the patients before the treatment, and to be informed about the side effects of the treatments. The severity of toxicities observed in treatments is usually graded according to assessment methods such as the National Cancer Institute Common Terminology Criteria for Adverse Events (NCI-CTCAE) [53]. Approaches such as discontinuation, postponement, dose reduction, as well as specific approaches specific to toxicity are made depending on the type and degree of toxicity observed.

10.6 Side Effects Management of Somatostatin Analogs

Octreotide and lanreotide are currently used as somatostatin analogs. The side effects profiles of both drugs are similar. Octreotide inhibits gallbladder contractility and reduces bile secretion. The risk increases when used for more than 12 months. It is thought to be a dose-dependent side effect [3, 18–20]. 62% of biliary tract dysfunctions such as jaundice, gallstones, gallbladder sludge, and dilatation were observed at 18 months of use, and 24% new gallstones were observed in the study conducted on patients with carcinoid tumors [54]. However, only about 1% of patients developed acute abdominal signs requiring cholecystectomy. It is recommended to follow up patients with abdominal ultrasonography and to perform prophylactic cholecystectomy if they undergo abdominal surgery in this respect [55].

Other common side effects of treatment with somatostatin analogs include nausea, abdominal cramps, mild steatorrhea (possibly due to temporary inhibition of pancreatic exocrine secretion), and swelling. These symptoms begin in the first hours after subcutaneous injection, are dose-dependent, and usually resolve spontaneously within the first few weeks of treatment. Injection site pain and erythema may occur locally. Impaired glucose tolerance or even diabetes mellitus (resulting from transient inhibition of insulin secretion) has also been observed during treatment with somatostatin analogs [56]. A very rare side effect is gastric atony [57]. Hypothyroidism has also been reported in very rare cases. Administration of the short-acting formulation is recommended prior to administration of the intramuscular storage formulation due to these adverse events [3, 6, 18–20].

One of the important side effects of octreotide use is bradycardia. Electrocardiogram was performed only in patients with carcinoid syndrome receiving storage form octreotide and 19% of patients with carcinoid syndrome developed sinus bradycardia, 9% conduction disorder, and 3% arrhythmia. The direct association of these events with octreotide acetate could not be established because most of these patients were reported to have a history of underlying cardiac disease [54].

10.7 Side Effects Management of Targeted Molecular Therapies

Sunitinib is the most widely used anti-VEGF TKI among molecular-based targeted therapies today. The most common adverse reactions were diarrhea (59%), nausea (45%), vomiting (34%), fatigue (32%), neutropenia (29%), skin and hair color change (29%), hypertension (26%), and hand-foot syndrome (23%) in the phase 3 study of sunitinib in patients with pNET. More rarely, thyroid dysfunction and QT prolongation are also described [58]. It is important to take precautions to prevent side effects from developing. Blood pressure control, evaluation of thyroid function tests, dietary recommendations for diarrhea, and moisturizing recommendations for hand-foot syndrome are required and movements requiring extreme heat and vibration should be avoided before starting treatment in this sense [6, 25, 26, 53, 58–61].

Antidiarrheal agents (such as loperamide) may be recommended in patients who develop diarrhea after infectious causes are excluded. Generally, there is no need to discontinue therapy for grade 1–2 diarrhea, a break is required for grades 3–4, fluid and electrolyte balance should be well evaluated in these patients, and replacements should be performed with hospitalization if necessary (Table 10.1) [53].

Neutropenia is usually low grade and does not require additional treatment. Generally, it does not reach the level that G-CSF is required. However, caution should be exercised in elderly patients [59, 60].

It is generally recommended to continue treatment by adding antihypertensive agents in patients who develop hypertension. ACE inhibitors and calcium channel blockers can be used even though they are not optimal agents for antihypertension. Treatment may be interrupted in grade 3–4 toxicities and may be resumed after blood pressure control is achieved [61].

Regular monitoring of TSH levels during the treatment of antiangiogenic TKIs is recommended in terms of hypothyroidism, initial evaluation of thyroid function tests, and subsequent and every 4–12 weeks monitoring in symptomatic patients. Symptomatic patients with hypothyroidism should receive thyroid hormone

Table 10.1 Diarrhea NCI-CTCAE v5.0 [53]

Adverse event	Grade 1	Grade 2	Grade 3	Grade 4	Grade 5
Diarrhea	<4 increase in daily defecation relative to baseline	4–6 increase in daily defecation relative to baseline	≥7 increase in daily defecation relative to baseline; requiring hospitalization	Life-threatening results; requiring urgent intervention	Death
	Moderate increase in stool coming from ostomy relative to baseline	Moderate increase in stool coming from ostomy relative to baseline	Severe increase in stool coming from ostomy relative to baseline; limitation of self-care		

NCI CTCAE, National Cancer Institute Common Terminology Criteria for Adverse Events support. No discontinuation of the agent causing toxicity and no dose modification is usually necessary. Temporary thyrotoxicosis is usually seen before hypothyroidism and does not require intervention [60].

Everolimus, one of the mTOR inhibitors, is another commonly used drug in the NETs. The most common adverse reactions with everolimus at all grades are stomatitis (70%), skin toxicity-rash (59%), diarrhea (50%), fatigue (45%), nausea (32%), and less frequent but clinically relevant non-infectious pneumonitis (17%). Only sodium-containing mouthwashes are recommended and treatment is continued, and analgesic and/or corticosteroid topical treatments and mouthwashes can be added according to the symptoms of the patients as the toxicity level increases in low-grade toxicities for stomatitis. Treatment is completely discontinued in grade 4 toxicities [42, 43, 62].

Recommendations have also been made according to the degree of toxicity of everolimus for pneumonitis, a rare but life-threatening serious side effect (Table 10.2) [62].

Table 10.2 Dose adjustment and side effect management of everolimus according to side effects [62]

Non-infectious pneumonitis/grade	Dose adjustment and side effect management
Grade 1 asymptomatic, only radiographic signs	No dose adjustment necessary, appropriate follow-up
Grade 2 symptomatic, ADL is not affected	Interrupt treatment, exclude infection, administer corticosteroid treatment until symptoms are ≤grade 1 Then resume at lower dose, discontinue treatment if no improvement within 4 weeks
Grade 3 symptomatic, ADL is affected, O_2 is needed	Interrupt drug administration until symptoms ≤ grade 1, exclude infection, administer corticosteroid therapy. Then resume at lower dose, discontinue treatment if toxicity grade 3 recurs
Grade 4 life-threatening, ventilation is needed	Completely discontinue treatment, exclude infection, administer corticosteroid therapy

ADL: Activity of Daily Living

10.8 Side Effects Management of Systemic Chemotherapies

The combination of temozolomide, an alkylating agent, and capecitabine, an antimetabolite, is generally pancreatic NET and can be preferred more primarily in patients with high tumor burden or rapidly progressing disease [44, 45]. The main side effects of temozolomide include nausea (41%), vomiting (34%), and malaise (23%), more commonly with alopecia, lymphocytopenia, neutropenia, thrombocytopenia, hepatic failure, peripheral edema, and fever [46, 47].

Main side effects of capecitabine include palmar-plantar erythrodysesthesia (hand-foot syndrome) (53–57%), diarrhea (49–57%), malaise (32–41%), nausea (38–53%), mucositis (25%), hematological toxicity (anemia 80%, lymphopenia 94%), peripheral edema, hyperbilirubinemia, and fever. In addition, its interaction with warfarin is also emphasized. Early and life-threatening toxicities may occur in patients with deficiency in dihydropyrimidine dehydrogenase enzyme involved in the metabolism of capecitabine [48, 49].

Hand-foot syndrome is a drug reaction accompanied by dry, red, numbness, and tingling, which can be accompanied by swelling of the palms of the hands and soles of the feet. Severe pain or ulceration occurs. The exact mechanism of the reaction is not known. It is usually seen in the early stages of treatment but it can also be seen in later periods. Symptoms usually improve with discontinuation of capecitabine. It is recommended that capecitabine treatment be discontinued immediately and resumed with a dose reduction after toxicity has decreased to 0–1° if a grade 2 or higher hand-foot skin reaction (pain-associated skin changes, but not affecting function) occurs. There are limited data in the prevention and treatment of hand-foot syndrome. However, measures such as avoiding tight-fitting shoes, avoiding strenuous activities that create pressure on the hands and feet, and frequent application of creams with lanolin to the affected areas are recommended [48, 49].

The combination of these two drugs increases the risks of nausea, vomiting, and hematological

Table 10.3 Hematological toxicity NCI-CTCAE v5.0 [53]

Blood element	Grade 1	Grade 2	Grade 3	Grade 4	Grade 5
Neutrophils	Between LLN and 1500/microL	1000–1500/microL	500–1000/microL	<500/microL	
Platelets	Between LLN and 75,000/microL	50,000–75,000/microL	25,000–50,000/microL	<25,000/microL	
Hemoglobin	Between LLN and 10.0 g/dL	8.0–10.0 g/dL	<8.0 g/dL	Life-threatening consequences; requiring urgent intervention	Death
Febrile neutropenia			Absolute number of neutrophils <1000 microL and presence of body temperature > 38.30 °C at a single measurement or ≥ 38.00 °C lasting longer than 1 h	Life-threatening consequences; requiring urgent intervention	Death

NCI CTCAE, National Cancer Institute Common Terminology Criteria for Adverse Events; LLN, lower limit of normal; Cell/microL, cell/mm^3 or cell × 10^9/L

Table 10.4 Acute kidney injury, creatinine increase NCI-CTCAE v5.0 [53]

Adverse event	Grade 1	Grade 2	Grade 3	Grade 4	Grade 5
Acute kidney injury			Requiring hospitalization	Life-threatening outcomes; Requiring dialysis	Death
Creatinine increase	ULN to 1.5 × ULN	Increase of 1.5–3.0 × baseline; Increase of >1.5–3.0 × ULN	Increase of >3.0 × baseline; Increase of >3.0–6.0 × ULN	Increase of >6.0 × ULN	

NCI CTCAE, National Cancer Institute Common Terminology Criteria for Adverse Events; ULN, upper limit of normal

toxicity. Antiemetics may be added for nausea and vomiting. The patient should be followed up with a complete blood count at certain intervals, treatment should be interrupted, and G-CSF should be added when necessary for hematological toxicities (Table 10.3) [53].

Platinum/etoposide combination is commonly used as systemic treatment in poorly differentiated NECs. Side effects of cisplatin include major nausea, vomiting, nephrotoxicity, autotoxicity, and peripheral neuropathy. In addition, arterial spasms can lead to electrolyte abnormalities and cardiac rhythm disorders. Hematological toxicity and hypersensitivity are more prominent side effects in carboplatin. Anemia, thrombocytopenia, leukopenia, neutropenia, and neutropenic fever may be observed due to hematological toxicity (Tables 10.1, 10.3, and 10.4) [51, 53].

The main side effects of etoposide include hematological toxicity and hypersensitivity, and hematological toxicity may lead to anemia, thrombocytopenia, leukopenia, neutropenia, and neutropenic fever. Apart from these, it also carries a lower risk of alopecia, weakness, loss of appetite, nausea, vomiting, cardiac, hepatic, renal toxicity, and secondary leukemia [52].

References

1. National Comprehensive Cancer Network (NCCN) Website. NCCN Clinical practice guidelines in oncology. Available at: https://www.nccn.org/professionals/physician_gls/pdf/neuroendocrine.pdf (Accessed on 12 October, 2018).
2. Uri I, Avniel-Polak S, Gross DJ, Grozinsky-Glasberg S. Update in therapy of advanced neuroendocrine tumors. Curr Treat Options Oncol. 2017;18(12):72. https://doi.org/10.1007/s11864-017-0514-9.
3. UpToDate website. Available at: https://www.uptodate.com/contents/metastatic-well-differentiated-gastrointestinal-neuroendocrine-carcinoid-tumors-systemic-therapy-options-to-control-tumor-growth-and-symptoms-of-hormone-hypersecretion.
4. Rindi G, Arnold R, Bosman FT, et al. Nomenclature and classification of neuroendocrine neoplasms of the digestive system. In: Bosman TF, Carneiro F, Hruban RH, Theise ND, editors. WHO Classification of tumours of the digestive system. 4th ed. Lyon: International Agency for Research on cancer (IARC); 2010. p. 13.
5. Panzuto F, Nasoni S, Falconi M, et al. Prognostic factors and survival in endocrine tumor patients: comparison between gastrointestinal and pancreatic localization. Endocr Relat Cancer. 2005;12(4):1083–92.
6. UpToDate website. Available at: https://www.uptodate.com/contents/metastatic-well-differentiated-pancreatic-neuroendocrine-tumors-systemic-therapy-options-to-control-tumor-growth-and-symptoms-of-hormone-hypersecretion.
7. Thulin L, Samnegard H, Tyden G, Long DH, Efendic S. Efficacy of somatostatin in a patient with carcinoid syndrome. Lancet. 1978;312(8079):43.
8. Bauer W, Briner U, Doepfner W, et al. SMS 201-995: a very potent and selective octapeptide analogue of somatostatin with prolonged action. Life Sci. 1982;31(11):1133–40.
9. Kvols LK, Moertel CG, O'Connell MJ, et al. Treatment of the malignant carcinoid syndrome. Evaluation of a long-acting somatostatin analogue. N Engl J Med. 1986;315(11):663–6.
10. di Bartolomeo M, Bajetta E, Buzzoni R, et al. Clinical efficacy of octreotide in the treatment of metastatic neuroendocrine tumors. A study by the Italian Trials in Medical Oncology Group. Cancer. 1996;77(2):402–8.
11. Saltz L, Trochanowski B, Buckley M, et al. Octreotide as an antineoplastic agent in the treatment of functional and nonfunctional neuroendocrine tumors. Cancer. 1993;72(1):244–8.
12. Rubin J, Ajani J, Schirmer W, et al. Octreotide acetate long-acting formulation versus open-label subcutaneous octreotide acetate in malignant carcinoid syndrome. J Clin Oncol. 1999;17(2):600–6.
13. Garland J, Buscombe JR, Bouvier C, et al. Sandostatin LAR (long-acting octreotide acetate) for malignant carcinoid syndrome: a 3-year experience. Aliment Pharmacol Ther. 2003;17(3):437–44.
14. Anthony L, Vinik AI. Evaluating the characteristics and the management of patients with neuroendocrine tumors receiving octreotide LAR during a 6-year period. Pancreas. 2011;40(7):987–94.
15. Rinke A, Müller HH, Schade-Brittinger C, et al. Placebo-controlled, double-blind, prospective, randomized study on the effect of octreotide LAR in the control of tumor growth in patients with metastatic neuroendocrine midgut tumors: a report from the PROMID Study Group. J Clin Oncol. 2009;27(28):4656–63.
16. Caplin ME, Pavel M, Ćwikła JB, et al. Lanreotide in metastatic enteropancreatic neuroendocrine tumors. N Engl J Med. 2014;371(3):224–33.
17. Sideris L, Dube P, Rinke A. Antitumor effects of somatostatin analogs in neuroendocrine tumors. Oncologist. 2012;17(6):747–55.
18. Sandostatin (octreotide solution) [prescribing information]. East Hanover, NJ: June 2018.
19. Sandostatin LAR Depot (octreotide suspension) [prescribing information]. East Hanover, NJ: Novartis; December 2018.
20. http://www.bccancer.bc.ca/drug-database-site/Drug%20Index/Octreotide_monograph.pdf
21. Kulke MH, Lenz HJ, Meropol NJ, et al. Activity of sunitinib in patients with advanced neuroendocrine tumors. J Clin Oncol. 2008;26(20):3403–10.
22. Hobday TJ, Rubin K, Holen J, et al. MC044h, a phase II trial of sorafenib in patients (pts) with metastatic neuroendocrine tumors (NET): A Phase II Consortium (P2C) study. J Clin Oncol. 2007;25. ASCO Annual Meeting Proceedings part I, abstract 4504
23. Phan AT, Halperin DM, Chan JA, et al. Pazopanib and depot octreotide in advanced, well- differentiated neuroendocrine tumours: a multicentre, single-group, phase 2 study. Lancet Oncol. 2015;16(6):695–703.
24. Grande E, Capdevila J, Castellano D, et al. Pazopanib in pretreated advanced neuroendocrine tumors: a phase II, open-label trial of the Spanish Task Force Group for Neuroendocrine Tumors (GETNE). Ann Oncol. 2015;26(9):1987–93.
25. Sutent (sunitinib) [product monograph]. Kirkland, QC: Pfizer Canada Inc; 2018.
26. http://www.bccancer.bc.ca/drug-database-site/Drug%20Index/Sunitinib_monograph.pdf
27. Votrient (pazopanib) [product monograph]. Dorval, QC: Novartis Pharmaceuticals Canada Inc; January 2018.
28. http://www.bccancer.bc.ca/drug-database-site/Drug%20Index/Pazopanib_monograph.pdf
29. Nexavar (sorafenib) [product monograph]. Toronto, ON: Bayer Inc.; May 2013.
30. http://www.bccancer.bc.ca/drug-database-site/Drug%20Index/Sorafenib_monograph.pdf
31. Kulke MH, Niedzwiecki D, Foster NR, et al. Randomized phase II study of everolimus versus everolimus plus bevacizumab in patients with locally advanced or metastatic pancreatic neuroendocrine tumors (pNET),CALGB 80701 (Alliance) (abstr). J Clin Oncol. 2015;33. (suppl; abstr 4005). Abstract available online at http://meetinglibrary.asco.org/

content/150169-156 (Accessed on September 04, 2015)
32. Yao JC, Guthrie KA, Moran C, et al. Phase III prospective randomized comparison trial of depot octreotide plus interferon Alfa-2b versus depot octreotide plus bevacizumab in patients with advanced carcinoid tumors: SWOG S0518. J Clin Oncol. 2017;35(15):1695–703.
33. Mir O, Coriat R, Cabanes L, et al. An observational study of bevacizumab-induced hypertension as a clinical biomarker of antitumor activity. Oncologist. 2011;16(9):1325–32.
34. Totzeck M, Mincu RI, Rassaf T. Cardiovascular adverse events in patients with cancer treated with bevacizumab: a meta-analysis of more than 20,000 patients. J Am Heart Assoc. 2017;6(8):e006278. https://doi.org/10.1161/JAHA.117.006278.
35. Nalluri SR, Chu D, Keresztes R, et al. Risk of venous thromboembolism with the angiogenesis inhibitor bevacizumab in cancer patients: a meta-analysis. JAMA. 2008;300(19):2277–85.
36. Avastin (bevacizumab) [product monograph]. Mississauga, ON: Hoffmann-La Roche Limited; June 2018.
37. http://www.bccancer.bc.ca/drug-database-site/Drug%20Index/Bevacizumab_monograph.pdf
38. Pavel ME, Hainsworth JD, Baudin E, et al. Everolimus plus octreotide long-acting repeatable for the treatment of advanced neuroendocrine tumours associated with carcinoid syndrome (RADIANT-2): a randomised, placebo-controlled, phase 3 study. Lancet. 2011;378(9808):2005–12.
39. Pavel ME, Baudin E, Öberg KE, et al. Efficacy of everolimus plus octreotide LAR in patients with advanced neuroendocrine tumor and carcinoid syndrome: final overall survival from the randomized, placebo-controlled phase 3 RADIANT-2 study. Ann Oncol. 2017;28(7):1569–75.
40. Yao JC, Fazio N, Singh S, et al. Everolimus for the treatment of advanced, non-functional neuroendocrine tumours of the lung or gastrointestinal tract (RADIANT-4): a randomised, placebo- controlled, phase 3 study. Lancet. 2016;387(10022):968–77.
41. Yao JC, Pavel M, Lombard-Bohas C, et al. Everolimus for the Treatment of Advanced Pancreatic Neuroendocrine Tumors: Overall Survival and Circulating Biomarkers From the Randomized, Phase III RADIANT-3 Study. J Clin Oncol. 2016;34(32):3906–13.
42. Afinitor and Afinitor Disperz (everolimus) [product monograph]. Dorval, QC: Novartis Pharmaceuticals Canada, Inc; November 2017.
43. http://www.bccancer.bc.ca/drug-database-site/Drug%20Index/Everolimus_monograph.pdf
44. Cives M, Ghayouri M, Morse B, et al. Analysis of potential response predictors to capecitabine/temozolomide in metastatic pancreatic neuroendocrine tumors. Endocr Relat Cancer. 2016;23(9):759–67.
45. Kunz PL, Catalano PJ, Nimeiri H, et al. A randomized study of temozolomide or temozolomide and capecitabine in patients with advanced pancreatic neuroendocrine tumors: A trial of the ECOG-ACRIN Cancer Research Group (E2211) (abstract). J Clin Oncol. 2018;36. (suppl; abstr 4004). Abstract available online at https://meetinglibrary.asco.org/record/160190/abstract (Accessed on June 19, 2018)
46. Temodal (temozolomide) [product monograph]. Kirkland, QC: Merck Canada Inc; June 2017.
47. http://www.bccancer.bc.ca/drug-database-site/Drug%20Index/Temozolomide_monograph.pdf
48. Xeloda (capecitabine) [product monograph]. Mississauga, Ontario: Hoffmann-La Roche Limited; August 2016.
49. http://www.bccancer.bc.ca/drug-database-site/Drug%20Index/Capecitabine_monograph.pdf
50. Fazio N, Spada F, Giovannini M. Chemotherapy in gastroenteropancreatic (GEP) neuroendocrine carcinomas (NEC): a critical view. Cancer Treat Rev. 2013;39(3):270–4.
51. http://www.bccancer.bc.ca/drug-database-site/Drug%20Index/Cisplatin_monograph.pdf
52. http://www.bccancer.bc.ca/drug-database-site/Drug%20Index/Etoposide_monograph.pdf
53. https://ctep.cancer.gov/protocoldevelopment/electronic_applications/docs/CTCAE_v5_Quick_Reference_8.5x11.pdf (Accessed on March 09, 2018).
54. https://www.pharma.us.novartis.com/sites/www.pharma.us.novartis.com/files/sandostatin_lar.pdf
55. Öberg LK, Caplin KM, et al. Consensus report on the use of somatostatin analogs for the management of neuroendocrine tumors of the gastroenteropancreatic system. Ann Oncol. 2004;15(6):966–73.
56. Lamberts SW, van der Lely AJ, de Herder WW, et al. Octreotide. N Engl J Med. 1996;334:246–54.
57. Behrus KE, Sarr MG. Diagnosis and management of gastric emptying disorders. Adv Surg. 1994;27:233–55.
58. Wiedmann MW, Mössner J. Safety and efficacy of sunitinib in patients with unresectable pancreatic neuroendocrine tumors. Clin Med Insights Oncol. 2012;6:381–93.
59. UpToDate website. Available at: https://www.uptodate.com/contents/cutaneous-side-effects-of-molecularly-targeted-therapy-and-other-biologic-agents-used-for-cancer-therapy.
60. UpToDate website. Available at: https://www.uptodate.com/contents/toxicity-of-molecularly-targeted-antiangiogenic-agents-non-cardiovascular-effects.
61. UpToDate website. Available at: https://www.uptodate.com/contents/toxicity-of-molecularly-targeted-antiangiogenic-agents-cardiovascular-effects.
62. https://www.accessdata.fda.gov/drugsatfda_docs/label/2012/022334s016lbl.pdf

Part IV

Clinical Information: Neuroectodermal Tumors

Radionuclide Therapy in Neuroectodermal Tumors

11

Zeynep Burak

Neurogenic tumors are used to identify a group of tumors that originate from the primitive neural crest tissue and have different clinical behaviors and pathological features. They can originate from the nerve sheath, sympathetic ganglia, paraganglion cells, and neuroectoderm, and they are subdivided according to their origin. Neural crest cells are pluripotent cells in embryogenesis and constitute sympathetic ganglion, autonomous ganglion, and adrenal medulla. The common features of these tissues are hormone and neurotransmitter synthesis in peptide structure called biogenic amine precursor uptake and decarboxylation (APUD) as well as intracytoplasmic storage granules. Childhood malignancies and adrenal gland tumors pheochromocytoma and paraganglioma are mentioned in this article even though there are many subtypes in pathological classification.

11.1 Pathology and Clinical Course Neuroblastoma

Neuroblastoma is an embryogenic tumor of the autonomic nervous system and originates from cells associated with precursor cells of neural crest tissue that have not completed differentiation [1]. 50% of neuroblastoma patients are under 2 years of age and 90% are children under 5 years of age since it is caused by developing tissues [2–4]. Neuroblastoma is the most common solid malignancy in childhood after brain tumors. It accounts for 8–10% of all childhood malignancies. The most common clinical origins are adrenal gland medulla and paraspinal ganglia. Unfortunately, 50–70% of the cases are metastatic at diagnosis. The most common sites of metastasis are lymph nodes, liver, bone, and bone marrow [5]. The most important parameters determining the prognosis are age, stage, and MYCN oncogene positivity. Being older than 12–18 months, MYCN positivity and metastatic disease at the time of diagnosis are consistent with poor prognosis. The prognosis is significantly good in low- and medium-risk cases compared to the high-risk group. The treatment approach is also based on risk assessment. This is important for survival and also to avoid the toxic effect of treatment. Patients with appropriate tumor biology and regional disease (low-risk) are treated only with surgery. Those with appropriate tumor biology and regional aggressive tumors (moderate risk) are treated with surgery and chemotherapy. The high-risk patient group is treated with multimodality therapy using agents such as 4–6 cycles of chemotherapy, surgical resection of the tumor mass, autologous stem cell transplantation, radiotherapy at the location of the primary tumor, monoclonal antibody therapy, and 13-cis-retinoic acid [2].

Z. Burak (✉)
Faculty of Medicine, Department of Nuclear Medicine, Ege University, Izmir, Turkey
e-mail: zeynep.burak@ege.edu.tr

R. Bekiş et al. (eds.), *Radionuclide Therapy*, https://doi.org/10.1007/978-3-030-97220-2_11

The clinical behavior of the disease is very variable and spontaneous regression, spontaneous differentiation to benign ganglioma, or rapid fatal progression can be observed [4]. The reason for this variation is essentially related to the age at which the disease occurs. Infants younger than 12 months of age have a good clinical course with chemotherapy and surgery, even if they have disseminated metastatic disease [4–8]. Conversely, children over 1 year of age constitute high-risk group and respond poorly to treatment. Nowadays, no improvement has been achieved for the prognosis even though the information related to the disease has increased.

The 3-year progression-free survival in patients over 1 year of age and with metastatic disease is below 35% [2–4]. The event-free survival rate was below 20% in patients who did not fully respond to induction therapy and who developed recurrence after bone marrow transplantation [9]. Disease-free survival in high-risk neuroblastoma is unfortunately less than 50% despite intensive treatment [5].

11.2 Pheochromocytoma and Paraganglioma

Paraganglioma and pheochromocytoma are rare tumors of neuroectodermal origin. The type originating from adrenal gland chromaffin cells is called pheochromocytoma; the non-adrenal type originating from sympathetic chromaffin cells or non-chromaffin parasympathetic cells is called paraganglioma. Their incidence rate is 0.1–0.8 per 100,000 [7]. Genetic mutations detected in pheochromocytoma and paraganglioma have been largely identified [10]. These are Cluster 1 (*SDHx, SDHAF2, HIF2A,* and *FH*) and Cluster 2 *(SRET, NF1, MAX,* and *TMEM127*), also known as tyrosine kinase pathway [11]. Determining the tumor phenotype is important for the application of targeted treatments due to these mutations. For example, SDHB mutations are more common in paragangliomas and increase the tendency of the tumor to metastasis [12]. It was shown in another study that tumors with SDHB mutation respond better to I-131 MIBG treatment [13].

Since these are rare tumors, the number of cases is low and the studies are retrospective. Today, the treatment of pheochromocytoma and paragangliomas are surgery, chemotherapy, tyrosine kinase inhibitors, and radionuclide therapy. The most commonly used chemotherapy regimen is cyclophosphamide, vincristine, and dacarbazine treatment [14]. Successful results have been reported in some studies with sunitinib, a tyrosine kinase inhibitor [15].

11.3 Medullary Thyroid Cancer

It originates from thyroid parafollicular C cells and accounts for approximately 3–10% of all thyroid cancers. One in third is familial and appears in the form of MEN IIA or MEN IIB. Medullary thyroid cancer manifests as a nodule or a mass in the thyroid [7]. High calcitonin levels in the blood are an important parameter reflecting tumor progression since parafollicular C cells secrete calcitonin. Medullary cancer is usually clinically silent, as calcitonin does not cause a clinical syndrome.

11.4 Neuroendocrine Cancers

These cancers originate from epithelial tissue in different parts of the body, called enterochromaffin or Kulchitsky cells. Their incidence rate is 0.1–0.14 per 100,000. Hormone-active tumors secrete various vasoactive peptides, leading to "carcinoid syndrome," which has clinical signs such as flushing, diarrhea, bronchospasm, and endocardial fibrosis. The characteristic product is serotonin. Biochemical diagnosis is done by 5-HIAA elevation in the urine which is a metabolite of serotonin [7].

11.5 Theragnostic Approach in Neuroectodermal Tumors

Studies conducted in the 1960s and 1970s investigated the role of labeled epinephrine for adrenal medulla imaging and later molecules that are analogs of ganglion-blocking drug guanidine were developed. Meta-iodobenzylguanidine (MIBG), a synthetic analog of norepinephrine, is one of them. The compound was developed by Wieland and Beierwaltes at the University of Michigan in 1979 [16].

Early animal studies have shown that MIBG accumulates in the adrenal gland medulla and in neuroectodermal tumors related to this tissue. MIBG labeled with radioactive iodine (I-123 or I-131) was first used as a molecular imaging agent in this context, and it was suggested that MIBG labeled with I-131 could be used for treatment purposes. A study showing that radioactive iodine-labeled MIBG can be used in the theragnostic approach was published, and I-131 MIBG was used for both imaging and treatment purposes in 8 cases diagnosed with pheochromocytoma in 1984 [17]. Results have supported that labeled MIBG can be administered for imaging and treatment in tumors associated with adrenal medulla, even though it does not show accumulation in the normal tissue. Then the use of I-131 MIBG for the treatment of neuroblastoma and other neuroendocrine tumors has been supported by other studies [18].

11.6 Uptake Mechanisms of Meta-iodobenzylguanidine

Studies in neuroblastoma cell cultures have shown that MIBG is specifically retained in these cells. A transmembrane protein called **norepinephrine transporter (NET)** is responsible for its uptake [19, 20]. NET is a protein responsible for transporting norepinephrine, a neurotransmitter, to sympathetic terminals in central and peripheral nervous system cells and neuroendocrine chromaffin cells. It is coded by the SLC6A2 gene, absolutely necessary for the reuptake of norepinephrine. The reuptake of norepinephrine is controlled by an active and saturable process (**uptake 1**) that requires energy. There is also an unsaturated passive diffusion mechanism that does not require energy. Norepinephrine is metabolized by monoamine oxidase in mitochondria or stored in vesicles by vesicular monoamine transporter (VMAT) after it is retained in the cell [21]. Many neuroendocrine-derived malignancies such as neuroblastoma, tumors originating from adrenal medulla chromaffin cells or non-adrenal paraganglioma tissue, or tumors originating from sympathetic neuronal precursors express NET.

The rate of meta-iodobenzylguanidine involvement in the cell is linearly correlated with the NET level [22]. A cell culture study has shown that neuroendocrine cells that do not normally show MIBG uptake begin to show MIBG uptake after being transfected with the NET gene [23]. MIBG, the synthetic guanethidine analog of norepinephrine, is taken up in neuroendocrine cells by a mechanism that involves both active (uptake 1) and passive diffusion mechanisms same as norepinephrine [24]. This event is inhibited by norepinephrine (competitive uptake) [19]. The majority of MIBG remains in the cytoplasm, and the rest is stored in vesicular granules via VMATs after being taken into the cell [25]. The rate of tumor involvement is proportional to the number of neurosecretory granules. Enzymes do not break down MIBG in the cell and MIBG does not bind to post-synaptic adrenergic receptors [26].

Experimental studies with chemotherapeutics have shown increased MIBG uptake in tumor cells in patients treated with cisplatin and doxorubicin [27, 28]. These two agents are used in the treatment of neuroblastoma. The reason for this effect may be the increase in the NET gene and therefore the receptor ratio during and after chemotherapy. These results support the premise that combined treatment models can be more successful.

11.7 Pharmacokinetics and Toxicity of MIBG Labeled with Radioactive Iodine

There is limited data about the elimination of MIBG in humans after IV injection, it is known that the molecule is rapidly removed from the blood, and the rate remaining in the blood after a few hours after injection drops below 10% [29].

The uptake of tumor tissue is faster compared to normal cells and peaks 6 h after injection. The unbound part is excreted in the urine. The half-life of excretion after 4 h of infusion is 10.6 h in individuals given 100–200 mCi (3.7–7.4 GBq) I-131 MIBG and is faster in children compared to adults [30].

It was shown that unlabeled MIBG up to 10 μmol level was not toxic when the effects of labeled and unlabeled MIBG on tumor cells were compared [31]. MIBG inhibits the growth of neuroblastoma cells by increasing intracellular oxidative stress in amounts above 10 μmol [32]. The cytotoxic effect of unlabeled MIBG is insignificant since the amount of MIBG used in clinical practice is below this value. The actual cytotoxic effect occurs when it is labeled with I-131. I-131 is a radionuclide emitting 606 keV beta emissions and 364 keV gamma rays with a half-life of 8.04 days. Approximately 90% of the cytotoxic effect is caused by beta radiation. Decay properties of I-131 with the release of high-energy particles penetrating the nucleus make it a suitable radionuclide in terms of treatment. In contrast, I-123's 13.3-hour half-life and 159 keV gamma rays make it ideal for imaging.

11.8 MIBG Scintigraphy Labeled with Radioactive Iodine

11.8.1 I-131/123 MIBG Imaging in Neuroblastoma

I-123/131 MIBG imaging is the gold standard in staging and treatment follow-up in neuroblastoma cases [33]. I-123 MIBG replaced I-131 MIBG today due to its shorter half-life, better image quality, and lower radiation dose despite the price disadvantage even though I-131 MIBG was used frequently in imaging in the past. MIBG imaging has 93–97% sensitivity in detecting the disease in patients with neuroblastoma. Therefore, it is recommended by the International Neuroblastoma Risk Group during the staging and treatment follow-up stages of neuroblastoma, especially in order to determine bone marrow involvement [34]. The method is more specific compared to magnetic resonance and has replaced bone scintigraphy. The sensitivity of I-123 MIBG is between 76% and 100% in staging or in relapsed disease [35, 36]. In a prospective multicenter study, the sensitivity and specificity of scintigraphy in diagnosis of disease was found as 88% and 83%, respectively [37]. Unexpected recurrences were shown in 82% of cases with I-123 MIBG, and no pathology was detected with other imaging methods in 27% of these cases.

Indications for I-131/123 MIBG imaging in the practice guidelines published by the European Association of Nuclear Medicine (EANM) are as follows [38]:

- In the diagnosis of neuroectodermal tumors (neuroblastoma, pheochromocytoma, paraganglioma).
- Staging the disease.
- Evaluation of the response to chemotherapy, especially in stage IV and IVS neuroblastomas.
- Before and after the primary tumor surgery.
- In the follow-up of treatment, in the investigation of recurrences that do not show any clinical sign such as bone marrow involvement, or in cases with a clinical suspicion of recurrence.
- Before MIBG treatment.

I-131/123 MIBG scintigraphy indications were expanded, and carcinoid tumor, medullary thyroid cancer, Merkel cell tumors, and MEN 2 syndrome were added to the indication list in the practice guide revised by the European Association of Nuclear Medicine in 2010 [39]. It is not recommended to be administered to pregnant patients as detailed in these guidelines.

Discontinuation of breastfeeding for 48 h is essential for breastfeeding patients. If I-131 MIBG is to be performed, lactation should be terminated. Oral stable iodine solution should be started one day before imaging and then continued for 1–2 days in order to prevent thyroid uptake of free iodine. The use of many drugs that may interact with MIBG uptake should be checked in advance. Bronchodilators commonly used especially in the pediatric group should be discontinued before imaging. A detailed list of drugs that interact with

MIBG is defined in the chapter covering patient preparation during MIBG treatment. If I-131 MIBG is administered, it is recommended to take whole-body, spot, SPECT, and SPECT-CT images, if any, after 2–3 days of I-131 MIBG and 24 h after I-123 MIBG injection.

The sites of physiological involvement are salivary glands, heart, liver, bladder, intestines, normal adrenal glands, and sometimes brown adipose tissue (Fig. 11.1). Thyroid uptake is observed if thyroid blockage is not sufficient. It is easy to detect metastatic disease since there is no physiological involvement in bone and bone marrow.

MIBG, with its very high sensitivity, helps accurately staging cases by showing primary tumors and/or metastases, evaluating the treatment response, and revealing recurrences in the follow-up process (Fig. 11.2). The absence of pathological signs in I-123 MIBG scintigraphy after chemotherapy is an indication that the prognosis will be good [40]. However, 24–41% of cases may have false-negative signs after treatment because chemotherapy leads to maturation and differentiation in the tumor, resulting in changes in the NET system and uptake mechanisms [41, 42].

Cases should be scanned with I-123 MIBG before I-131 MIBG treatment. The higher the rate of pathological involvement of MIBG compared to the liver, the higher the expectation of benefit from treatment. Foci that are not observed in planar examination can be detected in SPECT-CT images (Fig. 11.2). It is especially important to evaluate cases with stage 3 and 4 neuroblastoma with SPECT-CT [43]. The method increases the sensitivity especially in terms of detecting bone marrow metastases even though it

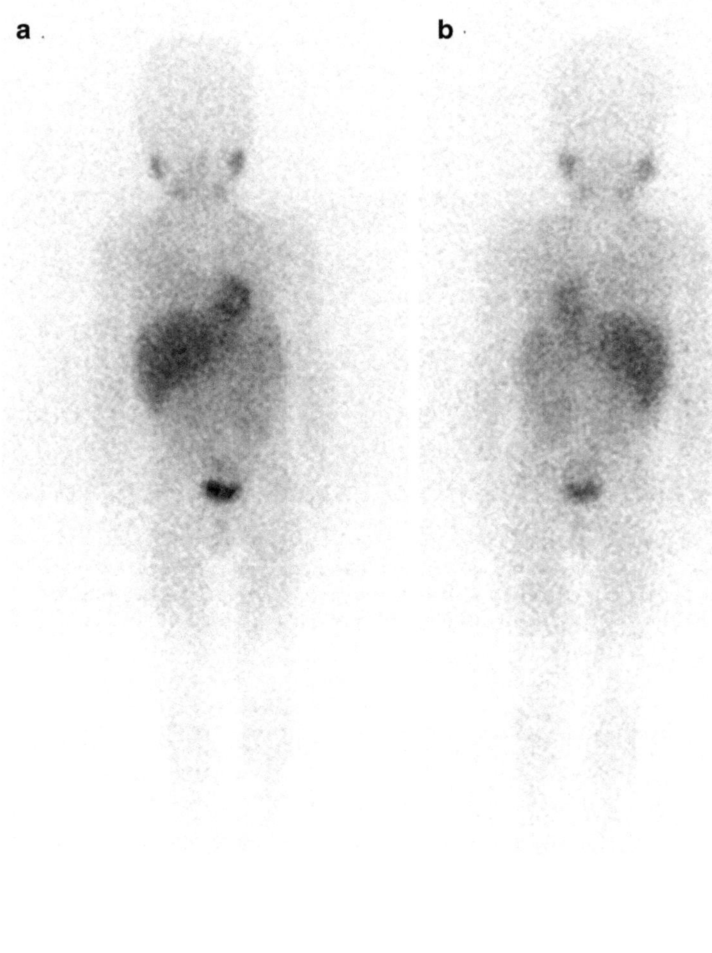

Fig. 11.1 I-123 MIBG images of a complete responsed neuroblastoma case after chemotherapy. (**a**) Anterior and (**b**) posterior images. Areas of physiological uptake are observed

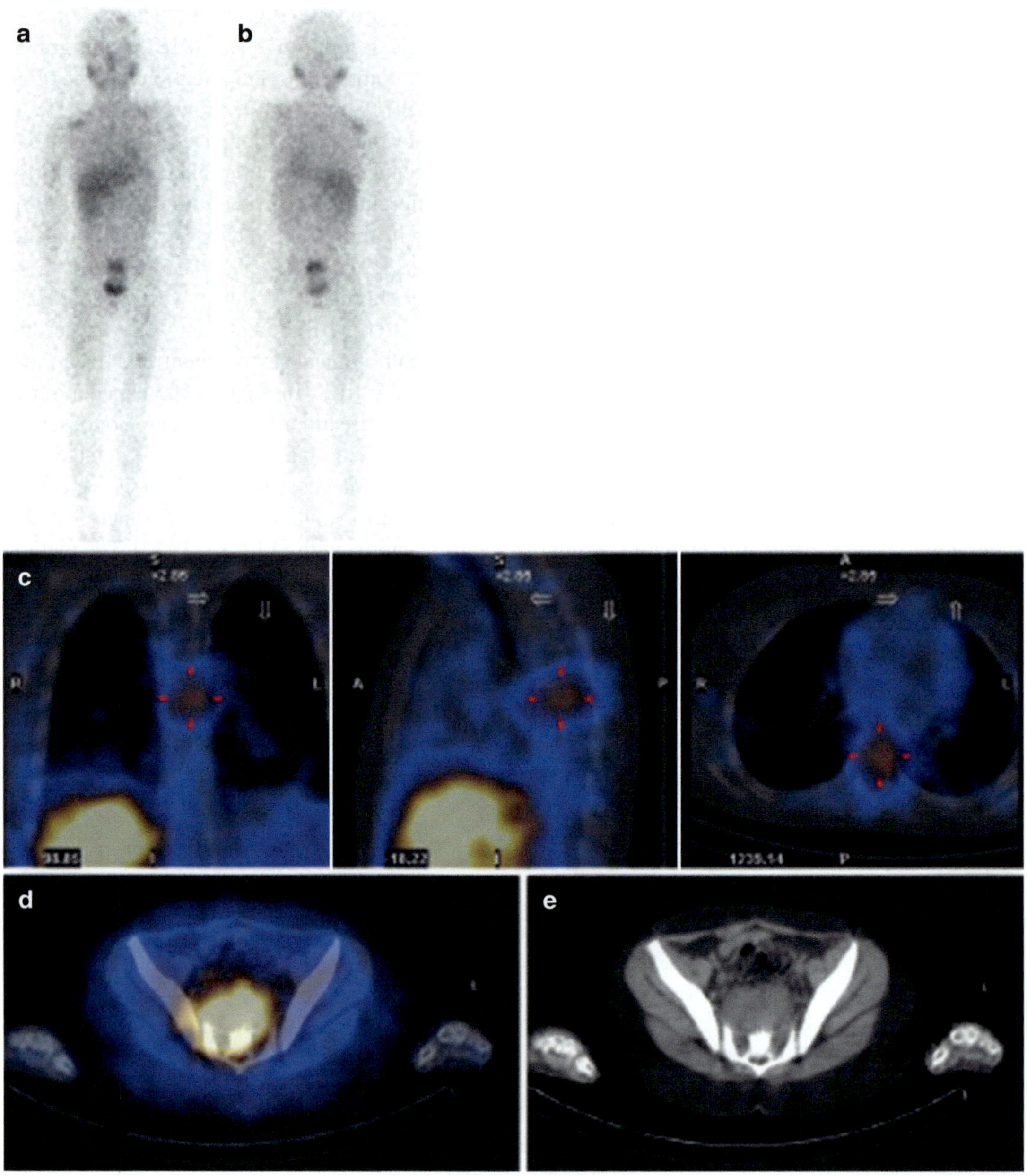

Fig. 11.2 Suspicious uptake in the posterior thorax and multiple bone/bone marrow involvement in the right shoulder and cranium were observed in anterior (**a**) and posterior (**b**) I-123 MIBG scintigraphy of a case, with diagnosis of paravertebral neuroblastoma. SPECT-CT was performed to evaluate the thoracic lesion and to examine the suspicious I-123 MIBG uptake visualized in the superior of the bladder. A large mass with extraosseous soft tissue was observed in the sacrum, which was not associated with the bladder (**d**) and (**e**) while SPECT-CT showed that the thoracic mass located in the bone (**c**). The case was diagnosed with high-risk neuroblastoma

is disadvantageous due to the longer imaging time in young children.

The evaluation of the distribution of the disease is also important in terms of the treatment plan. Cases with widespread disease are more suitable for systemic treatment while the presence of a large single mass in the abdomen with a few lesions in the soft tissue is consistent with surgical or local treatment [44]. Semi-quantitative scoring systems have been raised to increase the standardization in the evaluation of disease dissemination and therapy response after systemic treatment in neuroblastoma. These systems have been developed to determine the prognostic importance of tumor burden at the time of diagnosis and to evaluate the treatment response with standard treatment models in multicenter studies [45]. The first is the Curie score system proposed by Ady et al. in 1995 [46]. Nine diseased areas are selected from the whole body, and 0 to 3 points are given according to the intensity of involvement. Response to treatment is determined according to post-treatment total score. The modified Curie score system, which also includes soft tissue lesions, has proposed especially for multicenter studies [47]. Recently, the European Society of Pediatric Oncology Neuroblastoma Group (SIOPEN) recommends a repeatable and reliable scoring system consisting of 0–6 for the evaluation of skeletal and soft tissue involvement, especially in high-risk neuroblastoma patients [48]. Curie and SIOPEN scores and the rate of change after treatment have been shown to be prognostic. It has been emphasized that these systems are especially important in predicting treatment response after I-131 MIBG therapy.

11.8.2 I-131 MIBG Imaging in Pheochromocytoma and Paraganglioma

In these tumors, MIBG labeled with radioactive iodine is taken into the cell via NET and stored in vesicular granules with vesicular monoamine carriers (VMAT) as in neuroblastoma. The uptake of MIBG in these tumors is variable and the overall sensitivity is lower in those with liver involvement or nodal disease even though pheochromocytoma was the first disease in the history that I-131 MIBG was administered for imaging and therapy. This is probably because it is superposed by size and the physiological uptake. The sensitivity and specificity of I-123 MIBG imaging were reported to be 82–88% and 82–84%, respectively, in a prospective study involving 140 pheochromocytoma and paraganglioma patients [49]. NET expression in this type of tumors is variable and is associated with genotype. It has been reported that MIBG uptake is low in patients with SDHB mutation or pheochromocytoma associated with von Hippel-Lindau syndrome, possibly due to low NET expression [50]. In addition, the absence of VMAT1 expression has been proven in cases without MIBG uptake [51]. F-18 fluorodihydroxyphenylalanine (F-DOPA) PET-CT imaging is recommended if I-123-MIBG is negative in these cases.

Histologically malignant or benign distinction is not easy, even though most pheochromocytomas and paragangliomas are benign. When the cells of these tumors are detected in tissues that do not contain chromatin cells (lymph nodes, bones, internal organs), those cells are believed to be metastatic and malignant [52]. Benign and malignant differentiation of pheochromocytoma was tried to be made with a scoring system (PASS) using 12 different histological parameters [53]. Surgical removal is adequate when benign types are detected. Systemic treatment is not required in these cases. In contrast, chemotherapy, tyrosine kinase inhibitors, and radionuclide therapy (I-131 MIBG or Lu-177 PPRT) are treatment options in malignant types [14].

11.9 Other Radiopharmaceuticals Targeting Norepinephrine Transporter

PET radiopharmaceuticals targeting NET are investigated as an alternative to I-123 MIBG due to their superiority such as superior image quality and quantitative evaluation when necessary.

Bromine-76 (Br-76) labeled benzyl-guanidine analogs have been developed [54]. However, the labeling process is complex, and its effectiveness in large series has not been studied yet. MIBG labeled with I-124 was used in two neuroblastomas and one pheochromocytoma case [55, 56]. Among the reasons that limit the widespread usage of I-124 are its high-energy γ beams that cause problems in imaging, the long acquisition time after injection, and the high production cost. F-18-metafluorobenzylguanidine (F-18 MFBG), as one of the fluorine-18 labeled analogs has been evaluated in a prospective study involving cases with neuroectodermal tumors. It is defined as a promising radiopharmaceutical with good results in terms of target lesion involvement and image quality [57]. F-18 fluorodopamine (F-18 FDA) and F-18 fluoro-l-dihydroxyphenylalanine (F-18 DOPA), which are dopamine analogs, can detect pathological foci with 100% sensitivity in patients with SDHB mutations, especially in MIBG-negative pheochromocytoma and paragangliomas [58, 59]. However, none of these agents has yet entered routine clinical practice protocols. Their effectiveness should be evaluated in series with large number of patients.

11.10 I-131 MIBG Treatment in Neuroectodermal Tumors

In neuroectodermal tumors systemic treatment becomes a priority in metastatic, i.e., advanced stage cases while the first treatment is surgery when the disease is regional. Local radiotherapy that is administered to the surgical and primary disease site ensures the control of the regional disease while systemic disease is treated with multi-agent chemotherapy. Systemic treatment with I-131 MIBG has been suggested in metastatic cases who are resistant to initial treatment or developed recurrence at the end of treatment, since total body irradiation with radiotherapy is not applicable. In cases with positive uptake with I-123/131 MIBG imaging, the treatment of the same foci with high-dose I-131 MIBG is an example of theragnostic approach and internal radionuclide therapy.

I-131 MIBG is an ideal treatment agent because it is a radiopharmaceutical with a high affinity for tumor; it provides high levels of radiation to soft tissue, bone, and bone marrow; and its renal clearance is fast and metabolically stable. This treatment has been used since 1984 and more than 1000 patients have been treated worldwide. Its use as an induction therapy in newly diagnosed neuroblastoma patients is the subject of research, whereas generally cases with poor prognosis and resistance to treatment have been selected for I-131 MIBG treatment [45].

11.10.1 Indications

Indications for I-131 MIBG treatment have been defined according to the practice guideline published by the European Association of Nuclear Medicine (EANM) [60]. These indications are determined by accepting the precondition that I-123 MIBG imaging is applied before treatment and positive uptake(s) are detected.

- Inoperable pheochromocytoma, paraganglioma.
- Inoperable carcinoid tumor. (I-131 MIBG treatment was administered to reduce symptoms and hormone levels in metastatic neuroendocrine tumors.) Today, peptide receptor radionuclide therapy (PRRT) with Lu-177 is a much more successful alternative. I-131 MIBG treatment can be administered in cases with low peptide but high MIBG uptake and in conditions where PRRT cannot be administered [61].
- Stage III and IV neuroblastoma.
- Metastatic and recurrent medullary thyroid cancer.

11.10.2 Contraindications

- *Definitive contraindications*: Renal failure requiring dialysis, pregnancy, breastfeeding, life expectancy less than 3 months (except those with bone pain palliation).
- *Relative contraindications*: Incontinence, health problems causing isolation problems, glomerular filtration <30 ml/min, myelosuppression (White blood cell <3000 and platelets <100 thousand). Treatment can be applied by reducing the I-131 MIBG dose in cases with kidney and bone marrow problems.

11.10.3 Patient Preparation

The stage of the disease and the expectations from the treatment should be evaluated. The aim of I-131 MIBG therapy may be to achieve complete remission, to stop the progression of the disease or to reduce pain. Recent I-123 MIBG scintigraphy must be obtained before the treatment. In our department, the latest kidney and liver function tests and hemogram values are taken into consideration during the treatment planning.

11.10.4 Interaction with Drugs

If the drug interacting with MIBG is used, it should be discontinued for appropriate time [60]. Cardiovascular, neurological, and sympathomimetic drugs interacting with MIBG and when they should be discontinued are listed in Table 11.1. The most commonly used drugs that affect MIBG uptake and retention are alpha-beta adrenergic antagonists such as pseudoephedrine and labetalol [62]. Labetalol is especially used in neuroblastoma to control hypertension. It should be discontinued before treatment. The phenothiazine group sedatives should be discontinued prior to treatment also. In most cases with paraganglioma and pheochromocytoma, hypertension, tachycardia, and cardiomyopathy due to excessive catecholamine secretion are problems that may lead to death if not treated. Therefore, these catecholamines should be inhibited with an alpha-blocker before systemic treatment. Other drugs rarely used in children but important in adults are reserpine, tricyclic antidepressant, and cocaine. Antihypertensives such as phenoxybenzamine, nifedipine, and atenolol can be administered because they do not interact with MIBG. Diagnostic scan can be taken with I-123 MIBG to ensure drug interaction and uptake rate can be examined.

11.10.5 Thyroid Blockage

Protection of the thyroid gland from radiation is one of the most important steps in I-131 MIBG treatment. Serious quality control procedures are carried out before the administration to prevent free I-131 in the compound. However, preventing the thyroid gland from I-131 release as a result of de-iodination in the body after treatment is important for prevention of hypothyroidism that may develop in the future. Lugol's solution or oral potassium iodide tablets (100 mg for adults, 2 mg/kg for children) are started 24–48 h before radiopharmaceutical injection and continued for 10–15 days after treatment for this procedure [60]. It is also suggested that blockage will be effective even if administered a few hours before treatment because the mechanism of retention is rapid [63]. If the patient is allergic to iodine, potassium perchlorate at a dose of 8 mg/kg 3 times a day can be started 24 h before and then continued for 10 days.

11.10.6 Prevention of Early Side Effects

Nausea and vomiting are common side effects during and after the treatment and particularly are more common in patients with multiple liver metastases. Ondansetron is the first choice as an antiemetic drug. It is administered a few hours before starting treatment and continues for the next 3 days. Although rare, adult patients diagnosed with pheochromocytoma or paraganglioma may experience hypertensive crisis during radiopharmaceutical administration. For this reason, the blood pressure should be constantly under control during drug administration. Phentolamine, an alpha-adrenergic antagonist, should be available in the room. Hydration and frequent urination should be encouraged in terms of bladder protection.

11.10.7 Treatment Rooms and Personnel

Patients treated with I-131 MIBG are hospitalized in private rooms and treated with personnel trained in radiation protection like in other radionuclide therapies. The collaboration between the

Table 11.1 Drugs that interact with MIBG. (Source: Eur J Nucl Med Mol Imaging (2010) 37:2439-40)

Drug group	Drug name	Recommended discontinuation time
Cardiovascular and sympathomimetic drugs		
Antiarrhythmics	Amiodarone	(–)
Combined α/β blockers	Labetalol	72 h
Adrenergic blockers	Bretylium	48 h
	Guanethidine	48 h
	Reserpine	48 h
α Blockers	Phenoxybenzamine	15 days
Calcium channel blockers	Amlodipine	48 h
	Diltiazem	24 h
	Felodipine	48 h
	Lacidipine	48 h
	Nifedipine	24 h
	Nisoldipine	48 h
	Verapamil	48 h
Inotropic sympathomimetics	Dobutamine	24 h
	Dopamine	24 h
	Dopexamin	24 h
Vasoconstrictor sympathomimetics	Ephedrine	24 h
	Metaraminol	24 h
	Norepinephrine	24 h
	Phenylephrine	24 h
β2 stimulants (sympathomimetics)	Salbutamol	24 h
	Terbutaline	24 h
	Eformoterol	24 h
Systemic and local decongestants, common cold drugs	Pseudoephedrine	48 h
	Phenylephrine	48 h
	Ephedrine	24 h
	Oxymetazoline	24 h
Sympathomimetics used for glaucoma	Brimonidine	48 h
	Dipivefrine	48 h
Antipsychotic drugs:	Chlorpromazine	24 h
	Haloperidol	48 h/depot form 1 month
	Fluphenazine	24 h/depot form 1 month
	Clozapine	7 days
Tricyclic antidepressants	Amitriptyline	48 h
	Amoxapine	48 h
	Imipramine	24 h
Central nervous system stimulants	Cocaine	24 h
	Caffeine	24 h
	Amphetamine	48 h

referring clinic and nuclear medicine department is important for a successful treatment.

Treatment rooms should be lead-lined, with private toilets and bathrooms, where wastes are sent to special tanks.

Patients and their relatives should be informed in detail about the method of administration, follow-up, and side effects before the treatment, and written consent should be obtained in order not to encounter unnecessary questions during I-131 MIBG treatment. Since the treatment will be performed under the supervision of the child's caregiver, especially in the treatment of toddlers who need close attention, their parents should also be provided with radiation protection training and a digital pocket dosimeter should be attached. Disposal of the child's waste, length of stay in the room, and distance are determined. Doses of the patient's caregiver are supervised by the radiation safety officer. Urinary catheters should be inserted in babies without bladder control. Since more than 50% of the activity is excreted in the urine within the first 48 h, it is recommended to spend this time in the hospital. Patient's relatives should be trained about replacement of urinary bag and avoidance of activity contamination.

11.10.8 I-131 MIBG Administration

When the patient dose is prepared, quality control should be performed, and it should be documented that the free I-131 ratio is not more than 10%. I-131 MIBG is administered IV by slow infusion for 1–4 h to prevent side effects such as blood pressure changes caused by unlabeled MIBG. If I-131 MIBG with high specific activity is used, it can be administered faster. The radiopharmaceutical is administered through a lead-coated serum set and a three-way stopcock to a vein in order to reduce the dose of personnel and patient's relatives. Vital signs should be recorded by the personnel during the infusion. Patient follow-up should be performed more frequently in catecholamine-releasing tumors. Short-acting alpha or beta-blockers should be available at the patient's bedside. If the patient develops uncontrolled hypertension, temporarily stopping the infusion will resolve the problem. The intravenous route is retained open, and the serum is continued to be given after termination of the administration. This increases urinary excretion by providing hydration. Radiation safety rules should be followed in terms of transmission and environmental health due to urinary excretion of MIBG lasting 5 days after treatment. Tumor foci retaining I-131 MIBG are determined by taking the total body scan before the patient is discharged. In addition to the known sites of physiological uptake, cerebellum involvement not seen in diagnostic scintigraphy can be observed in the post-therapeutic image. More metastatic lesions than known are detected in 2/3 of the cases due to the higher dose in post-therapeutic scans.

Table 11.2 Acute, subacute, and late side effects in I-131 MIBG treatment. (AML, acute myelocytic leukemia, MDS, myelodysplasia)

Acute side effects (h/day)	Subacute side effects (weeks)	Late side effects (months)
Nausea, vomiting	Bone marrow suppression	AML, MDS
Hypertension	Liver and kidney dysfunction	Hypothyroidism
Parotitis	Venous thrombosis	Secondary tumors

11.10.9 Side Effects

Toxic effects that develop after treatment are divided into three as acute, subacute, and late side effects according to the time of development. Table 11.2 summarizes those side effects.

11.10.9.1 Acute Side Effects

- Acute toxicity observed in the first 8–12 h is usually nausea and vomiting. Nausea and vomiting are observed in 10–20% of cases and are more frequent in patients with diffuse liver metastases. Nausea and vomiting have been reported to be 11% and 21% in a series where I-131 MIBG is administered at doses of 4.2–21.7 mCi/kg [64]. It is recommended to start antiemetic drug before treatment and continue for 2 days after treatment since nausea and vomiting due to acute radiation gastritis are observed in some cases.
- The proportion of patients with hypertension-related problems within 48 h after I-131 MIBG infusion has been reported as 8% [65]. Hypertensive encephalopathy was observed in one case. The rate of hypertension requiring drug treatment in the pediatric group was 2.8% in another study [66]. Blood pressure should be monitored for 48 h in patients receiving treatment even though hypertension-related problems are rare.

- MIBG uptake may occur in the parotid glands within 48 h after treatment. Swelling and sialadenitis were detected in the parotid glands within the first 24 h in 50% of neuroblastomas given I-131 MIBG at doses of 12-18 mCi/kg [67].

11.10.9.2 Subacute Side Effects

- The most common side effect is hematological toxicity. Transient myelosuppression develops within 4–6 weeks after treatment in patients given doses below 200 mCi, although rare [60]. Isolated thrombocytopenia is more common, especially in children, due to the binding of MIBG to platelets. The risk of myelosuppression occurs more frequently in repeated treatments, in patients with diffuse bone marrow metastases, and in those receiving high-dose (> 12 mCi/kg) of I-131 MIBG. Grade 3 or 4 thrombocytopenia and leukopenia are observed in 83–87% of patients treated with I-131 MIBG of 15 mCi/kg and above. Platelet support and growth factor should be administered to these cases. However, few patients may have persistent myelosuppression at the level that stem cell transplantation is required [68].
- Temporary and mild impairment may occur in liver function and renal GFR. However, renal failure is a rare problem after I-131 MIBG therapy, compared to Lu-177 DOTATATE therapy even administered at repeated doses [69].
- Venous thrombosis in the liver is an important problem in the early period in patients undergoing myeloablative chemotherapy and stem cell transplantation following I-131 MIBG treatment [70]. This pathology is seen especially in cases with low glomerular filtration value. On the contrary venous thrombosis was not detected in patients treated with I-131 MIBG alone. It is suggested that the main cause of thrombosis is the decreased renal excretion of chemotherapeutics.

11.10.9.3 Late Side Effects

- Hypothyroidism is a common late complication despite thyroid blockade. The reason is that free I-131 is retained by the thyroid gland. Thyroid retention is observed in 10–25% of patients in post-therapeutic scans even though prophylaxis is performed with Lugol's solution [71]. Most of these patients develop asymptomatic TSH elevation in the future. Neuroblastoma patients treated with I-131 MIBG were followed up for a median of 15.5 years, and 50% of cases developed hypothyroidism requiring L-thyroxine treatment in a retrospective study reported from Denmark. Thyroid papillary cancer was detected in 2/9 cases [72].
- 2–4% of patients were reported to have acute myelocytic leukemia and 3% reported myelodysplastic syndrome 2 years after I-131 MIBG treatment [73]. Myelodysplasia and leukemia are more common in cases where I-131 MIBG treatment and chemotherapy are administered together. Secondary malignancies developed 5 years after treatment were below 4%. It is unlikely that secondary tumor development will be distinguished from the effect of chemotherapy in high-risk patients undergoing intensive chemotherapy. Tumors such as sarcoma, malignant schwannoma, and mesothelioma have been reported in a small number of cases 1.5–14 years after I-131 MIBG treatment [74]. The rate of secondary malignancy development in high-risk neuroblastoma cases at 10 years was 14.3% in a recent multicenter retrospective study [75]. The results were similar to the high-risk neuroblastoma group receiving standard regimen without I-131 MIBG treatment and revealed that the risk of developing secondary malignancy did not differ between the MIBG treated and non-MIBG groups.
- Primary ovarian insufficiency has been reported in two cases treated with I-131 MIBG [76].

11.11 I-131 MIBG Clinical Studies

11.11.1 Neuroblastoma

Systemic treatment scheme in high-risk group neuroblastoma includes the treatment of minimal residual disease with (1) induction therapy,

(2) consolidation with myeloablative therapy, and (3) immunotherapy and differentiation therapy. Surgery and radiotherapy are administered for regional disease. I-131 MIBG therapy has been administered alone (monotherapy) for approximately 30 years in metastatic neuroblastoma that does not respond to standard treatment protocol or has relapsed. The activity goes systemically to metastatic foci throughout the body with I-131 MIBG, and the dose reaching the tumor is much higher compared to radiotherapy. The total body radiation dose is 150 to 300 cGy while the median tumor dose is 30Gy in I-131 MIBG treatment [45].

11.11.1.1 Monotherapy

Most I-131 MIBG treatment studies were conducted in cases resistant to first-line chemotherapy. The most effective I-131 MIBG dose was investigated in refractory and relapsed neuroblastoma cases, starting from the 1980s. I-131 MIBG has been administered as monotherapy in refractory or relapsed patients for 20 years following the initial 1986 study [77] in which the objective response (complete or partial response) was reported to be between 0 and 66%.

Bone pain palliation was successful in cases with lower doses such as 1–5 mCi/kg, which will not cause bone marrow suppression at first, and the partial response was achieved in 33% of those cases [78]. However, the palliative response is short-termed and has no additional contribution to the survival. Phase 1 studies in chemotherapy-resistant neuroblastomas have shown that myelosuppression occurs, especially with administered doses above 444 MBq or 12 mCi/kg [79]. Severe myelosuppression has been detected at 18 mCi/kg or 666 MBq I-131 MIBG dose, and grade 4 thrombocytopenia has been reported to develop, especially at 4–sixth weeks, but the best response rate has been reported to be achieved at this dose [80].

Mattahey et al. reported the largest published series of I-131 MIBG monotherapy results in high-risk neuroblastoma patients with progressive, refractory, or recurrent disease in 2007 [81]. 148 patients received 18 mCi/Kg of I-131 MIBG dose and stem cell support while 16 patients received 12 mCi/Kg I-131 MIBG in this phase 2 study. Complete response (CR) + partial response (PR) rate was found to be 36% in this series. While the response rate in children over 12 years of age is 55%, this figure is 40% in children under 12 years. In addition, the response to radionuclide therapy was reported to be better in patients with soft tissue or bone metastasis alone compared to the group with both metastases. Factors affecting the response are the location of the disease and the number of previous chemotherapy protocols. However, the long-term contribution of I-131 MIBG to the disease is uncertain in this group of patients. The response rate with 12 mCi/kg monotherapy in the refractory or relapsed patient group ranges from 18% to 66%. The most prominent effect is usually observed in pain palliation even though there is a partial response in some cases. The objective response rate was reported to be 33–35% when lower doses were administered (9.5 mCi/Kg) to prevent bone marrow suppression [82]. In another study retrospectively evaluating 218 neuroblastoma patients, it was shown that the rate of progression-free survival after I-131 MIBG treatment was shorter in relapsed patients compared to primary refractory neuroblastoma patient group [83]. It is generally accepted that the 12 mCi/kg I-131 MIBG dose is the maximum tolerable dose that does not require stem cell support even though response rates are different. Stem cell support is required for administrations above this dose.

The Turkish Pediatric Oncology Group (TPOG) recommends I-131 MIBG treatment in neuroblastoma treatment protocol (NB2009), for relapsed or refractory neuroblastoma, before autologous stem cell transplantation or for pain palliation in disseminated metastatic cases (Figs. 11.3 and 11.4).

11.11.1.2 Consecutive Treatment Model

The modesty of the response to I-131 MIBG monotherapy has led to different strategies such as multiple dose administrations. Factors limiting these administrations are radiation safety limitations and insufficient tolerance to a single high dose [84]. Consequently, consecutive or fractionated dose administration has come up as an alternative. These protocols have been pro-

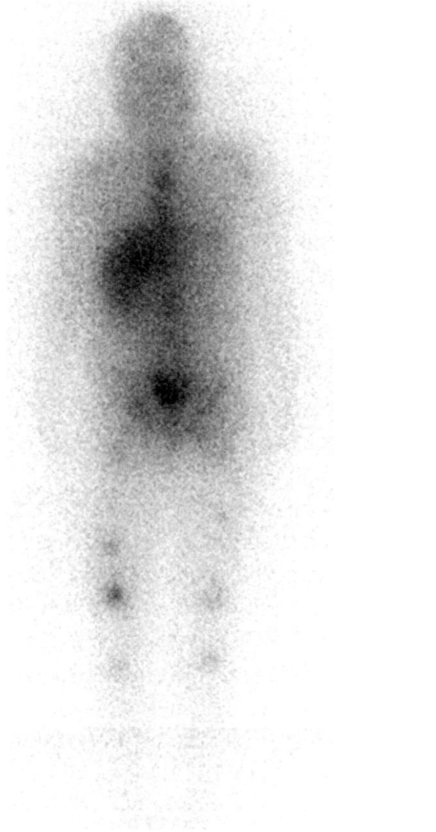

Fig. 11.3 I-131 MIBG treatment was planned to a high-risk neuroblastoma case (shown in Fig. 11.2) who is refractory to standard treatment. 200 m mCi I-131 MIBG treatment was administered, and bone and bone marrow metastases were visualized in both lower extremities as well as known lesions in the post-therapeutic image

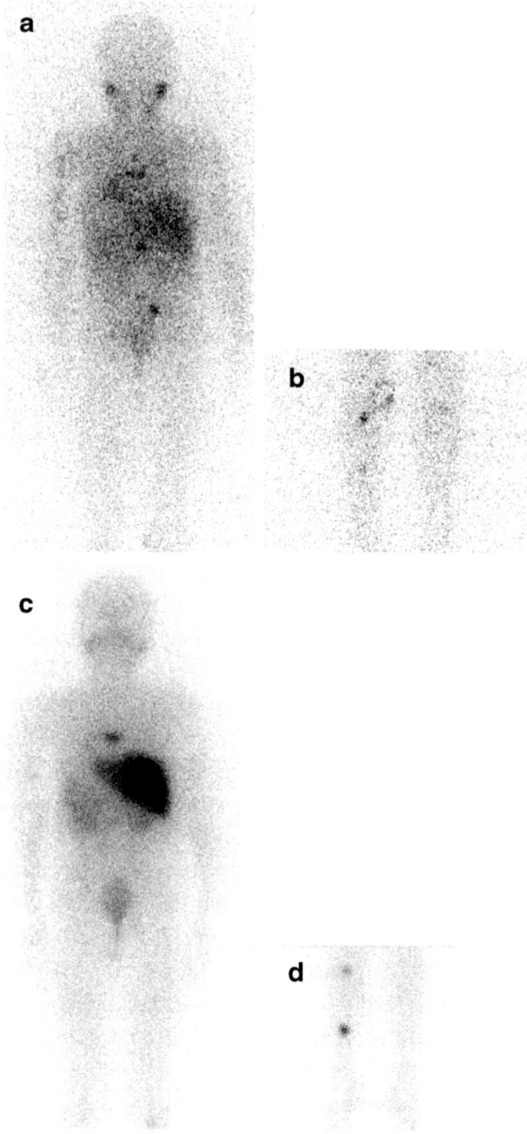

Fig. 11.4 Pathological I-123 MIBG uptakes in the thoracic and lumbar vertebrae, sacrum, and right tibia (**b**) were detected in posterior images (**a**) and relapse was diagnosed in I-123 MIBG scintigraphy taken due to right leg pain in a case diagnosed and treated with neuroblastoma. The patient was considered resistant to standard treatment, in the following process, 200 mCi I-131 MIBG treatment was administered for treatment and bone pain palliation. Post-therapeutic images (**c**) and (**d**) show multiple metastatic lesions

posed to fractionate the dose and prolong the anti-tumor effect preventing the toxic effect of a single high dose. Two or more I-131 MIBG treatments with 18-day intervals were administered to 28 patients at doses of 3–19 mCi/kg in 2005 [85]. A complete response was observed in 14 patients after the first infusion but thrombocytopenia was reported to be an important side effect limiting the dose. However, no significant change observed in response after the second dose suggested that the first dose was effective. Consecutive treatments administered at 2–12-week intervals were without any problems, but the response rates were below 40% and were not different from a single dose [44]. 30% objective response and 2% complete response were detected as a result of two consecutive doses administered at 3-month intervals [86]. Five-year event-free survival was 40% in the stage 4 patient group and 92% in the stage 3 patient group.

Refractory or recurrent 21 neuroblastoma patients were treated with two MIBG doses of 22 and 50 mCi/kg at 14 days intervals, and autologous stem cell transplantation (KHN) was performed after 14 days [87] in the phase 1 study of the New Approaches to Neuroblastoma (NANT) consortium. Response was observed in 45% of patients with soft tissue disease whereas response was observed in only 2 of 15 patients with bone marrow involvement. Myelotoxicity is minimal due to autologous SCT administration, but it has been reported that consecutive increased dose administration does not increase the objective response rate.

11.11.1.3 Chemotherapy + I-131 MIBG Treatment

Objective response rates are higher in studies where I-131 MIBG is administered with chemotherapeutics that increase radiation sensitivity such as cisplatin and cyclophosphamide. Cisplatin and cyclophosphamide were added to 200 mCi I-131 MIBG, and the objective response was reported to be 75% depending on the synergistic effect in a series reported by the Italian group [88]. Topoisomerase inhibitors are known to play a role in preventing the repair of radiation-related DNA damage. Accordingly, 24 patients with refractory or relapsed neuroblastoma were administered irinotecan, vincristine which are topoisomerase inhibitors, and I-131 MIBG at increasing doses of 8 and 18 mCi/kg, in phase 1 study conducted by the NANT consortium [89]. Overall survival was 25% and no significant adverse effects other than diarrhea were observed and phase 2 study was started. In addition, a phase 1 study investigating I-131 MIBG treatment with vorinostat, which is an inhibitor of "histone deacetylase" and increases its NET expression in neuroblastoma cells, is still being conducted by the same group (N2007-03).

NET expression is also known to be low in neuroblastoma patients with MYCN amplification. MYCN amplification is higher in the high-risk patient group. Clinical response has been reported in only 30% of children treated with I-131 MIBG in a recently published meta-analysis [90]. One of the factors that limit treatment effectiveness may be the decrease in NET expression. There are some studies in the literature aimed at increasing NET effectiveness based on this hypothesis. Methods such as corticosteroid therapy, gamma interferon, retinoic acid, cisplatin, doxorubicin, vorinostat, irinotecan and topotecan, hyperbaric oxygen therapy, gene therapy, and external radiotherapy have been investigated to increase NET expression [91]. These are studies with low evidence value, many of which have been conducted with a small number of cases even though promising.

11.11.1.4 I-131 MIBG Treatment and Autologous Stem Cell Transplantation (ASCT)

Many groups administered I-131 MIBG with high-dose chemotherapy and autologous stem cell support to increase the treatment effectiveness of I-131MIBG and to prevent the development of resistant tumor clones. The protocol was determined as I-131 MIBG treatment + carboplatin, etoposide, melphalan (CEM) chemotherapy + stem cell transplantation, I-131 MIBG was administered at 12 mCi/kg dose on -21st day, CEM treatment on -seventh and -fourth days, and OCHN was performed on 0th day [92]. Complete response or partial response was detected in 27% of patients, 3-year event-free survival was 31% ± 10%, and overall survival was 58% ± 10%. These results also showed that no additional toxicity developed when I-131 MIBG was added to standard treatment, and there was no problem in recovery after transplantation.

The same protocol was conducted in two groups in the NANT phase 2 study, which is the largest study conducted to date [93]. The first group consisted of 42 unresponsive or progressive patients, while the second group included 8 patients with partial response with 4 cycles of induction therapy. Three-year event-free survival was 38% in the second group, and overall survival was 75%, while 20% and 62% were observed in the other group. It has been reported that adding MIBG to treatment does not cause additional toxicity.

In TPOG Neuroblastoma treatment protocol (NB2009), in high-risk neuroblastoma cases, High Dose Chemotherapy (Megatherapy) + Autologous Stem Cell Transplantation (ASCT) group, in accordance with the NANT consortium, 12 mg/kg I-131 MIBG treatment is administered on the -21st day; melphalan, etoposide, carboplatin-containing megatherapy is administered in the week before ASCT; and on the 0th day ASCT is administered to every patient who receives 6-block megatherapy regardless of whether there is a tumor with or without I-131 MIBG. The maximum dose is 300 mCi in cases greater than 25 kg [94]. Three-year event-free survival was reported as 37%, and overall survival was 59% in the initial results of this ongoing study, differing from conventional treatment.

11.11.1.5 I-131 MIBG Induction Therapy

Successful treatment response in relapsed neuroblastoma patients has led to the investigation of the effectiveness of I-131 MIBG treatment in newly diagnosed neuroblastoma cases. However, there are few studies investigating the effectiveness of I-131 MIBG as an induction treatment. The reason for their low number is that the disease is mainly sensitive to chemotherapy, isolation problems for children with disseminated diseases and thrombocytopenia which develops after I-131 MIBG treatment.

De Kraker et al. reported the largest series [95]. Administering I-131 MIBG in addition to induction treatment aims to reduce the tumor burden and makes it suitable for surgery, to protect against toxicity caused by chemotherapy, and to reduce early drug resistance. Forty-four patients received a fixed dose of 200 mCi at the first and 100 mCi at the second infusion after 4 weeks. Partial response and tumor size reduction were observed in 66% of cases after two cycles of MIBG treatment. In addition, bone marrow metastases disappeared in 58% of cases. These results indicate that treatment can be used as neoadjuvant or in the initial stages of the disease. Grade 1–2 nausea, vomiting in 21%, grade 3 hepatotoxicity in 13%, and fever and neutropenia developed in 9% of the patients when I-131 MIBG was initially administered. There was no need for stem cell transplantation after treatment.

Evidence-based data are insufficient even though there are many studies on I-131 MIBG treatment in neuroblastoma. In a meta-analysis published in 2014 to determine the effective dose in I-131 MIBG treatment and to examine its reliability in light of available evidence, the articles published until 2012 were examined and common conclusions could not be reached due to the heterogeneity of the population, different follow-up periods, and lack of randomized controlled studies [90]. The median response rate is similar between the cases where I-131 MIBG is administered as monotherapy and with chemotherapy. Clinically objective tumor response was obtained, but the effect of this response on overall survival or event-free survival could not be demonstrated. However, a relationship between objective response and high cumulative dose has been shown in series with reported cumulative doses. Median response in recurrent or resistant cases is around 30%, even though response rates are variable.

The results show that I-131 MIBG treatment is ***a short-term active treatment*** in neuroblastoma. Its long-term effectiveness is uncertain. These are the problems that needed to be solved today: How effective is MIBG treatment compared to high-dose chemotherapy? Does co-administration of I-131 MIBG with chemotherapy contribute to survival instead of monotherapy? Is there a dose-dependent response, what is the optimal dose? Randomized, prospective, multicenter studies are needed to answer these questions. In general, it is seen that the data are heterogeneous due to their retrospective nature and the treatment schemes applied are different (single-dose, multiple-dose, etc.). There are also great differences in the definition of disease prevalence and clinical status. Response rates and response criteria are very different (overall response, overall survival, objective response, etc.) in the literature. Therefore, it is difficult to make a clear decision on the additive role of this treatment into clinical practice. High-dose I-131 MIBG treatment is still recommended especially with stem cell support in cases of chemotherapy-resistant neuroblastoma despite all these.

11.11.2 Pheochromocytoma and Paraganglioma

Curative treatment of pheochromocytoma (PHEO) and paraganglioma (Pg) is surgery. On the contrary, there is no curative treatment for metastatic disease. Most PHEO and Pg tumors are NETs, i.e., I-131 MIBG positive. I-131 MIBG treatment is generally preferred in progressive and metastatic disease. However, the number of patients in the literature is low, and there are no prospective studies examining treatment effectiveness and survival with increasing doses. The patient population in the literature is heterogeneous. Therefore, survival and response data are variable.

There are no systematic phase 1 studies comparing the effectiveness of low-, moderate-, or high-dose therapy in PHEO or Pg cases to date. Administrations can be performed empirically with the fixed-dose regimen or can be determined according to body weight. Low activity was defined as ≤200 mCi, moderate activity as ≤500 mCi, and high activity as 12–18 mCi/kg [52]. Low and medium doses of multiple-dose scheme are the most commonly used treatment modality. Stem cell transplantation is required above 12 mCi/kg.

When the articles published between 1983 and 1997 and containing 116 patients were examined, it was observed that the average dose of I-131 MIBG was 158 mCi, the average frequency of treatment was 3.3 times, and the cumulative dose was 2322 mCi [96]. The treatment response is evident in many of the studies even though the methodologies of these studies are different in retrospective nature. Complete response was reported as 4%, partial response was 26%, and stable disease was 57%. Complete biochemical response occurred in 13% and symptoms regressed in 76%. When the median 391 mCi I-131 MIBG dose was administered, the symptomatic response was reported to be 86%, the biochemical response was 60%, and the objective response was reported to be 38% in a retrospective study of 33 patients from Duke University [97].

It was noted in a prospective study with high dose I-131 MIBG treatment with a median activity of 818 mCi that the objective response was higher (57%) while the complete response was 8% [13].

The response rates were between 20% and 40% and similar when the objective response criteria of three studies with median I-131 MIBG doses of 200, 391, and 818 mCi are compared [13, 97, 98]. No significant difference was found in terms of objective response even though earlier response was obtained with higher doses in another study [99]. However, the authors recommend a higher dose >500 mCi in practice since the toxicity observed at high doses is moderate.

Treatment can be repeated every 3–6 months depending on the physical condition of the patient. There are no specific guidelines. The bone marrow takes longer to recover when high doses are administered. The growth rate of the tumor should also be taken into consideration when planning treatment intervals. It can be administered every 2.5–3 months in fast-growing tumors and every 6 months in slow-growing tumors. One to 11 treatment administrations have been reported in the literature [52, 98].

In general, clinical response is observed in PHEO patients after treatment. However, there is almost no complete response and there is a significant difference between the response rates reported in different studies [44]. Biological factors such as patient selection criteria, NET expression, dose of I-131 MIBG, frequency of administration, and duration of follow-up are likely to cause this. Objective response criteria were generally below 50%. The response rate was reported to be 25% in a meta-analysis of 17 studies covering 243 patients [99]. Success in symptom and hormone control is higher. Response rate in this disease does not appear to be directly related to dose increment. Factors determining the response rate are the type of disease (response in Pg is better compared to PHEO) and the location of the disease (response is better in soft tissue compared to bone). Objective response to treatment after the first dose of I-131 MIBG is prognostically important and indicates that it will be effective at subsequent doses.

The effect of I-131 MIBG treatment on overall survival in PHEO and Pg is unclear. Because even if they are metastatic, they are indolent diseases. Most patients usually survive for more than 10 years without anticancer treatment. Today, the accepted approach is to administer low or medium doses of treatment with multiple fractions without creating myelosuppression that requires stem cell support. It is administered at 8–12-week intervals for disease stabilization and symptom control. The palliative effect of the treatment is certain; disease-related pain and symptoms related to catecholamine secretion are controlled in 50–85% of the cases [97, 100]. In contrast, permanent objective response is rare. Therefore, I-131 MIBG treatment is not curative. There is no universally agreed treatment modality and dose scheme. Treatment has no place in some malignant subtypes of PHEO/Pg with SDHB mutation since there is no significant MIBG uptake. Consensus could not be reached on co-administration with other treatments.

As a result, prospective studies in PHEO and Pg are few and many are limited to ten cases. There is no evidence for this observation as comparative studies with fractionated low doses are insufficient even though the success rate has been reported to be high at doses above 500 mCi. However, the moderate toxicity compared to other treatments and the observation of symptomatic and biochemical response keep I-131 MIBG as a treatment option on the agenda in PHEO and Pg cases.

11.12 I-131 MIBG Treatment in Medullary Thyroid Cancer

Because medullary thyroid cancer is rare and tumors with I-131 MIBG uptake are also limited, the effectiveness of I-131 MIBG treatment in medullary thyroid cancer has been evaluated in a small number of patients [101].

The most important indication for this disease is palliative treatment in non-surgical metastatic disease. I-123 MIBG uptake was shown in 1/3 of the cases. Treatment protocol is similar to pheochromocytoma treatment, and 200–300 mCi I-131 MIBG is administered by slow infusion. The treatment is repeated at intervals of 3–6 months [102]. Objective response is around 30%.

11.13 MIBG Treatment in Neuroendocrine Tumors

I-131 MIBG treatment is only applied in a limited number of cases with negative somatostatin uptake and I-123 MIBG uptake with the introduction of Lu-177 DOTATATE PRRT. I-131 MIBG treatment has been reported to be administered especially in patients who cannot receive PRRT due to renal failure [70, 103].

11.14 Factors Increasing I-131 MIBG Uptake and Treatment Effectiveness

11.14.1 I-123/131 MIBG in High Specific Activity

I-131 MIBG, which is used in standard treatment, is produced by replacing stable I-127 bound to MIBG molecule with I-131. There are a large number of unlabeled MIBG molecules and the binding rate of the molecule with radionuclide is approximately 1/2000 in the radiopharmaceutical prepared by this method [104]. According to the hypothesis, unbound MIBG competes with radionuclide-bound MIBG during the receptor binding stage and treatment effectiveness decreases. I-131 MIBG specific activity in the standard method is 30–50 mCi/mg. Therefore, a total of 5–8.5 mg MIBG is injected for a 250 mCi treatment. This amount may cause a pharmacological effect in some patients.

Recently, I-131 MIBG, produced with high specific activity and no carrier has been shown to accumulate at a higher rate on tumor cells [104]. Different iodination methods compared to the standard method are developed for this. Specific activity greater than 1600 mCi per μmol can be obtained with these methods. Non-carrier added I-123 MIBG was shown to be retained at a higher rate in the heart and gastrointestinal tract in a phase 1 study [105]. Side effects such as nausea, vomiting, and hypertension have been reported to be less even though its contribution to clinical treatment is uncertain today [106]. Non-carrier MIBG was administered at doses of 12-15-18 mCi per kg in neuroblastoma cases, a similar response was obtained with standard treatment, and no dose-limiting toxicity was observed in the phase 1 study conducted by the NANT consortium [107]. Phase 2 work is currently ongoing.

11.14.2 Treatment Planning by Dosimetric Method

In dosimetric treatment models, the aim is to minimize the absorbed dose of normal organs while to maximize the dose to the target tumor tissue. The dose to be administered to the whole body or bone marrow is taken into account when planning the treatment dose in cases treated with a dosimetric approach. However, doses calculated from pre-treatment images with I-123 MIBG have been shown to be 20–30% different from doses obtained from post-therapeutic images [108]. 65% of the cases were administered a lower treatment dose than supposed to be in this case. When the whole-body absorption dose is considered, there are great differences from patient to patient in terms of treatment. I-131 MIBG treatments in neuroblastoma are generally applied with empirical approach and there are few studies with dosimetric treatment approach. There is a big difference in the whole-body dose calculations at varying doses from patient to patient, and this leads to problems in response and toxicity assessment. On the other hand, the optimum dose intended to reach the tumor is unknown.

Quantitative PET is a much better method for organ and lesion dosimetry. MIBG images labeled with I-124 with a half-life of 4.2 days are used for dosimetric approach. Pre-treatment images have been shown to be sufficient to evaluate the dissemination of the disease in neuroblastoma and PHEO patients [55]. Radiation dosimetry is appropriate, the average effective dose is 0.34 mSv/MBq in adults and 1.9–3.75 in children and infants according to the information obtained from animal images [109]. A dose of 20 Gy has been shown to reach the tumor with 52.8–206 MBq I-131 MIBG in a preclinical xenograft model [110]. The clinical benefit of dosimetric studies has not yet been established, but there are still phase 1–2 studies in neuroblastoma cases.

11.15 Alpha Emitters to Target Norepinephrine Transporter

Alpha emitters with a range of 50–80 μm and high linear energy transfer have higher cytotoxic effects in small tumors. Linear energy transfer is high, but the dose taken by the surrounding healthy tissues decreases due to its short range. Astatine-211 is an alpha emitter with a half-life of 7.2 h. They are labeled with MIBG analogs; At-211 meta-astrobenzylguanidine (MABG) and At-211 astatofluorobenzylguanidine (AFBG) are newly developed radiopharmaceuticals [111, 112]. Kit model has been developed for labeling. At-211 MABG showed high specific binding effectiveness in vitro. MABG shows dose-dependent toxicity, which is assumed to be effective due to its physical properties in cell culture studies. There are no clinical studies examining the effectiveness of treatment yet. It is unclear how to administer which dose in patients. However, it is assumed that radionuclide therapy will be more effective with alpha emitters that cause double-helical breaks in DNA.

11.16 Concluding Remarks

I-131 MIBG treatment, which is one of the first examples of the theragnostic approach and has been administered in certain centers all over the world for approximately 30 years, is a targeted internal radiotherapy application which is used in the treatment of metastatic, high-risk neuroectodermal tumors. The objective response in the advanced stage and refractory patient group is between 30% and 40% while the symptomatic response is significant. High-dose I-131 MIBG treatment in combination with megatherapy and stem cell transplantation in the high-risk patient group included in TPOG Neuroblastoma treatment protocol (NB2009) is carried out in a limited number of centers in Turkey since experienced personnel and equipped centers are required for this treatment.

The following questions on I-131 MIBG treatment are expected to be answered in the future: What is the optimal time and dose of treatment? Will response rates change when co-administered with radiation sensitizing chemotherapeutics? How effective is treatment with stable I-127-free labeled MIBG forms? What will be the treatment effectiveness with alpha emitters such as astatine-211? Ongoing and future research will provide answers to these questions.

References

1. Hoehner JC, Gestblom C, Hedborg F, Sandstedt B, Olsen L, Pahlman S. A developmental model of neuroblastoma: differentiating stroma-poor tumors' progress along an extra-adrenal chromaffin lineage. Lab Investig. 1996;75:659–75.
2. Matthay KK, Villablanca JG, Seeger RC, et al. Treatment of high-risk neuroblastoma with intensive chemotherapy, radiotherapy, autologous bone marrow transplantation, and 13-cis-retinoic acid. Children's Cancer Group. N Engl J Med. 1999;341(16):1165–73.
3. Berthold F, Boos J, Burdach S, et al. Myeloablative megatherapy with autologous stem-cell rescue versus oral maintenance chemotherapy as consolidation treatment in patients with high-risk neuroblastoma: a randomised controlled trial. Lancet Oncol. 2005;6(9):649–58.
4. Maris JM. Recent advances in neuroblastoma. N Engl J Med. 2010;362(23):2202–11.
5. Maris JM, Hogarty MD, Bagatell R, Cohn SL. Neuroblastoma. Lancet. 2007;369(9579):2106–20.
6. Evans AE, D'Angio GJ. Age at diagnosis and prognosis in children with neuroblastoma. J Clin Oncol. 2005;23(27):6443–4.
7. Howman-Giles R, Shaw PJ, Uren RF, Chung DK. Neuroblastoma and other neuroendocrine tumors. Semin Nucl Med. 2007;37(4):286–302.
8. George RE, London WB, Cohn SL, et al. Hyperdiploidy plus nonamplified MYCN confers a favorable prognosis in children 12 to 18 months old with disseminated neuroblastoma: a Pediatric Oncology Group study. J Clin Oncol. 2005;23(27):6466–73.
9. Ladenstein R, Philip T, Lasset C, et al. Multivariate analysis of risk factors in stage 4 neuroblastoma patients over the age of one year treated with megatherapy and stem-cell transplantation: a report from the European Bone Marrow Transplantation Solid Tumor Registry. J Clin Oncol. 1998;16(3):953–65.
10. Baysal BE, Willett-Brozick JE, Lawrence EC, et al. Prevalence of SDHB, SDHC, and SDHD germline mutations in clinic patients with head and neck paragangliomas. J Med Genet. 2002;39(3):178–83.
11. Dahia PLM. Pheochromocytoma and paraganglioma pathogenesis: learning from genetic heterogeneity. Nat Rev Cancer. 2014;14(2):108–19.
12. Timmers HJ, Kozupa A, Chen CC, et al. Superiority of fluorodeoxyglucose positron emission tomography to other functional imaging techniques in the evaluation of metastatic SDHB-associated pheochromocytoma and paraganglioma. J Clin Oncol. 2007;25(16):2262–9.
13. Gonias S, Goldsby R, Matthay KK, et al. Phase II study of high-dose [131I]metaiodobenzylguanidine therapy for patients with metastatic pheochromocytoma and paraganglioma. J Clin Oncol. 2009;27(25):4162–8.
14. Niemeijer ND, Alblas G, van Hulsteijn LT, Dekkers OM, Corssmit EP. Chemotherapy with cyclophosphamide, vincristine and dacarbazine for malignant paraganglioma and pheochromocytoma: systematic review and meta-analysis. Clin Endocrinol. 2014;81(5):642–51.
15. Ayala-Ramirez M, Chougnet CN, Habra MA, et al. Treatment with sunitinib for patients with progressive metastatic pheochromocytomas and sympathetic paragangliomas. J Clin Endocrinol Metab. 2012;97(11):4040–50.
16. Wieland DM, Wu J, Brown LE, Mangner TJ, Swanson DP, Beierwaltes WH. Radiolabeled adrenergic neuron-blocking agents: adrenomedullary imaging with [131I]iodobenzylguanidine. J Nucl Med. 1980;21(4):349–53.
17. Sisson JC, Frager MS, Valk TW, et al. Scintigraphic localization of pheochromocytoma. N Engl J Med. 1981;305(1):12–7.
18. Hoefnagel CA, Den Hartog Jager FC, Van Gennip AH, Marcuse HR, Taal BG. Diagnosis and treatment of a carcinoid tumor using iodine-131 meta-iodobenzylguanidine. Clin Nucl Med. 1986;11(3):150–2.
19. Iavarone A, Lasorella A, Servidei T, Riccardi R, Troncone L, Mastrangelo R. Biology of metaiodobenzylguanidine interactions with human neuroblastoma cells. J Nucl Biol Med. 1991;35(4):186–90.
20. Stöber G, Nöthen MM, Pörzgen P, et al. Systematic search for variation in the human norepinephrine

transporter gene: identification of five naturally occurring missense mutations and study of association with major psychiatric disorders. Am J Med Genet. 1996;67(6):523–32.
21. Mandela P, Ordway GA. The norepinephrine transporter and its regulation. J Neurochem. 2006;97(2):310–33.
22. Carlin S, Mairs RJ, McCluskey AG, et al. Development of a real-time polymerase chain reaction assay for prediction of the uptake of meta-[(131) I]iodobenzylguanidine by neuroblastoma tumors. Clin Cancer Res. 2003;9(9):3338–44.
23. Altmann A, Kissel M, Zitzmann S, et al. Increased MIBG uptake after transfer of the human norepinephrine transporter gene in rat hepatoma. J Nucl Med. 2003;44(6):973–80.
24. Lashford LS, Hancock JP, Kemshead JT. Meta-iodobenzylguanidine (mIBG) uptake and storage in the human neuroblastoma cell line SK-N-BE(2C). Int J Cancer. 1991;47(1):105–9.
25. Kölby L, Bernhardt P, Levin-Jakobsen AM, et al. Uptake of meta-iodobenzylguanidine in neuroendocrine tumours is mediated by vesicular monoamine transporters. Br J Cancer. 2003;89(7):1383–8.
26. Smets LA, Janssen M, Metwally E, Loesberg C. Extragranular storage of the neuron blocking agent meta-iodobenzylguanidine (MIBG) in human neuroblastoma cells. Biochem Pharmacol. 1990;39(12):1959–64.
27. Armour A, Cunningham SH, Gaze MN, Wheldon TE, Mairs RJ. The effect of cisplatin pretreatment on the accumulation of MIBG by neuroblastoma cells in vitro. Br J Cancer. 1997;75(4):470–6.
28. Meco D, Lasorella A, Riccardi A, Servidei T, Mastrangelo R, Riccardi R. Influence of cisplatin and doxorubicin on 125I-meta-iodobenzylguanidine uptake in human neuroblastoma cell lines. Eur J Cancer. 1999;35(8):1227–34.
29. Hickeson MP, Charron M, Maris JM, et al. Biodistribution of post-therapeutic versus diagnostic (131)I-MIBG scans in children with neuroblastoma. Pediatr Blood Cancer. 2004;42(3):268–74.
30. Wafelman AR, Nortier YL, Rosing H, et al. Renal excretion of meta-iodobenzylguanidine after therapeutic doses in cancer patients and its relation to dose and creatinine clearance. Nucl Med Commun. 1995;16(9):767–72.
31. Bruchelt G, Girgert R, Buck J, Wolburg H, Niethammer D, Treuner J. Cytotoxic effects of m- [131I]- and m-[125I]iodobenzylguanidine on the human neuroblastoma cell lines SK-N-SH and SK-N- LO. Cancer Res. 1988;48(11):2993–7.
32. Cornelissen J, Van Kuilenburg AB, Voûte PA, Van Gennip AH. MIBG causes oxidative stress and up-regulation of anti-oxidant enzymes in the human neuroblastoma cell line SK-N-BE(2c). Int J Cancer. 1997;72(3):486–90.
33. Kushner BH, Cheung NK. Exploiting the MIBG-avidity of neuroblastoma for staging and treatment. Pediatr Blood Cancer. 2006;47(7):863–4.
34. Brisse HJ, McCarville MB, Granata C, et al. Guidelines for imaging and staging of neuroblastic tumors: consensus report from the International Neuroblastoma Risk Group Project. Radiology. 2011;261(1):243–57.
35. Rufini V, Fisher GA, Shulkin BL, Sisson JC, Shapiro B. Iodine-123-MIBG imaging of neuroblastoma: utility of SPECT and delayed imaging. J Nucl Med. 1996;37(9):1464–8.
36. Jacobson AF, Deng H, Lombard J, Lessig HJ, Black RR. 123I-meta-iodobenzylguanidine scintigraphy for the detection of neuroblastoma and pheochromocytoma: results of a meta-analysis. J Clin Endocrinol Metab. 2010;95(6):2596–606.
37. Vik TA, Pfluger T, Kadota R, et al. (123)I-mIBG scintigraphy in patients with known or suspected neuroblastoma: Results from a prospective multicenter trial. Pediatr Blood Cancer. 2009;52(7):784–90.
38. Olivier P, Colarinha P, Fettich J, et al. Guidelines for radioiodinated MIBG scintigraphy in children. Eur J Nucl Med Mol Imaging. 2003;30(5):B45–50.
39. Bombardieri E, Giammarile F, Aktolun C, et al. 131I/123I-metaiodobenzylguanidine (mIBG) scintigraphy: procedure guidelines for tumour imaging. Eur J Nucl Med Mol Imaging. 2010;37(12):2436–46.
40. Matthay KK, Edeline V, Lumbroso J, et al. Correlation of early metastatic response by 123I-metaiodobenzylguanidine scintigraphy with overall response and event-free survival in stage IV neuroblastoma. J Clin Oncol. 2003;21(13):2486–91.
41. Feine U, Müller-Schauenburg W, Treuner J, Klingebiel T. Metaiodobenzylguanidine (MIBG) labeled with 123I/131I in neuroblastoma diagnosis and follow-up treatment with a review of the diagnostic results of the International Workshop of Pediatric Oncology held in Rome, September 1986. Med Pediatr Oncol. 1987;15(4):181–7.
42. Kushner BH, Yeh SD, Kramer K, Larson SM, Cheung NK. Impact of metaiodobenzylguanidine scintigraphy on assessing response of high-risk neuroblastoma to dose-intensive induction chemotherapy. J Clin Oncol. 2003;21(6):1082–6.
43. Černý I, Prášek J, Kašpárková H. Superiority of SPECT/CT over planar 123I-mIBG images in neuroblastoma patients with impact on Curie and SIOPEN score values. Nuklearmedizin. 2016;55(4):151–7.
44. Pandit-Taskar N, Modak S. Norepinephrine transporter as a target for ımaging and therapy. J Nucl Med. 2017;58(Suppl. 2):39S–53S.
45. Parisi MT, Eslamy H, Park JR, Shulkin BL, Yanik GA. 131I-Metaiodobenzylguanidine theranostics in neuroblastoma: historical perspectives; practical applications. Semin Nucl Med. 2016;46(3):184–202.
46. Ady N, Zucker JM, Asselain B, et al. A new 123I-MIBG whole body scan scoring method—application to the prediction of the response of metastases to induction chemotherapy in stage IV neuroblastoma. Eur J Cancer. 1995;31A(2):256–61.
47. Messina JA, Cheng SC, Franc BL, et al. Evaluation of semi-quantitative scoring system for metaiodo-

benzylguanidine (mIBG) scans in patients with relapsed neuroblastoma. Pediatr Blood Cancer. 2006;47(7):865–74.
48. Lewington V, Lambert B, Poetschger U, et al. 123I-mIBG scintigraphy in neuroblastoma: development of a SIOPEN semi-quantitative reporting ,method by an international panel. Eur J Nucl Med Mol Imaging. 2017;44(2):234–41.
49. Wiseman GA, Pacak K, O'Dorisio MS, et al. Usefulness of 123I-MIBG scintigraphy in the evaluation of patients with known or suspected primary or metastatic pheochromocytoma or paraganglioma: results from a prospective multicenter trial. J Nucl Med. 2009;50(9):1448–54.
50. Huynh TT, Pacak K, Brouwers FM, et al. Different expression of catecholamine transporters in phaeochromocytomas from patients with von Hippel-Lindau syndrome and multiple endocrine neoplasia type 2. Eur J Endocrinol. 2005;153(4):551–63.
51. Fottner C, Helisch A, Anlauf M, et al. 6-18F-fluoro-L-dihydroxyphenylalanine positron emission tomography is superior to 123I-metaiodobenzyl-guanidine scintigraphy in the detection of extraadrenal and hereditary pheochromocytomas and paragangliomas: correlation with vesicular monoamine transporter expression. J Clin Endocrinol Metab. 2010;95(6):2800–10.
52. Carrasquillo JA, Pandit-Taskar N, Chen CC. I-131 Metaiodobenzylguanidine therapy of pheochromocytoma and paraganglioma. Semin Nucl Med. 2016;46(3):203–14.
53. Szalat A, Fraenkel M, Doviner V, Salmon A, Gross DJ. Malignant pheochromocytoma: predictive factors of malignancy and clinical course in 16 patients at a single tertiary medical center. Endocrine. 2011;39(2):160–6.
54. Watanabe S, Hanaoka H, Liang JX, Iida Y, Endo K, Ishioka NS. PET imaging of norepinephrine transporter-expressing tumors using 76Br-meta-bromobenzylguanidine. J Nucl Med. 2010;51(9):1472–9.
55. Cistaro A, Quartuccio N, Caobelli F, et al. 124I-MIBG: a new promising positron-emitting radiopharmaceutical for the evaluation of neuroblastoma. Nucl Med Rev Cent East Eur. 2015;18(2):102–6.
56. Hartung-Knemeyer V, Rosenbaum-Krumme S, Buchbender C, et al. Malignant pheochromocytoma imaging with [124I]mIBG PET/MR. J Clin Endocrinol Metab. 2012;97(11):3833–4.
57. Pandit-Taskar N, Zanzonico P, Staton KD, et al. Biodistribution and dosimetry of 18F-meta-fluorobenzylguanidine: a first-in-human PET/CT ımaging study of patients with neuroendocrine malignancies. J Nucl Med. 2018;59(1):147–53.
58. Ilias I, Chen CC, Carrasquillo JA, et al. Comparison of 6-18F-fluorodopamine PET with 123I- metaiodobenzylguanidine and 111in-pentetreotide scintigraphy in localization of nonmetastatic and metastatic pheochromocytoma. J Nucl Med. 2008;49(10):1613–9.
59. Kauhanen S, Seppänen M, Ovaska J, et al. The clinical value of [18F]fluoro- dihydroxyphenylalanine positron emission tomography in primary diagnosis, staging, and restaging of neuroendocrine tumors. Endocr Relat Cancer. 2009;16(1):255–65.
60. Giammarile F, Chiti A, Lassmann M, Brans B, Flux G. EANM procedure guidelines for 131I-metaiodobenzylguanidine (131I-mIBG) therapy. Eur J Nucl Med Mol Imaging. 2008;35(5):1039–47.
61. Postema EJ, McEwan AJ. Radioiodinated metaiodobenzylguanidine treatment of neuroendocrine tumors in adults. Cancer Biother Radiopharm. 2009 Oct;24(5):519–25.
62. Babich JW, Graham W, Fischman AJ. Effect of adrenergic receptor ligands on metaiodobenzylguanidine uptake and storage in neuroblastoma cells. Eur J Nucl Med. 1997;24(5):538–43.
63. Zanzonico PB, Becker DV. Effects of time of administration and dietary iodine levels on potassium iodide (KI) blockade of thyroid irradiation by 131I from radioactive fallout. Health Phys. 2000;78(6):660–7.
64. Bleeker G, Schoot RA, Caron HN, et al. Toxicity of upfront ^{131}I-metaiodobenzylguanidine (^{131}I-MIBG) therapy in newly diagnosed neuroblastoma patients: a retrospective analysis. Eur J Nucl Med Mol Imaging. 2013;40(11):1711–7.
65. Kosmin MA, Bomanji JB, Cork NJ, Shankar A, Gaze MN. Hypertension complicating 131I-meta- iodobenzylguanidine therapy for neuroblastoma. Eur J Nucl Med Mol Imaging. 2012;39(4):597–601.
66. Wong T, Matthay KK, Boscardin WJ, Hawkins RA, Brakeman PR, DuBois SG. Acute changes in blood pressure in patients with neuroblastoma treated with ^{131}I-metaiodobenzylguanidine (MIBG). Pediatr Blood Cancer. 2013;60(9):1424–30.
67. Modak S, Pandit-Taskar N, Kushner BH, et al. Transient sialoadenitis: a complication of 131I-metaiodobenzylguanidine therapy. Pediatr Blood Cancer. 2008;50(6):1271–3.
68. Matthay KK, Panina C, Huberty J, et al. Correlation of tumor and whole-body dosimetry with tumor response and toxicity in refractory neuroblastoma treated with (131)I-MIBG. J Nucl Med. 2001;42(11):1713–21.
69. Vöö S, Bucerius J, Mottaghy FM. I-131-MIBG therapies. Methods. 2011;55(3):238–45.
70. Kayano D, Kinuya S. Iodine-131 metaiodobenzylguanidine therapy for neuroblastoma: reports so far and future perspective. Scientific World J. 2015;2015:189135.
71. van Santen HM, de Kraker J, Vulsma T. Endocrine late effects from multi-modality treatment of neuroblastoma. Eur J Cancer. 2005;41(12):1767–74.
72. Clement SC, van Eck-Smit BL, van Trotsenburg AS, Kremer LC, Tytgat GA, van Santen HM. Long- term follow-up of the thyroid gland after treatment with

131I-Metaiodobenzylguanidine in children with neuroblastoma: importance of continuous surveillance. Pediatr Blood Cancer. 2013;60(11):1833–8.
73. Weiss B, Vora A, Huberty J, Hawkins RA, Matthay KK. Secondary myelodysplastic syndrome and leukemia following 131I-metaiodobenzylguanidine therapy for relapsed neuroblastoma. J Pediatr Hematol Oncol. 2003;25(7):543–7.
74. Garaventa A, Gambini C, Villavecchia G, et al. Second malignancies in children with neuroblastoma after combined treatment with 131I-metaiodobenzylguanidine. Cancer. 2003;97(5):1332–8.
75. Huibregtse KE, Vo KT, DuBois SG, et al. Incidence and risk factors for secondary malignancy in patients with neuroblastoma after treatment with (131)I-metaiodobenzylguanidine. Eur J Cancer. 2016;66:144–52.
76. Clement SC, Kraal KC, van Eck-Smit BL, et al. Primary ovarian insufficiency in children after treatment with 131I-metaiodobenzylguanidine for neuroblastoma: report of the first two cases. J Clin Endocrinol Metab. 2014 Jan;99(1):E112–6.
77. Treuner J, Klingebiel T, Feine U, et al. Clinical experiences in the treatment of neuroblastoma with 131I-metaiodobenzylguanidine. Pediatr Hematol Oncol. 1986;3(3):205–16.
78. Klingebiel T, Berthold F, Treuner J, et al. Metaiodobenzylguanidine (mIBG) in treatment of 47 patients with neuroblastoma: results of the German Neuroblastoma Trial. Med Pediatr Oncol. 1991;19(2):84–8.
79. Lashford LS, Lewis IJ, Fielding SL, et al. Phase I/II study of iodine 131 metaiodobenzylguanidine in chemoresistant neuroblastoma: a United Kingdom Children's Cancer Study Group investigation. J Clin Oncol. 1992;10(12):1889–96.
80. DuBois SG, Messina J, Maris JM, et al. Hematologic toxicity of high-dose iodine-131-metaiodobenzylguanidine therapy for advanced neuroblastoma. J Clin Oncol. 2004;22(12):2452–60.
81. Matthay KK, Yanik G, Messina J, et al. Phase II study on the effect of disease sites, age, and prior therapy on response to iodine-131-metaiodobenzylguanidine therapy in refractory neuroblastoma. J Clin Oncol. 2007;25(9):1054–60.
82. Kang TI, Brophy P, Hickeson M, et al. Targeted radiotherapy with submyeloablative doses of 131I-MIBG is effective for disease palliation in highly refractory neuroblastoma. J Pediatr Hematol Oncol. 2003;25(10):769–73.
83. Zhou MJ, Doral MY, DuBois SG, Villablanca JG, Yanik GA, Matthay KK. Different outcomes for relapsed versus refractory neuroblastoma after therapy with (131)I-metaiodobenzylguanidine ((131)I- MIBG). Eur J Cancer. 2015;51(16):2465–72.
84. Kraal KC, Bleeker GM, van Eck-Smit BL, et al. Feasibility, toxicity and response of upfront metaiodobenzylguanidine therapy therapy followed by German Pediatric Oncology Group Neuroblastoma 2004 protocol in newly diagnosed stage 4 neuroblastoma patients. Eur J Cancer. 2017;76:188–96.
85. Howard JP, Maris JM, Kersun LS, et al. Tumor response and toxicity with multiple infusions of high dose 131I-MIBG for refractory neuroblastoma. Pediatr Blood Cancer. 2005;44(3):232–9.
86. Johnson K, McGlynn B, Saggio J, et al. Safety and efficacy of tandem 131I- metaiodobenzylguanidine infusions in relapsed/refractory neuroblastoma. Pediatr Blood Cancer. 2011;57(7):1124–9.
87. Matthay KK, Quach A, Huberty J, et al. Iodine-131-metaiodobenzylguanidine double infusion with autologous stem-cell rescue for neuroblastoma: a new approaches to neuroblastoma therapy phase I study. J Clin Oncol. 2009;27(7):1020–5.
88. Mastrangelo S, Tornesello A, Diociaiuti L, et al. Treatment of advanced neuroblastoma: feasibility and therapeutic potential of a novel approach combining 131-I-MIBG and multiple drug chemotherapy. Br J Cancer. 2001;84(4):460–4.
89. DuBois SG, Chesler L, Groshen S, et al. Phase I study of vincristine, irinotecan, and ^{131}I- metaiodobenzylguanidine for patients with relapsed or refractory neuroblastoma: a new approaches to neuroblastoma therapy trial. Clin Cancer Res. 2012;18(9):2679–86.
90. Wilson JS, Gains JE, Moroz V, Wheatley K, Gaze MN. A systematic review of 131I-meta iodobenzylguanidine molecular radiotherapy for neuroblastoma. Eur J Cancer. 2014;50(4):801–15.
91. Streby KA, Shah N, Ranalli MA, Kunkler A, Cripe TP. Nothing but NET: a review of norepinephrine transporter expression and efficacy of 131I-mIBG therapy. Pediatr Blood Cancer. 2015;62(1):5–11.
92. Matthay KK, Tan JC, Villablanca JG, et al. Phase I dose escalation of iodine-131- metaiodobenzylguanidine with myeloablative chemotherapy and autologous stem-cell transplantation in refractory neuroblastoma: a new approaches to Neuroblastoma Therapy Consortium Study. J Clin Oncol. 2006;24(3):500–6.
93. Yanik GA, Villablanca JG, Maris JM, et al. 131I-metaiodobenzylguanidine with intensive chemotherapy and autologous stem cell transplantation for high-risk neuroblastoma. A new approaches to neuroblastoma therapy (NANT) phase II study. Biol Blood Marrow Transplant. 2015;21(4):673–81.
94. Aksoylar S, Varan A, Vergin C, et al. Treatment of high-risk neuroblastoma: National protocol results of the Turkish Pediatric Oncology Group. J Cancer Res Ther. 2017;13(2):284–90.
95. de Kraker J, Hoefnagel KA, Verschuur AC, van Eck B, van Santen HM, Caron HN. Iodine-131-metaiodobenzylguanidine as initial induction therapy in stage 4 neuroblastoma patients over 1 year of age. Eur J Cancer. 2008;44(4):551–6.
96. Loh KC, Fitzgerald PA, Matthay KK, Yeo PP, Price DC. The treatment of malignant pheochromocytoma with iodine-131 metaiodobenzylguanidine (131I-MIBG): a comprehensive review

of 116 reported patients. J Endocrinol Investig. 1997;20(11):648–58.
97. Safford SD, Coleman RE, Gockerman JP, et al. Iodine –131 metaiodobenzylguanidine is an effective treatment for malignant pheochromocytoma and paraganglioma. Surgery. 2003;134(6):956–62.
98. Gedik GK, Hoefnagel CA, Bais E, Olmos RA. 131I-MIBG therapy in metastatic phaeochromocytoma and paraganglioma. Eur J Nucl Med Mol Imaging. 2008;35(4):725–33.
99. van Hulsteijn LT, Niemeijer ND, Dekkers OM, Corssmit EP. (131)I-MIBG therapy for malignant paraganglioma and phaeochromocytoma: systematic review and meta-analysis. Clin Endocrinol. 2014;80(4):487–501.
100. Shilkrut M, Bar-Deroma R, Bar-Sela G, Berniger A, Kuten A. Low-dose iodine-131 metaiodobenzylguanidine therapy for patients with malignant pheochromocytoma and paraganglioma: single center experience. Am J Clin Oncol. 2010;33(1):79–82.
101. Castellani MR, Alessi A, Savelli G, Bombardieri E. The role of radionuclide therapy in medullary thyroid cancer. Tumori. 2003;89(5):560–2.
102. Castellani MR, Seghezzi S, Chiesa C, et al. (131) I-MIBG treatment of pheochromocytoma: low versus intermediate activity regimens of therapy. Q J Nucl Med Mol Imaging. 2010;54(1):100–13.
103. Grünwald F, Ezziddin S. 131I-metaiodobenzylguanidine therapy of neuroblastoma and other neuroendocrine tumors. Semin Nucl Med. 2010;40(2):153–63.
104. Vaidyanathan G, Zalutsky MR. No-carrier-added meta-[123I]iodobenzylguanidine: synthesis and preliminary evaluation. Nucl Med Biol. 1995;22(1):61–4.
105. Chin BB, Kronauge JF, Femia FJ, et al. Phase-1 clinical trial results of high-specific-activity carrier-free 123I-iobenguane. J Nucl Med. 2014;55(5):765–71.
106. Owens J, Bolster AA, Prosser JE, et al. No-carrier-added 123I-MIBG: an initial clinical study in patients with phaeochromocytoma. Nucl Med Commun. 2000;21(5):437–40.
107. Matthay KK, Weiss B, Villablanca JG, et al. Dose escalation study of no-carrier-added 131I- metaiodobenzylguanidine for relapsed or refractory neuroblastoma: new approaches to neuroblastoma therapy consortium trial. J Nucl Med. 2012;53(7):1155–63.
108. Fielding SL, Flower MA, Ackery DM, Kemshead J, Lashford LS, Lewis IJ. The treatment of resistant neuroblastoma with 131I-mIBG: alternative methods of dose prescription. Radiother Oncol. 1992;25(1):73–6.
109. Lee CL, Wahnishe H, Sayre GA, et al. Radiation dose estimation using preclinical imaging with 124I-metaiodobenzylguanidine (MIBG) PET. Med Phys. 2010;37(9):4861–7.
110. Ott RJ, Tait D, Flower MA, Babich JW, Lambrecht RM. Treatment planning for 131I-mIBG radiotherapy of neural crest tumours using 124I-mIBG positron emission tomography. Br J Radiol. 1992;65(777):787–91.
111. Vaidyanathan G, Zalutsky MR. 1-(m-[211At]astatobenzyl) guanidine: synthesis via astato demetalation and preliminary in vitro and in vivo evaluation. Bioconjug Chem. 1992;3(6):499–503.
112. Vaidyanathan G, Affleck DJ, Alston KL, et al. A kit method for the high level synthesis of [211At] MABG. Bioorg Med Chem. 2007;15(10):3430–6.

12 Systemic Treatments and Related Side Effects in Neuroectodermal Tumors

Hüseyin Salih Semiz and İlhan Öztop

Primitive neuroectodermal tumors (PNETs) were defined by the World Health Organization (WHO) in 1980 to describe a group of tumors that develop from embryonic cells, have common biochemical and genetic characteristics, and are usually seen in childhood and young adults. These tumors are rare especially in adults and can be located in the central nervous system (CNS) or can be seen in many organs [1]. CNS-located PNETs were among the embryological tumors in the WHO brain tumor classification published in 2016 [2]. This group includes medulloblastoma, neuroblastoma, ganglioneuroblastoma, medulloepithelioma, ependymoblastoma, and atypical teratoid/rhabdoid tumors. Most of the PNETs are located outside the CNS are from Ewing family of tumors.

12.1 Ewing Family Tumors

This family includes extraosseous Ewing's sarcoma (ES), PNET, Askin's tumor (developing in the thoracic region), and atypical ES. Many studies show that they develop from a single stem cell even though these tumors exhibit some different clinicopathological features. The typical feature of ES is that the EWS gene in chromosome 22q12 forms fusion with one of the ETS gene family members. This fusion most often occurs with the FLI1 gene found in chromosome 11. This fusion occurs in 85–90% of cases [3]. An important feature of ES is that it intensively expresses the MIC2 (CD99) molecule on the cell surface [4]. ES can develop in both bone and soft tissue. ES occurring in the bone is usually seen in pelvic bones and long bones. The site most commonly involved in the long bone is diaphysis and may cause a typical radiological appearance resulting from a periosteal reaction called onion skin appearance. ES seen in soft tissue is more common in older and female patients compared to typical ES. ES family tumors have a very aggressive course. The most important prognostic factors are the location of the tumor, LDH value, and whether there is metastatic disease at the time of diagnosis. ES located in sacrum and vertebral column has a worse prognosis compared to other sites [5]. The most common sites of metastasis are the lungs and bone. The survival of patients with isolated lung metastases is better compared to patients with metastases to other organs. Bone metastases also most commonly occur in the vertebral column. Bone marrow involvement is common in ES. Therefore, some clinics recommend performing a bone marrow biopsy during staging and repeating the biopsy to evaluate the post-treatment tumor response. MRI or CT for the primary tumor site, CT and bone scintigraphy,

H. S. Semiz (✉)
Ministry of Health, Tepecik Training and Research Hospital, Izmir, Turkey
e-mail: huseyinsalih.semiz@deu.edu.tr

İ. Öztop
Dokuz Eylül University, Institute of Oncology, Izmir, Turkey
e-mail: ilhan.oztop@deu.edu.tr

R. Bekiş et al. (eds.), *Radionuclide Therapy*, https://doi.org/10.1007/978-3-030-97220-2_12

or PET/CT are recommended to exclude systemic metastases in staging. CT and MRI are equally sensitive, but MRI is more successful in showing local spread and vascular-nerve involvement. Therefore, MRI is usually performed to evaluate the primary area in ES [1].

Almost all of Ewing's sarcoma recurs when treated with local treatment options without systemic therapy. Chemotherapy has a very important role in this disease for this reason. The widespread use of systemic treatments in ES has also led to another review of prognostic factors.

Because these factors have generally been described only in patients receiving local treatment. In addition, the response to treatment has also taken its place among the prognostic factors with the widespread use of chemotherapy. Five-year overall survival (OS) reached 80% with the addition of chemotherapy to local treatments. Osseous ES and extraosseous ES have been shown to be sensitive to ifosfamide-containing treatment regimens, and these two tumors have similar responses [6–8].

12.1.1 Local Therapies

Surgical treatment is one of the main treatment methods for localized disease in ES, as with many malignancies. However, it may not always be appropriate to perform surgery as the first-line treatment in ES. Performing organ-protective surgery becomes even more important since ES is mostly seen in adolescents and young adults. It is widely accepted today to perform surgery after systemic neoadjuvant chemotherapy and radiotherapy in necessary cases if tumors requiring extensive resection, loss of organ function, or amputation. Definitive radiotherapy can only be evaluated in cases where surgical treatment is not possible. It would be more appropriate to use systemic chemotherapy before definitive radiotherapy in these cases, if possible. Although there is no definite indication today, except for the positivity of the surgical margin, where postoperative radiotherapy is applied as a standard, there are also authorities recommending postoperative adjuvant radiotherapy. In addition, patients who were given neoadjuvant therapy but did not achieve a good histological response are also candidates for postoperative radiotherapy. Past experience with Ewing's sarcoma shows that the vast majority of patients will relapse unless systemic therapy is added to surgery alone, radiotherapy alone, or a combination of these. For this reason, almost no patient is left with only local treatments, and systemic treatment should be added [1, 6, 7]. Surgery and radiotherapy can also be administered for palliation of metastatic disease except for adjuvant and neoadjuvant applications.

12.1.2 Systemic Therapies

Only local treatments are inadequate because Ewing family of tumors have very high recurrence rates. OS has increased dramatically after the widespread use of chemotherapy in ES. Systemic treatments are widely used today before and after local treatments. Five-year OS was around 10–30% with only local treatments in the past; it has reached 70–75% levels as a result of the combined use of chemotherapy, surgery, and radiotherapy [9]. The number of studies conducted in adults is fairly limited since ES is mostly seen in adolescents and young adults. It was revealed in a retrospective study conducted by Ahmed et al. on 102 adult patients diagnosed with ES (aged 18 years or older) that there may be similar survival outcomes with the pediatric age group [10]. Although different systemic treatments have been used previously for ES developing in bone and soft tissue, many studies suggest that the same regimens may be equally effective in these two ES groups and that ES developing in soft tissue may have a better prognosis than ES developing in bone. For this reason, it would be appropriate to treat ES developing in bone and soft tissue within the same principles [11].

12.2 Localized Disease

The first systemic treatment regimen showing a survival advantage in ES is the combination of vincristine, actinomycin D, and cyclophosphamide (VAC). Subsequently, addition of doxorubicin to this regimen (VACA regimen) has been shown to increase survival. There are also studies showing that this regimen is superior to total-lung irradiation with the VAC regimen [6]. Then, the effect of increasing the dose intensity of doxorubicin on survival was investigated. It was shown that increasing the dose intensity significantly increased toxicity but also significantly increased survival in the European study investigating this effect (intergroup study IESS-II) [7]. Due to the poor survival, especially in the high-risk group, searches have continued to increase the effectiveness of treatment. As a result of these searches, Grier et al. randomized patients with both metastatic and localized ES to VACA and VACA alternating with ifosfamide+etoposide (IE) arms. It was concluded in this study that adding IE to VACA combination increased 5-year disease-free survival in localized disease from 54% to 69%. However, the same survival benefit could not be demonstrated in metastatic disease [8]. Another maneuver to increase survival is to increase the dose intensity or increase the frequency of administration. This practice was abandoned by demonstrating that increasing the dose of alkylating agents (ifosfamide) does not provide survival benefits and increases the risk of developing secondary malignancy [12]. An event-free survival (EFS) advantage of 8% was obtained in another study investigating the benefit of reducing the frequency of administration from 3 weeks to 2 weeks. In addition, it is widely accepted that the same regimen (VACA/IE alternate regimen) is administered every 2 weeks [13].

These treatments are generally used peroperatively (both before and after local treatment). The general approach is to give 4–6 cycles of treatment before surgery and to complete the treatment to 48 weeks after surgery. Since severe hematological toxicities occur in treatments applied every 2 weeks, it is important that these treatments are given with colony-stimulating factor (CSF).

12.3 Metastatic Disease

The prognosis is fairly poor in metastatic ES. Only patients with lung metastases have a better prognosis compared to patients with bone and other organ metastases. It is possible to obtain cures in some patients even if they are diagnosed in the metastatic stage. Moreover, it is possible to achieve long survival with intensive multimodality treatments in patients without cure. Therefore, the treatment objective should be curative for patients with initial metastatic disease, as should early-stage patients. However, some intensive treatment regimens that are effective at an early stage do not provide superiority over conventional regimens in metastatic disease. High-dose chemotherapy and autologous bone marrow transplantation have also been evaluated in many studies in this patient group. Some studies have shown benefits whereas many studies have not yielded the same results.

The first-line treatment commonly used in metastatic disease is a combination of doxorubicin, vincristine, cyclophosphamide, ifosfamide, etoposide, and actinomycin D. Among these, VAC/IE, EVAIA (ifosfamide, doxorubicin, etoposide, actinomycin D, vincristine), VDC, and VAI (vincristine, ifosfamide, doxorubicin) regimens are the most commonly used. However, a significant survival advantage of VAC and altered IE regimen in metastatic disease could not be demonstrated as mentioned earlier. The effectiveness of cyclophosphamide+topotecan, docetaxel+gemcitabine, irinotecan+temozolomide, ifosfamide, etoposide, and platinum combinations has been demonstrated in patients progressing with first-line treatment [1, 9].

The main side effects of chemotherapeutic drugs commonly used in the treatment of Ewing family of tumors are summarized below. In general, the severity of toxicities caused by these drugs is graded according to assessment methods such as the National Cancer Institute Common Terminology Criteria for Adverse Events (NCI-CTC) [14]. Approaches such as discontinuation, postponement, dose reduction, as well as specific approaches specific to toxicity are made depending on the type and degree of toxicity observed.

The main side effects of vincristine include neurotoxicity (peripheral, autonomic, central), hearing loss, constipation, alopecia, hyperuricemia, visual abnormalities, and gonadal suppression. Of these, especially neurotoxicity side effects are a common side effect and have

Table 12.1 Neurotoxicity NCI-CTCAE v5.0 [14]

Adverse event	Grade 1	Grade 2	Grade 3	Grade 4	Grade 5
Paresthesia	Moderate symptoms	Moderate symptoms; limiting daily life	Severe symptoms; limiting self-care		
Peripheral motor neuropathy	Asymptomatic; based on clinical or diagnostic observation only	Moderate symptoms; limiting daily life	Severe symptoms; limiting self-care	Life-threatening outcomes; urgent intervention indicated	Death
Peripheral sensory neuropathy	Asymptomatic	Moderate symptoms; limiting daily life	Severe symptoms; limiting self-care	Life-threatening outcomes; urgent intervention indicated	

NCI CTCAE, National Cancer Institute Common Terminology Criteria for Adverse Events

dose-limiting properties. It may cause fatal damage to the liver when administered with abdominal radiotherapy (Tables 12.1 and 12.2) [14, 15].

The main side effects of doxorubicin include cardiotoxicity, myelosuppression, alopecia, secondary malignancy, amenorrhea, infertility, mucositis, abdominal pain, anorexia, and urinary discoloration. A rare but severe side effect affecting the treatment with doxorubicin is dose-dependent cardiotoxicity. The cardiotoxicity side effect is usually irreversible and patients should be monitored by regular echocardiography at the beginning of treatment and during treatment [16, 17].

The main side effects of actinomycin D include hematological toxicity (such as anemia, thrombocytopenia, leukopenia, neutropenic fever), secondary malignancy, nausea, vomiting, mucositis, rash, hepatotoxicity, and hepatic veno-occlusive disease [18].

The main side effects of ifosfamide include hematological toxicity (such as anemia, thrombocytopenia, leukopenia, neutropenic fever), neurotoxicity, encephalopathy, hemorrhagic cystitis, nausea, vomiting, mucositis, rash, hepatotoxicity, secondary malignancy, and arrhythmia. It is administered with mesna, a uroprotective drug, to prevent bladder toxicity. It is not recommended for use in patients with severe leukopenia, thrombocytopenia, severe renal or hepatic impairment, cystitis, and urinary obstruction due to the risk of life-threatening toxicity. Encephalopathy induced by ifosfamide is another serious toxicity. It occurs between days 1 and 4 after treatment and sometimes lasts for up to a month. Discontinuation of ifosfamide and administration of supportive treatments are recommended in this case. Methylene blue is also reported to be useful [19].

The main side effects of etoposide include hematological toxicity and hypersensitivity, and hematological toxicity may lead to anemia, thrombocytopenia, leukopenia, neutropenia, and neutropenic fever. Neutrophil decline usually occurs between 7 and 14 days after etoposide administration. Earlier and deeper hematological toxicities may occur in patients who have received prior intensive therapy or combined therapy (Table 12.3) [14, 20]. Apart from these, it also carries a lower risk of alopecia, weakness, loss of appetite, nausea, vomiting, cardiac, hepatic, renal toxicity, and secondary leukemia [20].

Table 12.2 Hepatobiliary toxicity NCI-CTCAE v5.0 [14]

Adverse event	Grade 1	Grade 2	Grade 3	Grade 4	Grade 5
ALP increase	If baseline is normal, ULN to 2.5 × ULN If baseline is abnormal, 2–2.5 × baseline	If baseline is normal, 2.5–5 × ULN If baseline is abnormal, 2.5–5 × baseline	If baseline is normal, 5–20 × ULN If baseline is abnormal, 5–20 × baseline	If baseline is normal, >20 × ULN If baseline is abnormal, >20 × baseline	
ALT increase	If baseline is normal, ULN to 3 × ULN If baseline is abnormal, 1.5–3 × baseline	If baseline is normal, 3–5 × ULN If baseline is abnormal, 3–5 × baseline	If baseline is normal, 5–20 × ULN If baseline is abnormal, 5–20 × baseline	If baseline is normal, >20 × ULN If baseline is abnormal, >20 × baseline	
AST increase	If baseline is normal, ULN to 3 × ULN; if baseline is abnormal, 1.5–3 × baseline	If baseline is normal, 3–5 × ULN; if baseline is abnormal, 3–5 × baseline	If baseline is normal, 5–20 × ULN; if baseline is abnormal, 5–20 × baseline	If baseline is normal, >20 × ULN; if baseline is abnormal, >20 × baseline	
Serum bilirubin increase	If baseline is normal, ULN to 1.5 × ULN; if baseline is abnormal, 1–1.5 × baseline	If baseline is normal, 1.5–3 × ULN; if baseline is abnormal, 1.5–3 × baseline	If baseline is normal, 3–10 × ULN; if baseline is abnormal, 3–10 × baseline	If baseline is normal, >10 × ULN; if baseline is abnormal, >10 × baseline	
GGT increase	If baseline is normal, ULN to 2.5 × ULN; if baseline is abnormal, 2–2.5 × baseline	If baseline is normal, 2.5–5 × ULN; if baseline is abnormal, 2.5–5 × baseline	If baseline is normal, 5–20 × ULN; if baseline is abnormal, 5–20 × baseline	If baseline is normal, >20 × ULN; if baseline is abnormal, >20 × baseline	
Liver failure			Asterixis, moderate encephalopathy, liver injury due to the drug, limitation of self-care	Life-threatening outcomes moderate-severe encephalopathy, coma	Death
Portal hypertension		Decrease in portal vein flow	Reverse/retrograde portal vein flow with varicose and/or acid	Life-threatening outcomes, requiring urgent intervention	Death

NCI CTCAE, National Cancer Institute Common Terminology Criteria for Adverse Events; ULN, upper limit of normal; ALP, alkaline phosphatase; ALT, alanine aminotransferase; AST, aspartate aminotransferase; GGT, gamma-glutamyl transpeptidase

Table 12.3 Hematological toxicity NCI-CTCAE v5.0 [14]

Blood element	Grade 1	Grade 2	Grade 3	Grade 4	Grade 5
Neutrophils	Between LLN and 1500/ microL	1000–1500/ microL	500–1000/microL	<500/microL	
Platelets	Between LLN and 75,000/ microL	50,000–75,000/ microL	25,000–50,000/microL	<25,000/ microL	
Hemoglobin	Between LLN and 10.0 g/dL	8.0–10.0 g/dL	<8.0 g/dL	Life-threatening consequences; requiring urgent intervention	Death
Febrile neutropenia			Absolute number of neutrophils <1000 microL and presence of body temperature >38.30 °C at a single measurement or ≥38.00 °C lasting longer than 1 h	Life-threatening consequences; requiring urgent intervention	Death

NCI CTCAE, National Cancer Institute Common Terminology Criteria for Adverse Events; LLN, lower limit of normal; cell/microL, cell/mm^3 or cell × 10^9/L

References

1. National Cancer Institute (web site) Available at: https://www.cancer.gov/publications/dictionaries/cancer-terms/def/primitive-neuroectodermal-tumor. Accessed March 12, 2018.
2. Louis DN, Perry A, Reifenberger G, et al. The 2016 World Health Organization Classification of Tumors of the Central Nervous System: a summary. Acta Neuropathol. 2016;131(6):803–20.
3. Delattre O, Zucman J, Melot T, et al. The Ewing family of tumors—a subgroup of small-round-cell tumors defined by specific chimeric transcripts. N Engl J Med. 1994;331(5):294–9.
4. Ambros IM, Ambros PF, Strehl S, et al. MIC2 is a specific marker for Ewing's sarcoma and peripheral primitive neuroectodermal tumors. Evidence for a common histogenesis of Ewing's sarcoma and peripheral primitive neuroectodermal tumors from MIC2 expression and specific chromosome aberration. Cancer. 1991;67(7):1886–93.
5. Cotterill SJ, Ahrens S, Paulussen M, et al. Prognostic factors in Ewing's tumor of bone: analysis of 975 patients from the European Intergroup Cooperative Ewing's Sarcoma Study Group. J Clin Oncol. 2000;18(17):3108–14.
6. Nesbit ME Jr, Perez CA, Tefft M, et al. Multimodal therapy for the management of primary, nonmetastatic Ewing's sarcoma of bone: an Intergroup Study. Natl Cancer Inst Monogr. 1981;56:255–62.
7. Burgert EO Jr, Nesbit ME, Garnsey LA, et al. Multimodal therapy for the management of nonpelvic, localized Ewing's sarcoma of bone: intergroup study IESS-II. J Clin Oncol. 1990;8(9):1514–24.
8. Grier HE, Krailo MD, Tarbell NJ, et al. Addition of ifosfamide and etoposide to standard chemotherapy for Ewing's sarcoma and primitive neuroectodermal tumor of bone. N Engl J Med. 2003;348(8):694–701.
9. Balamuth NJ, Womer RB. Ewing's sarcoma. Lancet Oncol. 2010;11(2):184–92.
10. Ahmed SK, Robinson SI, Okuno SH, Rose PS, Laack NN. Adult Ewing sarcoma: survival and local control outcomes in 102 patients with localized disease. Sarcoma. 2013;2013:681425. https://doi.org/10.1155/2013/681425. Epub 2013 Jun 11
11. Cash T, McIlvaine E, Krailo MD, et al. Comparison of clinical features and outcomes in patients with extraskeletal versus skeletal localized Ewing sarcoma: a report from the Children's Oncology Group. Pediatr Blood Cancer. 2016;63(10):1771–9.
12. Granowetter L, Womer R, Devidas M, et al. Dose-intensified compared with standard chemotherapy for nonmetastatic Ewing sarcoma family of tumors: A Children's Oncology Group Study. J Clin Oncol. 2009;27(15):2536–41.
13. Subbiah V, Anderson P, Lazar AJ, et al. Ewing's sarcoma: standard and experimental treatment options. Curr Treat Options Oncol. 2009;10(1-2):126–40.
14. https://ctep.cancer.gov/protocoldevelopment/electronic_applications/docs/CTCAE_v5_Quick_Reference_8.5x11.pdf. Accessed on March 09, 2018.
15. http://www.bccancer.bc.ca/drug-database-site/Drug%20Index/Vincristine_monograph.pdf
16. Doxorubicin [product monograph]. Caledon, ON: Panda Pharmaceuticals, Inc; August 2017.
17. http://www.bccancer.bc.ca/drug-database-site/Drug%20Index/Doxorubicine_monograph.pdf
18. http://www.bccancer.bc.ca/drug-database-site/Drug%20Index/Dactinomycin_monograph.pdf
19. http://www.bccancer.bc.ca/drug-database-site/Drug%20Index/Ifosfamide_monograph.pdf
20. http://www.bccancer.bc.ca/drug-database-site/Drug%20Index/Etoposide_monograph.pdf

Part V

Clinical Information: Liver Tumors

13 Radionuclide Therapy in Liver Tumors

M. Fani Bozkurt

The majority of malignant tumors of the liver, the largest solid organ in the human body, are metastases originating from other organs. The main reason for this is the presence of intense vascular connections of the liver with many organs, especially the gastrointestinal tract, and the fact that the liver is an organ that plays an important role in almost all metabolic pathways. The intraarterial radionuclide therapy of liver tumors is mainly based on the unique vascular system of the liver. The hepatocytes, which are the main building blocks of the liver, provide vascular nutrition from veins called portal venous system rather than arterially, unlike other organs. The metabolic functions of the liver, especially related to the digestive system, are carried out in this way. In contrast, primary neoplastic cells that develop in the liver or all other malignant cells that are metastasized to the liver provide their nutrition predominantly through the hepatic arterial route. From this point of view, tumor cells can be directly targeted, and healthy liver cells are protected from the possible side effects and complications due to radiation to a great extent when the hepatic arterial intervention is performed.

Therefore, it is possible to deliver therapeutic radiation-emitting pharmaceuticals through the intraarterial route to the liver tumors and to perform internal radiation treatment, thanks to the dual circulatory system, which is a unique feature of the liver.

Systemic radionuclide therapy (e.g., peptide receptor radionuclide therapy in diffuse metastatic neuroendocrine tumor including the liver or I-131-MIBG treatment in neuroectodermal tumor liver metastases, etc.) is also applied depending on the suitability of the tumor type that metastasizes the liver apart from hepatic intraarterial radionuclide therapy. However, only intraarterial hepatic radionuclide therapies will be mentioned within the scope of this chapter.

13.1 History of Hepatic Intraarterial Therapies

The first administration of selective arterial radionuclide therapy based on arterial nutrition of tumors in the liver dates back to the 1960s. Ariel defined the way in which microspheres labeled with yttrium-90 (Y-90) were given selectively to tumors through transfemoral arterial intervention and celiac trunk level through hepatic artery in 1964 in four liver cancer and six pancreatic cancer patients for the first time in the literature [1]. However, Y-90 microsphere treatment did not become widespread until the development of Y-90 resin and Y-90 glass microspheres since side effects and complications were observed more frequently in these first administrations due to

M. F. Bozkurt (✉)
Faculty of Medicine, Department of Nuclear Medicine, Hacettepe University, Ankara, Turkey
e-mail: muratfani.bozkurt@hacettepe.edu.tr

R. Bekiş et al. (eds.), *Radionuclide Therapy*, https://doi.org/10.1007/978-3-030-97220-2_13

both nonoptimal microsphere size and free Y-90 isotope leakage from the liver due to in vivo stability deficiency [2, 3].

13.2 Microspheres Used in Intraarterial Radionuclide Therapies

Radioactive-labeled microspheres used to treat hepatic tumors should have some basic characteristics for treatment effectiveness and safe use:

1. Microspheres should have the same or close density as blood density so that they do not adhere to and aggregate to the vascular wall at the time of injection.
2. Since the mechanism of uptake of microspheres in the tumor is embolization at the arteriolar level, their size should not be smaller than the arteriole dimensions in the tumor microcirculation. The arteriole diameters that feed liver tumors are on average 15–35 μm in size in humans, while larger-diameter microspheres do not reach the capillary bed, and smaller-diameter microspheres can progress from arterioles to distal and pass to adjacent organs, especially the lungs, through capillary web circulation. The fact that microspheres are spherically shaped also prevents them from adhering to each other in the peripheral vessels. It is preferred for this reason that the microspheres to be used in internal radionuclide therapy are produced in 25–30 μm diameter and in global morphology [4, 5].
3. Microspheres should be labeled with radionuclides such as high-energy beta emitter. The physical half-lives and tissue ranges of these radionuclides should be sufficient to penetrate deep into the major tumor foci.
4. The specific activities (activity amount/microsphere) of the microspheres should be high.
5. It should be easy to prepare and accessible.
6. Microspheres should be produced in a structure resistant to radiation damage. From this point of view, glass is a relatively more suitable material for microspheres, especially molecular weight loss and deformation due to neutron irradiation can be seen in microspheres produced from resin and polymeric-based material [6].
7. Radionuclide impurities in labeled microspheres should be as low as possible and in vivo stability should be high.
8. Microspheres to be used in intraarterial radionuclide therapy should be compatible with biological systems and ideally have high in vivo stability, but it should also be possible to biodegrade to a reasonable extent [7, 8].
9. It is preferred that the biodistribution of the labeled microspheres be predictable and traceable using imaging methods.

Although none of the different types of commercially produced microspheres that are licensed for use in many countries has all the ideal microsphere properties alone, they are presented for clinical use because they have most of the abovementioned properties (Table 13.1).

13.3 Radionuclides Used in Hepatic Intraarterial Radionuclide Therapy

Y-90 is the leading beta-emitting radionuclide for labeling the microspheres with the suitable energy to be used for the radionuclide therapy. Y-90 has an average beta energy of 0.94 MeV, an average tissue penetration of 2.5 mm, a maximum tissue penetration of 11 mm, and a physical half-life of 2.67 days.

Currently, two different radiomicrospheres are commercially and widely available: Y-90 resin microspheres (SIR-Spheres®, SIRTEX Australia) and Y-90 glass microspheres (TheraSphere®, BTG-Boston Scientific Canada). Y-90 resin microsphere received FDA approval in the USA for the treatment of unresectable liver metastases of colorectal cancer; Y-90 glass microsphere received FDA approval for the intraarterial treatment of unresectable hepatocellular cancer or neoadjuvant treatment before surgery and transplantation. There is a CE certificate that allows use in both primary liver tumors and metastatic liver tumors for both microsphere types in Europe [9, 10].

Table 13.1 Some characteristics of commercial microspheres used in the treatment of hepatic intraarterial tumors

	Resin microsphere (SIR-Spheres®)	Glass microsphere (TheraSphere®)	Poly-L-lactic acid (QuiremSpheres®)
Radionuclide and labeling method	Y-90; through ion exchange with Na to resin matrix	Y-90; through neutron activation in nuclear reactor	Ho-166; through neutron activation in nuclear reactor
Biodegradation	No	No	Yes
In vivo/in vitro radionuclide decomposition	Urinary excretion in trace amounts in the first 24 h (25–50 kBq/L)	In vivo unknown, in vitro, < 0.13% as a result of incubation for 6 weeks in water or saline	Stability after 72 hours in human plasma: 93.5%; in vitro, 0.3% after 270 h in isotonic buffer
Radionuclide impurity	For reactor-product Y-90: Y-88 (T1/2 = 106 days) Y-91 (T1/2 = 58.5 days) For generator-product Y-90: Sr-90 (T1/2 = 28.78 years)	Y-88 ve Y-91 depending on the neutron bombardment of Y-89 And depending on the neutron bombardment of impurities in the glass Eu-154 (*T*1/2 = 8.8 years) E-152 (*T*1/2 = 136 years) Co-57 (*T*1/2 = 271 days) Co-60 (*T*1/2 = 5.3 years)	Ho-166 m (1200 years)
Diameter	20–60 μm	20–30 μm	15–60 μm
Specific activity (at the time of calibration)	75 Bq/μCi	2500 Bq/μCi	Max. 450 Bq/μCi
Density (1.05 g/mL for blood)	1.6 g/mL	3.6 g/mL	1.4 g/mL
Microsphere count/vial	40 million	1.2 million (3 GBq vial)	33 million
Activity per vial	3 GBq	3, 5, 7, 10, 15, 20 GBq and interval doses with increments of 0.5 GBq on request	On request, max. 15 GBq
Liquid media compatible with microsphere	Sterile water for injection or 5% dextrose + water for injection mixture	Saline	Saline
Dose fractionation	Possible	Not possible	Not possible
CE commercial document date	2002	2014	2015

Even though both microsphere types have different characteristics, there is yet not any randomized study comparing two different microsphere types in terms of treatment effectiveness. However, there is a common sense that treatment effectiveness and safety will be ensured as long as the recommended patient selection and preparation steps for both types of microspheres are appropriately applied.

There are still some aspects of Y-90 microsphere therapy that cannot be fully explained even though the hepatic intraarterial radionuclide therapy approach using Y-90 resin microspheres and Y-90 glass microspheres has been reported to have very successful results in clinical studies. Among these, the most discussed topics are the embolic distribution profiles, microdosimetric differences of Y-90 microspheres, and the "real" dosimetric distributions that can be understood after administration. Microspheres labeled with rhenium-186 (Re-186), Re-188, and holmium-166 (Ho-166), which are also gamma-emitting radionuclides, as opposed to pure beta-emitting Y-90 radionuclides, have also been produced to give different insights into these controversial issues in Y-90 microspheres. The advantageous features of Ho-166 microspheres compared to other microspheres are that they can be visualized

Table 13.2 Some characteristics of radionuclides used in the treatment of hepatic intraarterial tumors

Radionuclide	Physical t1/2 (h)	Method of degradation and probability	Mean/maximum beta energy (MeV)	Mean/maximum in tissue	Imaging method
Y-90	64.2	99.9% β 0.003% Positron	0.94/2.28	2.5/11	Bremsstrahlung planar/ SPECT, PET
Re-186	89.3	91% β 9% γ (147 keV)	0.35/1.08	1/4.5	Planar/SPECT
Re-188	17	84.9% β 15.1% γ (155 keV)	0.76/2.12	3.8/11	Planar/SPECT
Ho-166	26.8	93.3% β 6.7% γ (81 keV)	0.66/1.85	2.2/10.2	Planar/SPECT, MRI

with SPECT and MRI due to both gamma radiation and paramagnetic properties [11].

The advantage of Re-186- and Re-188-labeled microspheres over Y-90 microspheres is that they allow SPECT imaging depending on gamma radiation. Re-188 has also lower production cost as it can be obtained from the tungsten-188 (W-188)/Re-188 generator [12].

The comparative properties of the three radionuclides used in microsphere labeling are given in Table 13.2.

13.4 Pretreatment Patient Assessment

Patient selection and compliance assessment steps should be performed with extreme care in order for intraarterial Y-90 microsphere therapy to be an effective and reliable treatment in primary and metastatic tumors of the liver that cannot be operated. The planning and implementation of intraarterial Y-90 microsphere therapy require a multidisciplinary approach. Nuclear medicine and interventional radiology as being the main disciplines that apply the therapy as well as other relevant clinical disciplines, especially medical oncology, gastroenterology, and general surgery, should play an active role in the assessment of the suitability for treatment of the patient as the disciplines that direct the patient to this treatment in this approach.

Pretreatment eligibility assessment is a two-step process. The general condition, performance, physical examination, and laboratory and imaging results of the patient are reviewed in detail during the first evaluation phase. Hepatic angiography and hepatic artery perfusion scintigraphy are performed in the same session, and the treatment is rehearsed in a sense in the second evaluation phase.

13.5 First Evaluation Phase

The liver functional reserve must be at a level that can sustain the life of the patient after the treatment in order to provide Y-90 microsphere therapy to eligible patients after multidisciplinary assessment. Serum albumin level should be greater than 3 g/dl, total bilirubin level should be lower than 2 g/dL, and liver transaminases ALT (SGPT)/AST (SGOT) should be lower than 5 times their upper limit. Computed tomography (CT) or magnetic resonance imaging (MRI) scans are performed to evaluate the degree of tumor vascularization, liver invasion, invasion of the vascular and biliary system, and the degree to which tumor foci are adjacent to major vascular structures and large bile ducts in addition to blood biochemistry. The prevalence and stage of the disease are evaluated by using whole-body F-18 fluorodeoxyglucose positron emission tomography (FDG-PET/CT) imaging if the indication is appropriate. Ga-68 DOTA-peptide components in well-differentiated neuroendocrine tumors, which are relatively silent tumors in terms of glycolytic metabolism, and Ga-68 prostate-specific membrane antigen (PSMA) PET/CT imaging in somatostatin receptor PET/CT, or prostate cancer liver metastases, have an important role in pretreatment evaluation.

Treatment should not be preferred in patients with excessive extrahepatic tumor burden or in patients with a life expectancy of less than 3 months according to general acceptance, except in very special cases specific to that case as a result of these evaluations. Simultaneously with these evaluations, the advantages and possible risks of Y-90 microsphere therapy compared to other alternative interventional treatments are evaluated in detail by the interventional radiology department whether intraarterial intervention to the tumor is appropriate in the first stage. Issues such as whether the patient has the chance of surgical treatment in a multidisciplinary manner and evaluating the treatment priority in patients requiring systemic treatment in addition to the local treatment approach should be clarified in the first evaluation phase in parallel with these evaluations [9, 10, 13].

13.6 Second Evaluation Phase

The second phase of the evaluation begins if the decision on the applicability of treatment has been made as a result of the multidisciplinary examinations mentioned above in the first phase. This phase includes hepatic angiography performed in the interventional radiology department and intraarterial hepatic artery perfusion scintigraphy performed in the nuclear medicine department on the same day.

13.6.1 Hepatic Angiography

Hepatic angiography shows the vascular anatomy of the liver in detail. Arterial feeding of the liver is provided by the celiac trunk in 55–65% of the cases. The celiac trunk is divided into three branches as the splenic artery, left gastric artery, and common hepatic artery in most cases. The gastroduodenal artery exits the common hepatic artery in approximately 90% of the cases and is named hepatic artery proper after this branching. Arterial vascularization of the entire lobe or the relevant segment of the liver, due to some embryonal developmental anomalies, may be via a source other than hepatic artery proper, and this artery is called the "replaced hepatic artery." Although a part of the liver has blood supply from the same lobe or segment hepatic artery proper, it may also be fed from an aberrant artery, which is called an "accessory artery." If Y-90 microspheres are directed to a lobe or selectively to a segment in the liver, it is possible to leak to the gastrointestinal tract due to nutrition from the accessory arteries. Therefore, a very detailed evaluation of the vascular anatomy of the liver during hepatic angiography and an arterial mapping study are very important. Angiography is started by entering through femoral or brachial artery and evaluating all vascular structures likely to supply blood to the liver in the abdomen. Subsequently, it is planned where the treatment should be performed by entering the arteries that feed the lobe, segment, or more distal subsegment to be treated. At this stage, embolization of some accessory arteries such as gastroduodenal, right gastric artery can be performed with coiling to prevent possible leakage of radiomicrosphere into the gastrointestinal system and to prevent some treatment-related complications such as gastroduodenal ulcer. The success of coil embolization is tested after the procedure, and it is ensured that there is no contrast transition to the gastrointestinal system or lungs [9, 10, 13].

13.6.2 Hepatic Artery Perfusion Scintigraphy

After the artery feeding the region as the lobe, segment, or segments to be treated with hepatic angiography is detected and coil embolization is performed on the accessory vessels to prevent possible leaks to the gastrointestinal region, Tc-99 m-macroaggregated albumin (MAA) in a volume of 5 cc at a dose of 3–5 mCi is injected intraarterially from the same region. The patient should be imaged in the nuclear medicine department within 1 hour at the latest after the injection.

The main purpose of hepatic artery perfusion scintigraphy is to both visualize the distribution of radioactivity in the liver and predict the biodistribution of Y-90 microspheres to be administered in the same way during treatment and to detect possible radioactivity leakage to the gastrointestinal region and lungs. Spot planar torso or half-body planar image and abdomen, mostly involving the thorax and abdomen, and, in addition, single-photon emission computed tomography (SPECT) or SPECT/CT hybrid cross-sectional imaging methods are preferred in scintigraphic imaging (Fig. 13.1a, b). The acquired images are visually evaluated and the gastrointestinal region is examined for radioactivity shunting. The presence of gastrointestinal shunting, regardless of its amount and location, constitutes a contraindication for treatment (Fig. 13.2). Hepatic angiography is performed again if deemed appropriate, and the presence of an accessory vessel causing leakage and without coil embolization in the previous study is investigated, and the leakage is tried to be prevented by coil embolization in this case. If it is determined by the interventional radiologist that coil embolization of all possible accessory arteries is performed for that particular patient and it is not possible to find any other arteries that may cause shunting, Y-90 microsphere therapy is discontinued, and the patient is directed to alternative treatments. Semiquantitative evaluation is performed in addition to visual evaluation in hepatic artery perfusion scintigraphy. The probable radioactivity shunt ratio (hepatopulmonary shunt) from the liver to bilateral lungs is determined numerically by semiquantitative evaluation. Areas of interest for torso or half-body imaging are drawn on images taken from anterior and posterior projection to the liver and bilateral lungs for this purpose. The lung shunt ratio is calculated using the following formula [9, 10, 13, 14]:

$$\begin{aligned}\text{Lung shunt ratio} = \text{Geometric mean of lung counts} \\ (\text{anterior and posterior}) / \text{Geometric mean of lung} \\ + \text{Liver counts}(\text{anterior and posterior}) \times 100\end{aligned}$$

When Y-90 resin microspheres are used, a lung shunt ratio of 20% or more constitutes a contraindication for the treatment (Fig. 13.3a, b). A shunt rate of less than 10% indicates that the entire calculated dose can be administered to the patient, while a shunt rate of between 10% and 20% is recommended to be treated by reducing the dose as follows (Table 13.3) [9].

13.6.3 Optimization of Hepatic Artery Perfusion Scintigraphy

Hepatic artery perfusion scintigraphy plays a key role in Y-90 microsphere therapy suitability assessment, treatment planning, and treatment activity calculation. This imaging process must be performed and interpreted in the most optimal conditions for this reason.

Tc-99 m MAA used in hepatic artery perfusion scintigraphy may show a misleading biodistribution pattern due to in vivo decomposition when imaging is performed more than 1 h after injection. Free Tc-99m may circulate and undergo secretion from the mucosa after in vivo decomposition. Gastric uptake, especially due to gastric mucosa secretion, may mislead the appearance of radioactivity shunting from the liver to stomach. There are several ways to distinguish real vascular gastrointestinal shunts from mucosal secretion of free Tc-99m, which is secreted. The first way is to examine whether the patient has thyroid and kidney uptake of the

a

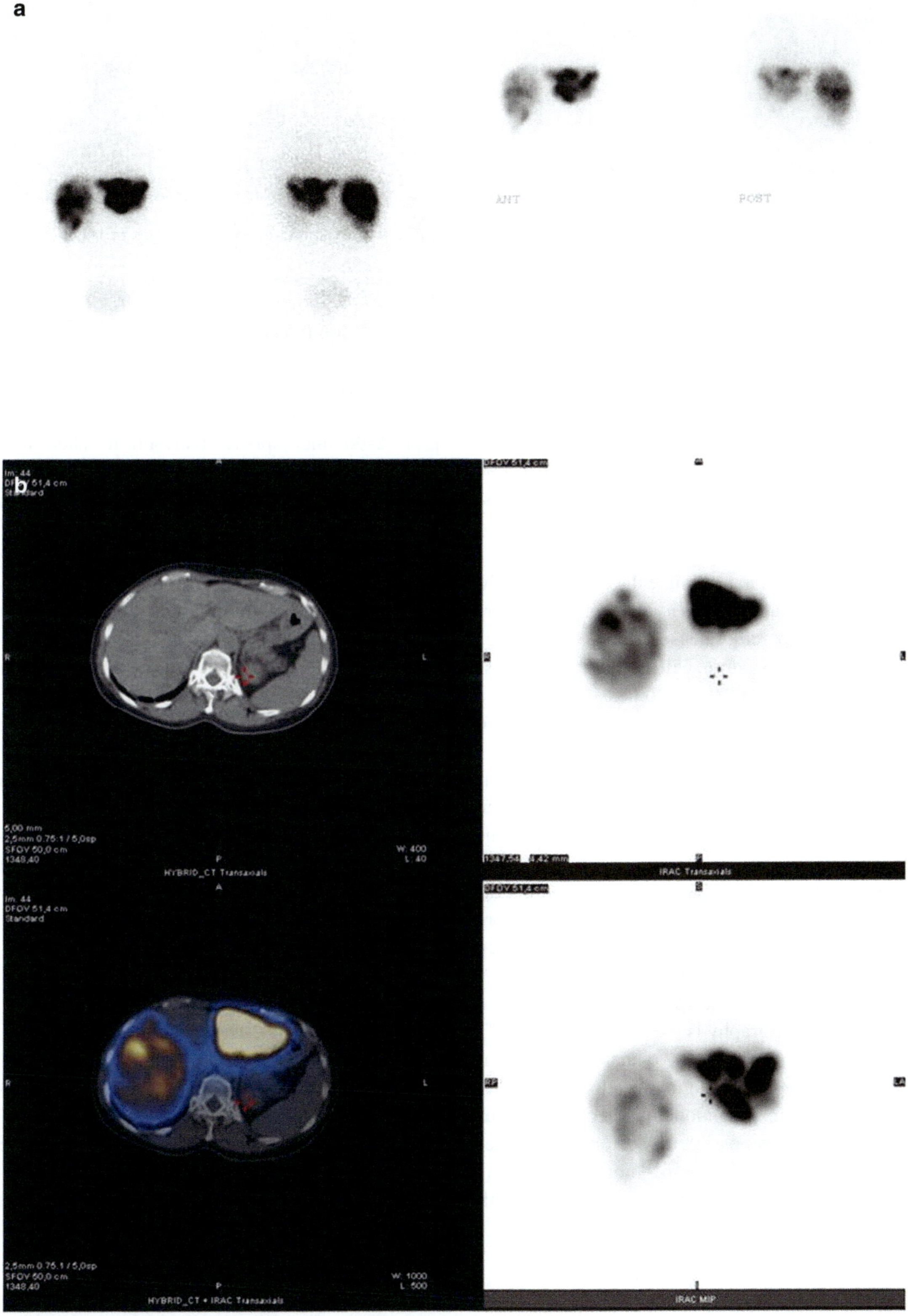

Fig. 13.1 (**a**) Whole-body anterior and posterior (left) and abdomen spot planar hepatic artery perfusion scintigraphy images in a patient scheduled for right and left liver lobe treatment. (**b**) Hepatic artery perfusion scintigraphy SPECT/CT cross-sectional imaging of the same patient

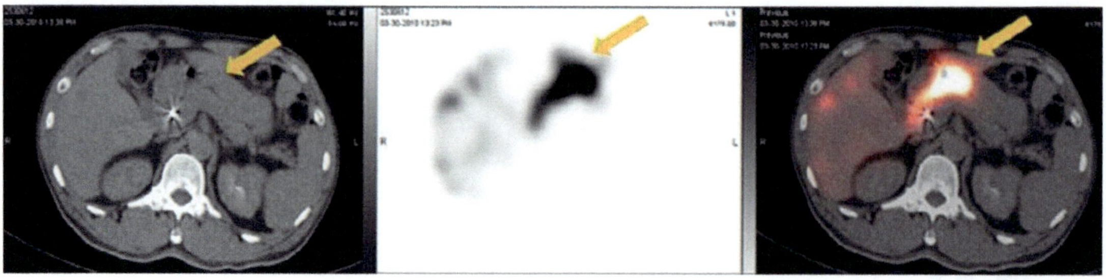

Fig. 13.2 Gastric Tc-99 mm MAA shunt (arrows) in SPECT/CT transaxial cross-sectional images of hepatic artery perfusion scintigraphy

radiopharmaceutical along with mucosal secretion. Free Tc-99m due to in vivo decomposition will show uptake in the thyroid as well as kidneys due to its excretion pathway. However, it is also possible that both gastrointestinal activity shunting and mucosal uptake due to in vivo decomposition may occur in some cases although that is a rare situation.

Therefore, imaging should be done within a maximum of 1 h to minimize the effect of in vivo Tc-99m decomposition. In addition, administration of oral perchlorate solution to the patient prior to the procedure will reduce the mucosal uptake of free Tc-99m due to possible decomposition depending on competitive inhibition. For this purpose, 200 ml perchlorate solution is administered orally to the patient a few hours before hepatic angiography and hepatic artery perfusion scintigraphy procedures. Gastric and intestinal mucosal secretion that will give the same appearance as gastrointestinal shunting due to in vivo decomposition can be adequately prevented, thanks to this simple preprocedural preparation [15].

Another method for optimizing hepatic artery perfusion scintigraphy is the addition of SPECT/CT hybrid imaging to planar scintigraphy. SPECT/CT hybrid imaging is more successful than SPECT imaging alone to detect gastrointestinal shunts. It is possible to perform a complete anatomical localization of non-liver activity involvements in the gastrointestinal tract, thanks to the CT component of SPECT/CT hybrid imaging (Fig. 13.4a, b).

Another benefit of SPECT/CT hybrid imaging is that it allows to anatomically evaluate intrahepatic Y-90 microsphere distribution. Therefore, SPECT/CT hybrid imaging is recommended whenever available in hepatic artery perfusion scintigraphy.

Biodistribution of Tc-99 m-MAA in hepatic artery perfusion scintigraphy can serve to determine the treatment dose and to predict treatment response as well as to evaluate suitability for treatment. Studies have been reported to support a relationship between the degree of Tc-99 m-MAA uptake in liver tumor foci in hepatic artery perfusion scintigraphy and Y-90 microsphere treatment success even though Tc99m-MAA and Y-90 microspheres do not have exactly the same physical characteristics [14]. Therefore, optimization of hepatic artery perfusion scintigraphy is very important.

13.7 Determination of the Treatment Activity

After the patient is found suitable for Y-90 microsphere therapy, the treatment activity is determined. There are different methods to determine treatment activity according to the type of radiomicrosphere used.

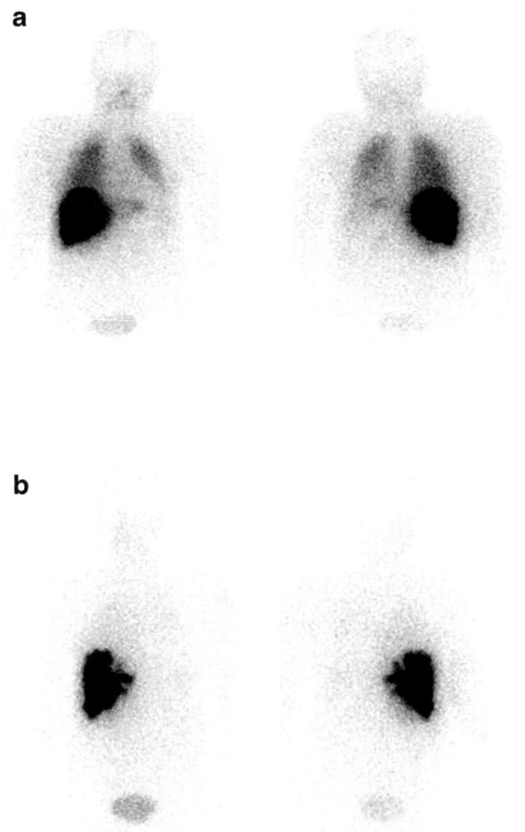

Fig. 13.3 (**a**) Hepatic artery perfusion scintigraphy anterior (left) and posterior (right) planar imaging of a patient with the diagnosis of HCC resulted with a pulmonary shunt ratio of 32% in bilateral lungs. The patient was not found suitable for treatment due to high pulmonary shunting. (**b**) Anterior (left) and posterior (right) planar images of hepatic artery perfusion scintigraphy of the same patient performed after coil embolization of the vessels causing pulmonary shunting on repeated angiography ended up with a lung shunt ratio of 5%, and the patient became eligible for treatment

Table 13.3 Recommended treatment dose reduction percentages according to the calculated lung shunt ratio for Y-90 resin microsphere therapy

Calculated lung shunt ratio	Therapeutic dose reduction recommendation
<10%	No need
10–15%	20%
15–20%	40%

13.7.1 Determination of the Treatment Activity for Y-90 Glass Microspheres

Y-90 glass microspheres are considered to have a fairly homogeneous distribution in the liver, and a treatment activity calculation formula based on the liver volume is recommended. Even though the actual target radiation dose for the tumor is not fully known in this calculation method, it is aimed to calculate the activity that will give 100–120 Gy radiation to minimize the risk of hepatic fibrosis. The recommended formula for determining therapy activity for Y-90 glass microspheres is as follows:

$$\text{Activity}\left(\text{GBq}\right) = \text{Dose}\left(\text{Gy}\right) \times \text{Liver mass}\left(\text{kg}\right) / 50$$

A practical method based on a simple internal dosimetric approach based on liver lobe and/or segment volume and hepatopulmonary shunt ratio is commonly used in routine practice to determine therapy activity in Y-90 glass microspheres. The treatment dose can be calculated practically by using a specific software which requires the liver volume and hepatopulmonary shunt ratio obtained from the hepatic artery perfusion scintigraphy predicting that the mean radiation dose to be administered to the tissue will be 120 Gy [10].

13.7.2 Determination of the Treatment Activity for Y-90 Resin Microsphere

Determination of the therapy activity for Y-90 resin microspheres is performed by a series of calculations based on "body surface area" and "partition model" methods.

Determining Dose Depending on the Body Surface Area: Calculation based on body surface area is a very simple and practical calculation method compared to the other method and is determined by the following formula based on the body

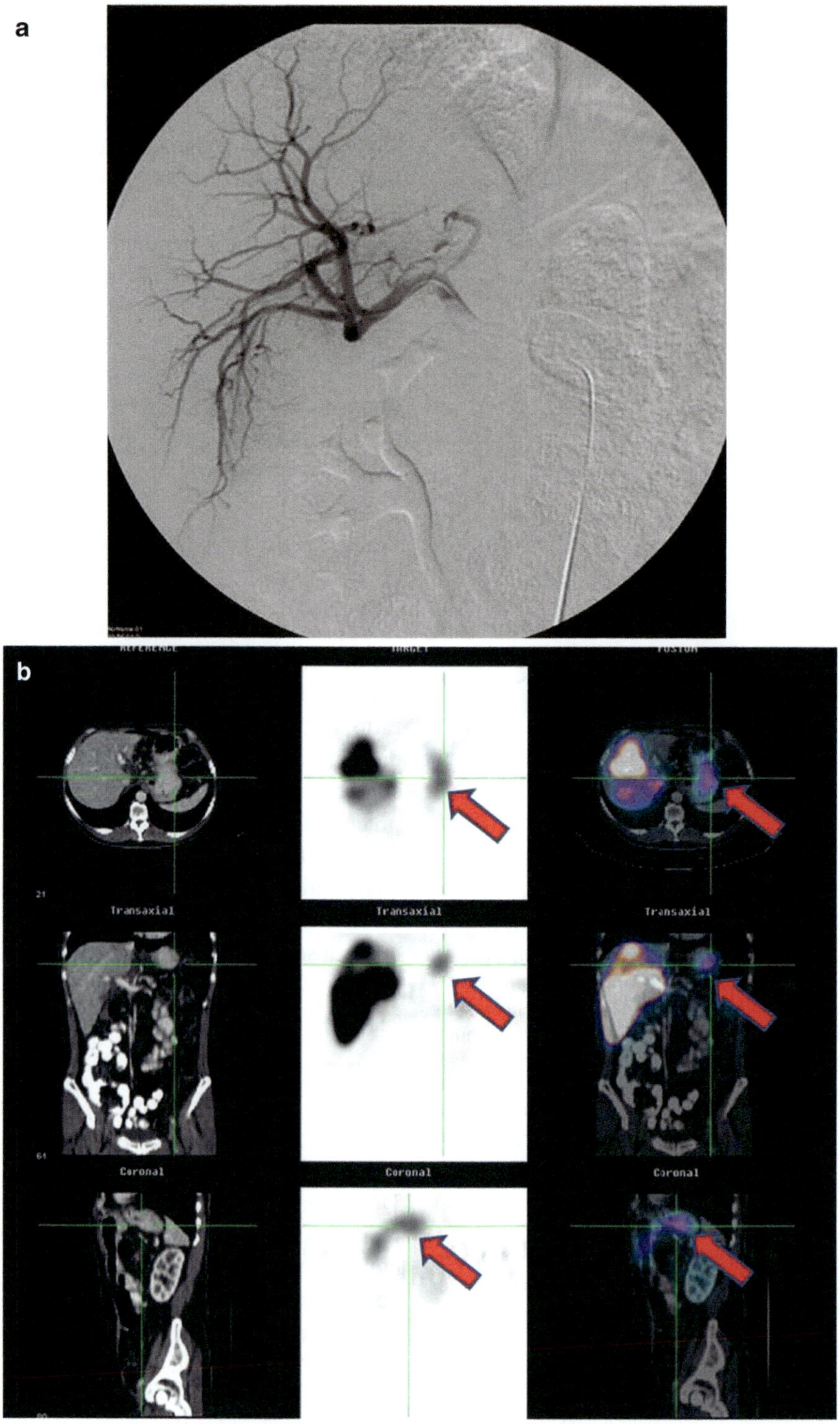

Fig. 13.4 (**a**) The pretreatment planning angiography of the patient scheduled for Y-90 microsphere therapy does not show any contrast flow in favor of gastrointestinal shunting. (**b**) Gastric shunting (arrows) not detected in angiography was detected with SPECT/CT cross-sectional images of hepatic artery perfusion scintigraphy performed in the same patient. The gastric localization of the activity shunting has been easily confirmed, thanks to the CT component of imaging

surface area calculated from the patient's height and body weight and the tumor's volumetric invasion rate in the liver (tumor/liver ratio) data:

$$\text{Activity}\left(\text{GBq}\right) = \left(\text{Body surface area}\left(\text{m2}\right) - 0.2\right) + \text{Tumor volume} / \text{Tumor volume} + \text{Liver volume}$$

Liver and tumor volumes in this formula can be calculated from CT, MRI, or SPECT/CT imaging performed in the suitability for treatment evaluation of the patient. It is recommended to reduce the calculated dose by 10–20% in patients with borderline liver function in Y-90 resin microsphere therapy dose calculation method based on body surface area. In addition, it is recommended to make necessary dose reductions according to the rate of hepatopulmonary shunt (Table 13.3) [9].

Determining Therapy Activity Based on Partition Model: This method aims to give the lowest possible dose to the liver parenchyma other than the tumor while giving the maximum intensity dose to the tumor. This method is based on the theoretical basis of the "medical internal radiation dose" (MIRD) and takes into account the tumor and non-tumor liver tissue separately. The Y-90 microsphere therapy dose is calculated in the partition model as follows:

1. Tumor and non-tumor liver volumes are calculated using CT, MRI, or SPECT/CT methods.
2. The activity rate (T/N) to be taken by tumor and non-tumor liver tissue is calculated using SPECT or SPECT/CT images of Tc-99 m-MAA hepatic artery perfusion scintigraphy: *T*/*N* = (Tumor activity/Tumor mass)/(Liver activity/Liver mass).
3. Lung (hepatopulmonary) shunt ratio is calculated using planar Tc-99 m-MAA hepatic artery perfusion scintigraphy.

   The treatment dose is calculated according to the partition model for Y-90 resin microspheres using the following formula when these parameters are calculated:

$$A\left(\text{GBq}\right) = D\,\text{liver}\left(\left(T/N \times \text{tumor mass}\right) + \text{liver mass}\right) / 49670\left(1 - \text{lung shunt\%} / 100\right)$$

D liver: It is the nominal dose in Gy for the liver.

The *D* value should not exceed 80 Gy in non-tumor liver parenchyma in patients with sufficient liver reserve and 70 Gy for non-tumor liver in cirrhotic patients when the partition model is used. A 40% reduction in the calculated dose is also recommended. The radiation dose to be administered to the lungs should not exceed 25 Gy. There is no upper limit for the dose to be administered to the tumor [7, 13, 16].

13.8 Y-90 Microsphere Therapy Administration

Y-90 resin and glass microsphere therapy requires a specifically designed "dose administration set" for each microsphere type (Fig. 13.5a, b). It includes methacrylate casing, dose vial, catheter connection set, and appropriate needles even though the dose set varies depending on the type of microsphere used. The patient-specific treatment dose for Y-90 microsphere therapy is emptied into the treatment vial placed in the administration set with 5 ml volume injectors. Glass microspheres are compatible with saline, and resin microspheres are compatible with water for sterile injection and dextrose mixture. The radiation dose is measured and recorded by the radiation physicist in the nuclear medicine department with a dose counter at an equal distance from the four sides of the methacrylate casing. This record is a practical method to indirectly understand whether the entire treatment dose is given after the end of the treatment dose infusion. The connection set of the dose vial placed in the administration set is connected to the outer end of the angiography catheter when the patient was intervened through the femoral artery and injected with Tc-99mMAA and confirmed with contrast angiography in the interventional radiology department.

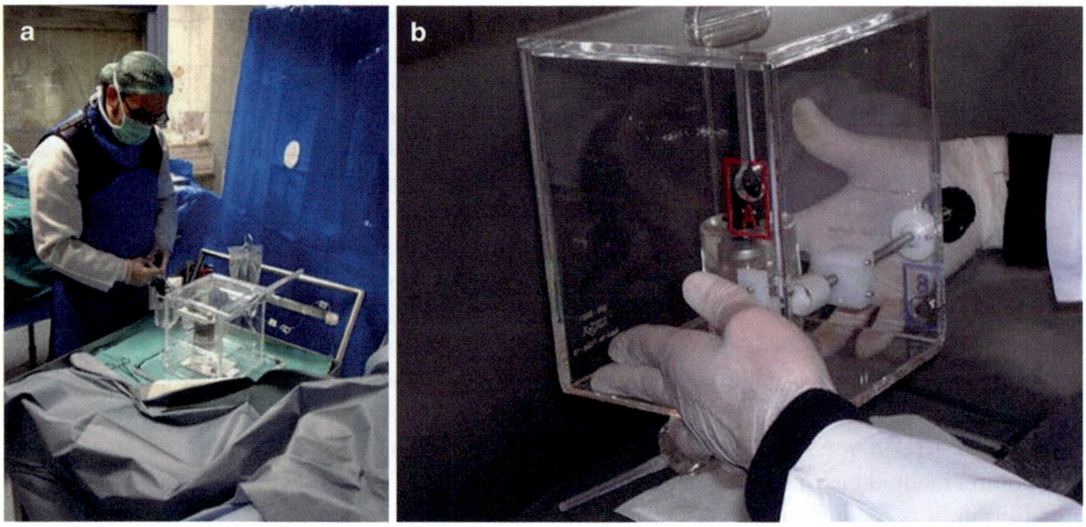

Fig. 13.5 (**a**) Y-90 glass microsphere administration set. (**b**) Y-90 resin microsphere administration set

In Y-90 resin microsphere therapy, radiomicrospheres are administered with slow infusion, contrast agent and water for injection are also infused occasionally, and microspheres are directed to the liver avoiding any obstruction in the set. In Y-90 glass microsphere therapy, 20 cc of the saline solution placed in the administration set is withdrawn, and the microspheres are directed from the catheter to the liver by slow infusion for approximately 2–3 minutes. The infusion is terminated by washing with 20 cc saline solution 2 times after the procedure is completed. It is very important for the treatment efficacy that the entire calculated dose is appropriately directed to the liver, and whether the entire treatment dose is given can be easily understood during administration of Y-90 glass microspheres with the dose counter, which is a component of the administration set.

However in Y-90 resin microsphere administration, since there is no attached dose counter and the administration is not continuous unlike Y-90 glass microspheres, the completeness of the dose administration can be estimated by radiation dose measurements at the equal distances from four sides of the administration set, and compare this measurement with pre-administration measurements. The activity delivered to the patient can be indirectly calculated by measuring the radiation dose with the radiation counter and proportioning it to the pretreatment dose in any case requiring discontinuation of the infusion during treatment. It is recommended to determine the actual amount of activity delivered to the patient by counting the treatment vial directly in the dose calibrator after the procedure. It is necessary to work very carefully especially against internal contamination during administration since Y-90 is a pure beta-emitting radionuclide. For this reason, it is recommended that especially radiopharmacists and/or radiochemists who provide dose withdrawal and set connection with double gloves touch the vial not with direct hand contact but with tongs and make it a habit to work with checklist method in order not to skip any steps in the process. The hands of the practitioners must be measured and recorded by the health physicist with a Geiger-Müller counter capable of measuring radiation levels of less than 0.1 mR/h in order to determine possible radioactivity contaminations of the administration room and waste after the procedure. The catheter connection of the dose administration set is disconnected after treatment administration preferably by an interventional radiologist who also applies groin compression to prevent bleeding. It is recommended that radiation measurements are made and recorded from the liver region over the skin and at a distance of 1 meter after these procedures are completed [13].

13.9 Bremsstrahlung and PET/CT Imaging After Therapy

It is very important to perform imaging immediately after treatment to ensure that Y-90 microspheres are delivered to the desired region in the liver and that there are no undesirable activity shunts in extrahepatic tissues. Since Y-90 is a pure-beta emitter, X-rays formed due to Bremsstrahlung can be used for imaging with gamma camera. Bremsstrahlung imaging can be performed without collimator, or the more preferred method is to take planar images similar to Tc99M-MAA hepatic artery perfusion scintigraphy in 20% windows set to an average of 80 keV energy if a low-energy collimator is placed or 20% windows set to an average of 159 keV if a medium-energy collimator is used (Fig. 13.6a). It is recommended to perform imaging within the first 24 h after treatment [13, 16].

Posttreatment biodistribution of Y-90 microspheres can be imaged with PET/CT imaging as an alternative to Bremsstrahlung imaging in recent years (Fig. 13.6b). Y-90 is a pure beta-emitting radionuclide and approximately 1 in 32 million

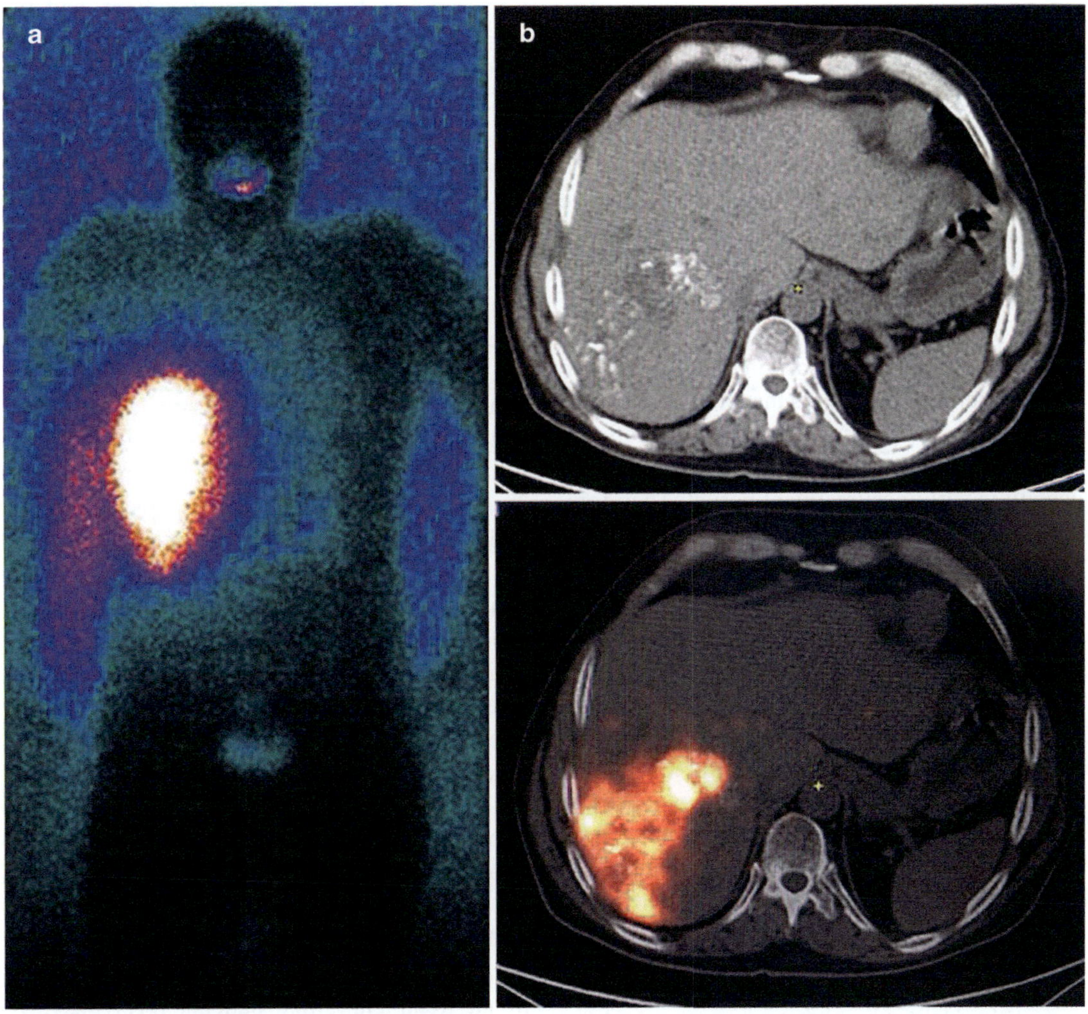

Fig. 13.6 (**a**) Activity uptake confirming the administration of treatment in the right lobe of the liver in the anterior Bremsstrahlung imaging performed after treatment in HCC patient who received Y-90 glass microsphere therapy in the right lobe of the liver. No evidence of extrahepatic activity shunting is observed. (**b**) Posttreatment Y-90 PET/CT of a 65 year-old patient with metastatic liver tumor from colorectal cancer in whom radiation segmentectomy to segment VIII with Y-90 glass microspheres was performed. The transaxial CT (upper) and the fused PET/CT (lower) images show adequate biodistribution of Y-90 microspheres following the procedure

positron decay occurs in radioactive decay. Patients can be imaged directly in the PET/CT unit after treatment based on this feature. However, it is recommended to perform imaging for at least 30 minutes per bed position and to place a 2.5 mm thick copper ring in the gantry to prevent the detectors from saturating in order to obtain a good-quality image [17]. The state-of-art PET/CT scanners of the new technology may not need such copper ring to obtain good-quality images. Bremsstrahlung imaging is routinely preferred to PET/CT since this requirement is not met in most centers even though it does not provide very good-quality images.

13.10 Patient Management in Early Posttreatment Period

It is not necessary to take a special radiation safety measure in patients after treatment since Y-90 is a pure beta-emitting radionuclide and is a locally administered treatment to the liver. The patient can be discharged after a few hours of follow-up for bleeding control, just like in the planning angiography procedure. However, since the vast majority of patients may have some additional health problems, most centers prefer to hospitalize their patients in order to monitor adequately in early posttreatment period. Therefore, patients are hospitalized for at least 1 day after treatment and followed up in most centers. It is recommended that antipyretic, antiemetic and antacid drugs should be given to the patient on the day of treatment against nausea, vomiting, and high fever, which are early side effects of the treatment. The same drugs are continued after the treatment, and the complete blood count and blood biochemical values of the patients are monitored. Patients can mostly be discharged on the next day without any serious symptoms.

Complete blood count and blood biochemistry control are performed weekly for 1 month. PET/CT imaging with FDG or other radiopharmaceuticals appropriate for that particular tumor type is performed to determine early treatment response at 4–6 weeks after treatment. Treatment response evaluation is also performed by CT and/or MRI at preferably 2–3 months after treatment [13].

13.11 Side Effects and Complications of Y-90 Microsphere Therapy

Intraarterial Y-90 microsphere therapy is a safe local treatment method in primary and metastatic liver tumors due to its highly selective and effective features. Therefore, side effects and complications are less common compared to systemic treatments and other similar local treatments. Treatment-related side effects are mostly seen in the acute period and the majority are mild and self-limited. Severe side effects and complications are less frequent after treatment, and the majority of them are subacute and chronic effects that occur after 3 months [2–10]. Y-90 microsphere therapy delivers radiomicrospheres intraarterially to the tumor vascular system and gives radiation damage to the tumor through embolization, and the main mechanism of action of this treatment is not embolization but internal radiation damage. Therefore, embolization syndrome observed in the treatment of similarly administered transarterial chemoembolization (TACE) is not an expected side effect for Y-90 microsphere therapy. However, side effects such as fever, abdominal pain, nausea, and vomiting may be observed in the first hours of treatment due to systemic endothelial damage response in patients depending on an intravascular intervention. It is possible to prevent these side effects by premedication of patients with appropriate antipyretics, analgesics, and antacid-antiemetic drugs and maintaining them with the same drugs in the first week after treatment even though most of these effects are self-limiting and of low to moderate severity. The most common side effect in patients is loss of appetite and fatigue. These constitutional effects may persist for 4–6 weeks after treatment. Regular oral nutrition and hydration of the patients in the posttreatment period along with resting are recommended and these symptoms mostly improve without the need for additional treatment. Most patients receiving Y-90 microsphere therapy may experience transient elevations in liver transaminases that start in the first 4–6 weeks and may persist for 2–3 months in some cases. This increase is mostly low-medium and has a self-limiting character. It is recommended to check the blood biochemistry values of the patients for the first 4–6 weeks after treatment. Particularly thrombocytopenia may be observed in blood count in the first 3 months after Y-90 microsphere therapy. This effect is thought to be due to inadequate production of some blood proteins in the liver due to liver damage and temporary insufficiency rather than directly affecting bone marrow due to the local administration of Y-90 microsphere and being a highly in vivo stable radiopharmaceutical. Therefore, it is recommended to monitor the blood counts of the patients during the first few months. Cholecystitis may develop within the first 4–6 weeks after treatment in Y-90 microsphere therapy apart from these effects. Cholecystitis develops mostly in patients without cystic artery coil embolization, which is an accessory artery, due to radiomicrosphere leak into the gallbladder. There may be a leak to the gallbladder due to reflux flow caused by vasospasm during treatment in some patients. Cholecystitis due to Y-90 microsphere therapy gives clinical signs of cholecystitis due to other causes, and its treatment does not differ. Temporary obstruction of the intrahepatic bile ducts may develop due to tissue edema caused mostly by radiation damage due to treatment.

Symptoms and signs such as increased biochemical values showing bile functions such as ALP and GGT, sudden and increased jaundice, abdominal distension, and severe abdominal pain may be observed in this case. Anti-edema treatments are primarily administered with cholecystomimetics and medical treatments that increase bile function. A temporary stent may also be placed in the biliary tract if the patient is unresponsive to these medical treatments.

The most serious complication of Y-90 microsphere treatment is "radioembolization-induced liver disease." Radioembolization-induced liver disease is a sudden and excessive increase in total bilirubin values without significant increase in liver transaminases in the third month after treatment, sudden decrease in albumin value and sudden-onset ascites, jaundice, and progressive liver failure in the patient. It is thought to be inflammation due to radiation damage and fibrosis developing in the following process even though the exact mechanism is not known. The patient is given supportive treatments for liver functions and anti-inflammatory and anti-edema treatments in radioembolization-induced liver disease. Fulminant hepatitis and related death may be observed in patients who do not respond to treatment. Studies have reported that the incidence of radioembolization-induced liver disease after Y-90 microsphere therapy is approximately 3% at maximum [18].

Another serious complication of Y-90 microsphere treatment is lung fibrosis. This serious complication is very rarely seen currently, thanks to pre-therapy lung shunt ratio calculation and treatment dose adjustment accordingly when needed [9, 10].

13.12 The Position of Y-90 Microsphere Therapy in Treatment Algorithms

Y-90 microsphere therapy is predominantly seen as a palliative treatment in primary and metastatic liver malignancies that are not surgically possible in internationally approved treatment algorithms. It mostly entered treatment algorithms in the form of salvage therapy in patients who received all possible systemic and local treatments before and still had disease progression in the years when the treatment was first applied. There was no significant difference between Y-90 microsphere therapy administered as salvage treatment and TACE therapy, another type of local therapy administered in similar fashion, in terms of progression-free survival and/or total survival. In addition, Y-90 microsphere therapy is reported to be more advantageous than TACE in terms of treatment-related side effects and complications. While there may be a high rate of abscess development after TACE in very large tumor foci, this rate is very low in Y-90 microsphere therapy. Post-embolization syndrome can be seen in almost all patients after administration since embolization is the treatment mechanism in TACE; this complication is almost never seen since embolization is not the therapeutic mechanism of Y-90 microsphere therapy.

Therefore, Y-90 microsphere therapy is preferred to TACE among the local treatments recommended for salvage therapy, especially in patients with multiple and large tumor foci, even though they have the same recommendation in algorithms [19–21].

Another use of Y-90 microsphere therapy is the preparation for surgery and transplantation. Theoretically, radical and curative treatment of liver malignancies is transplantation in surgical and/or appropriate patients. Radiofrequency ablation (RFA) therapy is also recommended as an alternative to surgery in case of limited disease to a small area among therapies administered for curative purposes. However, RFA is generally not recommended in cases with extensive metastasis that does not fit the definition of oligometastatic case or in lesions close to large vascular structures or bile ducts, even though it is a limited disease. Y-90 microsphere therapy can be applied in these cases in order to reduce the tumor burden and to make the patient suitable for surgery. Surgeries to be performed after Y-90 microsphere therapy may be segmentectomy or lobectomy, as well as transplantation in appropriate patients [22].

Even though Y-90 microsphere therapy is positioned as an alternative therapy among the therapies administered for palliative purposes in algorithms, its administrations for curative purposes in suitable patients have begun to be included in the literature in recent years. The radiation dose given to the tumor is much higher compared to the planned dose, and it is aimed to develop radiation necrosis in that segment in cases where other curative therapies are not appropriate in a segment limited disease. This method of administration is called radiation segmentectomy approach. Radiation segmentectomy can only be performed in patients with malignant disease that covers one segment or part of the segment and where it is possible to administer Y-90 microspheres only through the artery that feeds that region. Y-90 microsphere therapy administered in this way has a curative purpose as it allows very high radiation doses to be administered from the inside to a limited area [23].

13.12.1 Y-90 Microsphere Therapy in Primary Liver Tumors

Y-90 microsphere therapy is most commonly used in hepatocellular cancer (HCC) and less frequently in cholangiocellular cancer in primary liver tumors.

13.13 Y-90 Microsphere Therapy in Hepatocellular Cancer

Hepatocellular cancer (HCC) is the most common primary liver tumor and ranks second in cancer-related deaths worldwide. Cirrhosis, alcohol consumption, and viral hepatitis infection due to chronic liver disease are the most common risk factors for HCC development. Only less than 10% of patients have a chance of curative therapy even though radical therapy of HCC is curative surgery. Other treatment approaches, including Y-90 microsphere therapy, can be useful for patients in whom surgical treatment is not possible. HCC being a hypervascular tumor and 80–100% arterial nutrition of tumors have brought local therapy approaches through the hepatic artery to the forefront. HCC is a tumor that is naturally sensitive to radiation, and the dose of radiotherapy administered externally should be 70 Gy and above to achieve a tumoricidal effect. However, external radiotherapy has no practical role in HCCs since severe radiation-related liver injury is observed in humans at radiation doses of 35 Gy and above externally. Tumor doses that are never possible to be achieved with external radiotherapy can be reached since targeted radiotherapy can be performed intraarterially with Y-90 microsphere therapy.

It should be preferred to establish a council or a board consisting of gastroenterologists, surgeons, medical oncologists, interventional radiologists, and nuclear medicine physicians for the treatment decision of HCC patients. Treatment suitability should be given after evaluating the patients in terms of all alternative treatment methods. The location of Y-90 microsphere therapy in patients diagnosed with HCC according to the Barcelona Clinical Liver Cancer Staging System (BCLC) recommendations has not been determined very precisely. However, Y-90 microsphere therapy is recommended as the first treatment option in patients in whom TACE treatment is not appropriate in moderately advanced disease according to BCLC [24, 25].

Many studies in the literature have reported that Y-90 microsphere therapy is an alternative to TACE and sorafenib therapy and that patients can be directed to curative treatments such as surgery or transplantation by reducing the tumor burden to be obtained with Y-90 microsphere therapy for palliative purposes [20, 24, 25]. It was reported in a prospective study by Salem et al. including 291 HCC patients that the cases who benefited the most from Y-90 microsphere therapy were Child-Pugh A patients and whether there was vascular invasion did not change the treatment response for this group [26]. Fifty-seven percent of the patients were reported to have fatigue as the most frequent side effect, and grade 3 and 4 bilirubin toxicity was reported to be 19% in the same study. Y-90 microsphere therapy was administered to 43 patients, TACE was administered to 35 patients, and the time from T3 to T2 progression (TTP) was significantly higher in patients receiving Y-90 microsphere therapy in the study conducted by Lewandovski et al. involving 78 in-op T3 HCC patients. Access to longer TTP with this treatment approach has saved time for transplantation and surgical treatments [21]. Median survival was reported to be 13 months, and it was reported that patients with more than 5 lesions, bilobar disease, and alpha-fetoprotein >52 IU/mL had less treatment responses and had worse prognosis in a study on 72 HCC patients published by Inarrairaegui et al. [27] Studies have also been published reporting that Y-90 microsphere therapy is successful in the presence of portal vein thrombosis in HCC patients. Kulik et al. reported that Y-90 microsphere therapy provided approximately 3 months of survival advantage (10.1 months versus 13.4 months) in patients with portal vascular invasion in their study in which HCC patients with lung and adrenal metastasis were accepted as contraindications to treatment [28]. Y-90 microsphere therapy was administered to advanced-stage patients with portal vein thrombosis without portal venous thrombosis and compensated cirrhosis where other treatments could not be given in a prospective phase 2 study conducted by Mazzafero et al. on 52 patients. The mean overall survival was 13 months in those with portal venous thrombosis after Y-90 microsphere therapy, 18 months in those without portal vein thrombosis, and 15 months in the whole group in this study [29]. Kooby et al. reported that both treatment methods showed similar progression-free survival rates in HCC patients in their study comparing chemoembolization and Y-90 microsphere therapy [19]. Carr et al. published in their retrospective cohort study comparing HCC patients diagnosed with advanced stage and inoperable biopsy in North America that both treatment methods were close to each other [20]. A significant reduction in tumor burden is achieved after Y-90 microsphere therapy in patients diagnosed with HCC, the possibility of surgery or transplantation is also born in some patients, and treatment in appropriate centers serves this purpose [21, 22].

Y-90 microsphere therapy can also be administered in the form of radiation segmentectomy in patients diagnosed with HCC. Riaz et al. reported in 84 disease studies that the average tumor dose reached in this way was 1214 Gy, the overall survival of the patients was 26.9 months, and none of the patients developed radiation-related liver disease complications [23]. Similar results regarding the use of Y-90 microsphere therapy in HCC for radiation segmentectomy were also obtained in a multicenter study by Vouche et al. [30]. Serum alpha-fetoprotein levels and radiological imaging methods are preferred in patients diagnosed with HCC in the monitoring of Y-90 microsphere therapy. Riaz et al. reported that a > 50% decrease in alpha-fetoprotein levels after treatment showed a correlation with the treatment response [31].

FDG-PET/CT imaging in patients diagnosed with HCC is only limited in determining treatment response since it is considered to be beneficial in patients with positive FDG uptake before treatment. However, it has been reported that non-FDG radiopharmaceuticals such as carbon-11 acetate and FDG-PET imaging administered by PET/MR hybrid imaging can also play an important role in the treatment response in HCC [32].

13.14 Y-90 Microsphere Therapy in Cholangiocellular Cancer

In addition to HCC, Y-90 microsphere therapy provides useful results in eligible patients in cholangiocellular cancers, one of the primary liver tumors. The median survival of the cases was reported as 15.5 months, and the partial response rate was reported as 28%, and stable disease as 54% in the treatment responses evaluated by radiological methods in a meta-analysis study by Al-Adra et al. investigating a total of 12 studies on the effectiveness of Y-90 microsphere therapy in patients diagnosed with cholangiocellular cancer. It was emphasized in the same study that Y-90 microsphere therapy provides much better survival rates in cholangiocellular cancers compared to all other treatments [33]. Soydal et al. investigated the effectiveness of Y-90 microsphere therapy in patients with intrahepatic cholangiocellular cancer and pointed out the prognostic importance of FDG uptake, tumor burden, and tumor size and reported that patients with low tumor burden, FDG-PET/CT negative, and small tumor showed a longer survival profile [34].

FDG-PET/CT imaging in patients diagnosed with HCC is only beneficial in patients with positive FDG uptake before treatment. On the other hand, FDG-PET/CT imaging may be preferred to demonstrate early treatment response at 4–6 weeks after treatment, as FDG hypermetabolism is observed in most patients with cholangiocellular cancer.

13.14.1 Y-90 Microsphere Therapy in Metastatic Liver Tumors

The majority of liver malignancies are metastatic cancers originating from other primary tumors. The liver is the organ most commonly metastasized after lymph nodes. The most common cancers that metastasize to the liver include colorectal cancer, pancreatic cancer, breast cancer, and neuroendocrine tumors. In addition, recurrences can be seen in ocular malignant melanoma with liver metastases even years later. The first method to be preferred is mostly surgical treatment if resection is possible in liver metastatic disease. Five-year survival can increase to 40% with surgical treatment in colorectal cancer metastases. Similar results are also present in neuroendocrine tumor-induced metastases. However, Y-90 microsphere therapy is preferred over other treatments, regardless of the histopathology and behavior of the primary tumor that metastasizes, if eligibility criteria are met in patients with liver metastasis with surgical contraindications or unresectable characteristics [35].

13.15 Y-90 Microsphere Therapy in Colorectal Cancer

Approximately 20% of patients with colorectal cancer have liver metastasis at diagnosis. Approximately 50% of patients develop liver metastasis during disease, whereas the liver is the only metastatic site in 1/3 of patients [36]. Approximately 80% of cases diagnosed with colorectal cancer with liver metastasis die due to hepatic failure. Therefore, the presence of liver metastases in colorectal cancer is even more important compared to primary tumor in terms of clinical morbidity and life expectancy. The first treatment for liver metastases in colorectal cancer is surgery. Liver or other organ metastases develop in approximately 60% of patients in the future even though a 5-year survival rate of approximately 40% is possible with surgical treatment [37].

Y-90 microsphere therapy in the treatment of liver metastases that are not surgically possible in patients with colorectal cancer can be administered with chemotherapy, after chemotherapy or as salvage therapy in advanced disease, as neoadjuvant therapy, or as surgical adaptation therapy, taking into account existing clinical studies and ESMO (European School of Medical Oncology) guidelines in the literature [38]. Y-90 microsphere therapy administered with first-line chemotherapy, whether or not there is additional metastasis other than liver, strengthens the systemic chemotherapy response in patients diagnosed with colorectal cancer with liver metastasis without surgical chance [38, 39]. Gray et al. compared chemotherapy with Y-90 microsphere therapy versus chemotherapy as the first-line treatment in 75 patients with colorectal cancer liver metastasis and reported that the median survival in the Y-90 microsphere added group was prolonged to 17 months [40]. Van Hazel et al. reported in their study that Y-90 microsphere therapy added to the 5-fluorouracil/leucovorin chemotherapy protocol at the third month significantly increased the quality of life compared to the chemotherapy group alone [41]. Studies have also been published reporting that Y-90 microsphere therapy is an effective and reliable treatment approach when administered alone or in combination with radiosensitizing chemotherapy regimen as salvage therapy in chemotherapy-resistant metastatic advanced stage patients [42, 43]. Kennedy et al. published a study in which 208 colorectal cancer patients with liver metastasis showed a reduction in tumor size in 35.5% of the patients and a stable response in 55% of the patients with CT imaging at 3 months, while 85% of the patients had a good metabolic response with PET imaging [44].

PET/CT shows treatment response much earlier compared to radiological imaging (Fig. 13.7a, b). Even though all chemotherapy regimens have been tried, Y-90 microsphere therapy is administered to patients with colorectal cancer who continue to have metastatic disease in the liver and have or do not have metastasis in other regions, and the burden of metastatic disease is reduced, and it is possible to perform other treatment methods such as surgical treatment or radiofrequency ablation therapy [45].

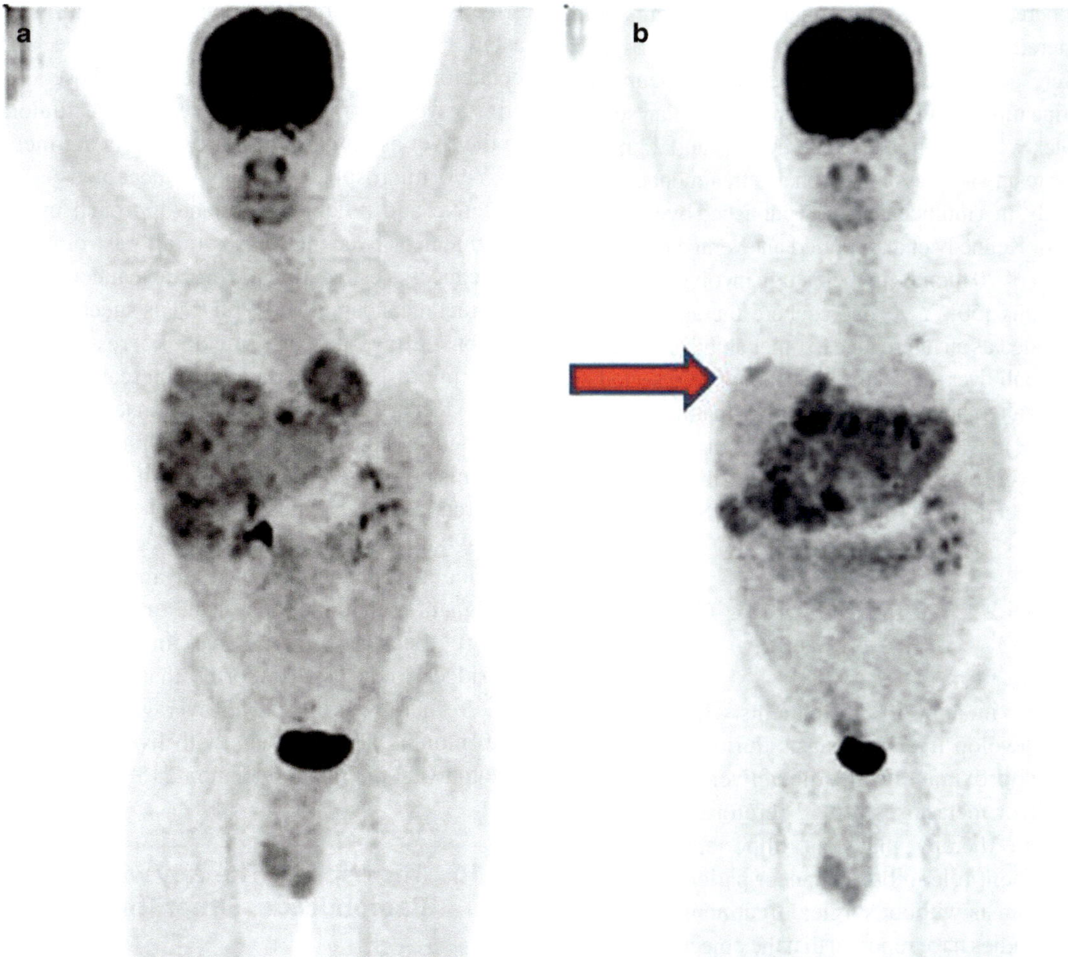

Fig. 13.7 (**a**) FDG uptake consistent with widespread liver metastases, more commonly in the right lobe of the liver, in baseline FDG-PET/CT imaging performed before Y-90 microsphere therapy in a 55-year-old male patient with the diagnosis of colon cancer. (**b**) Decreased FDG uptake (arrow) in metastatic foci in favor of complete partial metabolic response in the right lobe of the liver in FDG-PET/CT imaging following Y-90 microsphere therapy administered to the right lobe of the liver in the same patient

13.15.1 Y-90 Microsphere Therapy in Neuroendocrine Tumor Metastases

Approximately 13% of patients diagnosed with neuroendocrine tumors also have liver metastases. Surgical treatment of liver metastases in neuroendocrine tumors is still a controversial issue, and alternative local treatment methods are therefore needed [46]. Y-90 microsphere therapy in neuroendocrine tumor liver metastases has been emphasized to be a well-tolerated and highly effective therapy option especially to provide symptomatic improvement in some extensive clinical studies [47, 48]. The objective response rate was found to be 50% for Y-90 resin microspheres and 54% for Y-90 glass microspheres when Y-90 resin microspheres were administered to 20 patients and Y-90 glass microspheres were administered to 22 patients with neuroendocrine tumor liver metastasis, and the median survival rates were reported to be 28 months and 22 months for resin and glass microspheres treatments, respectively, in a multicenter study published by Rhee et al. [49]. Kennedy et al. reported an average overall survival of 70 months in their study involving 148 NET patients [50]. Y-90 microsphere therapy is recommended as an alternative to other ablative treatments in small liver metastases that cannot be resected and as an alternative to local palliative treatments such as TACE in widespread metastatic disease according to the current guidelines of the European Neuroendocrine Tumor Society (ENETS) [51].

13.15.2 Y-90 Microsphere Therapy in Breast Cancer

Approximately 50% of patients with breast cancer develop liver metastasis during their illness, and approximately 60% die of liver failure caused by liver metastases [46]. Therefore, Y-90 microsphere therapy plays an important alternative treatment role in breast cancer patients with liver metastasis without surgical treatment.

Studies have reported that the objective response rates (complete response + partial response + stable disease) of Y-90 microsphere therapy in patients with breast cancer are between 92% to 96% and the disease control rates are between 39% to 61% in patients with progressive liver metastases refractory to chemotherapy regimens [52–54]. Eichbaum et al. reported in their study that reducing tumor burden with Y-90 microsphere therapy in liver metastases in addition to systemic chemotherapy in breast cancer provided a significant increase in median survival compared to systemic chemotherapy alone [55]. Cianni et al. reported the objective response rate as 56% in 52 patients who received Y-90 microsphere therapy as salvage therapy [56].

13.15.3 Y-90 Microsphere Therapy in Liver Metastases of Other Malignant Tumors

Intraarterial Y-90 microsphere therapy offers an effective and reliable treatment option in all metastatic tumors, regardless of tumor type and behavior, as it provides a selectivity based on arterial vascularization characteristics of tumors in the liver as long as eligibility criteria are met.

Y-90 microsphere therapy is accepted as an effective and reliable treatment approach in the treatment of liver metastases in all gastrointestinal cancers, especially pancreatic cancer, as in colorectal cancers. FDG-PET/CT is successful in demonstrating the early metabolic response of Y-90 microsphere therapy in pancreatic cancer (Fig. 13.8a, b). Objective response rate was reported as 64.3% in Y-90 microsphere therapy administered by Michl et al. as salvage therapy in pancreatic cancer patients [57].

Y-90 microsphere therapy has been reported to provide a significant survival advantage in uveal malignant melanoma, one of the tumors that frequently metastasize to the liver, in the literature. Eldridge-Hindy et al. reported that Y-90 microsphere therapy provided an average survival of 23.9 months in 71 patients with liver metastasis due to uveal malignant melanoma [58].

13.16 Microsphere Therapy with Radionuclides Other Than Y-90

13.16.1 Rhenium-188 (Re-188) Microsphere Therapy

Re-188 is a high-energy beta- and low-energy gamma-emitting radionuclide obtained from the

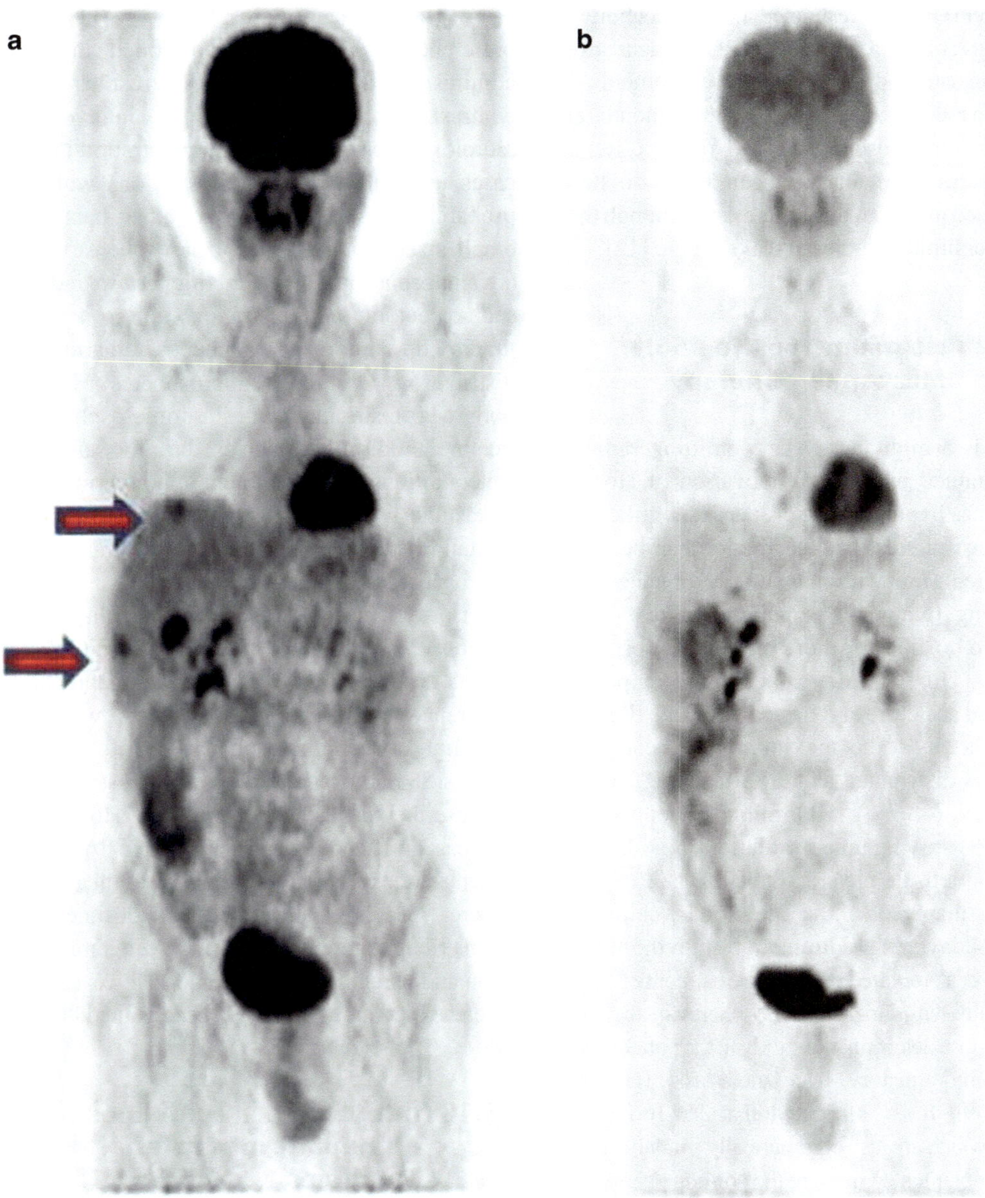

Fig. 13.8 (**a**) FDG uptake (arrows) consistent with multiple metastases in the liver in basal FDG-PET/CT imaging performed before Y-90 microsphere therapy in a 47-year-old male patient diagnosed with pancreatic cancer (**b**) Decreased FDG uptakes in metastatic foci in favor of partial metabolic response in the right lobe of the liver in FDG-PET/CT imaging at 1 month following Y-90 microsphere therapy administered to the right lobe of the liver in the same patient

Tungsten-188/Re-188 generator. Its physical half-life is 16.9 hours. Maximum beta energy of Re-188 is around 2.12 MeV and maximum 10 mm similar to soft tissue range Y-90.

The most important feature that distinguishes Re-188 from Y-90 is that it also has low-energy gamma radiation. The energy of the gamma ray is 155 keV, which is very close to the energy of Technetium-99m (Tc99m), the most commonly used radionuclide in diagnostic studies in nuclear medicine. Its availability from the generator provides a great advantage for Re-188, unlike Y-90 produced in the reactor. It is possible to obtain about 6 months of Re-188 from a generator. This leads to a lower Re-188 microsphere production cost compared to Y-90 microspheres.

Nowicki et al. investigated the applicability of Re-188 microsphere therapy in the patient group with primary and metastatic liver tumors and reported a median overall survival of 7.1 months and a progression-free survival of 5.1 months. Re-188 microspheres have not yet been found to be as widely used as Y-90 microspheres even though there are similar limited studies in the literature [12].

13.16.2 Holmium-166 (Ho-166) Microsphere Therapy

Ho-166 is a high-energy beta-emitting radionuclide obtained by neutron activation of Ho-165. Ho-166 has paramagnetic properties, unlike other radiomicrospheres. Biodistribution can be monitored in real time with magnetic resonance imaging during treatment as paramagnetic contrast agent and dosimetry studies can be performed in this way. Ho-166 microspheres are in poly-L-lactic acid structure and have an average diameter of 30 microns. The maximum beta energy of Ho-166 is distributed as 1.85 MeV (50.0%) and 1.77 MeV (48.7%). Holmium-166 emits low-energy (81 keV) gamma radiation in addition to beta radiation. Its physical half-life is 26.8 days, and more than 90% of the radiation is scattered in the first 4 days after administration to the liver.

Smits et al. reported promising treatment effectiveness results with Ho-166 microspheres in their preliminary dose determination study in the patient group with chemorefractory liver metastasis (HEPAR1 study) [59]. It is anticipated that Ho-166 microspheres, which are also commercially available today, will be implemented more in the coming years.

13.17 Microsphere-Type Selection in Clinical Practice

Currently, the worldwide commercially available microsphere types are Y-90 resin and Y-90 glass microspheres. Ho-166 microspheres are also commercially produced but are not yet as widely used as Y-90 microspheres. Re-188 microspheres require the supply of Re-186/Re-188 generator and its use is limited.

The unique characteristics of each microsphere type mentioned in detail earlier may give relative priority to another microsphere type in clinical preference. For example, controlled injectable administration of Y-90 resin microspheres with contrast may be preferred by the interventional radiologist performing the administration in some cases in small vessel administrations with high probability of reflux. On the other hand, it is emphasized that Y-90 glass microspheres may be advantageous by some practitioners in radiation segmentectomy administrations due to its ability to provide a more homogeneous radiation dose distribution with fewer microspheres. However, both Y-90 resin and Y-90 glass microspheres are treatment tools that can be used for the same clinical conditions in the treatment of both primary and metastatic liver tumors considering the accepted guidelines; there is no guide indicating a single microsphere type and emphasizing its clinical superiority. Thus, Y-90 resin and Y-90 glass microspheres are considered to have similar clinical effects if appropriate patient selection and careful adherence to the preparation steps, which are essential for each microsphere type [60–65].

Re-188 microspheres offer a low cost advantage because they are generator products. However, its use has not become widespread. Ho-166 microspheres are expected to be superior to other microsphere types especially in terms of dosimetry and biodistribution monitoring due to their gamma radiation and paramagnetic properties. However, widespread experience has not yet been gained [12, 59].

13.18 International Guidelines on Hepatic Intraarterial Therapies

Currently, there are some international guidelines which emphasize the impact of Y-90 microsphere therapy for primary and metastatic tumors of the liver. Through detailed examination of such guidelines, it can be stated that the ones published especially in earlier years are mostly written in the form of procedural guidelines where the details of the procedure are explained. Relatively more up-to-date guidelines mostly focus on the position of Y-90 microsphere therapy in algorithms and its changing indications over time in both primary tumors and metastatic tumors as the expert experience increases. Table 13.4 shows the

Table 13.4 Comparison of some comprehensive international guidelines on Y-90 microsphere therapy

Guideline name	Year published	Guideline content and fundamental message	Level of evidence	Access link
EANM procedure guidelines for the treatment of liver cancer and liver metastases	2011	Procedural guideline: Y-90 microsphere therapy is indicated in both primary and metastatic liver tumors	Not specified	http://eanm.org/publications/guidelines/EANM_liver_treatment_guidelines_2012.pdf
EASL-EORTC clinical practice guidelines, management of HCC	2012	Y-90 microsphere therapy in HCC is not acceptable as an alternative to TACE and sorafenib unless there are randomized studies	Not specified	https://www.ncbi.nlm.nih.gov/pubmed/22424438
ESMO-ESDO clinical practice guidelines	2012	Y-90 microsphere therapy may compete with sorafenib and TACE in HCC only in the following subgroups of patients: previously failed TACE, macrovascular invasion, patients with good liver function, and patients without extrahepatic disease	III/C	http://www.esmo.org/Guidelines/Gastrointestinal-Cancers/Hepatocellular-Carcinoma
NET Liver Metastases Consensus Kennedy	2014	Y-90 microsphere therapy can be administered in any NET liver metastasis (single/multiple, etc.) requiring palliation	Low/C2	https://www.ncbi.nlm.nih.gov/pmc/articles/PMC4266438/
NICE advice (SIR-spheres for treating in operable HCC)	2016	Y-90 resin microspheres are indicated in in-op HCC therapy. It may be an alternative to TACE, drug-emitting TACE, and systemic drug therapy to reduce tumor size, reduce symptoms, and prepare for surgery/transplant	Not specified	https://www.nice.org.uk/advice/mib63/chapter/technology-overview
NCCN clinical practice	2017	Y-90 microsphere therapy is useful in unresectable and liver-limited disease	Not specified	https://www.nccn.org/professionals/physician_gls/f_guidelines.asp

characteristics of the main international guidelines considered to be the most comprehensive in this field [60–65]. Novel guidelines, position papers and expert reports are expected to be published in the literature as the practice and experience in intraarterial radionuclide treatments increase.

13.19 Concluding Remarks

Hepatic intraarterial treatments are based on differential circulation system of the liver which implies the arterial feeding of the malignant cells in contrast to portal venous feeding of healthy hepatocytes. Therefore, tumor selectivity is reached.

Intraarterial administration of high-beta radiation-emitting microspheres allows very high radiation doses within the tumor that cannot be reached with external radiotherapy, while normal liver cells are largely protected from the harmful effects of radiation due to the selective distribution.

Hepatic intraarterial radionuclide therapy is mainly an internal radiation therapy and its embolizing effect is insignificant.

It is indicated if adequate liver reserve is provided in patients with primary and metastatic liver tumors that cannot be surgically treated.

Intraarterial Y-90 microsphere therapy can also be used with intent to prepare the unresectable patient for surgery and/or transplantation treatments that provide cure by reducing tumor burden and also with a directly curative intent such as radiation segmentectomy. Such approaches have become more popular in recent years in selected group of patients.

As an alternative to Y-90 resin microspheres and Y-90 glass microspheres, which are internationally approved for clinical use, Re-188 microspheres, which have relatively low cost due to being a generator product, and Ho-166 microspheres, which are predicted to provide an advantage due to their gamma radiation and paramagnetic properties, have also been introduced for clinical use.

References

1. Ariel IM. Ann Surg. 1965;162(2):267–78.
2. Burton MA, Gray BN, Klemp PF, Kelleher DK, Hardy N. Selective internal radiation therapy: distribution of radiation in the liver. Eur J Cancer Clin Oncol. 1989;25(10):1487–91.
3. Lau WY, Ho S, Leung TWT, Chan M, Ho R, Johnson PJ, Li AKC. Selective internal radiation therapy for nonresectable hepatocellular carcinoma with intraarterial infusion of 90Yttrium microspheres. Int Radiat Oncol Biol Phys. 1998;40(3):583–92.
4. Van de Wiele C, Maes A, Brugman E, D'asseler Y, De Spiegeleer B, Mees G, Stellamans K. SIRT of liver metastases: physiological and pathophysiological considerations. Eur J Nucl Med Mol Imaging. 2012;39:1646–55.
5. Laurent A. Microspheres and nonspherical particles for embolization. Tech Vasc Interv Rad. 2007;10:248–56.
6. Nijsen JFW, Zonnenberg BA, Woittiez JRW, Rook DW, Swildens-van Woudenberg IA, van Rijk PP, van het Schip AD. Holmium-166 poly lactic microspheres applicable for intra-arterial radionuclide therapy of hepatic malignancies: effects of preparation and neutron activation techniques. Eur J Nucl Med. 1999;26:699–704.
7. Cremonesi M, Ferrari M, Bartolomei M, Orsi F, Bonomo G, Aricò D, et al. Radioembolization with 90Y-microspheres: dosimetric and radiobiological investigation for multi-cycle treatment. Eur J Nucl Med Mol Imaging. 2008;35(11):2088–96.
8. Wunderlich G, Schiller E, Bergmann R, Pietzsch HJ. Comparison of the stability of Y-90-, Lu-177- and Ga-68- labeled human serum albumin microspheres (DOTA-HSAM). Nucl Med Biol. 2010;37:861–7.
9. Sirtex medical training manual, training program physicians and institutions. Sirtex Medical Limited, Australia. Available at: http://www.sirtex.com/usa/_data/page/549/TRN-US- 0320for20 US1.pdf.
10. TheraSphere yttrium-90 glass microspheres users manual. MDS Nordion, Ottawa, ON, Canada. http://www.nordion.com/therasphere/physicians-package-insert/package-insert-eu-en.pdf.
11. Van de Maat GH, Seevinck PR, Elschot M, Smits MLJ, de Leeuw H, van het Schip AD, et al. MRI-based biodistribution assessment of holmium-166 poly (L-lactic acid) microspheres after radioembolization. Eur Radiol. 2013;23:827–35.
12. Nowicki ML, Cwikla JW, Sankowski AJ, et al. Initial study of radiological and clinical efficacy: Radioembolisation using Re-188 HSA microspheres in patients with progressive, unresectable primary and secondary liver cancers. Med Sci Monitor. 2014;20:1353–62.
13. Bozkurt MF, Salanci BV, Uğur Ö. Intra-arterial radionuclide therapies for liver tumors. Semin Nucl Med. 2016 Jul;46(4):324–39. https://doi.org/10.1053/j.semnuclmed.2016.01.008.Review.

14. Volkan-Salancı B, Bozkurt MF, Peynircioğlu B, Cil B, Uğur O. The relation between perfusion pattern of hepatic artery perfusion scintigraphy and response to y-90 microsphere therapy. Mol Imaging Radionucl Ther. 2013;22(3):98–102. https://doi.org/10.4274/Mirt.77487. Epub 2013 Dec 10
15. Sabet A, Ahmadzadehfar H, Muckle M, Haslerud T, Wilhelm K, Biersack HJ, Ezziddin S. Significance of oral administration of sodium perchlorate in planning liver-directed radioembolization. J Nucl Med. 2011;52(7):1063–7. https://doi.org/10.2967/jnumed.110.083626. Epub 2011 Jun 16
16. Sangro B, Bilbao JI, Boan J, Martinez-Cuesta A, Benito A, Rodriguez J, Panizo A, Gil B, Inarrairaegui M, Herrero I, Quiroga J, Prieto J. Radioembolization using 90Y-resin microspheres for patients with advanced hepatocellular carcinoma. Int J Radiat Oncol Biol Phys. 2006;66(3):792–800. Epub 2006 Aug 14
17. Lhommel R, Goffette P, Van den Eynde M, Jamar F, Pauwels S, Bilbao JI, Walrand S. Yttrium-90 TOF PET scan demonstrates high-resolution biodistribution after liver SIRT. Eur J Nucl Med Mol Imaging. 2009;36(10):1696. https://doi.org/10.1007/s00259-009-1210-1. Epub 2009 Jul 18
18. Kuo JC, Tazbirkova A, Allen R, Kosmider S, Gibbs P, Yip D. Serious hepatic complications of selective internal radiation therapy with yttrium-90 microsphere radioembolization for unresectable liver tumors. Asia Pac J Clin Oncol. 2014;10(3):266–72.
19. Kooby DA, Egnatashvili V, Srinivasan S, Chamsuddin A, Delman KA, Kauh J, et al. Comparison of yttrium-90 radioembolization and transcatheter arterial chemoembolization for the treatment of unresectable hepatocellular carcinoma. J Vasc Interv Radiol. 2009;21(2):224–30.
20. Carr BI, Kondragunta V, Buch SC, Branch RA. Therapeutic equivalence in survival for hepatic arterial chemoembolization and yttrium 90 microsphere treatments in unresectable hepatocellular carcinoma: a two-cohort study. Cancer. 2010;116(5):1305–14.
21. Lewandowski RJ, Kulik LM, Riaz A, et al. A comparative analysis of transarterial downstaging for hepatocellular carcinoma: chemoembolization versus radioembolization. Am J Transplant. 2009;9(8):1920–8.
22. Wright GP, Marsh JW, Varma MK, Doherty MG, Bartlett DL, Chung MH. Liver resection after selective internal radiation therapy with Yttrium-90 is safe and feasible: a bi-institutional analysis. Ann Surg Oncol. 2017;24(4):906–13. https://doi.org/10.1245/s10434-016-5697-y. Epub 2016 Nov 22
23. Riaz A, Gates VL, Atassi B, et al. Radiation segmentectomy: a novel approach to increase safety and efficacy of radioembolization. Int J Radiat Oncol Biol Phys. 2011;79(1):163–71.
24. Llovet JM, Di Bisceglie AM, Bruix J, et al. Design and endpoints of clinical trials in hepatocellular carcinoma. J Natl Cancer Inst. 2008;100(10):698–711.
25. Yang T, Lau WY, Zhang H, et al. Grey zone in the Barcelona Clinic Liver Cancer Classification for hepatocellular carcinoma: surgeons' perspective. World J Gastroenter. 2015;21(27):8256–61.
26. Salem R, Lewandowski RJ, Mulcahy MF, Riaz A, Ryu RK, Ibrahim S, et al. Radioembolization for hepatocellular carcinoma using Yttrium-90 microspheres: a comprehensive report of long- term outcomes. Gastroenterology. 2010;138(1):52–64.
27. Inarrairaegui M, Martinez-Cuesta A, Rodriguez M, Bilbao JI, Arbizu J, Benito A, et al. Analysis of prognostic factors after Yttrium-90 Radioembolization of advanced hepatocellular carcinoma. Int J Radiat Oncol Biol Phys. 2010;77(5):1441–8.
28. Kulik LM, Carr BI, Mulcahy MF, Lewandowski RJ, Atassi B, Ryu RK, et al. Safety and efficacy of (90) Y radiotherapy for hepatocellular carcinoma with and without portal vein thrombosis. Hepatology. 2007;47(1):71–81.
29. Mazzaferro V, Sposito C, Bhoori S, Romito R, Chiesa C, Morosi C, Maccauro M, Marchiano A, Bongini M, Lanocita R, Civelli E, Bombardieri E, Camerini T, Spreafico C. Yttrium90 radioembolization for intermediate-advanced hepatocarcinoma: a phase II study. Hepatology. 2013;57:1826–37.
30. Vouche M, Habib A, Ward TJ, et al. Unresectable solitary hepatocellular carcinoma not amenable to radiofrequency ablation: multicenter radiology-pathology correlation and survival of radiation segmentectomy. Hepatology. 2014;60(1):192–201.
31. Riaz A, Ryu RK, Kulik LM, Mulcahy MF, Lewandowski RJ, Minocha J, et al. Alpha-fetoprotein response after locoregional therapy for hepatocellular carcinoma: oncologic marker of radiologic response, progression, and survival. J Clin Oncol. 2009;27(34):5734–42.
32. Lam MGEH, Kwee TC, Basu S, Alavi A. Underestimated role of F-18 FDG PET for HCC evaluation and promise of FDG PET/MR imaging in this setting. J Nucl Med. 2013;54(8):1510–1.
33. Al-Adra DP, Gill RS, Axford SJ, Shi X, Kneteman N, Liau SS. Treatment of unresectable intrahepatic cholangiocarcinoma with yttrium-90 radioembolization: a systematic review and pooled analysis. Eur J Surg Oncol. 2015;41(1):120–7.
34. Soydal C, Kucuk ON, Bilgic S, Ibis E. Radioembolization with (90)Y resin microspheres for intrahepatic cholangiocellular carcinoma: prognostic factors. Ann Nucl Med. 2016;30(1):29–34. https://doi.org/10.1007/s12149-015-1026-y. Epub 2015 Sep 14
35. Kawada K, Hasegawa S, Murakami T, et al. Molecular mechanisms of liver metastasis. Int J Clin Oncol. 2011;16:464–72.
36. Weiss L, Grundmann E, Torhost J, et al. Haematogenous metastatic patterns of colonic carcinoma : an analysis of 1541 necropsies. J Pathol. 1986;150:195–203.
37. De Jong MC, Pulitano C, Ribero D, et al. Rates and pattern of recurrence following curative intent sur-

gery for colorectal liver metastases: an international multiinstitutional analysis of 1669 patients. Ann Surg. 2009;250:440–8.
38. Van Cutsem E, Cervantes A, Adam R, Sobrero A, Van Krieken JH, Aderka D, et al. ESMO consensus guidelines for the management of patients with metastatic colorectal cancer. Ann Oncol. 2016;27:1386–422.
39. Sofocleous CT, Garcia AR, Pandit-Taskar N, Do KG, Brody LA, Petre EN, et al. Phase I trial of selective internal radiation therapy for chemorefractory colorectal cancer liver metastases progressing after hepatic arterial pump and systemic chemotherapy. Clin Colorectal Cancer. 2014;13(1):27–36.
40. Gray B, Van Hazel G, Hope M, Burton M, Moroz P, Anderson J, et al. Randomised trial of SIR-spheres plus chemotherapy vs. chemotherapy alone for treating patients with liver metastases from primary large bowel cancer. Ann Oncol. 2001;12(12):1711–20.
41. Van Hazel G, Blackwell A, Anderson J, Price D, Moroz P, Bower G, et al. Randomised phase 2 trial of SIR-spheres plus fluorouracil/leucovorin chemotherapy versus fluorouracil/leucovorin chemotherapy alone in advanced colorectal cancer. J Surg Oncol. 2004;88(2):78–85.
42. Van den Eynde M, Flamen P, El Nakadi I, Liberale G, Delatte P, Larsimont D, et al. Inducing resectability of chemotherapy refractory colorectal liver metastasis by radioembolization with yttrium-90 microspheres. Clin Nucl Med. 2008;33:697–9.
43. Kennedy A, Nag S, Salem R, Murthy R, McEwan AJ, Nutting C, et al. Recommendations for radioembolization of hepatic malignancies using yttrium-90 microsphere brachytherapy: a consensus panel report from the radioembolization brachytherapy oncology consortium. Int J Radiat Oncol Biol Phys. 2007;68:13–23.
44. Kennedy AS, Coldwell D, Nutting C, Murthy R, Wertman DE Jr, Loehr SP, et al. Resin 90Ymicrosphere brachytherapy for unresectable colorectal liver metastases: modern USA experience. Int J Radiat Oncol Biol Phys. 2006;65:412–25.
45. Hoffmann RT, Jakobs TF, Kubisch CH, Stemmler HJ, Trumm C, Tatsch K, et al. Radiofrequency ablation after selective internal radiation therapy with Yttrium90 microspheres in metastatic liver disease-Is it feasible? Eur J Radiol. 2010;74(1):199–205.
46. Page AJ, Weiss MJ, Pawlik TM, et al. Cancer. 2014;15:3111–21.
47. Kennedy AS, Dezarn WA, McNeillie P, Coldwell D, Nutting C, Carter D, et al. Radioembolization for unresectable neuroendocrine hepatic metastases using resin 90Y-microspheres: early results in 148 patients. Am J Clin Oncol. 2008;31:271–9.
48. Kalinowski M, Dressler M, König A, El-Sheik M, Rinke A, Höffken H, et al. Selective internal radiotherapy with Yttrium-90 microspheres for hepatic metastatic neuroendocrine tumors: a prospective single center study. Digestion. 2009;79:137–42.
49. Rhee TK, Lewandowski RJ, Liu DM, Mulcahy MF, Takahashi G, Hansen PD, et al. 90Y Radioembolization for metastatic neuroendocrine liver tumors: preliminary results from a multi-institutional experience. Ann Surg. 2008;247:1029–35.
50. Kennedy A, Bester L, Salem R, Sharma RA, Parks RW, Ruszniewski P. NET-Liver-Metastases Consensus Conference. Role of hepatic intra-arterial therapies in metastatic neuroendocrine tumors (NET): guidelines from the NET-liver-metastases consensus conference. HPB (Oxford). 2015;17(1):29–37. https://doi.org/10.1111/hpb.12326.
51. Pavel M, O'Toole D, Costa F, Capdevila J, Gross D, Kianmanesh R, Krenning E, Knigge U, Salazar R, Pape UF, Öberg K. Vienna Consensus Conference participants. ENETS Consensus Guidelines update for the management of distant metastatic disease of intestinal, pancreatic, bronchial neuroendocrine neoplasms (NEN) and NEN of unknown primary site. Neuroendocrinology. 2016;103(2):172–85. https://doi.org/10.1159/000443167. Epub 2016 Jan 5
52. Coldwell DM, Kennedy AS, Nutting CW. Use of yttrium-90 microspheres in the treatment of unresectable hepatic metastases from breast cancer. Int J Radiat Oncol Biol Phys. 2007;69:800–4.
53. Bangash AK, Atassi B, Kaklamani V, Rhee TK, Yu M, Lewandowski RJ, et al. 90Y radioembolization of metastatic breast cancer to the liver: toxicity, imaging response, survival. J Vasc Interv Radiol. 2007;18:621–8.
54. Jakobs TF, Hoffmann RT, Fischer T, Stemmler HJ, Tatsch K, La Fougere C, et al. Radioembolization in patients with hepatic metastases from breast cancer. J Vasc Interv Radiol. 2008;19:683–90.
55. Eichbaum MH, Kaltwasser M, Bruckner T, deRossi TM, Schneeweiss A, Sohn C. Prognostic factors for patients with liver metastases from breast cancer. Breast Cancer Res Treat. 2006;96:53–62.
56. Cianni R, Pelle G, Notarianni E, Saltarelli A, Rabuffi P, Bagni O, et al. Radioembolisation with (90)Y-labelled resin microspheres in the treatment of liver metastasis from breast cancer. Eur Radiol. 2013;23(1):182–9. https://doi.org/10.1007/s00330-012-2556-5.
57. Michl M, Haug AR, Jakobs TF, Paprottka P, Hoffmann RT, Bartenstein P, et al. Radioembolization with Yttrium-90 microspheres (SIRT) in pancreatic cancer patients with liver metastases: efficacy, safety and prognostic factors. Oncology. 2014;86(1):24–32. https://doi.org/10.1159/000355821.
58. Eldredge-Hindy H, Ohri N, Anne PR, Eschelman D, Gonsalves C, Intenzo C, et al. Yttrium-90 microsphere brachytherapy for liver metastases from uveal melanoma: clinical outcomes and the predictive value of Fluorodeoxyglucose positron emission tomography. Am J Clin Oncol. 2016;39(2):189–95. https://doi.org/10.1097/COC.0000000000000033.

59. Smits ML, Nijsen JF, van den Bosch MA, et al. Holmium-166 radioembolisation in patients with unresectable, chemorefractory liver metastases (HEPAR 1 trial):a phase 1 dose escalation study. Lancet Oncol. 2012;13:1025–34.
60. Giammarile F, Bodei L, Chiesa C, Flux G, Forrer F, Kraeber-Bodere F, et al. EANM procedure guideline for the treatment of liver cancer and liver metastases with intra-arterial radioactive compounds. Eur J Nucl Med Mol Imaging. 2011;38(7):1393–406. https://doi.org/10.1007/s00259-011-1812-2.
61. European Association for The Study Of The Liver, European Organisation for Research and Treatment Of Cancer. EASL-EORTC clinical practice guidelines: management of hepatocellular carcinoma. J Hepatol. 2012;56:908–43.
62. Verslype C, Rosmorduc O, Rougier P. Hepatocellular carcinoma: ESMO-ESDO clinical practice guidelines. Ann Oncol. 2012;23:vii41–8.
63. Kennedy A, Bester L, Salem R, Sharma RA, Parks RW, Ruszniewski F. Role of hepatic intra-arterial therapies in metastatic neuroendocrine tumours (NET): guidelines from the NET- Liver-Metastases Consensus Conference. HPB (Oxford). 2015;17:29–37.
64. NICE Organization Website. Available at: https://www.nice.org.uk/advice/mib63/chapter/technology-overview. Accessed online 20.04.2018.
65. NCCN Guidelines Website: Available at: https://www.nccn.org/professionals/physician_gls/f_guidelines.asp. Accessed online 20.04.2018.

14 Systemic Treatments and Related Side Effects in Liver Tumors

Hüseyin Salih Semiz and İlhan Öztop

Mass formation in the liver is a common condition, but most of these masses are benign. Benign formations in the liver may include mass formations originating from the liver parenchyma such as focal nodular hyperplasia, nodular regenerative hyperplasia, hepatocellular adenoma, and regenerative and dysplastic nodules, as well as mass formations originating from the bile ducts such as simple cyst, biliary hamartoma, biliary adenoma, or biliary cystadenoma. Vascular benign masses originating from mesenchymal tissues can also be observed [1, 2].

Most malignant tumors observed in the liver are metastatic masses. It is one of the most common distant organs infiltrated by metastases in the malignancy of many organs due to the intense vascular circulation and receptor expression of the liver. The most common tumors that metastasize to the liver include colon, stomach, pancreas, breast, and lung cancer and malignant melanoma. Primary tumors of the liver are less common. These tumors include hepatocellular carcinoma, cholangiocellular carcinoma, primary liver lymphoma, mesenchymal tumors such as hepatoblastoma and angiosarcoma, and epithelioid hemangioendothelioma [1–4].

H. S. Semiz (✉)
Ministry of Health, Tepecik Training and Research Hospital, Izmir, Turkey
e-mail: huseyinsalih.semiz@deu.edu.tr

İ. Öztop
Dokuz Eylül University, Institute of Oncology, Izmir, Turkey
e-mail: ilhan.oztop@deu.edu.tr

14.1 Liver Metastases of Colorectal Cancers

Colorectal cancers (CRC) rank third in both genders in terms of incidence and cancer-related deaths [5]. The incidence of CRC has been reported to decrease by around 3% every year since 1990, and mortality due to CRC has also decreased gradually [6]. Approximately 20% of CRC cases have metastatic disease at diagnosis. The likelihood of developing liver metastasis during the follow-up period of patients diagnosed with CRC varies according to the stage of the disease and can reach high rates such as 50–70% [4]. The liver may be the only metastasis site in 30–40% of cases [7]. While only 20–25% of cases with liver metastasis due to CRC can be cured, this rate is expected to increase further with the development of systemic chemotherapy regimens, local treatment options, and liver surgery techniques [8]. Colorectal cancers and neuroendocrine tumors are of particular importance in this sense, while liver metastasis is an inoperability criterion for many tumors. This area has a special place since the experience gained over many years in patients with liver metastases due to colon cancer shows that longer survival can be achieved by metastasectomy [9]. However, the important point here is to determine whether a patient with liver metastasis will benefit from curative treatments. It is vitally important to choose the patients who are candidates for metastasectomy correctly in this sense. Many

R. Bekiş et al. (eds.), *Radionuclide Therapy*, https://doi.org/10.1007/978-3-030-97220-2_14

parameters such as patient-related factors [patient performance status (ECOG) and accompanying diseases] and tumor-related factors (anatomical location of the tumor, biological characteristics, etc.) are considered in patient selection. Tumor biology is one of the most important prognostic factors. There are scoring systems that estimate prognosis according to clinicopathological characteristics for patients scheduled for liver metastasectomy. The scoring system developed by Fong et al. is one of the first examples of this study investigating the results of metastasectomy in liver metastases due to CRC involving 1001 cases from Memorial Sloan Kettering Cancer Center (MSKCC).

Poor prognostic factors after metastasectomy were accepted as presence of metastasis greater than 5 cm, presence of multiple metastases, disease-free survival less than 1 year, primary tumor having lymph node metastasis, and carcinoembryogenic antigen (CEA) level more than 200 according to this system. Five-year survival was 60% in patients with no risk factor, while survival was 14% in patients with five risk factors according to the number of these risk factors [10]. It is important to consider these prognostic factors in patients undergoing metastasectomy in terms of the optimal patient selection. Starting with systemic chemotherapy in high-risk patients may allow the selection of patients who will progress in a short time and will not benefit from metastasectomy.

Successful results have been reported with conversion chemotherapy for cases that are not resectable at the time of diagnosis. Specifically, targeted molecules such as bevacizumab (antibody against vascular endothelial growth factor) and cetuximab and panitumumab (antibody against epidermal growth factor) may be added to conventional chemotherapies, allowing some patients to achieve a chance of resection. However, there is no standard approach to which treatment regimen will be used for this purpose. The addition of bevacizumab to conventional chemotherapy increases response rates but brings about wound healing problems. Therefore, it is recommended that the surgical procedure should be performed at least 4 weeks after the last bevacizumab dose or even 6–8 weeks if possible. Bevacizumab has a half-life of approximately 20 days. In addition, increased thromboembolic events, bowel perforation, and bleeding are among other possible side effects. It should be kept in mind that it may lead to loss of surgical chance even though the incidence of these side effects is low [11]. There are studies in which higher response rates are obtained with the FOLFOXIRI regimen in young patients and patients with good performance status even though a standard for the chemotherapy regimen to be administered before surgery in unresectable patients has not yet been described. A response rate of around 70% can be achieved, while resection rates can be around 20% with this regimen combining 5-fluorouracil (5-FU) and oxaliplatin and irinotecan [12]. An alternative for initially unresectable patients is the combination of hepatic intraarterial chemotherapy (HIAC) and systemic chemotherapy. HIAC is the administration of a chemotherapeutic agent, such as fluorodeoxyuridine, through the hepatic artery. This treatment aims to reduce systemic side effects and to ensure that chemotherapeutics reach high concentrations in the liver. The main logic of this method is that most of the metastases are fed through the hepatic artery and approximately half of the recurrences occur in the liver after metastasectomy.

Neoadjuvant systemic chemotherapy is available for subjects with initially resectable metastases. The main purpose of this administration is to eliminate systemic micrometastases and to select patients who will progress in the early period and will not benefit from surgery. Both NCCN (National Comprehensive Cancer Network) and ESMO (European Society for Medical Oncology) guidelines recommend oxaliplatin-based treatments even though there is no standard treatment regimen in neoadjuvant treatment [13, 14]. There is no significant difference between irinotecan-containing regimens and oxaliplatin-containing regimens except for toxicity profile in practice. One of the main concerns in neoadjuvant treatment is liver toxicity that may occur due to oxaliplatin and irinotecan. Both agents can cause steatohepatitis and sinusoidal damage. Therefore, it is recommended that neoadjuvant treatment should be retained as short as possible and patients should be referred to surgery after 6–8 weeks of treatment. Another problem with neoadjuvant therapy is that it may cause an increase in postoperative complication rates. However, it does not create a significant increase in mortality.

Therefore, it is useful to take these issues into consideration when selecting patients.

It is stated that adjuvant chemotherapy provides only disease-free survival (DFS) advantages after surgical treatment of liver metastases due to CRC, and its contribution to overall survival (OS) is not significant. For example, in the study of the European Organization for Research and Treatment of Cancer (EORTC) group using the FOLFOX regimen (oxaliplatin, 5-FU, folinic acid), patients were randomized to follow-up arm only after metastasectomy and a total of 6 months of systemic chemotherapy before and after metastasectomy. The advantages of progression-free survival (PFS) were shown in the group receiving chemotherapy in the 3-year follow-up results of this study, whereas this advantage was eliminated after 5-year follow-up [15]. In another study using the FOLFIRI regimen (irinotecan, 5-FU, folinic acid), 321 patients were included. Patients were divided into two groups after metastasectomy. 5-FU and folinic acid treatment was administered to one group, and irinotecan was administered to the other group in addition to this regimen. There was no DFS difference between the two groups [16]. The benefit of irinotecan in adjuvant therapy in stage 2 and 3 colorectal cancer patients has not been demonstrated. Therefore, all international guidelines agree that oxaliplatin is the agent to be added to 5-FU-based treatments. The regimen to be chosen for the post-resection treatment of metastatic patients should be a chemotherapy regimen containing oxaliplatin.

Unfortunately, up to 80% of patients are not suitable for metastasectomy, while the primary preference for liver metastases due to CRC is metastasectomy in eligible patients. Many local treatment options have also been tried to increase survival in these patients, while palliative systemic chemotherapy is the main approach for patients who cannot undergo surgery. These options include hyperthermic coagulation (radiofrequency ablation [RFA], microwave ablation, laser ablation), radionuclide therapies (yttrium-90 microsphere), ethanol injection, HIAC, radiotherapy (RT), and transarterial chemoembolization (TACE). The order in which systemic chemotherapy should be given with local treatments for the liver has not been clarified yet due to the lack of a sufficient number and size of randomized studies. Local treatments can be applied as the first-line treatment option to prolong the time to start systemic chemotherapy. However, the more widely adopted practice today is to evaluate local treatment options in patients who develop progression with systemic chemotherapy.

Chemotherapeutics commonly used in the treatment of metastatic colorectal cancer include 5-fluorouracil, capecitabine, oxaliplatin, and irinotecan. The main toxicities caused by these drugs are summarized below. The severity of toxicities is usually graded according to assessment methods such as the National Cancer Institute Common Terminology Criteria for Adverse Events (NCI-CTCAE) [17]. Approaches such as discontinuation, postponement, dose reduction, as well as specific approaches specific to toxicity are made depending on the type and degree of toxicity observed.

Main side effects of capecitabine include mucositis, diarrhea, palmar-plantar erythrodysesthesia (hand-foot syndrome), malaise, nausea, hematological toxicity, peripheral edema, hyperbilirubinemia, and fever. In addition, its interaction with warfarin is also emphasized. Early and life-threatening toxicities may occur in patients with deficiency in dihydropyrimidine dehydrogenase enzyme involved in the metabolism of capecitabine [18]. Main side effects of 5-fluorouracil include mucositis, diarrhea, palmar-plantar erythrodysesthesia (hand-foot syndrome), dermatitis, hematological toxicity, malaise, coronary spasm, angina pectoris, arrhythmia, acute cerebellar syndrome, cerebrovascular event, mesenteric ischemia, and nail changes. In addition, it interacts with warfarin.

Neutrophil decline as a hematological toxicity usually occurs between 9 and 14 days after 5-fluorouracil administration (Table 14.1) [17]. Nowadays, toxicities are relatively less common due to the preference of infusion 5-FU regimens rather than bolus regimens [19]. 5-FU toxicity increases unpredictably in individuals with dihydropyrimidine dehydrogenase (DPD) predominance who are responsible for 5-FU metabolism. The frequency of this enzyme deficiency in the society is less than 1%, but severe neutropenia, severe diarrhea, and severe mucositis may occur in these patients. In fact, these side effects can be fatal. The toxicities that may occur are related to the level of enzyme deficiency. Partial deficiency is seen at 3–15%, while complete loss of enzyme is seen at 0.1–0.5%. This approach is not accepted all over the world even though routine screening of this enzyme deficiency is recommended by some authorities [20]. However, patients who develop unexpected levels of toxicity should be kept in mind.

Main side effects of oxaliplatin include peripheral neuropathy, nausea, vomiting, diarrhea, pharyngolaryngeal dysesthesia, cold intolerance, infusion reaction, hematological toxicity, liver enzyme increase, and fever. It can also cause hypersensitivity reaction. Of these, peripheral neuropathy can be dose-limiting (Table 14.2) [17]. Neutrophil decline between hematological toxicities usually occurs between 9 and 14 days after oxaliplatin administration [21].

Main side effects of irinotecan include diarrhea, cholinergic syndrome, abdominal pain, nausea, vomiting, hematological toxicity, hepatotoxicity, bilirubin increase, alopecia, and malaise. Diarrhea can occur in two ways: early and late onset. Early-onset diarrhea occurs within the first 24 hours after irinotecan administration and is accompanied by cholinergic symptoms such as hypersalivation, flashing, and abdominal cramps. This side effect is usually treated with atropine. Blood pressure and heart rate should be monitored during atropine treatment. Late-onset diarrhea usually occurs 24 hours after irinotecan administration and may last longer. It can lead to life-threatening dehydration and electrolyte imbalance (Table 14.3) [17]. Late-onset diarrhea is actively treated with loperamide, diphenoxylate-atropine after exclusion of infectious factors, as well as fluid-electrolyte replacement [22]. Somatostatin analogs may be considered in treatment-resistant cases [23]. An important issue related to irinotecan is the increased toxicity in

Table 14.1 Hematological toxicity NCI-CTCAE v5.0 [17]

Blood element	Grade 1	Grade 2	Grade 3	Grade 4	Grade 5
Neutrophils	Between LLN and 1500/microL	1000–1500/microL	500–1000/microL	<500/microL	
Platelets	Between LLN and 75,000/microL	50,000–75,000/microL	25,000–50,000/microL	<25,000/microL	
Hemoglobin	Between LLN and 10.0 g/dL	8.0–10.0 g/dL	<8.0 g/dL	Life-threatening consequences; requiring urgent intervention	Death
Febrile neutropenia			Absolute number of neutrophils <1000 microL and presence of body temperature >38.30 °C at a single measurement or ≥38.00 °C lasting longer than 1 h	Life-threatening consequences; requiring urgent intervention	Death

NCI-CTCAE, National Cancer Institute Common Terminology Criteria for Adverse Events; LLN, lower limit of normal; cell/microL, cell/mm^3 or cell × 10^9/L

Table 14.2 Neurotoxicity NCI-CTCAE v5.0 [17]

Adverse event	Grade 1	Grade 2	Grade 3	Grade 4	Grade 5
Paresthesia	Moderate symptoms	Moderate symptoms; limiting daily life	Severe symptoms; limiting self-care		
Peripheral motor neuropathy	Asymptomatic; based on clinical or diagnostic observation only	Moderate symptoms; limiting daily life	Severe symptoms; limiting self-care	Life-threatening consequences; urgent intervention indicated	Death
Peripheral sensory neuropathy	Asymptomatic	Moderate symptoms; limiting daily life	Severe symptoms; limiting self-care	Life-threatening outcomes; urgent intervention indicated	

NCI-CTCAE, National Cancer Institute Common Terminology Criteria for Adverse Events

Table 14.3 Diarrhea NCI-CTCAE v5.0 [17]

Adverse event	Grade 1	Grade 2	Grade 3	Grade 4	Grade 5
Diarrhea	Increase of <4 defecations per day compared to basal; moderate increase in amount from ostomy compared to basal	Increase in the number of daily defecations compared to basal between 4 and 6; moderate increase in the amount from ostomy compared to basal	Increase of ≥7 defecations per day compared to basal; significant increase in amount from ostomy compared to basal; restriction of self-care	Life-threatening outcomes; urgent intervention indicated	Death

NCI-CTCAE, National Cancer Institute Common Terminology Criteria for Adverse Events

patients with UGT1A1 deficiency, an enzyme responsible for the metabolism of this agent. The likelihood of toxicity is very high especially in homozygous loss of UGT1A1*28 allele. Severe neutropenia and prolonged and severe diarrhea may occur in these cases. Therefore, irinotecan should be used by dose reduction in cases with UGT1A1 deficiency [24].

14.2 Primary Malignant Liver Tumors

14.2.1 Hepatocellular Carcinoma

Hepatocellular carcinoma (HCC) is the most common primary malignant tumor of the liver, usually developing based on chronic hepatitis or liver cirrhosis. It is less common compared to metastatic liver tumors. It usually has a poor clinical course and very short survival times. Its incidence is around 6 in 100,000 and ranks ninth among all cancers. Its frequency is gradually increasing in the last three decades, and it is thought that this increase may be due to the increase in the frequency of hepatitis C (HCV) infection [25]. Its distribution in the world is closely related to the prevalence of hepatitis B. It is most common in Asia and Africa, whereas it is least common in Australia, the United States, and Europe [26]. Hepatitis B (HBV) infection is one of the most important risk factors. Other risk factors include HCV infection, exposure to environmental toxic substances such as aflatoxin, nonalcoholic fatty liver, chronic alcohol use, smoking, family history, diabetes and obesity, hemochromatosis, and alpha-1 antitrypsin deficiency.

HCC is one of the tumors that has been shown to provide survival benefits of a number of screening programs. Therefore, it is recommended to include high-risk patients in these screening programs in terms of HCC development. Diagnosing HCC can sometimes be fairly difficult. Therefore, it is often necessary to use several diagnostic methods together. Radiological methods such as CT and MRI and nuclear medicine methods such as FDG-PET are used in this sense. FDG-PET makes a more important contribution especially in terms of distant metastasis scan [27]. The final pathological diagnosis is obtained by biopsy.

The staging of HCC is slightly different from other solid organ tumors. Most HCC patients cannot undergo surgery. Therefore, the TNM (tumor, node, metastasis) system, which performs staging according to pathological factors, is not reliable enough for HCC since it only considers tumor size, the presence of lymph node metastasis, and the presence of distant metastasis. In addition, this staging system has important deficiencies in terms of evaluation because it does not include parameters such as the functional capacity of the liver or the presence of acid with prognostic significance, serum albumin level, and bilirubin level for patients with cirrhosis.

These deficiencies can be eliminated by other staging systems. The best known of these are the Okuda system, the CLIP (Cancer of the Liver Italian Program) system, and the Barcelona staging system. Patients are divided into three stages according to tumor size, acid presence, and serum albumin and bilirubin levels in the Okuda system. A positive finding is considered if the tumor size is more than 50% of the liver size in cross-sectional measurements, albumin < 3 mg/dl, bilirubin > 3 mg/dl, or clinically significant ascites is present. If all results are negative, stage 1; if one or two results are positive, stage 2; if three or four results are positive, stage 3 is accepted. There are no prognostic results such as portal vein invasion and lymph node metastasis in this staging system as can be seen [28]. Child-Pugh score, tumor morphology, AFP level, and presence of portal vein thrombosis are taken into account in CLIP scoring. At least 0 point, at most 2 points, at least 0 point, and at most 1 point are given according to tumor morphological characteristics and Child score, portal vein thrombosis, and AFP level. The patient's score is obtained by adding these scores. OS was found to be 36, 22, 9, 7, and 3 months for patients with CLIP scores between 0, 1, 2, 3, and 4–6 in a study conducted according to the scores obtained in this way [29]. Patients are divided into four stages considering the spread of the tumor, the patient's performance status, vascular invasion and extrahepatic spread, Okuda stage, and the presence of constitutional symptoms in the Barcelona (BCLC= Barcelona Clinic Liver Cancer) system. Stage A to stage D survival deteriorates gradually. The Barcelona system is not only prognostic but also an important system in directing treatment [30]. Today, the best prognostic system is considered to be the TNM system in patients with HCC who have undergone surgical treatment, while the use of other systems in patients who are unsuitable for surgery and whose liver functions are poor may be a more appropriate approach.

The main treatment method for HCC is surgery in early-stage disease. There is no method that has been shown to be superior to surgical resection in local disease yet. Surgical treatment can be performed as tumor resection or liver transplantation. However, the number of patients suitable for surgery is unfortunately fairly limited since the disease is usually diagnosed at advanced stages. Generally, Child A and B patients are eligible for tumor resection, whereas Child C patients are eligible for organ transplantation. Patients suitable for resection are generally considered to have a single tumor, sufficient liver reserve, no major vascular invasion, no portal hypertension, no distant metastasis, and good performance apart from the Child score. It is stated that patients with tumor size over 5 cm may also be surgical candidates provided that they are performed in experienced centers even though tumor size (>5 cm) is seen as an obstacle for surgical resection for some clinics [31].

Another important surgical method in HCC treatment is liver transplantation. There are internationally accepted Barcelona criteria and Milan criteria for transplantation. Guidelines such as EASL and AASLD also accept these criteria. Liver transplant candidates are patients with a single tumor of 5 cm or less, patients with a maximum of three tumors of 3 cm or less, and patients without major vascular invasion and no extrahepatic involvement according to Milan criteria. The EASL guideline recommends reevaluation for transplantation in patients who do not meet these criteria and do not have metastasis if Milan criteria are met after tumor reduction by local or systemic treatment methods. One of the most important problems for patients who meet the criteria to be transplant candidates is their long waiting times until the appropriate donor comes out. International guidelines emphasize that other local treatments can be administered during this waiting period, thus reducing the risk of developing metastatic disease [32–34].

Treatment options in patients unsuitable for surgery include transarterial chemoembolization (TACE), radiofrequency ablation (RFA), cryoablation, injection of ethanol from the wig, SBRT, radioembolization (TARE), systemic chemotherapy, and tyrosine kinase inhibitors such as sorafenib or regorafenib.

Systemic treatment options should be evaluated in patients inappropriate for local treatments or patients with metastatic HCC. These treatment options include sorafenib, regorafenib, lenvatinib, and cabozantinib, a multikinase inhibitor with anti-vascular endothelial growth factor (VEGF). Today, systemic chemotherapies are not preferred as a treatment of HCC. These treatments do not provide a survival advantage and are toxic treatments. Furthermore, HCC is generally considered to be a chemoresistant tumor. Sorafenib was considered the first-line treatment option in HCC after Llovet et al. showed in the SHARP study published in 2008 that it provided a 3-month OS and radiological PFS advantage compared to the best supportive care [35]. Suitable patients for sorafenib can be summarized as metastatic, progressive after local treatments or unsuitable for local treatments, patients with Child A cirrhosis, and patients with adequate organ function and performance. Sorafenib is not recommended for use in Child C patients as it causes intense toxicities and an increase in mortality rates. The survival advantage is very limited, and the toxicity-benefit ratio shifts toward toxicity in Child B patient. Lenvatinib is also an option in first-line treatment. Lenvatinib was found to be non-inferior to sorafenib in patients with unresectable or metastatic HCC who had not received systemic treatment before in the REFLECT study published by Kudo et al. Lenvatinib is a first-line treatment option such as sorafenib [36]. Regorafenib after progression with sorafenib is one of the options. Regorafenib was superior in terms of OS, objective response rates, and disease control rates compared to placebo in patients who progressed with sorafenib in the RESORCE study conducted by Bruix et al. [37]. Another alternative to second-line therapy is nivolumab, a monoclonal antibody that specifically inhibits the PD-1 molecule involved in inhibiting T-cell immune response. Objective response rates with nivolumab were found between 15 and 20%, and median survival was found around 15 months. Phase 3 studies of nivolumab, the toxicity profile of which is quite different from tyrosine kinase inhibitors, are still ongoing [38].

14.2.2 Side Effects of TKIs Used in the Treatment of Hepatocellular Carcinoma

Main side effects of sorafenib and lenvatinib include malaise, diarrhea, hypertension, hand-foot syndrome, myelosuppression, bleeding, thyroid dysfunction, arterial thromboembolism, and QT prolongation [39–42]. Side effects of nivolumab, an anti-PD1 agent, include myelosuppression, thyroid dysfunction (hypo-hyperthyroidism), diarrhea, nausea, elevated transaminase, and immune-related events such as hepatitis, pneumonitis and itching, rash, and erythema [43].

Expert advice from an international reconciliation group is available for hand-foot syndrome (HFSR) which occurs with sorafenib. The most important of these recommendations are the removal of existing hyperkeratotic areas and calluses using appropriately sterilized tools, avoiding exposure of hands and feet to hot water, and avoiding excessive friction on the skin in daily activities. It should be emphasized that severe exercises that exert excessive stress especially on the palms and/or soles of the feet should be avoided, especially during the first treatment period. It should be recommended to wear padded soles throughout treatment to reduce foot pressure. Patients should be warned to wear thick cotton gloves or socks to prevent injury and to keep palms and soles dry [44, 45].

The following management strategies are recommended for patients who develop HFSR while receiving sorafenib [44, 46].

No dose adjustment is required for mild (grade 1) symptoms. Hot water should be avoided and the use of topical softeners should be encouraged. Keratolytics such as topical urea (20–40%) or salicylic acid (6–10%) may be recommended.

Treatment for grade 2 HFSR should continue as in grade 1 HFSR, but with topical corticosteroids (clobetasol 0.05% ointment) added to erythematous areas twice daily. Topical analgesics such as 2% lidocaine may be sufficient. If necessary, the dose of sorafenib may be temporarily reduced by up to 50% for at least 7 days until HFSR grade 0 or 1 is reached, and then the full dose can be resumed. For grade 3 HFSR, treatment according to grade 1 or 2 HFSR should be provided upon temporary discontinuation of the drug for at least 7 days until grade 1 or 2. Treatment should continue up to 50% of the dose. Dose increase can be attempted if the side effect is not repeated [44–46].

Sorafenib is also associated with cutaneous squamoproliferative lesions, including keratoacanthomas (KA) and squamous cell carcinomas (SCC) [47, 48]. Twenty-two squamoproliferative lesions were seen in 13 patients within 9 months of initiation in a series after starting sorafenib. One was reported as classic invasive SCC, 5 as KA-like SCC, and 16 as classic KA [47, 48]. Squamoproliferative lesions that develop during treatment with sorafenib should be treated in a similar manner to lesions that develop in patients who have not taken any drug (usually with complete surgical excision). There is no definite evidence to continue against discontinuation of sorafenib in patients who develop SCC or KA during treatment. Close clinical follow-up is required during treatment [46].

Thyroid dysfunction appears more frequently in patients receiving sunitinib for metastatic RCC, but can be seen in patients treated with sorafenib [49]. In general, these agents are stated to have a class effect [50–52, 53]. Regular monitoring of TSH levels at baseline and during treatment is recommended in patients treated with antiangiogenic TKIs due to the high frequency of hypothyroidism, initial evaluation of thyroid function tests, and subsequent and every 4 to 12 weeks monitoring in symptomatic patients. Symptomatic patients with hypothyroidism should receive thyroid hormone support. No discontinuation of the agent causing toxicity and no dose modification are usually necessary [3, 13, 53].

Nausea (all grades) was reported in 23% to 58% of patients treated with antiangiogenic TKIs in clinical trials. Sunitinib-, lenvatinib-, and cabozantinib-treated patients had the highest rates. Vomiting of any grade was reported in 10% to 48% of patients treated with pazopanib and sorafenib with the lowest and sunitinib, lenvatinib, and cabozantinib with highest rates [54–57]. Nausea and vomiting are rarely severe and are usually controlled with oral antiemetics. However, caution should be exercised in combining vandetanib, lenvatinib, sunitinib, and sorafenib with serotonin antagonists such as granisetron and ondansetron due to QTc interval prolongation and torsades de pointes (especially with BRAF inhibitors) [53].

Infections should be treated in accordance with their degree after being excluded in addition to performing fluid-electrolyte replacement in case of diarrhea. It is generally sufficient to prevent food and supplements that increase symptomatic management and gastrointestinal motility with an oral antidiarrheal agent such as loperamide in the treatment of grade 1 or 2 diarrhea. Treatment should be discontinued for grade 3 or 4 diarrhea, and dose modifications may be required to control diarrhea if the drug is continued [58].

Sorafenib-induced hepatitis can be accompanied by hepatocellular hepatic injury, which is a significant increase in transaminases that can result in hepatic failure and death (Table 14.4) [17]. There may also be increases in bilirubin and INR. It is recommended to exclude the causes

Table 14.4 Hepatobiliary toxicity NCI-CTCAE v5.0 [17]

Adverse event	Grade 1	Grade 2	Grade 3	Grade 4	Grade 5
ALP increase	If baseline is normal, ULN to 2.5 × ULN; if baseline is abnormal, 2–2.5 × baseline	If baseline is normal, 2.5–5 × ULN; if baseline is abnormal, 2.5–5 × baseline	If baseline is normal, 5–20 × ULN; if baseline is abnormal, 5–20 × baseline	If baseline is normal, >20 × ULN; If baseline is abnormal, >20 × baseline	
ALT increase	If baseline is normal, ULN to 3 × ULN; if baseline is abnormal, 1.5–3 × baseline	If baseline is normal, 3–5 × ULN; if baseline is abnormal, 3–5 × baseline	If baseline is normal, 5–20 × ULN; if baseline is abnormal, 5–20 × baseline	If baseline is normal, >20 × ULN; if baseline is abnormal, >20 × baseline	
AST increase	If baseline is normal, ULN to 3 × ULN; if baseline is abnormal, 1.5–3 × baseline	If baseline is normal, 3–5 × ULN; if baseline is abnormal, 3–5 × baseline	If baseline is normal, 5–20 × ULN; if baseline is abnormal, 5 to 20 x baseline	If baseline is normal, >20 × ULN; if baseline is abnormal, >20 × baseline	
Serum bilirubin increase	If baseline is normal, ULN to 1.5 × ULN; if baseline is abnormal, 1–1.5 × baseline	If baseline is normal, 1.5–3 × ULN; if baseline is abnormal, 1.5–3 × baseline	If baseline is normal, 3–10 × ULN; if baseline is abnormal, 3–10 × baseline	If baseline is normal, >10 × ULN; if baseline is abnormal, >10 × baseline	
GGT increase	If baseline is normal, ULN to 2.5 × ULN; if baseline is abnormal, 2–2.5 × baseline	If baseline is normal, 2.5–5 × ULN; if baseline is abnormal, 2.5–5 × baseline	If baseline is normal, 5–20 × ULN; if baseline is abnormal, 5–20 × baseline	If baseline is normal, >20 × ULN; if baseline is abnormal, >20 × baseline	
Liver failure			Asterixis, moderate encephalopathy, liver injury due to the drug, limitation of self-care	Life-threatening outcomes, moderate-severe encephalopathy, coma	Death
Portal hypertension		Decrease in portal vein flow	Reverse/retrograde portal vein flow with varicose and/or acid	Life-threatening outcomes, requiring urgent intervention	Death

NCI-CTCAE, National Cancer Institute Common Terminology Criteria for Adverse Events; ULN, upper limit of normal; ALP, alkaline phosphatase; ALT, alanine aminotransferase; AST, aspartate aminotransferase; GGT, gamma-glutamyl transpeptidase

such as viral hepatitis or progressive malignancy first and to discontinue the drug considering drug-related hepatotoxicity in case of a significant increase in transaminases [53, 59]. In general, liver function tests (LFTs) should be periodically evaluated at baseline and during treatment in patients treated with any of the TKIs.

Evaluation of liver function tests is recommended, especially for patients treated with pazopanib, at baseline and at weeks 3, 5, 7, 9, 12, and 16 and periodically thereafter, and interruption or complete discontinuation of treatment is recommended in patients with bilirubin levels 3 times and above [60, 61].

Another problem encountered during the use of antiangiogenic TKIs is hypertension. Recommendations in this regard include risk assessment for potential cardiovascular complications, identification and treatment of existing hypertension before using these agents, active monitoring of blood pressure during treatment, more frequent measurements in the first few weeks of treatment, and lower blood pressure in those with preexisting cardiovascular risk factors such as diabetes or chronic kidney disease [62]. Patients who develop hypertension during treatment (defined as hypertension; blood pressure ≥140/90 mmHg or 20 mmHg increase in diastolic blood pressure compared to basal) should be treated with antihypertensives. Agent selection should be based on the severity of hypertension and the urgency of blood pressure control. It is very important to avoid from verapamil or diltiazem that undergoes partial metabolism with cytochrome p450 such as sunitinib/sorafenib even though it is not an optimal antihypertensive agent recommendation [63].

There is also an increase in the risk of venous and arterial thromboembolism with antiangiogenic TKIs. Both prevention and rapid management of arterial thromboembolic (ATE) events are important. Cardiovascular risk factors (e.g., hypertension, hyperlipidemia, and diabetes) should be predetermined and aggressively managed prior to initiating treatment with antiangiogenic TKIs. Basal blood pressure should be monitored, and the drug should preferably not be administered within 6–12 months in patients with severe cardiovascular events. Low-dose aspirin prophylaxis is appropriate in patients with ATE or other high-risk patients [62, 64, 65]. Antiangiogenic treatment should be discontinued, and ATE should be managed as in other patients who develop ATE while receiving antiangiogenic TKI.

Left ventricular (LV) function may decrease in patients treated with any of the VEGF-targeted treatments. Therefore, screening of LVEF of patients with ECHO or MUGA and evaluation with ECG are recommended. Some sources have suggested that patients receiving these drugs should be treated as "stage A" heart failure patients (but without structural heart disease or symptoms, i.e., at risk of heart failure) [66]. The American Heart Association guideline states that it may be reasonable to consider those who receive potentially cardiotoxic agents for LV dysfunction as stage A heart failure in 2013 [67].

Another important toxicity associated with VEGF receptor tyrosine kinase inhibitors is QT prolongation on ECG. The risk of other VEGFR-TKIs, including sorafenib and pazopanib, is lower, while vandetanib and sunitinib are more associated with QTc prolongation [68, 69]. Specific guidelines for the evaluation and monitoring of the QTc interval and recommendations for managing the toxicities are available, especially for vandetanib and lenvatinib. Guidelines for other antiangiogenic TKIs are not yet available. Concomitant drugs should be carefully reviewed; especially drugs that increase QTc should be evaluated for any patient receiving treatment with antiangiogenic TKI. Those with a history of QT interval prolongation, a history of arrhythmia, and preexisting heart disease, bradycardia, or electrolyte disorder may be more prone to develop QTc prolongation. Dose reduction for TKI may be required if antiangiogenic TKIs are to be taken concomitantly with strong CYP3A4 inhibitors that may increase plasma concentrations. Patients who develop arrhythmia should be evaluated and treated separately with cardiological consultation according to the definition of arrhythmia [41, 62].

References

1. Bahirwani R, Reddy KR. Review article: the evaluation of solitary liver masses. Aliment Pharmacol Ther. 2008;28(8):953–65.
2. Paredis V. Benign liver tumors: an update. Clin Liver Dis. 2010;14(4):719–29.
3. Assy N, Nasser G, Djibre A, et al. Characteristics of common solid liver lesions and recommendations for diagnostic workup. World J Gastroenterol. 2009;15(26):3217–27.
4. Göksoy E, Kapan M. İ.Ü. Cerrahpaşa Tıp Fakültesi Sürekli Tıp Eğitimi Etkinlikleri. Hepato-Bilier Sistem ve Pankreas Hastalıkları. Sempozyum Dizisi. No: 28, Ocak 2002; s. 183–190.
5. American Cancer Society. Cancer facts & figures 2018. Atlanta: American Cancer Society; 2018.
6. Jemal A, Ward EM, Johnson CJ, et al. Annual report to the nation on the status of cancer, 1975–2014, featuring survival. J Natl Cancer Inst. 2017;109(9)
7. Hugh TJ, Kinsella AR, Poston GJ. Management strategies for colorectal liver metastases—Part I. Surg Oncol. 1997;6:19–30.
8. Robertson DJ, Stukel TA, Gottlieb DJ, Sutherland JM, Fisher ES. Survival after hepatic resection of colorec-

tal cancer metastases: a national experience. Cancer. 2009;115(4):752–9.
9. Tomlinson JS, Jarnagin WR, DeMatteo RP, et al. Actual 10-year survival after resection of colorectal liver metastases defines cure. J Clin Oncol. 2007;25:4575–80.
10. Fong Y, Fortner J, Sun RL, et al. Clinical score for predicting recurrence after hepatic resection for metastatic colorectal cancer: analysis of 1001 consecutive cases. Ann Surg. 1999;230:309–18. discussion 318–321
11. Walter H, Thomas AL. Liver resection following FOLFOXIRI plus bevacizumab: a detailed pathological review. Br J Cancer. 2013;108(12):2417–8.
12. Masi G, Loupakis F, Pollina L, et al. Long-term outcome of initially unresectable metastatic colorectal cancer patients treated with 5-fluorouracil/leucovorin, oxaliplatin, and irinotecan (FOLFOXIRI) followed by radical surgery of metastases. Ann Surg. 2009;249(3):420–5.
13. National Comprehensive Cancer Network (NCCN) website. NCCN Clinical practice guidelines in oncology. Available at: https://www.nccn.org/professionals/physician_gls/pdf/colon.pdf (Accessed on 30 January, 2019).
14. Van Cutsem E, Cervantes A, Adam R, et al. ESMO Consensus Guidelines for the management of patients with metastatic colorectal cancer. Ann Oncol. 2016;8:1386–422.
15. Nordlinger B, Sorbye H, Glimelius B, et al. Perioperative FOLFOX4 chemotherapy and surgery versus surgery alone for resectable liver metastases from colorectal cancer (EORTC 40983): long-term results of a randomised, controlled, phase 3 trial. Lancet Oncol. 2013;14:1208–15.
16. Portier G, Elias D, Bouche O, et al. Multicenter randomized trial of adjuvant fluorouracil and folinic acid compared with surgery alone after resection of colorectal liver metastases: FFCD ACHBTH AURC 9002 trial. J Clin Oncol. 2006;24:4976–82.
17. https://ctep.cancer.gov/protocoldevelopment/electronic_applications/docs/CTCAE_v5_Quick_Reference_8.5x11.pdf (Accessed on March 09, 2018).
18. http://www.bccancer.bc.ca/drug-database-site/Drug%20Index/Capecitabine_monograph.pdf
19. http://www.bccancer.bc.ca/drug-database-site/Drug%20Index/Fluorouracil_monograph.pdf
20. Loriot MA, Ciccolini J, Thomas F, et al. Dihydropyrimidine déhydrogenase (DPD) deficiency screening and securing of fluoropyrimidine-based chemotherapies: update and recommendations of the French GPCO-Unicancer and RNPGx networks. Bull Cancer. 2018;105(4):397–407.
21. http://www.bccancer.ca/drug-atabasesite/Drug%20Index/Oxaliplatin_monograph_1Dec2016.pdf
22. http://www.bccancer.bc.ca/drug-database-site/Drug%20Index/Irinotecan_monograph.pdf
23. Saliba F, Hagipantelli R, Misset JL, et al. Pathophysiology and therapy of irinotecan-induced delayed-onset diarrhea in patients with advanced colorectal cancer: a prospective assessment. J Clin Oncol. 1998;16(8):2745.
24. Hu Z-Y, Yu Q, Pei Q, Guo C. Dose-dependent association between UGT1A1*28 genotype and irinotecan-induced neutropenia: low doses also increase risk. Clin Cancer Res. 2010;15:3832–42. https://doi.org/10.1158/1078-0432.CCR-10-1122.
25. El-Serag HB, Kanwal F. Epidemiology of hepatocellular carcinoma in the United States: where are we? Where do we go? Hepatology. 2014;60:1767.
26. Ferlay J, Soerjomataram I, Dikshit R, Eser S, Mathers C, Rebelo M, Parkin DM, Forman D, Bray F. Cancer incidence and mortality worldwide: sources, methods and major patterns in GLOBOCAN 2012. Int J Cancer. 2015;136(5):E359–86. Epub 2014 Oct 9
27. Trojan J, Schroeder O, Raedle J, Baum RP, Herrmann G, Jacobi V, Zeuzem S. Fluorine-18 FDG positron emission tomography for imaging of hepatocellular carcinoma. Am J Gastroenterol. 1999;94(11):3314–9.
28. Okuda K, Ohtsuki T, Obata H, et al. Natural history of hepatocellular carcinoma and prognosis in relation to treatment. Study of 850 patients. Cancer. 1985;56(4):918–28.
29. Farinati F, Rinaldi M, Gianni S, Naccarato R. How should patients with hepatocellular carcinoma be staged? Validation of a new prognostic system. Cancer. 2000;89(11):2266–73.
30. Llovet JM, Brú C, Bruix J. Prognosis of hepatocellular carcinoma: The BCLC Staging Classification. Semin Liver Dis. 1999;19(3):329–38.
31. Liu JH, Chen PW, Asch SM, Busuttil RW, Ko CY. Surgery for hepatocellular carcinoma: does it improve survival? Ann Surg Oncol. 2004;11(3):298–303.
32. National Comprehensive Cancer Network (NCCN) website. NCCN Clinical practice guidelines in oncology. Available at: https://www.nccn.org/professionals/physician_gls/pdf/hepatobiliary.pdf (Accessed on 30 January, 2019).
33. Vogel A, Cervantes A, Chau I, et al. Hepatocellular Carcinoma: ESMO Clinical Practice Guidelines for diagnosis, treatment and follow-up. Ann Oncol. 2018;29(Suppl. 4):iv238-iv255.
34. Heimbach JK, Kulik LM, Finn RS, et al. AASLD guidelines for the treatment of hepatocellular carcinoma. Hepatology. 2018;67(1):358–80.
35. Llovet JM, Ricci S, Mazzaferro V, SHARP Investigators Study Group, et al. Sorafenib in advanced hepatocellular carcinoma. N Engl J Med. 2008;359(4):378–90.
36. Kudo M, Finn RS, Qin S, et al., Kudo M, et al. Lenvatinib versus sorafenib in first-line treatment of patients with unresectable hepatocellular carcinoma: a randomised phase 3 non-inferiority trial. Lancet. 2018;391(10126):1163–73.
37. Bruix J, Qin S, Merle P, et al. Regorafenib for patients with hepatocellular carcinoma who progressed on sorafenib treatment (RESORCE): a randomised, double-blind, placebo-controlled, phase 3 trial. Lancet. 2017;389(10064):56–66.

38. El-Khoueiry AB, Sangro B, Yau T, et al. Nivolumab in patients with advanced hepatocellular carcinoma (CheckMate 040): an open-label, non-comparative, phase 1/2 dose escalation and expansion trial. Lancet. 2017;389(10088):2492–502.
39. Nexavar (sorafenib) [product monograph]. Toronto, ON: Bayer Inc.; May 2013.
40. http://www.bccancer.bc.ca/drug-database-site/Drug%20Index/Sorafenib_monograph.pdf
41. Lenvima (lenvatinib) [product monograph]. Mississauga, ON: Eisai Limited; December 2018.
42. http://www.bccancer.bc.ca/drug-database-site/Drug%20Index/Lenvatinib_monograph.pdf
43. http://www.bccancer.bc.ca/drug-database-site/Drug%20Index/Nivolumab_monograph.pdf
44. Lacouture ME, Wu S, Robert C, et al. Evolving strategies for the management of hand-foot skin reaction associated with the multitargeted kinase inhibitors sorafenib and sunitinib. Oncologist. 2008;13(9):1001–11.
45. Boone SL, Jameson G, Von Hoff D, et al. Blackberry-induced hand-foot skin reaction to sunitinib. Invest New Drugs. 2009;27(4):389–90.
46. UpToDate website. Available at: https://www.uptodate.com/contents/cutaneous-side-effects-of-molecularly-targeted-therapy-and-other-biologic-agents-used-for-cancer-therapy
47. Arnault JP, Wechsler J, Escudier B, et al. Keratoacanthomas and squamous cell carcinomas in patients receiving sorafenib. J Clin Oncol. 2009;27(23):e59. Epub 2009 Jul 13
48. Dubauskas Z, Kunishige J, Prieto VG, et al. Cutaneous squamous cell carcinoma and inflammation of actinic keratoses associated with sorafenib. Clin Genitourin Cancer. 2009;7(1):20–3.
49. Feldt S, Schüssel K, Quinzler R, et al. Incidence of thyroid hormone therapy in patients treated with sunitinib or sorafenib: a cohort study. Eur J Cancer. 2012;48(7):974–81.
50. Fujiwara Y, Kiyota N, Chayahara N, et al. Management of axitinib (AG-013736)-induced fatigue and thyroid dysfunction, and predictive biomarkers of axitinib exposure: results from phase I studies in Japanese patients. Invest New Drugs. 2012;30(3):1055–64.
51. Figlin RA, de Souza P, McDermott D, et al. Analysis of PTEN and HIF-1alpha and correlation with efficacy in patients with advanced renal cell carcinoma treated with temsirolimus versus interferon-alpha. Cancer. 2009;115(16):3651–60.
52. Sternberg CN, Davis ID, Mardiak J, et al. Pazopanib in locally advanced or metastatic renal cell carcinoma: results of a randomized phase III trial. J Clin Oncol. 2010;28(6):1061–8.
53. UpToDate website. Available at: https://www.uptodate.com/contents/toxicity-of-molecularly-targeted-antiangiogenic-agents-non-cardiovascular-effects
54. Schlumberger M, Tahara M, Wirth LJ, et al. Lenvatinib versus placebo in radioiodine-refractory thyroid cancer. N Engl J Med. 2015;372:621–30.
55. Smith DC, Smith MR, Sweeney C, et al. Cabozantinib in patients with advanced prostate cancer: results of a phase II randomized discontinuation trial. J Clin Oncol. 2013;31:412–9.
56. Raymond E, Dahan L, Raoul JL, et al. Sunitinib malate for the treatment of pancreatic neuroendocrine tumors. N Engl J Med. 2011;364:501.
57. Motzer RJ, Hutson TE, Tomczak P, et al. Overall survival and updated results for sunitinib compared with interferon alfa in patients with metastatic renal cell carcinoma. J Clin Oncol. 2009;27:3584–90.
58. Eisen T, Sternberg CN, Robert C, et al. Targeted therapies for renal cell carcinoma: review of adverse event management strategies. J Natl Cancer Inst. 2012;104:93–113.
59. Ghatalia P, Je Y, Mouallem NE, et al. Hepatotoxicity with vascular endothelial growth factor receptor tyrosine kinase inhibitors: a meta-analysis of randomized clinical trials. Crit Rev Oncol Hematol. 2015;93:257–76.
60. Shibata SI, Chung V, Synold TW, et al. Phase I study of pazopanib in patients with advanced solid tumors and hepatic dysfunction: a National Cancer Institute Organ Dysfunction Working Group study. Clin Cancer Res. 2013;19:3631–9.
61. Shibata S, Longmate J, Chung VM, et al. A phase I and pharmacokinetic single agent study of pazopanib in patients with advanced malignancies and varying degrees of liver dysfunction (Abstract 2571). J Clin Oncol. 2010;28:221s.
62. UpToDate website. Available at: https://www.uptodate.com/contents/toxicity-of-molecularly-targeted-antiangiogenic-agents-cardiovascular-effects
63. Sica DA. Angiogenesis inhibitors and hypertension: an emerging issue. J Clin Oncol. 2006;24:1329–31.
64. Patrono C, Coller B, FitzGerald GA, et al. Platelet-active drugs: the relationships among dose, effectiveness, and side effects: the Seventh ACCP Conference on Antithrombotic and Thrombolytic Therapy. Chest. 2004;126:234S.
65. Tran H, Anand SS. Oral antiplatelet therapy in cerebrovascular disease, coronary artery disease, and peripheral arterial disease. JAMA. 2004;292:1867–74.
66. Chintalgattu V, Patel SS, Khakoo AY. Cardiovascular effects of tyrosine kinase inhibitors used for gastrointestinal stromal tumors. Hematol Oncol Clin N Am. 2009;23:97–107.
67. Yancy CW, Jessup M, Bozkurt B, et al. 2013 ACCF/AHA guideline for the management of heart failure: a report of the American College of Cardiology Foundation/American Heart Association Task Force on Practice Guidelines. J Am Coll Cardiol. 2013;62:e147–239.
68. Shah RR, Morganroth J, Shah DR. Cardiovascular safety of tyrosine kinase inhibitors: with a special focus on cardiac repolarisation (QT interval). Drug Saf. 2013;36:295–316.
69. Ghatalia P, Je Y, Kaymakcalan MD, et al. QTc interval prolongation with vascular endothelial growth factor receptor tyrosine kinase inhibitors. Br J Cancer. 2015;112:296–305.

Part VI

Clinical Information: Prostate Cancer

15 Radionuclide Therapy in Prostate Cancer

Emine Acar, Recep Bekiş, and Berna Polack

15.1 Incidence, Epidemiology, and Etiology of Prostate Cancer

Prostate cancer is the second most common disease in Turkey and in the world after lung cancer in men according to Turkey's cancer statistics 2017 report. Prostate cancer is the most common type of cancer in the member countries of the international cancer agency, Europe, and the United States in men. The rate of incidence in Turkey varies between 32.9 and 39.2 in 100,000 people [1].

Hypertension alone or waist circumference >102 cm is an increased risk factor for prostate cancer. The risk of high-grade prostate cancer increases in the presence of obesity. However, the presence of three or more metabolic syndrome components is a reduced risk factor for prostate cancer. Excessive use of alcohol and both high and low serum vitamin D levels were found to be associated with the development of prostate cancer [2].

Five-year survival in metastatic disease decreases to 31% even though 5-year survival is 100% in localized prostate cancer [3].

E. Acar (✉) · R. Bekiş · B. Polack
Faculty of Medicine, Department of Nuclear Medicine, Dokuz Eylul University, Izmir, Turkey
e-mail: emine.acar@kenthospital.com; recep.bekis@deu.edu.tr; berna.degirmeci@deu.edu.tr

15.1.1 Genetics in Prostate Cancer

Familial prostate cancer is the presence of prostate cancer in three or more relatives of the person, who were at least diagnosed before the age of 55 [2]. The incidence of prostate cancer increases by more than 4 times in people with prostate cancer in the first-degree relative before the age of 60 compared to the normal population. If a person is diagnosed with prostate cancer, they are 50% more likely to have prostate cancer in a monozygotic twin than in a dizygotic twin. Five percent of familial prostate cancers are associated with BRCA1, BRCA2, ATM, HOXB13, MMR, NBS1, and CHEK2. Seventy-seven single nucleotide polymorphisms in more than 20 genes in 30% have been reported to be associated with prostate cancer. However, 65% of familial prostate cancer cases cannot be genetically explained. Prostate cancer patients with the BRCA2 mutation have a higher Gleason score and a worse prognosis compared to those without it [2, 4].

15.1.2 Carcinogenesis and Molecular Subclassification

It is possible to detect gene rearrangement with the routine introduction of next-generation DNA sequencing. Gene rearrangement detection may provide insight into carcinogenesis, clonal hierarchy characterization, and androgen-dependent ETS gene expression. The pres-

R. Bekiş et al. (eds.), *Radionuclide Therapy*, https://doi.org/10.1007/978-3-030-97220-2_15

ence of ETS gene fusion alone is not sufficient to create cancer. In addition, the PI3K/AKT pathway must be activated, and PTEN loss is also required [5]. The PI3K/AKT/mTOR pathway is responsible for cell survival, apoptosis, cell proliferation, autophagy, metabolism, and protein synthesis. PI3K can be activated by various growth factors (EGFR, IGF-1R, FGFR, PDGFR) and signal pathways [6].

ETS status can be different from each other even in the lobes of cancer in the same prostate gland. PTEN and TP53 mutation or loss, which are tumor suppressor genes, are most commonly observed in prostate cancer. SPINK1, a serine protease inhibitor, is highly expressed in 5–10% of prostate cancers.

Cancers with SPINK1 expression were ETS negative. SHELF, RAS, and FGFR mutations have also been identified in prostate cancer even though it is less frequent. Mutation is seen in the SPOP gene accumulated in the binding area of the encoded protein in 5–10% of prostate cancers. CHD1 mutation and homozygous deletion are seen in 5–15% of prostate cancers [5].

Androgen suppression therapy is used in prostate cancer because androgens direct prostate cancer cells to grow. Androgen suppression therapy is not sufficient in some tumors even though an increase in survival is observed with androgen suppression therapy. This occurs secondary to the loss of androgen sensitivity of the cells. Androgen receptor genes may undergo amplification independent of feedback mechanisms or increase tumor cell androgen receptor mRNA expression [6].

All these steps described above allow the prostate cancer cell to grow and metastasize. The most important step in the metastatic process is epithelial-mesenchymal transition. The tumor cell loses its epithelial properties, gains mesenchymal cell properties, and makes intravasation, and tumor cells are released into the circulation, make extravasation in the area where they will metastasize, then lose mesenchymal cell properties in the metastatic area, regain epithelial properties, and start to multiply.

15.2 Diagnosis of Prostate Cancer

Prostate-specific antigen (PSA) monitoring is the most important biochemical marker in diagnosing prostate cancer. PSA is specific to prostate tissue, not prostate cancer; thus an increase is also observed in non-cancer cases (benign prostate hyperplasia, prostatitis) [7]. PSA follow-up diagnoses early prostate cancer and reduces mortality. On the other hand, PSA may bring unnecessary prostate biopsies in case of PSA elevation due to its nonspecificity to the cancer cell. PSA threshold value for prostate cancer is used as 4 ng/mL. It causes overdiagnosis in 30–50% of patients, while this value leads to unnecessary biopsy in 75% of patients [5]. One in two people has prostate cancer when PSA value is >10 ng/mL, while one in four people is diagnosed with prostate cancer at PSA values of 4–10 ng/mL [8].

It was reported in the European randomized prostate cancer scan study (ERSPC) that prostate cancer-related mortality decreased in healthy subjects followed up with PSA scan for 9–11 years. On the other hand, the scan causes overdiagnosis and overtreatment in 40–50% of patients. These conditions disrupt patient comfort by causing side effects secondary to therapy (urinary, sexual, gastrointestinal problems) [9].

It is the first digital rectal examination to be performed in case of clinical suspicion of the patient or when PSA is above 4 ng/mL [5]. Because most tumors are localized in the peripheral zone, lesions ≥0.2 mL can be detected during digital rectal examination. Abnormal digital rectal examination result is associated with high Gleason score and is an indication for biopsy [2]. Rectal ultrasound (USG) can be performed, and prostate gland volume and suspicious lesions can be visualized after the examination. Biopsy of the palpable lesion or USG-guided lesion during examination increases the likelihood of diagnosis.

Serum-free/total PSA ratio can be used to differentiate benign prostate hypertrophy (BPH) from prostate cancer. If PSA value is between 4 and 10 ng/mL, there is no palpable result on digital rectal examination; if serum-free/total PSA ratio is <0.10 ng/mL, prostate cancer is diagnosed by biopsy at 56%; while if serum-free/total PSA ratio is >0.25 ng/mL, prostate cancer is diagnosed by biopsy at 8% [2].

Prostate cancer gene 3 (PCA3) is a prostate-specific, noncoding mRNA biomarker. It can be measured in urine sediment after massaging the prostate during digital rectal examination [2].

15.2.1 Prostate Cancer Biopsy

The need for prostate biopsy is determined by serum PSA value and/or digital rectal examination result. If prostate gland sizes are <30–40 mL, ≥8 cores biopsy should be performed; usually 10–12 cores biopsy is recommended [10]. Oral or intravenous antibiotics should be used to prevent post-biopsy infection. Biopsy complications are hematospermia, hematuria, rectal bleeding, prostatitis, fever, and epididymitis. Biopsies can be repeated when the conditions specified in the table below occur. National or internationally accepted terminologies must be followed to ensure interpersonal standardization. The terminology that should be included in the biopsy reports is shown in the table below.

Recurrent biopsy indications [2]
– Increased or persistent PSA level
– Suspected digital rectal exam
– Typical small acinar proliferation
– Intense high-grade prostatic intraepithelial neoplasia
– Intraductal carcinoma with solid results
– Positive multiparametric magnetic resonance (mpMR) imaging results

Recommended terminology in biopsy reporting [2]
– Benign/negative in terms of malignancy
– Active inflammation
– Granulomatous inflammation
– High-grade prostatic intraepithelial neoplasia (PIN)
– High-grade PIN with atypical gland, suspected for adenocarcinoma
– Suspected lesion in terms of atypical gland focus/adenocarcinoma/atypical small acinar proliferation, cancer suspected
– Adenocarcinoma
– Intraductal carcinoma

15.3 Classification and Staging of Prostate Cancer

Routine methods used in prostate cancer staging are tumor-lymph node-metastasis (TNM) staging (Table 15.1), anatomical and prognostic prostate

Table 15.1 Staging of TNM in prostate cancer

T staging	
Tx	Primary tumor could not be evaluated
T1	Tumor that cannot be detected clinically, cannot be detected by palpation and imaging
T1a	Tumor detected in less than 5% of the tissue sample by random histological examination
T1b	Tumor detected in more than 5% of the tissue sample by random histological examination
T1c	Tumor detected by needle biopsy due to high PSA
T2	Limited and palpable tumor into prostate[a]
T2a	Tumor in half or less of a lobe of the prostate
T2b	Tumor in more than half of one lobe of the prostate, but no tumor in both lobes
T2c	Tumor in both lobes of the prostate
T3	Tumor exceeding the prostate capsule[b]
T3a	Single or bilateral extracapsular extension
T3b	Tumor involving microscopic bladder neck
T4	Tumor holding seminal vesicle(s) Tumor involving adjacent organs other than seminal vesicles (external sphincter, rectum, levator muscles, pelvic wall)
N staging[c]	
Nx	Regional lymph nodes not evaluated
N0	No regional lymph node metastasis
N1	Regional lymph node metastases present
M staging[d]	
Mx	Distant metastasis not evaluated
M1	Distant metastasis is present
M1a	Non-regional lymph node(s) metastasis
M1b	Metastasis to bone(s)
M1c	Metastasis to other area(s)

[a]Invasion to the prostate apex or prostate capsule is classified as T2
[b]T2a-c is only available in the clinical classification. Pathological classification has only pT2
[c]Metastases not greater than 2 mm are called pNmi
[d]M1c terminology should be used if there is metastasis in more than one region

Table 15.2 Anatomical and prognostic prostate cancer staging

Stage	T	N	M	PSA	Gleason
I	T1a-c T2a T1–2a	N0 N0	M0 M0	PSA <10 PSA <10 PSA X	Gleason ≤6 Gleason ≤6 Gleason X
IIa	T1a-c T1a-c T2a T2b T2b	N0	M0	PSA <10 PSA ≥10 < 20 PSA < 20 PSA <20 PSA X	Gleason 7 Gleason ≤6 Gleason ≤7 Gleason ≤7 Gleason X
IIb	T2c T1–2 T1–2	N0	M0	Any PSA PSA ≥20 Any PSA	Any Gleason Any Gleason Gleason ≥8
III	T3a-b	N0	M0	Any PSA	Any Gleason
IV	T4 Any T Any T	N0 N1 Any N	M0	Any PSA Any PSA Any PSA	Any Gleason Any Gleason Any Gleason

cancer staging (Table 15.2), and International Society of Urological Pathology classification (Table 15.3). The Gleason score is given by the characteristics of the cancer cell in pathological preparations.

15.4 Diagnostic and Visual Staging, Restaging

Imaging methods include anatomical and functional imaging. Anatomical imaging includes direct radiography, ultrasound, computed tomography, and magnetic resonance imaging. Functional imaging includes bone scintigraphy, positron emission tomography/computed tomography (PET/CT), spectroscopy, and diffusion-weighted magnetic resonance imaging. The frequency of imaging varies according to personal risk, disease stage, androgen-suppressed PSA value, and Gleason score in disease follow-up.

PSA progression and tumor recurrence are observed in 15–40% of patients receiving curative therapy. The most common recurrence site is the prostate bed and local lymph nodes [11]. Biochemical recurrence classification (Table 15.4) and NCCN risk grouping (Table 15.5) can be used in localized and local advanced prostate cancer of

Table 15.3 Comparisons of Gleason score with International Society of Urological Pathology (ISUP) and histopathological grade

Gleason score	ISUP degree	Histopathologic degree
2–6	1	Good differentiated (low anaplasia)
7 (3 + 4)	2	
7 (4 + 3)	3	Moderate differentiated (moderate anaplasia)
8 (4 + 4 or 3 + 5 or 5 + 3)	4	Poorly differentiated/ undifferentiated (high anaplasia)
9–10	5	

Table 15.4 Biochemical recurrence risk groups in local and local advanced prostate cancer of the European Association of Urology

Low risk	Medium risk	High risk	
PSA <10 ng/mL and GS <7 (ISUP grade 1) and cT1–2a	PSA 10–20 ng/mL or GS 7 (ISUP grade 2/3) or cT2b	PSA >20 ng/mL or GS >7 (ISUP grade 4/5) or cT2c	Any PSA and any GS and cT3–4 or cN+ any ISUP grade
Local disease			**Locally advanced disease**

PSA, prostate-specific antigen; GS, Gleason score; ISUP, International Society of Urological Pathology

Table 15.5 NCCN risk groups for recurrence

Risk groups	
Very low risk	T1c, Gleason ≤6, PSA <10 ng/mL, <3 in each biopsy site presence of tumors in ≤50%
Low risk	T1–T2a, Gleason ≤6, PSA <10 ng/mL
Medium risk	T2b–T2c, Gleason 7, PSA 10–20 ng/mL
High risk	T3a, Gleason 8–10, PSA >20 ng/mL
Very high risk	T3b–T4, primary Gleason pattern 5 or > 4 at biopsy site Gleason 8–10

the European Association of Urology for recurrence classification.

Five-year survival is 11% if there is retroperitoneal lymph node metastasis in patients undergoing lymph node dissection, while this rate increases to 53% if there is no retroperitoneal lymph node metastasis [12].

15.4.1 Direct Graphy

It can be used to assess the symptomatic site area in the skeleton, but it is generally not possible to detect a metastatic lesion by direct radiography without loss of approximately 50% of bone mineral density.

15.4.2 Ultrasound (USG)

Endorectal USG can be used for transrectal biopsy. In addition, the prostate bed can be evaluated with USG in local recurrence disease.

15.4.3 Magnetic Resonance Imaging (MRI)

Multiparametric MRI (mpMRI) is the best imaging method for local staging, and the most useful images are T2-weighted images. 1.5 T MR has high specificity in T3 disease, while it has low sensitivity. MR images are very important in deciding neuroprotective surgery [4]. mpMR is not good at showing microscopic residual disease. Lymph node metastases larger than 1 cm can be easily detected by MRI, while the sensitivity of MRI is low in demonstrating subcentimetric lymph node metastasis. Diffusion-weighted MRI may detect metastatic lymph nodes, but the negative diffusion-weighted images do not rule out the possibility of metastasis [2]. mpMR is a very useful test in imaging the primary prostate cancer site in patients with elevated PSA levels despite negative biopsy. However, it may not always distinguish inflammation and hyperplasia clearly from the tumor, and it is also a nonspecific examination [11].

15.4.4 Computed Tomography (CT)

It is an examination that gives high anatomical information detail. It is a test used to demonstrate extracapsular invasion, local lymph node metastasis, or visceral organ metastasis. Its success in showing the primary lesion is not as good as MRI. CT is recommended in staging in patients with T3 and T4 tumors and in patients with T1 and T2 tumors and suspected lymph node metastasis. CT can be used for restaging if PSA rises after radical prostatectomy after reaching undetectable levels [4]. The probability of detecting microscopic lymph node metastasis by CT in a Gleason score < 8, PSA <20 ng/mL, or localized disease is <1% [2].

15.4.5 Bone Scintigraphy

Bone scintigraphy is the most commonly used method to demonstrate bone metastasis (Fig. 15.1). It can even show 10% bone loss in the bones. Its specificity is low due to its false positivity secondary to trauma and degeneration even though it is a very sensitive examination in detecting bone metastasis [13]. However, tomographic images are obtained by adding SPECT and CT images to the planar images, thus minimizing false-positive results. Bone scintigraphy should be performed if PSA is ≥20 ng/mL in T1 disease, PSA is ≥10 ng/mL in T2 disease, Gleason score is ≥8, and T3 and T4 diseases are present. In addition, bone scintigraphy should be performed if any PSA fluctuation is observed in

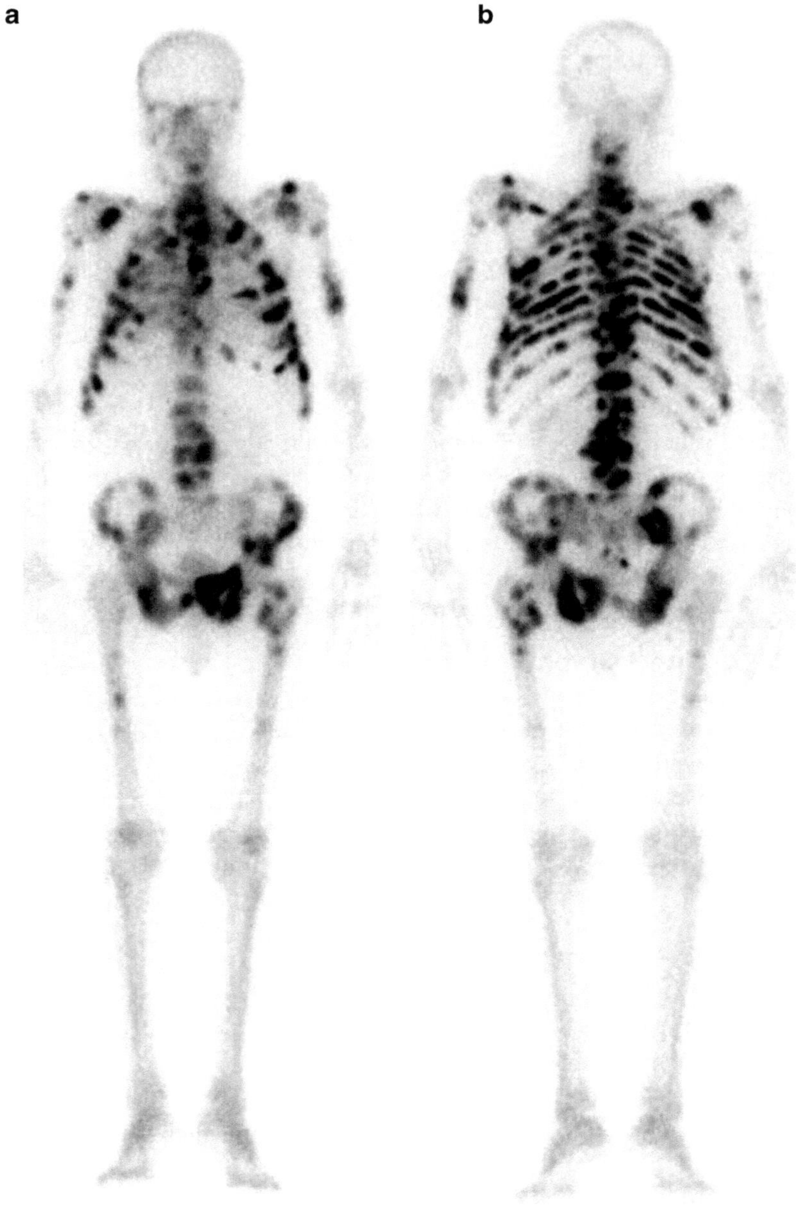

Fig. 15.1 Diffuse bone metastases of the patient diagnosed with prostate cancer and Tc-99 m MDP bone scintigraphy anterior (**a**) and posterior (**b**) images with superscan

the follow-up of patients with a PSA level of <0.2 ng/mL after radical prostatectomy or who have received local radiotherapy. Bone scintigraphy can be performed every 6–12 months in symptomatic patients [4].

Bone scintigraphy is recommended in symptomatic patients regardless of Gleason score, stage, and PSA level. Bone scintigraphy positivity was reported to be 2.3% in patients with PSA level < 10 ng/mL, 5.3% in patients with PSA level 10.1–19.9 ng/mL, and 16.2% in patients with PSA value 20–49.9 ng/mL in a study [2].

15.4.6 F-18 NaF PET/CT

It is one of the most sensitive tests in bone metastasis. It is taken to the cells with ion exchange, and blood flow is a speed-limiting step. High clearance from plasma increases image quality [14].

However, the specificity of the imaging method is low. It does not show metastatic sites other than bone. It is only a bone-specific examination and the cost is very high compared to bone scintigraphy.

15.4.7 Choline PET/CT

C-11 choline is a good way of distinguishing tumor tissue from benign tissue. Since the half-life of C-11 is 20 min, it requires onsite (within the imaging unit) cyclotron. It can be used in biochemical recurrence seen after the first therapy in localized disease. It is recommended to visualize the whole body in case of suspicion of metastatic disease [15]. C-11 choline PET/CT sensitivity is 85% and its specificity is 88% when used in restaging [4]. C-11 and F-18 choline PET/CT have high specificity in demonstrating lymph node metastasis, while their sensitivity is between 10 and 73% [2].

There are studies reporting that the sensitivity of PET/CT in detecting lymph node metastasis is higher, similar, and lower compared to diffusion-weighted MRI considering the results of studies conducted in moderate–/high-risk patients comparing diffusion-weighted MRI and choline PET/CT [16–19].

The chronic problem of choline PET/CT is false-positive results. Choline PET positivity is observed in cases such as BPH, prostatitis, and prostatic intraepithelial neoplasia (PIN) [11].

15.4.8 F-18 FDG PET/CT

F-18 FDG PET/CT may provide important information in prostate cancer metastases, but it is not recommended to be used routinely since it is a limited examination for prostate cancer (Fig. 15.2) [4]. However, it can be used in selected cases in aggressive tumors [20].

15.4.9 Ga-68 PSMA PET/CT

The Ga-68 is obtained from the Ge-68/Ga-68 generator. Eighty-nine percent is degraded by positron. Its half-life is 67.63 min. The prostate-specific membrane antigen (PSMA) is a densely

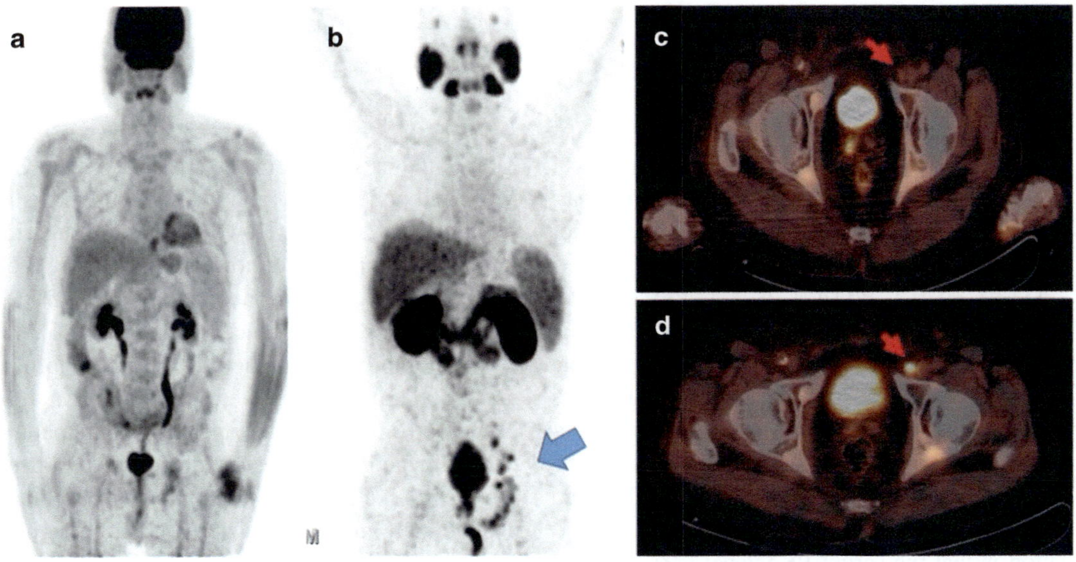

Fig. 15.2 F-18 FDG PET/CT MIP (**a**) and transverse (**c**) images of the patient followed up for metastatic prostate cancer show mild FDG uptake in the pelvic bones, and no FDG uptake is observed in the left inguinal lymph node (red arrow). Ga-68 PSMA PET/CT MIP image (**b**) performed 20 days later shows multiple lymph nodes (blue arrow) in the pelvis and PSMA expression in the non-FDG-avid lymph node in the transverse image (**d**) (red arrow)

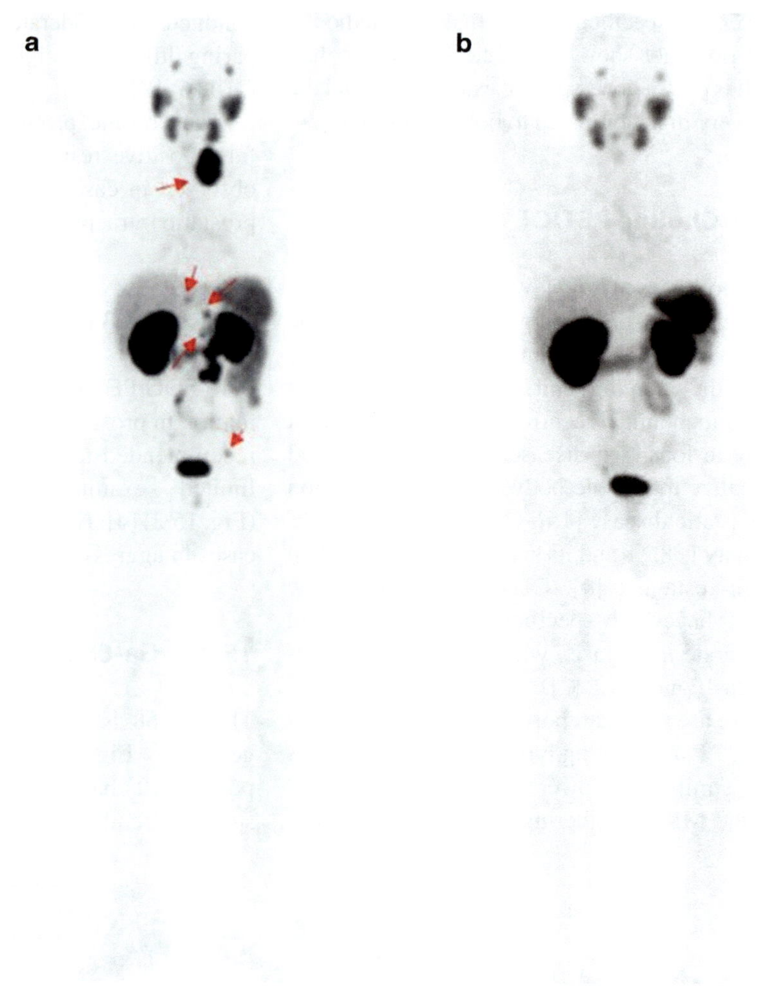

Fig. 15.3 A 62-year-old male, diagnosed with prostate cancer in 2016. There is a history of chemotherapy and hormone therapy. Ga-68 PSMA PET/CT MIP image (**a**) shows metastasis areas (red arrow) showing multiple PSMA expression when serum PSA value is 23.2 ng/mL. Ga-68 PSMA PET/CT MIP image (**b**) performed after four cycles of Lu-177 PSMA therapy shows complete response to therapy

produced transmembrane glycoprotein in prostate cancer cells. Ga-68 binds to the external part of PSMA and then internalizes into the tumor cell.

Ga-68 PSMA PET/CT is a high-resolution examination used in the diagnosis, staging, restaging, and response to therapy of prostate cancer (Fig. 15.3). Its use for diagnostic purposes in Turkey is not within the scope of reimbursement even though it has been reported in the EANM guideline and studies that it can be used in diagnosis. The highest benefit from the examination is that the serum PSA level is 0.2–10 ng/mL in recurrent disease [21].

It is recommended to be used routinely in Gleason >7, PSA >20 ng/mL, and T2c-3a tumors before operation and RT in primary staging. Many studies have shown superiority over CT, MRI, and bone scintigraphy in showing metastasis in primary staging. However, it is not superior to mpMR in primary tumor area imaging. Ga-68 PSMA PET/CT is false-negative in about 5% of patients with prostate cancer (Fig. 15.4) [21].

Whole-body image should be taken approximately 60 min after intravenous injection of 1.8–2.2 MBq (0.05–0.06 mCi) per kg for the patient to be imaged [21]. Lesion detection has been reported to increase at the second and third hours even though imaging between 50 and 100 min is acceptable [21, 22].

PSMA expression secondary to neovascularization is also observed in some solid tumors because it is expressed by endothelial cells during neovascularization, apart from PSMA pros-

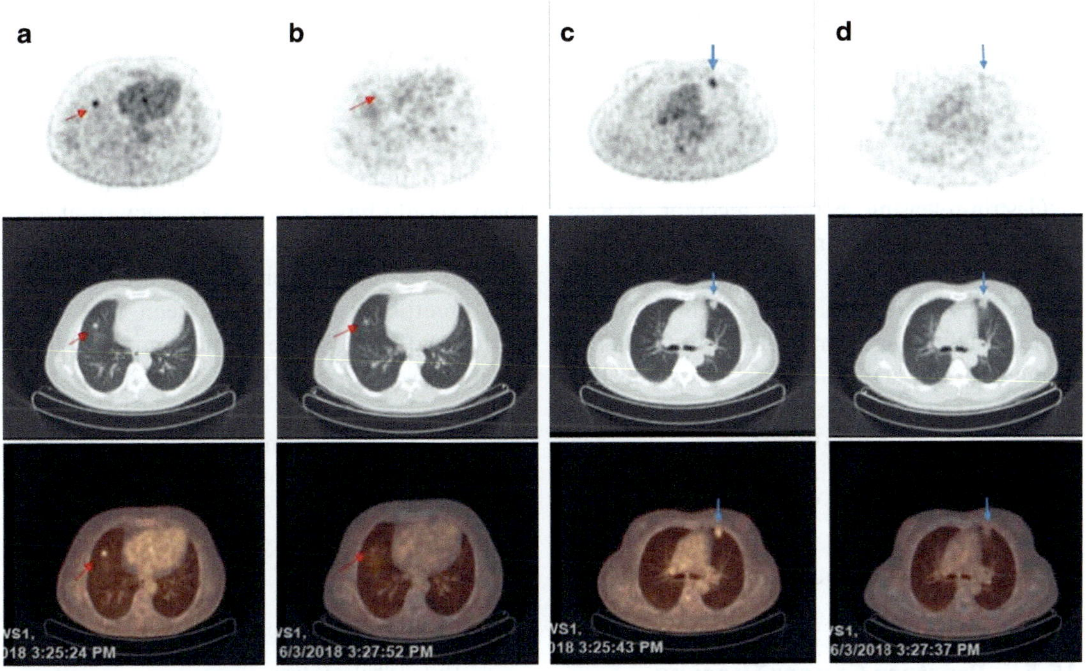

Fig. 15.4 Wedge resection was performed with the suspicion of metastasis, and metastatic prostate cancer was reported pathologically upon the observation of nodules in both lungs in CT images of the patient diagnosed with prostate cancer. F-18 FDG PET/CT images (**a**, **c**) performed on the patient show FDG-avid nodules, while Ga-68 PSMA PET/CT images (**b**, **d**) do not show PSMA expression in these nodules

tate cancer. Ga-68 PSMA PET/CT may be false-negative in small lesions and neuroendocrine differentiation, while it may show false-positive uptake in celiac ganglia and other neoplasms [8, 23].

There are three separate PSMA complexes labeled with Ga-68, commonly used in PET/CT imaging; PSMA-11, PSMA-617, and PSMA I&T. PSMA-617 and PSMA I&T are used in both imaging and therapy for theranostic purposes as Lu-177 can also be connected [24]. PSMA-11 is only used for imaging purposes.

It should be kept in mind that there will be activity in the lacrimal glands, salivary glands, liver, spleen, small intestine, colon, and kidneys due to PSMA expression during the evaluation of the images.

Recurrence was demonstrated with Ga-68 PSMA in 43.8% of patients considered to have recurrence but found to be negative with F-18 choline. In fact, the serum PSA value of some of these patients is <0.2 ng/mL [25].

Ga-68 PSMA PET/CT imaging performed in our routine practice revealed the presence of metastasis even in the 3 mm lymph node. These lymph nodes are reported not to be metastatic due to their small size in radiological examinations (if they do not have a prominent malignancy character).

Eiber et al. reported the sensitivity of mpMR as 66%, the sensitivity of PET as 92%, and the sensitivity of PET/MR as 98% in primary tumor detection in a patient-based study comparing Ga-68 PSMA PET, mpMR, and PET/MR. Hybrid imaging has a high sensitivity even though no statistically significant difference was observed between PET and PET/MR images [26].

15.4.10 Other PET/CT Scans

C-11 acetate, F-18 FACBC, F-18 FDHT, F-18 DCFBC, and F-18 DCFPyL are radiopharmaceuticals used for imaging with PET/CT in prostate cancer. However, studies have shown that PSMA-based PET/CT imaging is more sensitive compared to these images [11]. F-18-PSMA-1007 is a potential imaging agent that has been studied in vitro and in mice and started to be studied clinically [27, 28].

Gastrin-releasing peptide receptor (GRPR) expression is known in prostate cancer cells. Clinical imaging was performed with Ga-68 NeoBOMB1 PET/CT targeting this receptor, preclinical studies were conducted with Lu-177 for theranostic use, and translation into clinical use was aimed [29]. Prostate cancer areas that cannot be shown with F-18 FECH have also been reported to be shown with Ga-68 RM2 targeting the same receptor [30]. Table 15.6 shows molecules used for diagnosis, therapy, and theranostic purposes in prostate cancer.

15.5 Prostate Cancer Therapy

15.5.1 Localized Prostate Cancer Therapy

Localized prostate cancer therapy is decided by evaluating age, clinical tumor staging, serum PSA value, Gleason score, number of positive prostate biopsies, and cancer tissue site in biopsy together. Radical prostatectomy, external radiotherapy (RT), or brachytherapy can be used in local therapy. Cryotherapy, high-density focal ultrasound, and photodynamic therapy are no longer used.

The patient undergoing radical prostatectomy should have a life expectancy of at least 10 years and should not have severe comorbid diseases. Urinary incontinence is seen in 17%, and erectile dysfunction is seen in 81% of patients after radical prostatectomy [5]. It can be increased up to 80 Gy in moderate-high-risk patients, while the external RT dose (including or not seminal vesicles) is 75.6–79.2 Gy in low-risk patients.

Intensity-modulated radiotherapy (IMRT) is performed at 2.4–4 Gy fractionated doses for 4–6 weeks.

Recommended to report prostatectomy specimen [2]
– Histopathologic type
– Histological grade
– Tumor quantification (size of tumor/nodule and how much of the prostate gland it covers)
– Pathological TNM staging
– Surgical margin

Histopathological typing involves adenocarcinoma and squamous carcinoma. Adenocarcinoma variants are mucinous, signet ring cell, ductal,

Table 15.6 Prostate cancer targeted diagnosis, therapy, and theranostic molecules

Use	Molecular (radionuclide)	Mechanism	Reference
Diagnosis	Glucose (F^{18})	Glucose metabolism	[4]
	Acetate (C^{11})	Fatty acid de novo synthesis	[11]
	Choline (C^{11}, F^{18})	Phospholipid synthesis	[2, 31–34]
	FACBC (F^{18})	PSMA ligand; antibody	[11, 35, 36]
	MIP-1404 (Tc^{99m})	PSMA ligand; small-molecule inhibitor	[37, 38]
	MIP-1072 (I^{123})	PSMA ligand; small-molecule inhibitor	[38]
	DCFBC (F^{18})	PSMA ligand; small-molecule inhibitor	[11, 39]
	DCFPyL (F^{18})	PSMA ligand; small-molecule inhibitor	[11, 40]
	PSMA-11 (Ga^{68})	PSMA ligand; small-molecule inhibitor	[11, 24, 41]
	PSMA-1007 (F^{18})	PSMA ligand; small-molecule inhibitor	[42]
	RM2 (Ga^{68})	GRPR antagonist	[30]
Therapy	MIP-1466 (I^{131})	PSMA ligand; small-molecule inhibitor	
Theranostic	J591 (In^{111}, Cu^{64}, Zr^{89}, Y^{90}, Lu^{177})	PSMA ligand; antibody	[38]
	MIP-1095 (I^{123}, I^{124}, I^{131})	PSMA ligand; small-molecule inhibitor	[37, 43]
	PSMA-I&T (Ga^{68}, Lu^{177})	PSMA ligand; small-molecule inhibitor	[44]
	PSMA-617 (Ga^{68}, Sc^{44}, Y^{90}, Lu^{177}, Ac^{225})	PSMA ligand; small-molecule inhibitor	[24, 37, 42, 45]
	NeoBOMB1 (Ga^{68}, Lu^{177})	GRPR antagonist	[29]

adenosquamous, and small cell neuroendocrine carcinoma. Transitional cell carcinoma is considered a urethral tumor [4].

Seminal vesicle invasion is a predictor of local recurrence and widespread metastatic disease. Perineural invasion is associated with lymph node metastasis [2].

Most prostate cancer-related deaths occur in patients with metastatic disease and PSA >100 ng/mL [46].

15.5.2 Medical Therapy

Castration: Castration should be performed in patients with metastatic or PSA progression because androgen hormones trigger prostate cancer cells to grow. Castration is performed medically or surgically. Testosterone levels are expected to be <50 ng/dL in medical castration and 15 ng/dL on average in surgical castration [2]. Today, medical castration is more preferred compared to surgical castration [12].

Estrogen: It suppresses testosterone without causing bone loss. However, its use in first-line therapy is not recommended due to the side effect of thromboembolism [2].

LHRH agonists (goserelin, histrelin, leuprorelin, triptorelin): It is used as 1-, 2-, 3-, and 6-month or annual storage injection. Flare phenomenon occurs 2–3 days after the first injection and lasts for up to 1 week. The flare phenomenon is secondary to the temporary increase in LH and FSH. Cardiovascular deaths due to bone pain, acute bladder outlet obstruction, obstructive renal failure, spinal cord compression, and hypercoagulation may occur during the flare phenomenon process [2].

LHRH antagonists (degarelix): It binds directly to the LHRH receptor and reduces the LH and FSH levels without causing the flare phenomenon [2].

Antiandrogens: There are steroid (cyproterone acetate, megestrol acetate, medroxyprogesterone acetate) and nonsteroidal (nilutamide, flutamide, bicalutamide) forms, and they compete with androgens at the level of androgen respirators [2]. Antiandrogen therapy alone to suppress androgen is less effective compared to medical or surgical castration, so it is not recommended.

15.5.2.1 Only Used in Castration-Resistant Patients

Abiraterone acetate: It is an inhibitor of CYP17, causing a decrease in arachidonic acid, resulting in a decrease in intracellular testosterone at the adrenal level and cancer cell level. It should be used in combination with prednisone/prednisolone [2]. It received FDA approval in 2011. It increases survival by approximately 3–4 months. Side effects are weakness, peripheral edema, joint-back pain, diarrhea, loss of appetite, constipation, hypoplasia, hypophosphatemia, atrial fibrillation, flashing, urinary infection, cough, hypertension, nocturia, dyspepsia, AST-ALT increase, and cardiac disorders [4].

Enzalutamide: It is a high-affinity antiandrogen drug to the androgen receptor. It received FDA approval in 2012. It is administered orally as 160 mg daily.

Long-term use is difficult in most patients because androgen suppression therapy has many side effects such as cardiovascular, metabolic, musculoskeletal, sexual dysfunction, mood disorder, and depressive mode.

Patients who received androgen suppression therapy for 7 months in the cohort of 9346 patients were divided into 3 prognostic groups. The mean survival of patients with PSA <0.2 ng/mL in Group 1 was reported to be 75 months, the mean survival of patients with PSA <4 ng/mL in Group 2 was reported to be 44 months, and the mean survival of patients with PSA >4 ng/mL in Group 3 was reported to be 13 months [47].

15.5.2.2 Chemotherapy

The first combination to be used in the therapy of metastatic castration-resistant prostate cancer is docetaxel+prednisone. The option in the patient with progression is cabazitaxel + prednisone despite the docetaxel therapy.

Docetaxel toxicity without six-cycle prednisone is weakness, neuropathy, stomatitis, diarrhea, febrile, or nonfebrile neutropenia [4]. The side effect of cabazitaxel on peripheral neuropathy is lower compared to docetaxel.

15.5.2.3 Immunotherapy/Vaccine

The immunotherapy agent used in prostate cancer is sipuleucel-T. It is recommended in asymptomatic or minimally symptomatic patients, without liver metastasis, with a life expectancy >6 months, and with an ECOG performance of 0–1. It received FDA approval in 2010. It can cause chills/tremors, fever, and headache even though it can usually be tolerated well. It has been reported to reduce the risk of mortality by 22% in a phase III study [4]. It is given as three doses and each dose consists of three steps. White blood cells, especially antigen-presenting cells, are collected from the patient with first step leukapheresis, these leukocytes are incubated with PSA and GM-CSF fusion protein in second step, and activated blood is given back to the patient in the last step. Progression-free survival did not change and an average of 4-month increase in overall survival was observed [5]. Cost is high and not within the scope of reimbursement in Turkey.

15.5.2.4 Bone-Targeted Therapies

Zoledronic acid: It is a type of bisphosphate. It prevents osteoclast-associated bone resorption.

Denosumab: It is a monoclonal antibody against RANKL, which inhibits osteoclast function. It may cause osteonecrosis of the jaw [5].

Ra-223 osteoblastic bone metastasis therapy: Significant increases in survival were observed in patients with symptomatic bone metastasis and without visceral metastasis in patients with metastatic castration-resistant prostate cancer with alpha agent Ra-223 [14]. Its half-life is 11 days and tissue penetration is 100 µm. Ra-223 is different from other agents given for beta-emitting pain palliation (Sr-89, Sm-153). These agents are only used for pain palliation and do not have any therapeutic effects. However, the alpha rays emitted by Ra-223 cause double chain fractures in tumor DNA, resulting in the death of the tumor cell, due to the high linear energy transfer.

It is administered by intravenous injection as six doses every 4 weeks. Neutrophil count should be $\geq 1.5 \times 10^9$/L, platelets $\geq 100 \times 10^9$/L, and hemoglobin ≥ 10 g/dL in order to be treated [4].

15.5.3 Monitoring

T0-T2 localized prostate cancer patients were followed up for 15 years, only 13% of these patients developed metastasis, and 11% died due to prostate cancer in the study by Johansson et al. [48].

Nonmetastatic castration-resistant prostate cancer is associated with increased PSA levels despite castration and is used for situations where no metastatic focus can be found clinically. 1/3 of them have bone metastases within 2 years in these patients [2]. PSA doubling time can be predicted to be a slow-moving disease if it is >10 months, while secondary hormonal therapy methods may be required in patients with <10 months [4].

PSA level > 0.2 ng/mL in the patient with radical prostatectomy creates a suspicion of progression/recurrence disease. If there is a good response to therapy in metastatic patients, if there is a PSA response (<4 ng/mL), and if there is symptomatic improvement, the follow-up of the patient can be done every 3–6 months [2].

Therapies that increase survival in metastatic castration-resistant prostate cancer patients are docetaxel, cabazitaxel, enzalutamide, abiraterone, sipuleucel-T, and Ra-223. Docetaxel and cabazitaxel increased survival for a few months, while abiraterone provided a survival advantage of 3.9 months, 4.8 months in enzalutamide, and 3.6 months in Ra-223 [49]. Table 15.7 presents the European Association of Urology's recommendation for the therapy of metastatic prostate cancer.

Increased survival and PSA responses of up to 99.9% have been reported in almost all radioligand therapies for prostate cancer apart from these therapies [50, 51]. Rahbar et al. conducted a study in which 19.7-week survival was observed in patients receiving the best supportive care, while an average of 29.4-week survival was reported in patients receiving Lu-177 PSMA therapy [51]. Radioligand therapy in prostate cancer has not yet been included in prostate cancer guidelines in the routine management of the disease despite all these positive data. It is expected to be included soon.

15.6 Radionuclide Therapy in Prostate Cancer

Prostate cancer cells are radiation-sensitive. Radiosensitivity is associated with high metabolic rate, good nutrient intake, cleavage rate, and proliferation rate. The phase with the highest effect is G2 and M (mitosis) phase, while the phase with the lowest effect of radiation in the cell cycle is S (synthesis) phase. Radiosensitivity is not only dependent on the characteristics of the cell despite all this. It also depends on which type of radiation (alpha, beta, gamma) is used [12]. Alpha or beta particles are used extensively in the therapy. Alpha particles cause more intense ionization in the tissue through which they pass due to the high linear energy transfers (LET) (100 keV/μm). The LET of beta particles is approximately 0.2–0.3 keV/μm. High LET means that it will create more double DNA fractures [52]. Therefore, the biological effect of radiation with high LET is independent of cell cycle, tissue oxygenation, and absorbed dose.

Prostate-specific membrane antigen is a zinc-dependent, glycoprotein-structured glutamate carboxypeptidase II enzyme. This glycoprotein has a total of 3 parts: the first part consisting of 19 amino acids in the cell, the second part consisting of 24 amino acids, and finally the external part consisting of 707 amino acids. The enzyme is responsible for folate uptake, cell migration, proliferation, and survival [53]. It is called prostate-specific membrane antigen due to its intense expression in prostate cancer cells even though it is an enzyme originally found in the non-prostate-specific brain, salivary gland, tear gland, small intestine, kidney, and liver. 100–1000 times less PSMA expression is observed in non-prostate tissues than prostate cancer cells [54]. It is found in normal prostate cells in the cytosol, while it is found in cancerous prostate cells bound to the membrane [37]. PSMA expression is observed on the cell surface in prostate cancer and transparent cell renal cancer. PSMA expression secondary to neovascularization is also observed in some solid tumors (glioblastoma multiforme, colorectal cancers, gastric cancers, head and neck squamous cell cancers, etc.) even in some benign neoplasms, because PSMA is also produced in endothelial cells during neovascularization, apart from prostate cancer. It should be known that endothelial cells, not neoplastic cells, exhibit PSMA expression in these individuals [53].

PSMA expression in prostate cancer is positively associated with tumor stage and early recurrence. Following ligand binding to PSMA, PSMA internalizes into the cell with clathrin-mediated endocytosis [55].

7E11-C5.3 is the first anti-PSMA monoclonal antibody developed [56]. Subsequently, In-111 capromab pendetide, the first PSMA-based radionuclide prostate cancer imaging agent, was released by binding this antibody to In-111. It has only been damaged and accumulated in necrotic cells since this radiopharmaceutical binds to the internal part of PSMA. Therefore, there was no imaging agent at the desired activity [37]. The new focus of attention was the external part when the desired activity could not be created in the internal part of PSMA. The first monoclonal antibody developed against the external part is J591. J591 is immediately labeled with In-111. It binds to the living cell by binding to the external part of PSMA. Then, this monoclonal antibody was also labeled with Y-90 and Lu-177 for therapy purposes. Finally, radionuclide imaging and therapy, that is, a theranostic approach, where prostate cancer cells are targeted, has been created. It was possible to monitor the site treated with a theranostic approach. J591 monoclonal antibody was also used in PET/CT imaging by binding with Zr-89 [37]. The desired imaging and therapy capacity has not been achieved even though all these monoclonal antibody studies are exciting.

Table 15.7 European Association of Urology metastatic prostate cancer therapy recommendation

First-line therapy	Abiraterone Enzalutamide Docetaxel Sipuleucel-T
Second-line therapy	Cabazitaxel Abiraterone (after first-line docetaxel) Enzalutamide (after first-line docetaxel) Ra-223

Because monoclonal antibodies are large structures, nonspecific involvements can be observed due to their long plasma half-life, low tumor penetrations, and immunoglobulin. The long plasma half-lives bring about hematological toxicity.

Researchers turned to small-molecule inhibitors against PSMA in the absence of expected response from monoclonal antibodies. Small molecules being 1–2 kDa in size enabled them to be cleaned more easily from the circulation and taken into the cell faster, while monoclonal antibodies were about 150 kDa in size [38]. Thus, it became more possible to reach a high therapeutic dose within the cell. The first human imaging was performed with small-molecule PSMA inhibitors I-123-MIP-1972 and I-123-MIP-1095 in 2008. Human imaging was performed with Ga-68-PSMA-11 in 2011, and the first small-molecule PSMA inhibitor radioligand therapy was administered with I-131-MIP-1095. Afterward, the process of rapid spread and development of these imaging and therapies began. PET/CT imaging was performed with I-124-MIP-1095, and plans and SPECT imaging were performed with Tc-99 m-MIP-1404 and Tc-99 m-MIP-1405. Production of Ga-68-PSMA-11 has been reported to bind to the external part of PSMA in clinical trials and then intensify and exhibit excellent accumulation in tumor tissue. Lu-177-dependent PSMA therapies have entered our lives as of 2013. Theranostic administrations are performed in prostate cancer in more and more patients in more centers with each passing day.

PSMA-617 and PSMA are commonly used theranostic agents as they can be connected with both Ga-68 and Lu-177 via I&T chelator.

15.6.1 Lu-177 PSMA therapy

Lu-177 has a physical half-life of 6.65 days and beta decay with 497 keV (78.6%), 384 keV (9.1%), and 176 keV (12.2), while 113 keV (6.4%) and 208 keV (11%) make gamma radiation [57]. Therapy can be performed, and imaging can be performed, thanks to gamma rays with the beta radiation feature of radionuclide. The maximum tissue penetration of Lu-177 is <2 mm. The radiation effect on the intact tissue adjacent to tumor tissue is minimal due to the low tissue penetration.

15.7 Patient Selection

There are no strict criteria for patient selection. It is recommended in the therapy decision that the multidisciplinary team including urology, oncology, pathology, radiology, and nuclear medicine specialist make the decision. Lu-177 PSMA dose should be preferred according to the patient's general condition, hematological and nephrological parameters, ECOG and Karnofsky performance scale, and previous therapies. Blood transfusions can be performed before therapy in anemic patients.

Patients who have received therapy for metastatic castration-resistant prostate cancer due to the fact that Lu-177 PSMA therapy has not yet been included in the prostate cancer guidelines generally consist of a group of patients who have progressed despite receiving at least one or more of their chemotherapy, abiraterone, or enzalutamide therapies. This therapy is not very common in anamnesis yet due to the fact that Ra-223 bone metastasis therapy has no reimbursement in Turkey (for the first half of 2019). However, a group of patients has a history of Ra-223 therapy before Lu-177 PSMA therapy in therapies administered outside Turkey.

This therapy is predicted to be one of the first therapy modalities to be chosen in the therapy of metastatic castration-resistant prostate cancer when more experience is gained in Lu-177 PSMA therapy and randomized prospective publications are made compared with other therapies.

Patient file must include

–	Prostate cancer histological type
–	Castration history
–	Presence of metastatic disease
–	Presence of tumor progression (radiological, biochemical)
–	Androgen deprivation therapy history
–	History of hormonal/taxane therapy
–	History of chemotherapy (at least 6 weeks have passed)

–	History of Ra-223 therapy (at least 2–3 months have passed)
–	PSMA expression in tumor (Ga-68 PSMA with PET/CT)
–	Presence of postrenal obstruction (with MAG3 dynamic kidney scintigraphy)
–	Life expectancy (should be >6 months)
–	ECOG, Karnofsky performance scale
–	ECHO (the presence of possible heart failure should be known since the patient will be infused with fluid)
–	Hemoglobin value (> 5.5 mmol/L, >8.5 g/dL)
–	Leukocyte value (should be $>3.0\times10^9$/L)
–	Platelet value (should be $>75\times10^9$/L)
–	Biochemistry (liver enzyme tests, kidney function test, ALP, Ca, electrolyte)
–	Serum PSA value

15.8 Ga-68 PSMA PET/CT Administration

Ga-68 PSMA PET/CT imaging should be performed before therapy and PSMA expression of lesions should be examined. The absence of PSMA expression in the lesions means that Lu-177 will not reach that site either. It is known before the therapy that the patient will not benefit from the therapy in this case. Ga-68 lesions showing PSMA expression on PSMA PET/CT images may benefit from therapy, but radiopharmaceutical concentration of the lesion is important. While lesions with generally higher involvement than normal liver tissue respond better to therapy, therapy effectiveness will be lower in lesions with less involvement compared to normal liver tissue due to insufficient radiopharmaceutical accumulation. Involvement below normal liver tissue does not constitute a contraindication for therapy, while lesion involvement is expected to be above normal liver tissue in order to benefit from therapy. Therapy can also be administered to these patients according to the physician's preference, but it should be taken into consideration that the therapy effectiveness will be low in cases where there is no choice.

The areas where prostate cancer most metastasizes are the bone, lymph node, liver, and lung. The highest rate is bone metastases [58].

PSMA may not be visualized by PET/CT in 5% of metastatic castration-resistant prostate cancer patients because the tumor loses its PSMA expression feature or is dedifferentiated [59].

15.9 Lu-177 PSMA Therapy Administration

There is no evidence of hormonal agents affecting PSMA expression in metastasis. Therefore, hormonal agents do not need to be discontinued before or during therapy [60].

When Lu-177 PSMA therapy was first initiated, amino acid administration, which is commonly used for renal protection in radioligand therapy in neuroendocrine tumors, was used by some centers [57, 60, 61]. However, amino acid administration was discontinued in almost all centers since experience in Lu-177 PSMA therapy showed that amino acid solution did not affect renal protection [49, 62, 63]. Preclinical and clinical studies have shown decreased renal activity with 2-phosphate methylpentane dioxide acid (2-PMPA) [64, 65].

Studies suggest that the specific activity of Lu-177 to be bound to PSMA inhibitor should be >555 MBq/μg [57]. Patients should be well hydrated before therapy. Intravenous prednisone and antiemetic (e.g., ondansetron) can be administered before therapy [66]. It was recommended to administer radiopharmaceuticals diluted with saline in 5 mL as a slow intravenous injection in 30 s, while there were centers that injected radiopharmaceuticals in 10–30 min when the therapy was first started [60, 61, 67–69]. 3–8 GBq (81–216 mCi) Lu-177 PSMA infusion can be administered per therapy depending on the condition of the disease and the physician's preference [53, 70]. Therapy of 6–8 GBq (162–216 mCi) is recommended in patients with unexpected hematological toxicity. Patients with diffuse bone involvement should receive a low dose of therapy. The patient should continue to be hydrated at least 1000 cc intravenously after therapy. The patient should be informed that they should continuously empty their bladder. Diuretic injection can be used after the therapy, and laxative drugs can be used considering the patient's distress according to the preference of the clinic.

Cold/ice packs can be applied to the parotid and submandibular glands starting 30 min before therapy and continuing for 4 h after therapy [66, 71]. Vasoconstriction can be created in the vessels going to the salivary glands, and side effects can be reduced by providing less radioactivity to the glands with this application [3].

15.9.1 Post-therapy Imaging Protocol [66, 72]

- With medium energy collimator in 15% window range at 208 keV and 113 keV.
- Planar imaging; 1024 × 256 matrix, 2.4 × 2.4 mm pixel, 10 cm/min.
- SPECT; 128 × 128 matrix, 4.8 × 4.8 mm pixel, 20 s 128 projections (64 per collimator).
- CT; 130 kVp, 1 × 1 × 5 mm voxel.

Imaging is recommended only in patients who will undergo imaging after 24 h, while imaging is recommended at 1–4, 24, 48, and 72 h after therapy in patients who will undergo dosimetry. Radioligand excretion in the abdominal organs continues until 24–48 h, while radioligand uptake in the tumor increases until 24 h. The 24th hour is ideal if single imaging is to be performed for this reason [66]. Post-therapy images should be evaluated and compared with previous post-therapy images.

Image-based dosimetry is recommended for each patient to predict antitumor effect and organ toxicity. The renal critical radiation dose threshold with external radiotherapy information is 23 Gy. It has been reported in the literature that the critical radiation threshold can reach up to 28–40 Gy depending on the risk factors of the person even though there are not many studies in this field in internal radiotherapy [53]. However, the effect of late therapy on kidney damage remains unknown. Okamoto et al. reported that 28 Gy cumulative renal dose could be well tolerated by patients, but 50% of these patients expected severe renal damage within 5 years [73]. Dose-limiting organs in Lu-177 PSMA therapy are the kidney, lacrimal gland, parotid gland, and bone marrow [72]. The parotid gland is exposed to a dose of 0.55–1.90 mGy/MBq, salivary glands 0.10–1.48 mGy/MBq, lacrimal glands 2.82–3.80, bone marrow 0.01–0.05 mGy/MBq, kidney 0.53–0.99 mGy/MBq, and the whole body 0.02–0.06 mGy/MBq after therapy (Table 15.8).

Lu-177 PSMA therapy can achieve doses up to an average of 13.1 mGy/MBq in the tumor site (Table 15.8).

The optimal therapy dose and optimal therapy cycle for Lu-177 PSMA therapy have not yet been established. The number and cycle of therapies vary according to Gleason score, number and area of metastatic areas, PSMA expression of cells, general and hematological status of the patient, age, and renal functions [49]. Therapy should be discontinued if the patient cannot tolerate the therapy or if the patient does not want to receive therapy in the presence of progression. Therapy should be repeated every 8–10 weeks (at least 6 weeks) apart from these possibilities according to the literature and our individual clinical experience. At least three to four cycles of therapy should be given unless a complete metabolic response is observed even though there is no clear information about the upper limit of the number of therapies (Figs. 15.5 and 15.6). Up to eight cycles of therapy were given in our own experience and no side effects were observed in the patient, while up to six therapies were observed in the literature [68, 74]. However, we do not have sufficient information about the long-term side effects of Lu-177 PSMA therapy. Data will be generated on long-term side effects with Lu-177 PSMA therapy becoming available earlier in prostate cancer and increased preference rates. There is a need for randomized controlled prospective studies on this subject.

A patient with accidental subcutaneous injection of Lu-177 PSMA was monitored by scintigraphic examinations for 2 days. It has been reported that radiopharmaceutical is distributed to the body over time and adheres to tumor sites, and there is no medical problem in the subcutaneous site [78].

Table 15.8 Lu-177 PSMA therapy doses exposed to organs

Ligand	Author, year	N, NCT, activity* (GBq)	Parotid gland (mGy/MBq)	Salivary gland (mGy/MBq)	Lacrimal gland (mGy/MBq)	Bone marrow (mGy/MBq)	Kidney (mGy/MBq)	Whole body (mGy/MBq)	Tumor (mGy/MBq)
Lu177-PSMA-617	Delker, 2016 [66]	5, 5, 3.4–3.9	NR	0.1	NR	0.01	0.60	NR	13.1
	Hohberg, 2016 [75]	9, 9, 5.3–5.8	NR	0.72	2.82	NR	0.53	0.06	NR
	Kabasakal, 2015 [72]	7, 7, 0.2	1.17	NR	NR	0.03	0.88	0.06	NR
	Kabasakal, 2017 [76]	6, 6, 3.6–7.4	1.90	NR	NR	0.03	0.82	NR	NR
	Kratochwil, 2016 [70]	4, 8, 4.0–6.0	1.28	1.48	NR	0.03	0.75	NR	NR
	Yadav, 2017 [77]	26, 26, 1.1–5.5	NR	1.24	NR	0.05	0.99	0.02	11
Lu177-PSMA-I&T	Baum, 2016 [60]	30, 30, 6	1.30	NR	NR	NR	0.80	0.02	3.30
	Okamoto, 2017 [73]	18, 34, 7.4	0.55	0.64	3.8	NR	0.72	0.06	3.2

N, number of patients; NCT, number of cycles of therapy; *, average activity per cycle; NR, not reported

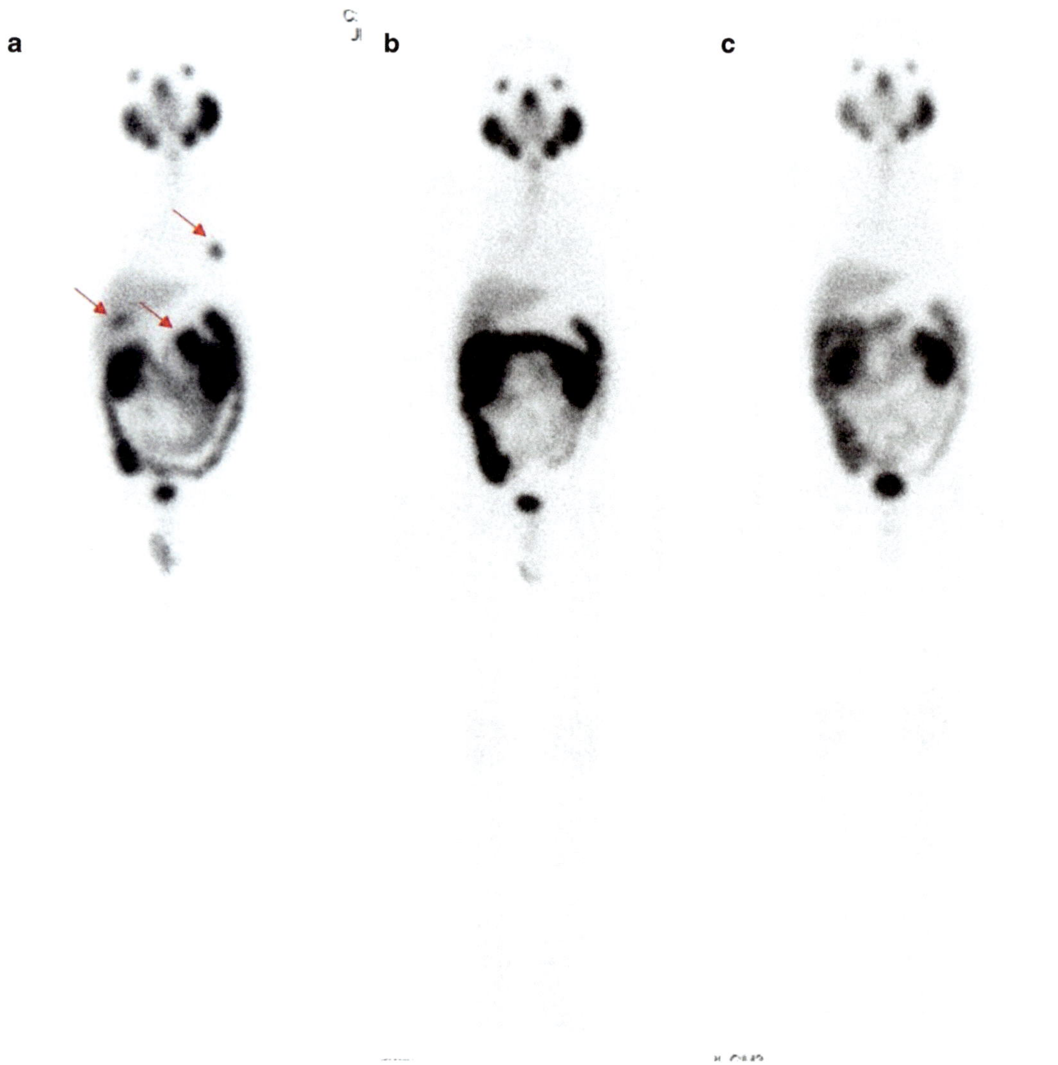

Fig. 15.5 A 62-year-old male patient diagnosed with prostate cancer 9 years ago with a Gleason score of 3 + 3 = 6 had metastases showing PSMA expression in the lung, liver, and left adrenal gland in the anterior image (**a**) after Lu-177 PSMA first therapy, while no metastasis was observed in the anterior image (**b**) after second therapy and in the anterior image (**c**) after third therapy While the serum PSA value of the patient was 58.7 ng/mL before the therapy, it was measured as <0.2 ng/mL after the third therapy

15.10 Therapy Response Evaluation

It is necessary to monitor patients with hemogram, GFR, and serum creatine values every 2–4 weeks after therapy. The likelihood of hematological toxicity should be closely monitored since 90% of patients with prostate cancer have metastatic bone disease. Grade 1–2 anemia was reported in 3–67% of the patients, grade 3–4 anemia in 0–19%, grade 1–2 leukopenia in 0–35%, grade 3–4 leukopenia in 0–3%, grade 1–2 thrombocytopenia in 0–44%, and grade 3–4 thrombocytopenia in 0–3% after Lu-177 PSMA therapy (Table 15.9). Toxicity was found to be high in some studies since basal hemogram values were not compared and only post-therapy values were used in toxicity in some studies. However, this elevation is not secondary to Lu-177 PSMA therapy. Lu-177 is the hematological toxicity that

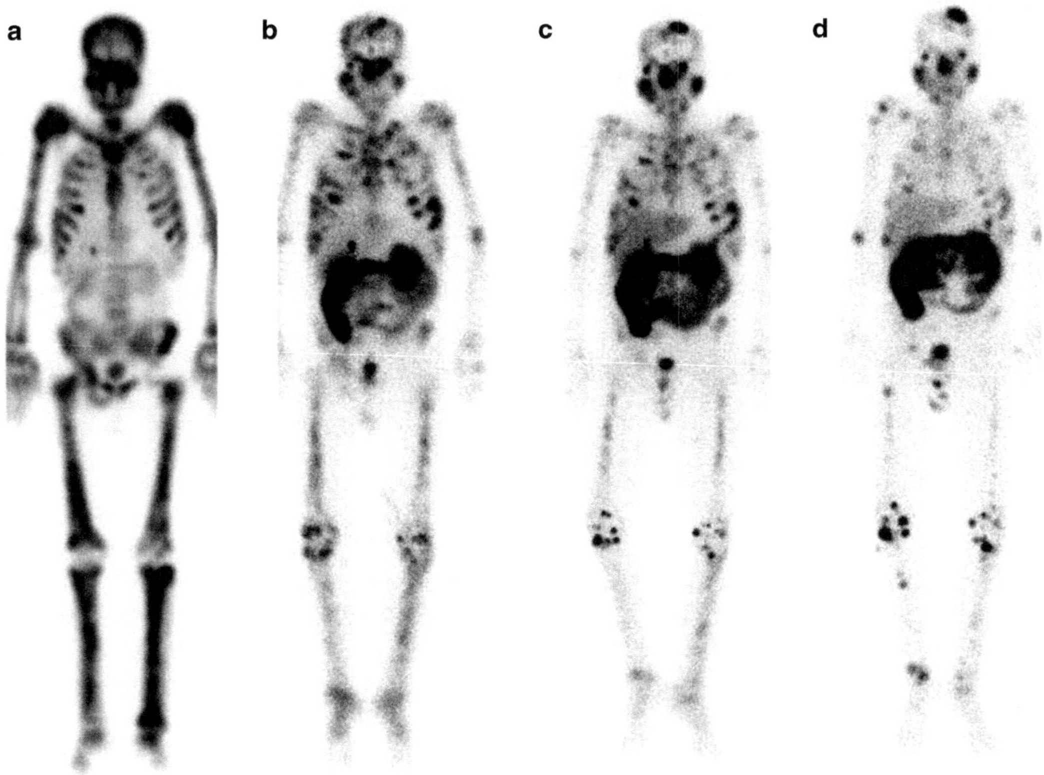

Fig. 15.6 A 67-year-old male, Gleason score 4 + 4 = 8, docetaxel, abiraterone therapies, first pre-therapy serum PSA value 11 ng/mL. The anterior image (**a**) of the patient after the first therapy shows diffuse bone metastases, while the anterior images of the patient after the second (**b**), third (**c**), and fourth (**d**) therapy show a significant therapy response in the metastatic lesions of the patient

Table 15.9 Lu-177 PSMA therapy hematotoxicity

Ligand	Author, year	N, NCT, *activity (GBq)	Grade 1–2 toxicity			Grade 3–4 toxicity		
			Hb	WBC	Plt	Hb	WBC	Plt
Lu^{177}-PSMA-617	Ahmad Zadehfar, 2016 [3]	24, 46, 4.1–7.1	29%	21%	17%	8%	0%	0%
	Bruer, 2017 [67]	59, 159, 5.9–6.3	67%	35%	44%	19%	3%	3%
	Rahbar, 2017 [71]	145, 248, 2–8	NR	NR	NR	8%	1%	2%
	Rahbar, 2016 [58]	74, 74, 5.9	30%	16%	21%	1%	0%	1%
	Rathke, 2017 [69]	40, 40, 4–9.3	3%	8%	5%	0%	3%	3%
	Yadav, 2017 [79]	31, 31, 1.1–5.5	29%	0%	3%	3%	0%	0%
Lu177-PSMA-I&T	Baum, 2016 [60]	56, 125, 3.6–8.7	0%	0%	0%	0%	0%	0%

N, number of patients; NCT, number of cycles of therapy; *, mean activity per cycle; Hb, hemoglobin; WBC, leukocyte; Plt, platelet; NR, not reported

exists before PSMA therapy in the patient secondary to previous therapies and stage of the disease.

Another follow-up as important as hemogram follow-up is follow-up of renal function tests due to intense PSMA expression in the proximal tubule. Lu-177 PSMA therapy has not been reported in the literature for grade 3–4 nephrotoxicity (Table 15.10). Other therapy-related toxicities include fatigue, nausea, dry mouth, and

Table 15.10 Lu-177 PSMA therapy nephrotoxicity and other toxicities

Ligand	Author, year	N, NCT, *activity (GBq)	Nephrological toxicity		Other toxicities
			Grades 1–2	Grades 3–4	
Lu^{177}-PSMA-617	Ahmad Zadehfar, 2016 [3]	24, 46, 4.1–7.1	13%	0%	17% fatigue, 13% nausea, 9% dry mouth
	Bruer, 2017 [67]	59, 159, 5.9–6.3	72%	0%	25% temporary dry mouth, 20% fatigue, 10% dry mouth, 2% dry eye
	Rahbar, 2017 [71]	145, 248, 2–8	NR	0%	8% mild dry mouth
	Rahbar, 2016 [58]	74, 74, 5.9	6%	0%	9% dry mouth
	Yadav, 2017 [79]	31, 31, 1.1–5.5	0%	0%	NR
	Yordanova, 2017 [74]	55, 165, 4–7.1	0%	0%	NR
Lu^{177}-PSMA-I&T	Baum, 2016 [60]	56, 125, 3.6–8.7	0%	0%	4% temporary dry mouth

N, number of patients; NCT, number of cycles of therapy; *, activity range per cycle; NR, not reported

dry eye (Table 15.10). In a recent publication, it was reported that Lu-177 PSMA therapy caused less grade 3–4 toxicity than cabazitaxel [80].

Serum PSA value should be used in the evaluation of therapy response. Lu-177 PSMA therapy has been reported to decrease >50% PSA in 19–63% of patients and > 75% PSA in 8–45% of patients in the literature. Stable PSA was observed in 0–27% of the patients, and progressive PSA was observed in 9–37% of the patients (Table 15.11). Table 15.11 provides a literature review of PSA response to Lu-177 PSMA therapy. The majority of patients have a high level of biochemical response to Lu-177 PSMA therapy as it is understood from the literature.

Ga-68 PSMA PET/CT should also be used to evaluate therapy response (Fig. 15.7). However, it is necessary to decide clinically when to administer it. It is performed after two cycles of therapy in some applications, while in some administrations it is performed after three to four cycles of therapy. In addition, it should be kept in mind that the metabolic response observed in Lu-177 whole-body scan images after therapy may provide information on continued therapy. Lu-177 PSMA therapy was observed in 50–80% of patients, while some studies reported complete molecular response and a high rate of symptomatic response in 33% of patients (Table 15.12). Table 15.12 provides a literature review of molecular and symptomatic response to Lu-177 PSMA therapy. Unfortunately, not all prostate cancer patients respond well to Lu-177 therapy. Approximately 1/3 of the patients have progression after therapy (Fig. 15.8). This may be secondary to various factors such as the emergence of new lesions and disease progression despite the fact that the lesions during the therapy keep radiopharmaceutical and respond to the therapy due to the lack of PSMA expression in the tumor, heterogeneity of PSMA expression, and high time of disease duplication.

Aggressive tumors express more PSMA and cause more radiopharmaceutical uptake. However, the therapy response may not be correlated with this high uptake [81]. Lymph node metastases and visceral organ metastases respond better than bone metastases in Lu-177 PSMA therapy [49, 60].

High serum GGT, LDH, CRP level before therapy, young age, low hemoglobin level before therapy, high Gleason score, and regular pain relief need are negatively effective in response to therapy [81]. Studies in the literature reported progression-free survival up to 54.8 weeks and overall survival up to 64 weeks with PSMA-targeted radioligand therapies (Table 15.13). Sartor et al. [82] showed similar results.

PSA response and therapy response are generally correlated. Based on our own experience, there is also a group of patients in whom we have detected progression with Ga-68 PSMA PET/CT,

Table 15.11 PSA response to Lu-177 PSMA therapy

Ligand	Author, year	N, NCT, activity (GBq)	PSA decline				S-PSA (±25%)	P-PSA (>25%)
			<25%	25–50%	>50%	>75%		
Lu^{177}-PSMA-617	Ahmad Zadehfar, 2016 [3]	24, 24, 4.1–7.1	12%	25%	38%	8%	20%	17%
		20, 40, 4.1–7.1	5%	10%	65%	30%	10%	15%
	Ahmad Zadehfar, 2017 [68]	32, 32, 4.0–7.2	37%		44%	NR	NR	NR
		32, 64, 4.2–6.9	44%		23%	NR	NR	NR
		32, 96, 4.2–6.6	35%		19%	NR	NR	NR
	Bruer, 2017 [67]	45, 159, 5.9–6.3	16%	22%	53%	31%	16%	9%
	Ferdinandus, 2016 [81]	40, 40, 4.1–7.1	35%		33%	NR	NR	NR
	Kratochwil, 2016 [70]	30, 30, 4.0–6.0	10%	10%	54%	13%	13%	23%
		11, 33, 4.0–6.0	0%	9%	73%	45%	0%	18%
	Rahbar, 2017 [71]	99, 99, 2–8	5%	8%	44%	27%	11%	37%
		61, 122, 2–8	3%	11%	57%	30%	7%	25%
	Rahbar, 2016 [58]	74, 74, 5.9	12%	19%	31%	12%	27%	23%
	Rathke, 2017 [69]	40, 40, 4–9.3	10%	30%	38%	18%	12%	20%
	Yadav, 2017 [79]	31, 31, 1.1–5.5	NR	71%		NR	10%	19%
Lu177-PSMA-I&T	Baum, 2016 [60]	56, 125, 3.6–8.7	12%	9%	59%	27%	21%	11

N, number of patients; NCT, number of cycles of therapy; *, activity range in the cycle; S-PSA, stable PSA; P-PSA, progressive PSA; NR, not reported

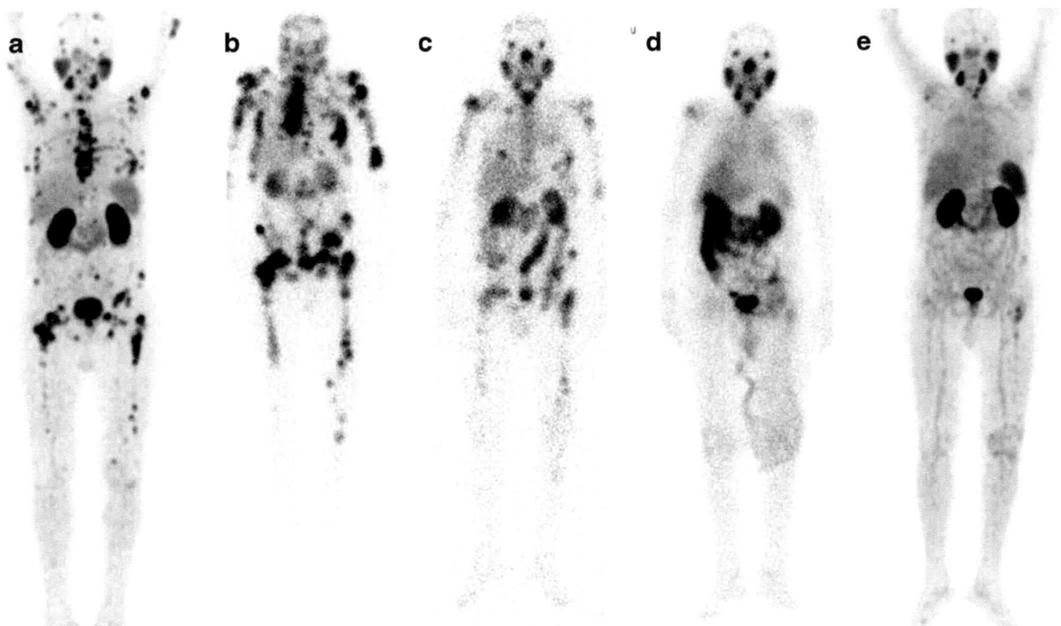

Fig. 15.7 Ga-68 PSMA PET/CT MIP image (**a**) before therapy shows diffuse metastatic disease, planar images (**b**, **c**, **d**) performed after three cycles of Lu-177 PSMA therapy, and Ga-68 PSMA PET/CT MIP image (**e**) shows significant metabolic response

Table 15.12 Molecular and symptomatic response to Lu PSMA therapy

Ligand	Author, year	N, NCT, activity (GBq)	Molecular response CR (%)	RD (%)	SD (%)	PD (%)	Symptomatic response CR (%)	RD (%)	SD (%)	PD (%)
Lu^{177}-PSMA-617	Ahmad Zadehfar, 2016 [3]	20, 40, 4.1–7.1	NR	80	0	20	NR	NR	NR	NR
	Baum, 2016 [60]	56, 125, 3.6–8.7	0	56	8	36	0	33	67	0
	Yadav, 2017 [79]	31, 31, 1.1–5.5	33	50	17	0	23	45	23	9

N, number of patients; NCT, number of cycles of therapy; *, average activity per cycle; CR, complete response; RD, regressed disease; SD, stable disease; PD, progressive disease; NR, not reported

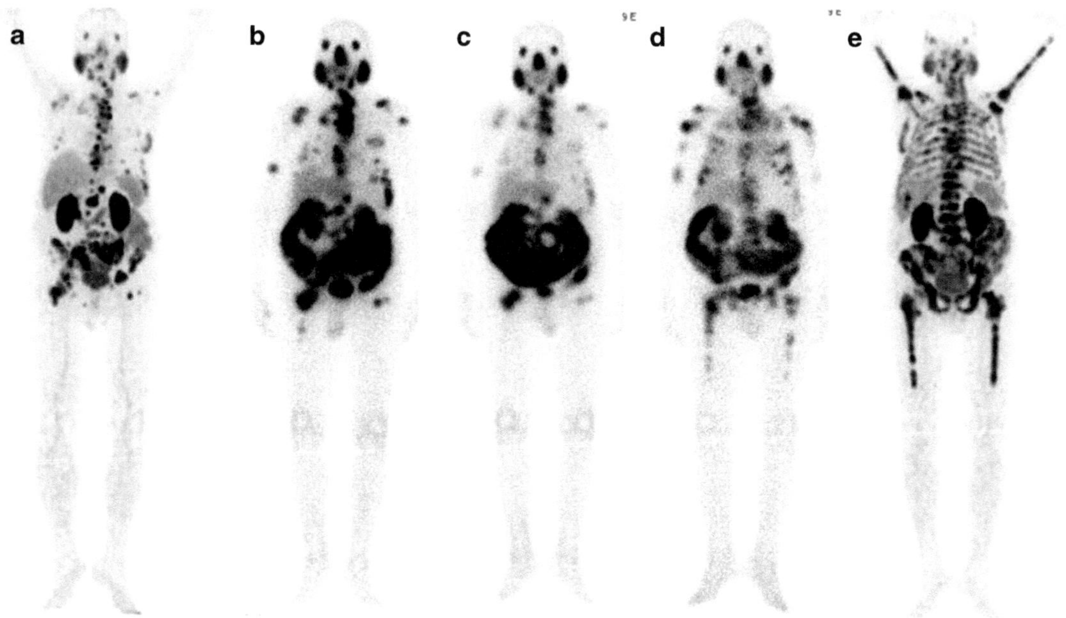

Fig. 15.8 Ga-68 PSMA PET/CT MIP image (**a**) performed before therapy shows metastasis areas showing diffuse PSMA expression. Patient's first pre-therapy serum PSA value is 43.1 ng/mL, second pre-therapy serum PSA value is 22.5 ng/mL, and third pre-therapy serum PSA value is 21.3 ng/mL. While diffuse metastatic disease was observed in the anterior image (**b**) after the first therapy, some therapy response was observed in the anterior image (**c**) after the second therapy, and new metastases were noted in the anterior image (**d**) after the third therapy and Ga-68 PSMA PET/CT MIP image (**e**) after the therapy There is progression in the disease due to the emergence of new lesions even though PSA response to therapy is observed and therapy is noteworthy in some of the initial lesions of the patient

Table 15.13 Lu-177 PSMA therapy progression-free and overall survival

Ligand	Author, year	N, NCT, activity (GBq)	Progression-free survival	Overall survival
Lu^{177}-PSMA-617	Ahmad Zadehfar, 2017 [68]	32, 190, 4.0–7.2	NR	60 (44–76) weeks
	Bruer, 2017 [67]	59, 159, 5.9–6.3	18 weeks	32 weeks
	Yadav, 2017 [79]	31, 31, 1.1–5.5	48 weeks	64 weeks
Lu^{177}-PSMA-I&T	Baum, 2016 [60]	56, 125, 3.6–8.7	54.8 weeks	62 weeks
Ac^{225}-PSMA-617	Kratochwil, 2018 [83]	40, 120, 100 kBq/kg	28 weeks	>48 weeks

N, number of patients; NCT, number of cycles of therapy; *, activity range in cycle; NR, not reported even though PSA response has reached very high rates (80–95%). It can be observed that new lesions emerge due to the fact that the disease has a very high duplication time and that these lesions could not be treated due to the fact that they did not reach radiopharmaceutical during therapy even though regression is observed in the tumor foci existing at the time of therapy in these patients. Therefore, it is not appropriate to monitor the disease only with serum PSA value. Radiological imaging methods and Ga-68 PSMA PET/CT also play an important role in evaluating therapy response.

15.11 Radiation Safety in Lu-177 PSMA Therapy

The patient should be informed about simple radiation safety before therapy, both valid for the duration of hospital stay and valid after leaving the hospital, and should be given in writing. Lu-177 PSMA therapy provides the highest dose per patient and this dose is approximately 6 μSv. Radiopharmacists receive 4 μSv per patient, while technicians receive 3 μSv, and physicists and physicians receive approximately 2 μSv. The highest dose of finger radiation during therapy is taken by radiopharmacists during drug preparation. While the finger dose of radiopharmacists was 31 μSv, it was 3 μSv in nurses [84].

Patients excrete approximately 45% of the injected dose in the first 6 h. The patient dose measured at a distance of 2 meters is <30 μSv at the first hour, whereas the patient dose measured at a distance of 1 meter is <30 μSv at the fifth hour, and < 20 μSv at the sixth hour after 7.4 GBq (200 mCi) Lu-177 PSMA therapy, so it is appropriate to give daily therapy according to the legal conditions of Turkey. The average cumulative dose of 4–5 days in relatives was approximately 202 μSv [84].

15.11.1 Other Radionuclide Therapies

The effectiveness of initial radionuclide therapy was reported to be higher than subsequent therapies in a study of 34 PSMA-targeted patients with I-131-MIP-1095. In other words, it is unlikely to receive therapy response from repeated therapies in the group of patients who did not respond to the first therapy [43]. Another study reported a significant biochemical response with I-131MIP-1095 (Table 15.14) [85]. Lu-177 PSMA therapy can be administered daily, while I-131-MIP-1095 therapy requires patient hospitalization. Specific radiopharmaceuticals (Lu-177 EDTMP) have been reported to be used as cocktails in the therapy of osteoblastic bone metastasis with Lu-177 PSMA in patients with diffuse visceral and bone metastasis [86].

Actinium-225 (Ac-225) PSMA-617 was used for alpha therapy in patients who were not hematologically eligible for Lu-177 PSMA therapy or who progressed despite Lu-177 PSMA therapy, and significant PSA decline and complete remission were even reported in patients with metastatic castration-resistant prostate cancer (Table 15.14) [70, 87, 88]. Then, bismuth-213 (Bi-213) PSMA-617 studies, another alpha agent, started, and a significant biochemical response was reported in these studies [89]. These studies are promising in theranostic therapy as an alternative to beta therapy regimens, even predicting that they will provide more benefits in some cases.

Preclinical studies have been published with I-125 aimed at PSMA and aimed at therapy with Auger electrons [90]. Preclinical studies have been conducted with analogs and antagonists of Lu-177-induced bombesin, and its high rate of involvement in prostate cancer tumor has been reported [91, 92]. In addition, preclinical studies are conducted with Lu-177-DOTA-AE105 targeted at uPAR [93]. There are also preclinical studies where I-131-MIP-1095 and chemotherapy are administered together and Lu-177-labeled radio-immunotherapies are administered [94, 95].

15.12 Concluding Remarks

Ga-68 PSMA PET/CT and Lu-177 PSMA therapy have shown very good clinical, biochemical, anatomical, and metabolic results in the imaging

Table 15.14 PSA response after I-131-MIP-1095 and Ac-225-PSMA-617 therapy

Ligand	Author, year	N, NCT, activity (GBq)	PSA decline <25%	25–50%	>50%	>75%	S-PSA (±25%)	P-PSA (>25%)
I^{131}-MIP-1095	Zechmann, 2014 [85]	25, 25, 2–7.2	8%	10%	64%	28%	10%	16%
	Afshar-Oromieh, 2017 [43]	34, 34, 1.9–7.2	9%	15%	70%	38%	9%	6%
		23, 46, 2.0–6.4	13%	22%	35%	9%	17%	30%
		3, 9, 1.5–3.5	33%	0%	0%	0%	33%	67%
Ac225-PSMA-617	Kratochwil, 2016 [87]	2, 6, 0.006–0.010	0%	0%	100%	100%	0%	0%
	Kratochwil, 2018 [83]	40, 40, 100 kBq/kg	10%	12%	60%	28%	13%	15%
		40, 80, 100 kBq/kg	3%	7%	58%	43%	7%	28%
		40, 120, 100 kBq/kg	5%	5%	45%	35%	10%	40%

N, number of patients; NCT, number of cycles of therapy; *, activity range in the cycle; S-PSA, stable PSA; P-PSA, progressive PSA; NR, not reported

and therapy of castration-resistant prostate cancer. The low levels of side effects of the therapy and its easy tolerance provide a great advantage. Lu-177 PSMA therapy is expected to be included in prostate cancer guidelines soon. Many theranostic agents for the therapy of prostate cancer continue to be developed in light of these results.

References

1. Türkiye Kanser İstatistikleri. 2017.; http://kanser.gov.tr/Dosya/ca_istatistik/2014-RAPOR._uzuuun.pdf.
2. Mottet N, van den Bergh RC, Briers E, et al. EAU-EANM-ESTRO-ESUR-SIOG guidelines on prostate cancer-2020 update. Part 1: Screening, diagnosis, and local treatment with curative ıntent. Eur Urol. 2021;79(2):243–62.
3. Ahmadzadehfar H, Eppard E, Kurpig S, et al. Therapeutic response and side effects of repeated radioligand therapy with 177Lu-PSMA-DKFZ-617 of castrate-resistant metastatic prostate cancer. Oncotarget. 2016;7(11):12477–88.
4. Prostate Cancer Version 2. 2017. NCCN Clin Pract Guidelines Oncol 2017.
5. Attard G, Parker C, Eeles RA, et al. Prostate cancer. Lancet (London, England). 2016;387(10013):70–82.
6. Lian F, Sharma NV, Moran JD, Moreno CS. The biology of castration-resistant prostate cancer. Curr Probl Cancer. 2015;39(1):17–28.
7. Tabayoyong W, Abouassaly R. Prostate cancer screening and the associated controversy. Surg Clin North Am. 2015;95(5):1023–39.
8. Pillai MRA, Nanabala R, Joy A, Sasikumar A, Russ Knapp FF. Radiolabeled enzyme inhibitors and binding agents targeting PSMA: effective theranostic tools for imaging and therapy of prostate cancer. Nucl Med Biol. 2016;43(11):692–720.
9. Schroder FH, Hugosson J, Roobol MJ, et al. Screening and prostate cancer mortality: results of the European Randomised Study of Screening for Prostate Cancer (ERSPC) at 13 years of follow-up. Lancet (London, England). 2014;384(9959):2027–35.
10. Litwin MS, Tan HJ. The diagnosis and treatment of prostate cancer: a review. JAMA. 2017;317(24):2532–42.
11. Lindenberg ML, Turkbey B, Mena E, Choyke PL. Imaging locally advanced, recurrent, and metastatic prostate cancer: a review. JAMA Oncol. 2017;3(10):1415–22.
12. Bernard B, Gershman B, Karnes RJ, Sweeney CJ, Vapiwala N. Approach to oligometastatic prostate cancer. Am Soc Clin Oncol Educ Book. 2016;35:119–29.
13. Bekiş R. Erkek Genital Sistem Kanserlerinde Nükleer Tıp Görüntüleme Yöntemleri. Turkiye Klinikleri J Med Oncol Spec Top. 2011;4(1):168–76.
14. Iagaru AH, Mittra E, Colletti PM, Jadvar H. Bone-targeted ımaging and radionuclide therapy in prostate cancer. J Nucl Med. 2016;57(Suppl 3):19s–24s.
15. Ceci F, Castellucci P, Graziani T, Schiavina R, Fanti S. PET/computed tomography in the ındividualization of treatment of prostate cancer. PET Clin. 2015;10(4):487–94.
16. Van den Bergh L, Lerut E, Haustermans K, et al. Final analysis of a prospective trial on functional imaging for nodal staging in patients with prostate cancer at high risk for lymph node involvement. Urol Oncol. 2015;33(3):109.e123–31.
17. Pinaquy JB, De Clermont-Galleran H, Pasticier G, et al. Comparative effectiveness of [(18) F]- fluorocholine PET-CT and pelvic MRI with diffusion-weighted imaging for staging in patients with high-risk prostate cancer. Prostate. 2015;75(3):323–31.

18. Heck MM, Souvatzoglou M, Retz M, et al. Prospective comparison of computed tomography, diffusion-weighted magnetic resonance imaging and [11C]choline positron emission tomography/computed tomography for preoperative lymph node staging in prostate cancer patients. Eur J Nucl Med Mol Imaging. 2014;41(4):694–701.
19. Budiharto T, Joniau S, Lerut E, et al. Prospective evaluation of 11C-choline positron emission tomography/computed tomography and diffusion-weighted magnetic resonance imaging for the nodal staging of prostate cancer with a high risk of lymph node metastases. Eur Urol. 2011;60(1):125–30.
20. Bekiş R. Prostat kanserinde pozitron emisyon tomografi. Üroonkoloji Bülteni. 2014;13(1):46–9.
21. Fendler WP, Eiber M, Beheshti M, et al. (68)Ga-PSMA PET/CT: Joint EANM and SNMMI procedure guideline for prostate cancer imaging: version 10. Eur J Nucl Med Mol Imaging. 2017;44(6):1014–24.
22. Afshar-Oromieh A, Hetzheim H, Kratochwil C, et al. The theranostic PSMA ligand PSMA-617 in the diagnosis of prostate cancer by PET/CT: biodistribution in humans, radiation dosimetry, and first evaluation of tumor lesions. J Nucl Med. 2015;56(11):1697–705.
23. Jadvar H. Targeted radionuclide therapy: an evolution toward precision cancer treatment. AJR Am J Roentgenol. 2017;209(2):277–88.
24. Benesova M, Schafer M, Bauder-Wust U, et al. Preclinical evaluation of a tailor-made DOTA-conjugated PSMA ınhibitor with optimized linker moiety for ımaging and endoradiotherapy of prostate cancer. J Nucl Med. 2015;56(6):914–20.
25. Bluemel C, Krebs M, Polat B, et al. 68Ga-PSMA-PET/CT in patients with biochemical prostate cancer recurrence and negative 18F-Choline-PET/CT. Clin Nucl Med. 2016;41(7):515–21.
26. Eiber M, Weirich G, Holzapfel K, et al. Simultaneous (68)Ga-PSMA HBED-CC PET/MRI ımproves the localization of primary prostate cancer. Eur Urol. 2016;70(5):829–36.
27. Cardinale J, Schafer M, Benesova M, et al. Preclinical evaluation of (18)F-PSMA-1007, a new prostate-specific membrane antigen ligand for prostate cancer ımaging. J Nucl Med. 2017;58(3):425–31.
28. Giesel FL, Cardinale J, Schafer M, et al. (18) F-Labelled PSMA-1007 shows similarity in structure, biodistribution and tumour uptake to the theragnostic compound PSMA-617. Eur J Nucl Med Mol Imaging. 2016;43(10):1929–30.
29. Nock BA, Kaloudi A, Lymperis E, et al. Theranostic perspectives in prostate cancer with the gastrin-releasing peptide receptor antagonist NeoBOMB1: preclinical and first clinical results. J Nucl Med. 2017;58(1):75–80.
30. Wieser G, Popp I, Christian Rischke H, et al. Diagnosis of recurrent prostate cancer with PET/CT imaging using the gastrin-releasing peptide receptor antagonist (68)Ga-RM2: Preliminary results in patients with negative or inconclusive [(18)F] Fluoroethylcholine- PET/CT. Eur J Nucl Med Mol Imaging. 2017;44(9):1463–72.
31. Umbehr MH, Muntener M, Hany T, Sulser T, Bachmann LM. The role of 11C-choline and 18F- fluorocholine positron emission tomography (PET) and PET/CT in prostate cancer: a systematic review and meta-analysis. Eur Urol. 2013;64(1):106–17.
32. Hernandez-Arguello M, Quiceno H, Pascual I, et al. Index lesion characterization by (11)C- Choline PET/CT and apparent diffusion coefficient parameters at 3 Tesla MRI in primary prostate carcinoma. Prostate. 2016;76(1):3–12.
33. Grosu AL, Weirich G, Wendl C, et al. 11C-Choline PET/pathology image coregistration in primary localized prostate cancer. Eur J Nucl Med Mol Imaging. 2014;41(12):2242–8.
34. Fanti S, Minozzi S, Castellucci P, et al. PET/CT with (11)C-choline for evaluation of prostate cancer patients with biochemical recurrence: meta-analysis and critical review of available data. Eur J Nucl Med Mol Imaging. 2016;43(1):55–69.
35. Ren J, Yuan L, Wen G, Yang J. The value of anti-1-amino-3-18F-fluorocyclobutane-1-carboxylic acid PET/CT in the diagnosis of recurrent prostate carcinoma: a meta-analysis. Acta Radiol (Stockholm, Sweden : 1987). 2016;57(4):487–93.
36. Odewole OA, Tade FI, Nieh PT, et al. Recurrent prostate cancer detection with anti-3- [(18)F]FACBC PET/CT: comparison with CT. Eur J Nucl Med Mol Imaging. 2016;43(10):1773–83.
37. Afshar-Oromieh A, Babich JW, Kratochwil C, et al. The rise of PSMA ligands for diagnosis and therapy of prostate cancer. J Nucl Med. 2016;57(Suppl 3):79s–89s.
38. Haberkorn U, Eder M, Kopka K, Babich JW, Eisenhut M. New strategies in prostate cancer: prostate-specific membrane antigen (PSMA) ligands for diagnosis and therapy. Clin Cancer Res. 2016;22(1):9–15.
39. Rowe SP, Gage KL, Faraj SF, et al. (1)(8)F-DCFBC PET/CT for PSMA-based detection and characterization of primary prostate cancer. J Nucl Med. 2015;56(7):1003–10.
40. Rowe SP, Drzezga A, Neumaier B, et al. Prostate-specific membrane antigen-targeted radiohalogenated PET and therapeutic agents for prostate cancer. J Nucl Med. 2016;57(Suppl. 3):90s–6s.
41. Perera M, Papa N, Christidis D, et al. Sensitivity, specificity, and predictors of Positive (68)Ga-prostate-specific membrane antigen positron emission tomography in advanced prostate cancer: a systematic review and meta-analysis. Eur Urol. 2016;70(6):926–37.
42. Kopka K, Benesova M, Barinka C, Haberkorn U, Babich J. Glu-Ureido-based inhibitors of prostate-specific membrane antigen: lessons learned during the development of a novel class of low-molecular-weight theranostic radiotracers. J Nucl Med. 2017;58(Suppl. 2):17s–26s.
43. Afshar-Oromieh A, Haberkorn U, Zechmann C, et al. Repeated PSMA-targeting radioligand therapy of

metastatic prostate cancer with (131)I-MIP-1095. Eur J Nucl Med Mol Imaging. 2017;44(6):950–9.
44. Weineisen M, Schottelius M, Simecek J, et al. 68Ga- and 177Lu-Labeled PSMA I&T: optimization of a PSMA-targeted theranostic concept and first proof-of-concept human studies. J Nucl Med. 2015;56(8):1169–76.
45. Eppard E, de la Fuente A, Benesova M, et al. Clinical translation and first in-human use of [(44) Sc]Sc-PSMA-617 for PET Imaging of metastasized castrate-resistant prostate cancer. Theranostics. 2017;7(18):4359–69.
46. Caicoya M. Prostate cancer screening in Europe. Lancet (London, England). 2015;385(9977):1507.
47. Hussain M, Tangen CM, Higano C, et al. Absolute prostate-specific antigen value after androgen deprivation is a strong independent predictor of survival in new metastatic prostate cancer: data from Southwest Oncology Group Trial 9346 (INT-0162). J Clin Oncol. 2006;24(24):3984–90.
48. Johansson JE, Holmberg L, Johansson S, Bergstrom R, Adami HO. Fifteen-year survival in prostate cancer. A prospective, population-based study in Sweden. JAMA. 1997;277(6):467–71.
49. Kulkarni HR, Singh A, Schuchardt C, et al. PSMA-Based radioligand therapy for metastatic castration-resistant prostate cancer: The Bad Berka experience since 2013. J Nucl Med. 2016;57(Suppl. 3):97s–104s.
50. Roll W, Bode A, Weckesser M, Bogemann M, Rahbar K. Excellent response to 177Lu-PSMA-617 radioligand therapy in a patient with advanced metastatic castration resistant prostate cancer evaluated by 68Ga-PSMA PET/CT. Clin Nucl Med. 2017;42(2):152–3.
51. Rahbar K, Bode A, Weckesser M, et al. Radioligand therapy with 177Lu-PSMA-617 as A novel therapeutic option in patients with metastatic castration resistant prostate cancer. Clin Nucl Med. 2016;41(7):522–8.
52. Elgqvist J, Timmermand OV, Larsson E, Strand SE. Radiosensitivity of prostate cancer cell lines for irradiation from beta particle-emitting radionuclide (1)(7)(7)Lu compared to alpha particles and Gamma rays. Anticancer Res. 2016;36(1):103–9.
53. Emmett L, Willowson K, Violet J, Shin J, Blanksby A, Lee J. Lutetium (177) PSMA radionuclide therapy for men with prostate cancer: a review of the current literature and discussion of practical aspects of therapy. J Med Radiat Sci. 2017;64(1):52–60.
54. Violet JA, Hofman MS. Prostate-specific membrane antigen from diagnostic to therapeutic target: radionuclide therapy comes of age in prostate cancer. BJU Int. 2017;120(3):310–2.
55. Fendler WP, Rahbar K, Herrmann K, Kratochwil C, Eiber M. (177)Lu-PSMA Radioligand therapy for prostate cancer. J Nucl Med. 2017;58(8):1196–200.
56. Troyer JK, Beckett ML, Wright GL Jr. Location of prostate-specific membrane antigen in the LNCaP prostate carcinoma cell line. Prostate. 1997;30(4):232–42.
57. Chakraborty S, Chakravarty R, Shetty P, Vimalnath KV, Sen IB, Dash A. Prospects of medium specific activity (177) Lu in targeted therapy of prostate cancer using (177) Lu-labeled PSMA inhibitor. J Label Compd Radiopharm. 2016;59(9):364–71.
58. Rahbar K, Schmidt M, Heinzel A, et al. Response and tolerability of a single dose of 177Lu- PSMA-617 in patients with metastatic castration-resistant prostate cancer: a multicenter retrospective analysis. J Nucl Med. 2016;57(9):1334–8.
59. Ferdinandus J, Violet J, Sandhu S, Hofman MS. Prostate-specific membrane antigen theranostics: therapy with lutetium-177. Curr Opin Urol. 2017;
60. Baum RP, Kulkarni HR, Schuchardt C, et al. 177Lu-Labeled prostate-specific membrane antigen radioligand therapy of metastatic castration-resistant prostate cancer: safety and efficacy. J Nucl Med. 2016;57(7):1006–13.
61. Das T, Guleria M, Parab A, et al. Clinical translation of (177)Lu-labeled PSMA-617: Initial experience in prostate cancer patients. Nucl Med Biol. 2016;43(5):296–302.
62. Rahbar K, Bogemann M, Ahmadzadehfar H. (177) Lu-PSMA-617 radioligand therapy of mCRPC: evaluation criteria of response. Eur J Nucl Med Mol Imaging. 2017;44(1):166–7.
63. Yadav MP, Ballal S, Tripathi M, Bal C. Reply to Rahbar K et al. Eur J Nucl Med Mol Imaging. 2017;44(1):168–9.
64. Chatalic KL, Heskamp S, Konijnenberg M, et al. Towards personalized treatment of prostate cancer: PSMA I&T, a promising prostate-specific membrane antigen-targeted theranostic agent. Theranostics. 2016;6(6):849–61.
65. Kletting P, Schuchardt C, Kulkarni HR, et al. Investigating the effect of ligand amount and injected therapeutic activity: a simulation study for 177Lu-labeled PSMA-targeting peptides. PLoS One. 2016;11(9):e0162303.
66. Delker A, Fendler WP, Kratochwil C, et al. Dosimetry for (177)Lu-DKFZ-PSMA-617: a new radiopharmaceutical for the treatment of metastatic prostate cancer. Eur J Nucl Med Mol Imaging. 2016;43(1):42–51.
67. Brauer A, Grubert LS, Roll W, et al. (177) Lu-PSMA-617 radioligand therapy and outcome in patients with metastasized castration-resistant prostate cancer. Eur J Nucl Med Mol Imaging. 2017;44(10):1663–70.
68. Ahmadzadehfar H, Wegen S, Yordanova A, et al. Overall survival and response pattern of castration-resistant metastatic prostate cancer to multiple cycles of radioligand therapy using [(177)Lu]Lu-PSMA-617. Eur J Nucl Med Mol Imaging. 2017;44(9):1448–54.
69. Rathke H, Giesel FL, Flechsig P, et al. Repeated Lu-177-PSMA-617 radioligand therapy using treatment activities up to 9.3 GBq. J Nucl Med. 2017;
70. Kratochwil C, Giesel FL, Stefanova M, et al. PSMA-Targeted radionuclide therapy of metastatic castration-resistant prostate cancer with 177Lu-labeled PSMA-617. J Nucl Med. 2016;57(8):1170–6.
71. Rahbar K, Ahmadzadehfar H, Kratochwil C, et al. German multicenter study investigating 177Lu-PSMA-617 radioligand therapy in

advanced prostate cancer patients. J Nucl Med. 2017;58(1):85–90.
72. Kabasakal L, AbuQbeitah M, Aygun A, et al. Pre-therapeutic dosimetry of normal organs and tissues of (177)Lu-PSMA-617 prostate-specific membrane antigen (PSMA) inhibitor in patients with castration-resistant prostate cancer. Eur J Nucl Med Mol Imaging. 2015;42(13):1976–83.
73. Okamoto S, Thieme A, Allmann J, et al. Radiation dosimetry for (177)Lu-PSMA I&T in metastatic castration-resistant prostate cancer: absorbed dose in normal organs and tumor lesions. J Nucl Med. 2017;58(3):445–50.
74. Yordanova A, Becker A, Eppard E, et al. The impact of repeated cycles of radioligand therapy using [(177) Lu]Lu-PSMA-617 on renal function in patients with hormone refractory metastatic prostate cancer. Eur J Nucl Med Mol Imaging. 2017;44(9):1473–9.
75. Hohberg M, Eschner W, Schmidt M, et al. Lacrimal glands may represent organs at risk for radionuclide therapy of prostate cancer with [(177)Lu]DKFZ-PSMA-617. Mol Imaging Biol. 2016;18(3):437–45.
76. Kabasakal L, Toklu T, Yeyin N, et al. Lu-177-PSMA-617 Prostate-specific membrane antigen inhibitor therapy in patients with castration-resistant prostate cancer: stability, bio- distribution and dosimetry. Mol Imaging Radionucl Ther. 2017;26(2):62–8.
77. Yadav MP, Ballal S, Tripathi M, et al. Post-therapeutic dosimetry of 177Lu-DKFZ-PSMA-617 in the treatment of patients with metastatic castration-resistant prostate cancer. Nucl Med Commun. 2017;38(1):91–8.
78. Schlenkhoff CD, Essler M, Ahmadzadehfar H. Possible treatment approach to an extravasation of 177Lu-PSMA-617. Clin Nucl Med. 2017;42(8):639–40.
79. Yadav MP, Ballal S, Tripathi M, et al. (177)Lu-DKFZ-PSMA-617 therapy in metastatic castration resistant prostate cancer: safety, efficacy, and quality of life assessment. Eur J Nucl Med Mol Imaging. 2017;44(1):81–91.
80. Hofman MS, Emmett L, Sandhu S, et al. [^{177}Lu] Lu-PSMA-617 versus cabazitaxel in patients with metastatic castration-resistant prostate cancer (TheraP): a randomised, open-label, phase 2 trial. Lancet. 2021;397:797–804.
81. Ferdinandus J, Eppard E, Gaertner FC, et al. Predictors of response to radioligand therapy of metastatic castrate-resistant prostate cancer with 177Lu-PSMA-617. J Nucl Med. 2017;58(2):312–9.
82. Sartor O, Bono J, Chi KN, et al. Lutetium-177-PSMA-617 for metastatic castration-resistant prostate cancer. N Engl J Med. 2021;385:1091–103.
83. Kratochwil C, Bruchertseifer F, Rathke H, et al. Targeted Alpha Therapy of mCRPC with (225) Actinium-PSMA-617: Swimmer-Plot analysis suggests efficacy regarding duration of tumor-control. J Nucl Med. 2018;
84. Demir M, Abuqbeitah M, Uslu-Besli L, et al. Evaluation of radiation safety in (177)Lu-PSMA therapy and development of outpatient treatment protocol. J Radiol Protect. 2016;36(2):269–78.
85. Zechmann CM, Afshar-Oromieh A, Armor T, et al. Radiation dosimetry and first therapy results with a (124)I/(131)I-labeled small molecule (MIP-1095) targeting PSMA for prostate cancer therapy. Eur J Nucl Med Mol Imaging. 2014;41(7):1280–92.
86. Bal C, Yadav MP, Ballal S. Cocktail therapy of 177Lu-PSMA-617 and 177Lu-EDTMP in patients with mCRPC: a proof-of-principle application. Clin Nucl Med. 2016;41(8):e386–7.
87. Kratochwil C, Bruchertseifer F, Giesel FL, et al. 225Ac-PSMA-617 for PSMA-targeted alpha-radiation therapy of metastatic castration-resistant prostate cancer. J Nucl Med. 2016;57(12):1941–4.
88. Kratochwil C, Bruchertseifer F, Rathke H, et al. Targeted alpha-therapy of metastatic castration-resistant prostate cancer with (225)Ac-PSMA-617: dosimetry estimate and empiric dose finding. J Nucl Med. 2017;58(10):1624–31.
89. Sathekge M, Knoesen O, Meckel M, Modiselle M, Vorster M, Marx S. (213)Bi-PSMA-617 targeted alpha-radionuclide therapy in metastatic castration-resistant prostate cancer. Eur J Nucl Med Mol Imaging. 2017;44(6):1099–100.
90. Kiess AP, Minn I, Chen Y, et al. Auger radiopharmaceutical therapy targeting prostate-specific membrane antigen. J Nucl Med. 2015;56(9):1401–7.
91. Lim JC, Cho EH, Kim JJ, et al. Biological evaluation of (177)Lu-labeled DOTA-Ala(SO3H)-Aminooctanoyl-Gln-Trp-Ala-Val-N methyl Gly-His-Statine-Leu-NH2 for gastrin-releasing peptide receptor-positive prostate tumor targeting. Nucl Med Biol. 2015;42(2):131–6.
92. Stott Reynolds TJ, Schehr R, Liu D, et al. Characterization and evaluation of DOTA-conjugated Bombesin/RGD-antagonists for prostate cancer tumor imaging and therapy. Nucl Med Biol. 2015;42(2):99–108.
93. Persson M, Juhl K, Rasmussen P, et al. uPAR targeted radionuclide therapy with (177)Lu- DOTA-AE105 inhibits dissemination of metastatic prostate cancer. Mol Pharm. 2014;11(8):2796–806.
94. Tesson M, Rae C, Nixon C, Babich JW, Mairs RJ. Preliminary evaluation of prostate-targeted radiotherapy using (131) I-MIP-1095 in combination with radiosensitising chemotherapeutic drugs. J Pharm Pharmacol. 2016;68(7):912–21.
95. van Rij CM, Frielink C, Goldenberg DM, et al. Pretargeted radioimmunotherapy of prostate cancer with an Anti-TROP-2xAnti-HSG bispecific antibody and a (177)Lu-labeled peptide. Cancer Biother Radiopharm. 2014;29(8):323–9.

16 Systemic Treatments and Related Side Effects in Prostate Cancer

Hüseyin Salih Semiz and İlhan Öztop

Prostate cancer is the most common cancer in the males. It ranks second in cancer-related deaths in the males [1]. The most common symptoms are frequent urination, difficulty in urinating, dysuria, nocturia, and hematuria even though most patients with early prostate cancer are asymptomatic. Pain in the pelvic region and bone pain may also occur at later stages. There are no symptoms specific to prostate cancer. However, it is necessary to suspect in patients who describe these symptoms. Digital rectal examination (DRE) and prostate-specific antigen (PSA) measurement are the two most important parameters in the diagnosis of prostate cancer. Prostate biopsy is required when these two parameters are abnormal. Prostate biopsy is performed with transrectal ultrasound (TRUS). Studies have been conducted to increase diagnostic accuracy with prostate biopsy accompanied by multiparametric MRI (mpMRI) [2]. It has been adopted by international guidelines that prostate biopsy should be taken from at least 12 quadrants [3]. Sometimes biopsy may be benign despite all efforts. Biopsy should be repeated if DRE suggests prostate tumor and PSA continues to increase in such cases.

H. S. Semiz (✉)
Ministry of Health, Tepecik Training and Research Hospital, Izmir, Turkey
e-mail: huseyinsalih.semiz@deu.edu.tr

İ. Öztop
Dokuz Eylül University, Institute of Oncology, Izmir, Turkey
e-mail: ilhan.oztop@deu.edu.tr

Patients with prostate carcinoma are divided into certain risk groups according to the pathological and radiological characteristics of the tumor and PSA values. Treatment is also planned according to these risk groups. Pathologically, the histological degree of the tumor is very important. Gleason score (GS) is used to determine this grade. This scoring system is based on evaluating the architecture of tumor cells and scoring on a scale of 5 points. Gleason score has been in use for many years. However, this system was modified by the International Society of Urological Pathology (ISUP), and a new grading system was developed in 2014. According to this system, grade groups were determined as follows: Grade group 1, GS ≤ 6; Grade group 2, GS $3 + 4 = 7$; Grade group 3, GS $4 + 3 = 7$; Grade group 4, GS $= 8$ ($4 + 4 = 8$, $3 + 5 = 8$, or $5 + 3 = 8$); and Grade group 5, GS 9–10 ($4 + 5$, $5 + 4$, or $5 + 5$). The risk of biochemical failure and prostate cancer-related death increases from Grades 1 to 5 [4]. The use of this system is becoming increasingly widespread all over the world. However, the original Gleason score is still not abandoned. Another parameter in determining the risk groups is the measured total PSA level. PSA levels <10 ng/mL, 10–20 ng/mL, or >20 ng/mL are used to stratify the patients. Another parameter is the number of involvements in these sites in the prostate biopsy and the percentage of tumors in these sites. The risk increases if the number of involvement sites is 3 or more and if the tumor is more than 50% of the site evaluated

R. Bekiş et al. (eds.), *Radionuclide Therapy*, https://doi.org/10.1007/978-3-030-97220-2_16

in the percentage involvement sites. The final parameter in determining the risk groups is the T stage of the tumor [3, 5].

Early-stage prostate cancer patients are divided into five risk groups considering all these factors. Active follow-up, prostatectomy, and curative radiotherapy options in very low- and low-risk patients have almost similar oncological results. Surgery (pelvic lymph node dissection in cases at risk of radical prostatectomy and lymph node metastasis) or radical radiotherapy may be considered in the moderate-risk group. Radiotherapy should be considered in addition to surgery in patients with additional risk factors (surgical margin positivity, seminal vesicle invasion, extracapsular extension, and presence of measurable PSA) detected by pathological evaluation after radical prostatectomy.

Patients with postoperative lymph node metastasis should also receive 6-month androgen deprivation therapy (ADT) in addition to radiotherapy [3]. The weighted approach is 2–3 years of ADT in addition to radiotherapy, while surgery remains an option in high- and very high-risk patients. Adding ADT to radiotherapy contributes to survival.

Local or local advanced prostate cancer may recur despite all these treatment methods. There are two ways in which recurrence can be detected. The first is the increase in PSA after definitive treatments, which is called biochemical recurrence (failure). The second is the detection of distant organ metastasis or local recurrence by imaging methods. Recurrence of disease after radical prostatectomy depends on the GS of the tumor, pathological T stage, PSA value, and other pathological parameters such as surgical margin positivity or perineural invasion.

The presence of distant metastasis should be investigated in patients who develop biochemical recurrence after radical treatments. Patients who develop recurrence after radical treatments are defined as castration-sensitive (CSPC). The situation is different in patients who develop progression while receiving adjuvant ADT. These patients are defined as castration-resistant (CRPC). Prostate cancer is highly sensitive to testosterone and its derivatives, and these hormones are necessary for prostate cancer cells to grow. Prostate cancer cells can obtain these hormones in several different ways. Sources for these hormones are testicles and adrenal glands. Prostate cancer cells, which need non-tumorous hormones in the early stages, develop different mechanisms over time and get rid of this addiction. Castration resistance develops in this case. Some of the mechanisms of this escape are androgen receptor (AR) mutation and amplification, mutations and overexpression in receptor co-activators, androgen-independent AR activation, and androgen production from alternative pathways. AR variants, whose importance has become increasingly better understood in recent years, have also been associated with castration resistance, poor prognosis, and poor response to treatment. Another mechanism whose importance has just begun to be understood is aberrant activation of receptor tyrosine kinases [6].

16.1 Castrate-Sensitive Metastatic Prostate Cancer

Factors affecting the prognosis of metastatic castration-sensitive prostate cancer (mCSPC) include sites of metastasis, time from radical treatments to relapse, PSA doubling time (PDT), duration of response to ADT for patients initially metastatic, and patient performance status. Approximately 20% of newly diagnosed prostate cancer patients are metastatic at diagnosis. Recurrence usually starts as an increase in PSA and progresses toward the metastatic process in other patients. Metastasis sites are important in determining disease burden. Accordingly, the disease is divided into low volume and high volume. High-volume disease is the presence of four or more bone metastases, at least one lesion outside of the vertebral column or pelvis, and/or the presence of solid organ metastases. The main purpose of mCSPC treatment is to reduce the serum testosterone level below 50 ng/mL due to the sensitivity of prostate cancer cells to testosterone and its derivatives. There are also studies in recent years that this level should be reduced below 20 ng/mL. Lowering testosterone levels (castration) can be done in two different ways: bilateral orchiectomy or LHRH analogs/antagonists. There is no clear difference between these two methods yet. Therefore, both methods can be administered by discussing with the patient [3].

Surgical castration is a relatively cheap and easy method. It can also be preferred in spinal cord compression due to metastases where testosterone level needs to be reduced rapidly or urinary obstructions that require urgent intervention. The main mechanism is the suppression of testosterone production from the testicles by suppression of the hypothalamic-pituitary axis in medical castration. Gonadotropin-releasing hormone (GnRH) agonists are usually used for this purpose. GnRH agonists suppress testicular testosterone production by reducing luteinizing hormone (LH) secretion. However, they may cause a temporary increase in testosterone at the beginning of treatment since these molecules are agonist. The patient's symptoms and PSA level may increase as a result of this increase. This is called as "flare phenomenon." Anti-androgen therapy is administered with GnRH analogs to prevent flare phenomenon [3]. These agents start 1 week before the first dose of GnRH analogs and are used up to 1 week after the first dose. GnRH analogs include leuprolide acetate, triptorelin, goserelin, and buserelin. Depot forms of these agents administered subcutaneously every 3 months are used in prostate cancer. There are also agents that do not cause the flare phenomenon. These agents are GnRH antagonists. The most common side effects of GnRH analogs include osteoporosis, cardiovascular toxicity, depression, malaise, gynecomastia, and sexual dysfunction [7].

After demonstrating the effectiveness of chemotherapy administrations in CRPC, it was thought that chemotherapy could provide survival benefits in CSPC. It has been suggested that chemotherapy can be used with ADT (chemohormonal treatment) based on this idea. In large randomized controlled studies such as CHAARTED (Chemohormonal Therapy versus Androgen Ablation Randomized Trial for Extensive Disease in Prostate Cancer), GETUG 15, and STAMPEDE performed for this purpose, it has been shown that docetaxel treatment in high-volume CSPC provides a survival advantage of up to 20 months compared to placebo [8]. Chemohormonal treatment has become the standard in high-volume CSPC today based on these large randomized controlled trials.

Another agent used to prolong survival in CSPC is abiraterone acetate. This molecule is a next-generation androgen synthesis inhibitor. The molecule that inhibits both gonadal and adrenal androgen synthesis strongly suppresses the CYP 17A enzyme, which is the main enzyme in the production of testosterone and its derivatives in steroidogenesis. Excessive activation occurs in the aldosterone synthesis step as a result of this suppression. Side effects such as edema and hypertension occur as a result. This is why abiraterone acetate (AA) is used with prednisone. In the LATITUDE, which showed the efficacy of AA in CSPC, the study was terminated in the interim analysis because the combination of AA and prednisolone versus ADT alone provided a significant survival advantage [9]. The success of abiraterone acetate and docetaxel in CSPC is highly promising. However, there are no randomized controlled trials comparing these agents. Therefore, it is not yet clear which of these two agents should be selected. CSPC passes to CRPC stage within 2–3 years on average despite all these efforts. Survival is around 30–35 months when CRPC occurs.

16.2 Castrate-Resistant Metastatic Prostate Cancer

Retrospective data suggest that there may be a survival advantage of up to 6 months even though there are no randomized controlled studies showing the survival benefit of continuing testosterone synthesis inhibition in patients who develop progression under ADT treatment [10]. Therefore, it is recommended to continue ADT in patients who develop progression under ADT [3, 11]. In addition, the fact that prostate cancer is a heterogeneous disease and that both hormone-sensitive and hormone-resistant clones can be found in the same tumor necessitates the continuation of ADT.

Survival was around 24 months once patients entered the CRPC stage, but this period reached up to 34 months with the development of new molecules. Treatment options in CRPC include anti-androgen therapies (abiraterone acetate, oteronel, seviteronel, galeterone), androgen receptor blockers (enzalutamide, apalutamide, darolutamide), taxanes (docetaxel, cabazitaxel), radionuclide therapies (Lu-177, Ra-223), immunotherapies (sipuleucel-T, pembrolizumab, durvalumab, ipilimumab), PARP inhibitors (olaparib), and multikinase inhibitors (cabozantinib) [3]. Among these treatments, enzalutamide, abiraterone, taxanes, sipuleucel-T, and Ra-223 treatments are used as standard, while most of the other agents are in clinical investigation.

16.2.1 Androgen Receptor Antagonists

Enzalutamide, which has been shown to be superior to anti-androgen treatments such as bicalutamide, has an important place in CRPC treatment [12]. Enzalutamide has three different mechanisms of action: inhibition of the binding of androgens to AR, inhibition of nuclear translocation of AR, and inhibition of AR-induced gene expression. Enzalutamide was first used in CRPC patients who developed progression after docetaxel treatment in the AFFIRM study. Up to 50% of the cases received 3 or more hormone therapies, and up to 25% received 2 or more chemotherapy regimens in this study of 1199 patients diagnosed with CRPC, in which enzalutamide was compared with placebo. OS was 18.4 months in patients receiving enzalutamide and 13.6 months in the placebo group in this study ($p < 0.001$). Enzalutamide was superior to placebo in all patients in the subgroup analysis of the study [13]. This agent has been tested in patients who have not received chemotherapy due to this OS advantage provided with enzalutamide. 1717 patients diagnosed with CRPC who did not receive docetaxel in the PREVAIL study were randomized to enzalutamide and placebo groups. Enzalutamide provided a 4-month OS advantage over placebo in the final analysis of the study ($p = 0.0002$).

Enzalutamide was superior to placebo in all patients in the subgroup analysis of the study [14]. Enzalutamide provided an OS advantage in both studies. However, the opposite group was placebo in both studies. There is no randomized controlled trial comparing enzalutamide with docetaxel or other agents yet. Therefore, there is no standard in which patients enzalutamide treatment should be preferred. However, the patient group in which enzalutamide treatment can be preferred may be patients without solid organ metastasis, who have not progressed for a long time with ADT, and who are not suitable for chemotherapy when the literature is reviewed. The most important side effects associated with enzalutamide treatment were weakness, transaminase elevation, musculoskeletal pain, diarrhea, headache, and pyrexia in both studies. The most feared side effect associated with enzalutamide was epileptic seizure. However, the proportion of patients who had seizures was below 1% for both studies. Caution should be exercised during enzalutamide use in patients with a history of seizures in this respect. Other side effects of enzalutamide include peripheral edema, hypertension, weakness, electrolyte imbalance, pyrexia, nausea, myalgia, ischemic heart disease, and lower and upper respiratory tract infections [15]. No standard recommendation is available for dose reduction when any toxicity develops. However, it has been reported in clinical and preclinical studies that adequate plasma levels of up to 80 mg/day can be achieved. The drug should be discontinued completely if any grade 4 side effects develop [16].

Successful results with enzalutamide led to the development of new molecules. Apalutamide and darolutamide are newly developed AR antagonists in this sense. Clinical trials with these agents are ongoing and promising.

16.2.2 Androgen Synthesis Inhibitors

One of the earliest examples of androgen synthesis inhibitors is ketoconazole, an adrenolytic antifungal. However, it is not preferred today due to its toxic effects and low effectiveness. Instead, abiraterone acetate was developed, which specifically inhibits 17 alpha-hydroxylase and 17,20-lyase, which are very important enzymes in testosterone synthesis in androgen synthesis steps. In the COU-AA-301 study, the first study of this agent, patients with CRPC who had previously received docetaxel and had progressed were randomized to the abiraterone acetate and placebo arms. Abiraterone must be used in combination with steroids to reduce its side effects due to increased aldosterone rebound. Therefore, prednisone was administered to both groups. Abiraterone acetate provided a 4.6-month advantage in terms of OS compared to placebo in this study [17]. A COU-AA-302 study was conducted in patients with CRPC who had not received docetaxel treatment afterward. Patients were also randomized to abiraterone+prednisone and placebo+prednisone groups in this study.

Abiraterone acetate made a 4.4-month difference compared to placebo when the results of the study were evaluated in terms of OS [18]. The most common side effects of abiraterone were fluid retention, hypertension, hypokalemia, cardiac toxicity, elevated transaminase, and atrial fibrillation in both studies. However, it was difficult to establish a standard treatment scheme since the opposite group was placebo in both studies. It is still unclear which hormone therapy should be preferred in which patients.

One of the biggest issues with hormonal therapies is the development of resistance. AR variants are an important mechanism in this resistance. Of these, AR-V7 is the most studied variant and is associated with hormone therapy resistance, poor prognosis, and, in part, poor response to chemotherapy. AR-V7 positivity was detected in 19–39% of patients treated with enzalutamide and abiraterone. Hormone therapy response is significantly poor in AR-V7-positive patients. This high rate means that almost one third of patients are primarily resistant to hormonal therapies. In addition, AR-V7 positivity may develop in AR-V7-negative patients after hormone therapy. Therefore, docetaxel and cabazitaxel treatments are thought to be less effective in patients receiving hormonal therapy compared to those not receiving hormonal therapy. This taxane resistance is thought to be related to the inhibition of microtubules by taxanes, which prevents leaf AR from being transported to the nucleus [19].

Today, there is no definitive rule on which hormone therapies should be preferred first in which patients. It is also unclear in which patients chemotherapy should be administered first and in which patients hormone therapy should be administered first. It will be more accurate to make individualized choices for each patient by evaluating the comorbidities of the patients, the course of the disease, PSA doubling time, the patient's performance, the duration of response to previous ADT, and the natural course of the disease when selecting these treatments.

16.2.3 Chemotherapeutics

Many chemotherapy agents were tested for prostate cancer several decades ago, but none of them had a survival advantage. The most effective chemotherapeutic drug before docetaxel was mitoxantrone. Mitoxantrone, an antimicrotubular agent, provided only symptom palliation and did not contribute to survival. In addition, dose-dependent cardiotoxicity was also an important problem. Subsequently, studies were conducted with docetaxel.

Firstly, Tannock et al. showed that docetaxel 75 mg/m^2 every 3 weeks provided 2.4-month OS advantage in patients diagnosed with CRPC [20]. There were three treatment groups in this study. There was mitoxantrone in the first arm, docetaxel 25 mg/m^2 weekly in the second arm, and docetaxel 75 mg/m^2 in the other arm for 3 weeks. It was shown that weekly docetaxel arm was not different from mitoxantrone, and docetaxel every 3 weeks arm was superior to the other two arms. Toxicities included neuropathy, myelosuppression, alopecia, nausea-vomiting, nail changes, fluid retention, loss of appetite, diarrhea, fever, and weakness, and these side effects were acceptable in the study [21]. Docetaxel 75 mg/m^2 every 3 weeks has become standard for CRPC treatment in line with this study.

Cabazitaxel is another chemotherapeutic that was developed after docetaxel and has been shown to be effective in docetaxel-resistant prostate carcinoma cell clones. Cabazitaxel is also a microtubule inhibitor of the taxane class. After showing its efficacy in a few prostate cancer cases in Basket studies, it was first studied in TROPIC study in patients with CRPC who had progressed after docetaxel treatment. In this study, neutropenia was observed to be the most important toxicity. Cabazitaxel provides a survival advantage of 2.4 months compared to mitoxantrone. In this study, 80% of patients developed neutropenia, and 8% developed neutropenic fever because prophylactic colony-stimulating factor (CSF) was not given as standard [22].

For this reason, cabazitaxel is currently applied with CSF support. Due to these survival results and the activity of cabazitaxel in docetaxel-resistant cell clones, the question of which taxane would be more beneficial to administer first came to mind. In the FIRSTANA study designed to answer this question, doses of 20 mg/m^2 and 25 mg/m^2 of cabazitaxel and 75 mg/m^2 of docetaxel were compared in a randomized controlled manner. In this study, it was concluded that all three arms were equally effective and cabazitaxel 20 mg/m^2 dose caused less toxicity [23].

Chemotherapeutic drugs commonly used in the treatment of metastatic prostate cancer include docetaxel and cabazitaxel. Main side effects of docetaxel include hypersensitivity, fluid retention, hematological toxicity, skin and nail changes, alopecia, and neurotoxicity. Side effects are much more common and more severe in patients with preexisting liver dysfunction and elevated enzymes. Premedication is routinely performed with steroids and antihistamines against hypersensitivity reaction. Patients who develop hypersensitivity despite premedication are intervened in line with the principles of approach to general hypersensitivity. Fluid retention is mostly associated with cumulative dose and manifests itself as progressive peripheral edema, weight increase, acid, pleural effusion, and pericardial effusion [21]. Main side effects of cabazitaxel include hematological toxicity, hypersensitivity reaction, diarrhea, malaise, alopecia, and nausea-vomiting. Age is an important factor in terms of toxicity and the risk of toxicity increases in patients aged 65 years and older. Today, it is routinely applied in G-CSF support to reduce the risk of neutropenia and related complications. Premedication is routinely performed with steroids and antihistamines against hypersensitivity reaction. However, patients who develop hypersensitivity reaction are intervened in line with the principles of approach to general hypersensitivity [24].The severity of toxicities is usually graded according to assessment methods such as the National Cancer Institute Common Terminology Criteria for Adverse Events (NCI-CTCAE) [25]. Approaches such as discontinuation, postponement, dose reduction, as well as specific approaches specific to toxicity are made depending on the type and degree of toxicity observed (Tables 16.1–16.3) [3, 11].

16.2.4 Immunotherapies

Prostate cancer is one of the tumors in which the immune response, namely, inflammation, is very low. Therefore, immunotherapy has not been included in prostate cancer until recently. One of the first immunotherapy trials in CRPC patients is sipuleucel-T treatment, a dendritic cell-based treatment. Sipuleucel-T has been developed to increase T cell response to prostatic acid phosphatase (PAP). PSA response and radiological response cannot be achieved with this treatment. It has not been shown to be useful in patients with solid organ metastases and symptomatic diseases. In the IMPACT study, patients diagnosed with CRPC who were previously treated and progressed with docetaxel or who were not eligible for docetaxel evaluating the efficacy of this agent. Patients were randomized 2:1 to placebo and sipuleucel-T groups. Sipuleucel-T contributed 4.1-month OS compared to placebo in this study. The most common side effects were infusion reactions and 3.5% cerebrovascular events were also observed [26]. Although this treatment (which is very difficult to apply and requires special laboratory conditions) provides a survival advantage, it cannot be used in many centers. The most common side effects of this treatment include chills, tremors, fever, back pain, nausea, anemia, and diarrhea [27].

Table 16.1 Hematological toxicity NCI-CTCAE v5.0 [25]

Blood element	Grade 1	Grade 2	Grade 3	Grade 4	Grade 5
Neutrophils	Between LLN and 1500/ microL	1000–1500/ microL	500–1000/microL	<500/microL	
Platelets	Between LLN and 75,000/ microL	50,000–75,000/ microL	25,000–50,000/microL	<25,000/microL	
Hemoglobin	Between LLN and 10.0 g/dL	8.0–10.0 g/ dL	<8.0 g/dL	Life-threatening consequences; requiring urgent intervention	Death
Febrile neutropenia			Absolute number of neutrophils <1000 microL and presence of body temperature >38.3 °C at a single measurement or ≥38.00 °C lasting longer than 1 h	Life-threatening consequences; requiring urgent intervention	Death

NCI-CTCAE, National Cancer Institute Common Terminology Criteria for Adverse Events; LLN, lower limit of normal; cell/microL, cell/mm^3 or cell × 10^9/L

Table 16.2 Neurotoxicity NCI-CTCAE v5.0 [25]

Adverse event	Grade 1	Grade 2	Grade 3	Grade 4	Grade 5
Paresthesia	Moderate symptoms	Moderate symptoms; limiting daily life	Severe symptoms; limiting self-care		
Peripheral motor neuropathy	Asymptomatic; based on clinical or diagnostic observation only	Moderate symptoms; limiting daily life	Severe symptoms; limiting self-care	Life-threatening outcomes; urgent intervention indicated	Death
Peripheral sensory neuropathy	Asymptomatic	Moderate symptoms; limiting daily life	Severe symptoms; limiting self-care	Life-threatening outcomes; urgent intervention indicated	

NCI-CTCAE, National Cancer Institute Common Terminology Criteria for Adverse Events

Apart from this, studies on ipilimumab, a CTLA-4 inhibitor; pembrolizumab, a PD-1 inhibitor; and their combination with chemotherapeutics and other agents are ongoing and have not yet been reflected in clinical practice.

16.3 Castrate-Resistant Nonmetastatic Prostate Cancer

The first sign of treatment failure in cases of local advanced or local prostate carcinoma (that is not metastatic at the time of diagnosis) is usually an increase in PSA values. The vast majority of these patients develop distant organ, bone, or lymph node metastasis. However, only some of the patients who develop biochemical recurrence and receive salvage therapies can proceed to the CRPC stage before metastasis develops during follow-up. There is no standard treatment approach in this group of patients. Clinical follow-up was performed in this group of patients from past to present until secondary hormonal manipulations or metastasis developed. However, recent studies with abiraterone acetate and apalutamide have shown that the time until metastasis develops in this patient group can be extended to 40 months [28, 29]. OS, which is around 24 months after the development of castration-

Table 16.3 Hepatobiliary toxicity NCI-CTCAE v5.0 [25]

Adverse event	Grade 1	Grade 2	Grade 3	Grade 4	Grade 5
ALP increase	If baseline is normal, ULN to 2.5 × ULN	If baseline is normal, 2.5–5 × ULN	If baseline is normal, 5–20 × ULN	If baseline is normal, >20 × ULN	
	If baseline is abnormal, 2–2.5 × baseline	If baseline is abnormal, 2.5–5 × baseline	If baseline is abnormal, 5–20 × baseline	If baseline is abnormal, >20 × baseline	
ALT increase	If baseline is normal, ULN to 3 × ULN If baseline is abnormal, 1.5–3 × baseline	If baseline is normal, 3–5 × ULN If baseline is abnormal, 3–5 × baseline	If baseline is normal, 5–20 × ULN If baseline is abnormal, 5–20 × baseline	If baseline is normal, >20 × ULN If baseline is abnormal, >20 × baseline	
AST increase	If baseline is normal, ULN to 3 × ULN If baseline is abnormal, 1.5–3 × baseline	If baseline is normal, 3–5 × ULN If baseline is abnormal, 3–5 × baseline	If baseline is normal, 5–20 × ULN If baseline is abnormal, 5–20 × baseline	If baseline is normal, >20 × ULN If baseline is abnormal, >20 × baseline	
Serum bilirubin increase	If baseline is normal, ULN to 1.5 × ULN	If baseline is normal, 1.5–3 × ULN	If baseline is normal, 3–10 × ULN	If baseline is normal, >10 × ULN	
	If baseline is abnormal, 1–1.5 × baseline	If baseline is abnormal, 1.5–3 × baseline	If baseline is abnormal, 3–10 × baseline	If baseline is abnormal, >10 × baseline	
GGT increase	If baseline is normal, ULN to 2.5 × ULN	If baseline is normal, 2.5–5 × ULN	If baseline is normal, 5–20 × ULN	If baseline is normal, >20 × ULN	
	If baseline is abnormal, 2–2.5 × baseline	If baseline is abnormal, 2.5–5 × baseline	If baseline is abnormal, 5–20 × baseline	If baseline is abnormal, >20 × baseline	
Liver failure			Asterixis, moderate	Life-threatening outcomes	Death
			Encephalopathy, liver injury due to the drug, limitation of self-care	Moderate-severe encephalopathy, coma	
Portal hypertension		Decrease in portal vein flow	Reverse/retrograde portal vein flow with varicose and/or acid	Life-threatening outcomes, requiring urgent intervention	Death

NCI-CTCAE, National Cancer Institute Common Terminology Criteria for Adverse Events; ULN, upper limit of normal; ALP, alkaline phosphatase; ALT, alanine aminotransferase; AST, aspartate aminotransferase; GGT, gamma-glutamyl transpeptidase

resistant metastatic disease in patients diagnosed with prostate carcinoma, is expected to progress to much better points in line with these developments.

16.3.1 Bisphosphonates

Bone is one of the most commonly involved regions in prostate cancer cases. Bone metastases are usually osteoblastic in prostate cancer. It is often located in the axial skeleton. Intensive efforts have been made in this regard due to the fact that bone metastases cause serious morbidities such as fractures and pain. Many bone-targeted radionuclide therapies such as Ra-223, sipuleucel-T, strontium, and samarium have been developed because of these efforts. In addition, surgery and radiotherapy options are used extensively in metastases leading to neurological symptoms and fractures. Other frequently used treatment options for bone metastases are bisphosphonates and denosumab, a monoclonal antibody developed against nuclear factor kappa beta (RANK) ligand (RANKL), which has been increasingly used in recent years [30]. Many studies have shown that bisphosphonate treatment has no effect on OS.

However, the main function of bisphosphonates is to reduce and delay bone-related events (fracture, surgery, radiotherapy requirement, etc.). Studies on ibandronic acid, zoledronic acid, clodronate, and pamidronate have been conducted in prostate carcinoma, and all these agents have been shown to prolong the time to the first skeletal-related event. Bisphosphonate treatment also has a palliation function of bone pain due to metastases. Denosumab, an osteoclast inhibitor, has been shown to significantly prolong time to the skeletal-related first event compared to zoledronic acid. In addition, zoledronic acid therapy requires dose adjustments in patients with impaired renal function. It is even contraindicated if creatinine clearance is <30 mL/min. However, no dose adjustments are required for denosumab in patients with renal failure. But, it should be kept in mind that deep hypocalcemia may develop in patients with renal failure [3, 11, 30].

References

1. American Cancer Society. Cancer facts & figures 2018. Atlanta: American Cancer Society; 2018.
2. Siddiqui MM, Rais-Bahrami S, Truong H, et al. Magnetic resonance imaging/ultrasound-fusion biopsy significantly upgrades prostate cancer versus systematic 12-core transrectal ultrasound biopsy. Eur Urol. 2013;64(5):713–9.
3. National Comprehensive Cancer Network (NCCN) Website. NCCN Clinical practice guidelines in oncology. Available at: https://www.nccn.org/professionals/physician_gls/pdf/prostate.pdf. Accessed 14 May 2018.
4. Epstein JI, Zelefsky MJ, Sjoberg DD, et al. A contemporary prostate cancer grading system: a validated alternative to the Gleason score. Eur Urol. 2016;69(3):428–35.
5. Afshar-Oromieh A, Malcher A, Eder M, et al. PET imaging with a [68Ga]gallium-labelled PSMA ligand for the diagnosis of prostate cancer: biodistribution in humans and first evaluation of tumour lesions. Eur J Nucl Med Mol Imaging. 2013;40(4):486–95.
6. Chandrasekar T, Yang JC, Gao AC, Evans CP. Mechanisms of resistance in castration-resistant prostate cancer (CRPC). Transl Androl Urol. 2015;4(3):365–80.
7. Prostate Cancer Trialists' Collaborative Group. Maximum androgen blockade in advanced prostate cancer: an overview of the randomised trials. Lancet. 2000;355:1491–8. [No authors listed]
8. Parimi S, Chi KN. Chemotherapy for metastatic castration-sensitive prostate cancer. Int J Urol. 2016;23:726–33.
9. Fizazi K, Tran N, Fein L, et al. Abiraterone plus prednisone in metastatic, castration-sensitive prostate cancer. N Engl J Med. 2017;377(4):352–60.
10. Taylor CD, Elson P, Trump DL. Importance of continued testicular suppression in hormone-refractory prostate cancer. J Clin Oncol. 1993;11(11):2167–72.
11. UpToDate website. Available at: https://www.uptodate.com/contents/overview of the treatment of castration-resistant prostate cancer (CRPC).
12. Shore ND, Chowdhury S, Villers A, et al. Efficacy and safety of enzalutamide versus bicalutamide for patients with metastatic prostate cancer (TERRAIN): a randomised, double-blind, phase 2 study. Lancet Oncol. 2016;17(2):153–63.
13. Scher HI, Fizazi K, Saad F, et al. Increased survival with enzalutamide in prostate cancer after chemotherapy. N Engl J Med. 2012;367(13):1187–97.
14. Beer TM, Armstrong AJ, Rathkopf DE, et al. Enzalutamide in metastatic prostate cancer before chemotherapy. N Engl J Med. 2014;371(5):424–33.
15. http://www.bccancer.bc.ca/drug-database-site/Drug%20Index/Enzalutamide_monograph.pdf
16. Scher HI, Beer TM, Higano CS, et al. Antitumour activity of MDV3100 in castration-resistant prostate cancer: a phase 1–2 study. Lancet. 2010;375(9724):1437–46. Published online 2010 Apr 14. https://doi.org/10.1016/S0140-6736(10)60172-9.
17. de Bono JS, Logothetis CJ, Molina A, et al. Abiraterone and increased survival in metastatic prostate cancer. N Engl J Med. 2011;364(21):1995–2005.
18. Ryan CJ, Smith MR, Fizazi K, et al. Abiraterone acetate plus prednisone versus placebo plus prednisone in chemotherapy-naive men with metastatic castration-resistant prostate cancer (COU- AA-302): final overall survival analysis of a randomised, double-blind, placebo-controlled phase 3 study. Lancet Oncol. 2015;16(2):152–60.
19. Antonarakis ES, Lu C, Wang H, et al. AR-V7 and resistance to enzalutamide and abiraterone in prostate cancer. N Engl J Med. 2014;371(11):1028–38.
20. Tannock IF, de Wit R, Berry WR, et al. Docetaxel plus prednisone or mitoxantrone plus prednisone for advanced prostate cancer. N Engl J Med. 2004;351(15):1502–12.
21. http://www.bccancer.bc.ca/drug-database-site/Drug%20Index/Docetaxel_monograph.pdf
22. de Bono JS, Oudard S, Ozguroglu M, et al. Prednisone plus cabazitaxel or mitoxantrone for metastatic castration-resistant prostate cancer progressing after

docetaxel treatment: a randomised open-label trial. Lancet. 376(9747):1147–54.
23. Oudard S, Fizazi K, Sengelov L, et al. Cabazitaxel versus docetaxel as first-line therapy for patients with metastatic castration-resistant prostate cancer: a randomized phase III trial-FIRSTANA. J Clin Oncol. 2017;35(28):3189–97.
24. http://www.bccancer.bc.ca/drug-database-site/Drug%20Index/Cabazitaxel_monograph.pdf
25. https://ctep.cancer.gov/protocoldevelopment/electronic_applications/docs/CTCAE_v5_Quick_Reference_8.5x11.pdf (Accessed on March 09, 2018).
26. Kantoff PW, Higano CS, Shore ND, et al. Sipuleucel-T immunotherapy for castration-resistant prostate cancer. N Engl J Med. 2010;363(5):411–22.
27. https://www.pbm.va.gov/clinicalguidance/drugmonographs/SipuleucelTDrugMonograph.doc
28. Ryan CJ, Crawford ED, Shore ND, et al. The IMAAGEN Study: effect of abiraterone acetate and prednisone on prostate specific antigen and radiographic disease progression in patients with nonmetastatic castration resistant prostate cancer. J Urol. 2018;200(2):344–52.
29. Smith MR, Saad F, Chowdhury S, et al. Apalutamide treatment and metastasis-free survival in prostate cancer. N Engl J Med. 2018;378:1408–18.
30. Fizazi K, Carducci M, Smith M, et al. Denosumab versus zoledronic acid for treatment of bone metastases in men with castration-resistant prostate cancer: a randomised, double-blind study. Lancet. 2011;377(9768):813–22.

Part VII

Clinical Information: Bone and Joint Diseases

17 Radionuclide Therapy in Joint Diseases: Radiosynovectomy

Cüneyt Türkmen

Radiosynovectomy is a minimally invasive and effective radionuclide therapy method in the treatment of resistant synovial inflammation. The effect of the therapy is obtained by fibrosing hypertrophic synovia with ionizing radiation emitted by colloidal form radionuclides injected locally into the joint. The most common indications are rheumatoid arthritis, hemophilic synovitis, and osteoarthritis [1].

The first radiosynovectomy was performed in 1963 with radioactive gold (Au-198) injection to the knee joint to treat resistant effusion in the literature [2]. However, yttrium-90 (Y-90) and phosphor-32 (P-32) have been used more commonly in radiosynovectomy since the 1970s due to the small particle size and high rates of extraarticular leakage of Au-198. Today, erbium-169 citrate (Er-169) in small joints, rhenium-186 (Re-186) sulfide, or P-32 colloid in medium-sized joints such as wrists, elbows, and shoulders and Y-90 citrate/silicate colloid in the knee joint are commonly used radiosynovectomy agents although accessibility varies in different regions (Table 17.1). There are radiosynovectomy agents such as dysprosium-165 ferric hydroxide, holmium-166 hydroxyapatite, and samarium-153 hydroxyapatite used in the studies although not common [3].

C. Türkmen (✉)
Istanbul Faculty of Medicine, Department of Nuclear Medicine, Istanbul University, Istanbul, Turkey
e-mail: cturkmen@istanbul.edu.tr

17.1 Mechanism of Action

The size of 2–5 μ colloidal particles injected into the joint space is small enough to be phagocytized by synovial cells but not large enough to enter the systemic circulation through capillaries. Radiopharmaceutical is phagocytized by type 2 synovial cells (synovial macrophages) after injection into the joint space (Fig. 17.1). Since more than 90% of beta radiation is effective at a penetration distance of 10 mm, most of it is absorbed by synovial tissue, synovial fluid, superficial cartilage, and articular capsule. Radiation exposure of subchondral bone and other paraarticular tissues is minimal [4]. Fibrotic changes develop in the synovial membrane, and occlusion develops in the superficial capillaries due to the effect of radiation. The regression of inflammation and synovial proliferation occurs clinically as decreased pain, effusion, and increased joint mobility in patients with signs of arthritis. The most prominent clinical effect is the decrease in the number of bleeding in hemophilic synovitis.

17.2 Indications and Contraindications

Interdisciplinary approach is very important in determining the indication for radiosynovectomy treatment. Evaluation of the patients by rheumatologist, orthopedist, hematologist, and nuclear

R. Bekiş et al. (eds.), *Radionuclide Therapy*, https://doi.org/10.1007/978-3-030-97220-2_17

Table 17.1 Radiopharmaceuticals used in radiosynovectomy

	Y-90	Re-186	Er-169
Physical half-life (days)	2.7	3.7	9.5
Maximum beta energy (MeV)	2.26	1.07	0.34
Gamma energy (KeV)	–	137	–
Maximum tissue penetration (mm)	11.0	3.7	1.0
Mean tissue penetration (mm)	2.8	1.0	0.3
Particle size (μm)	2	1–2	0.05–0.5
Joint	Knee	Shoulder, coxofemoral, wrist, ankle elbow	Small joints in hands and feet, acromioclavicular and temporomandibular
Dose/volume	185–222 MBq/3–5 ml	37–185 MBq/1–3 ml	10–40 MBq/0.5–1 ml

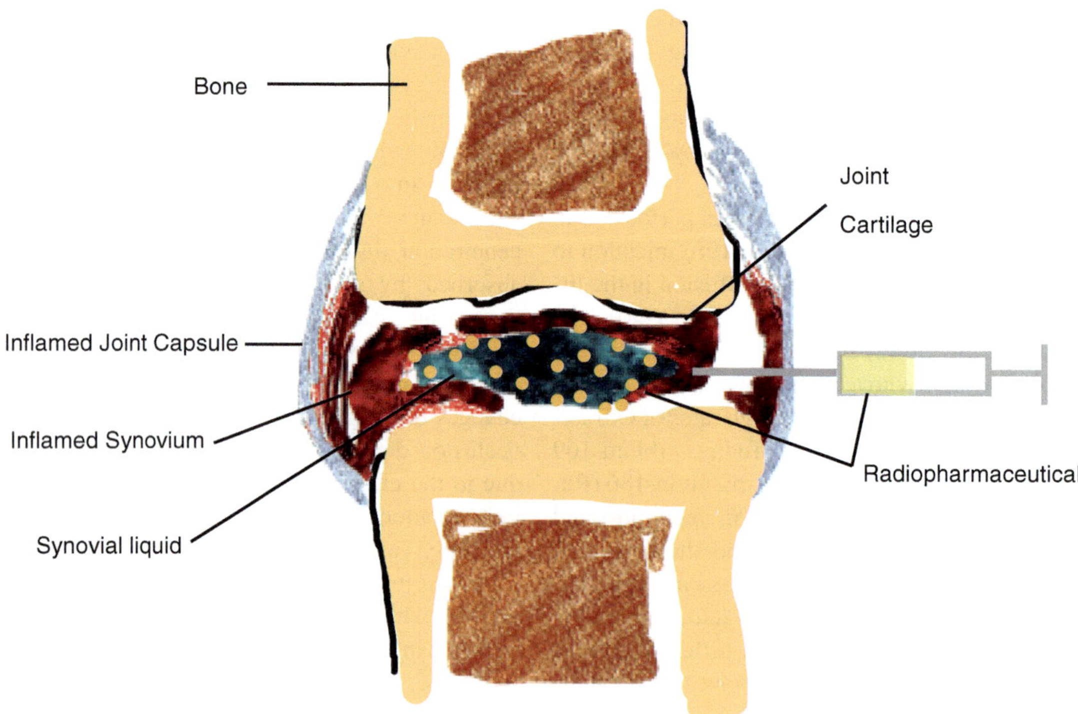

Fig. 17.1 Radiosynovectomy treatment

medicine specialist according to the indication is important in determining the group of patients who will benefit from the treatment. Radiosynovectomy is particularly effective in patients with evidence of active synovitis. Therefore, joint ultrasonography and three-phase bone scintigraphy are diagnostic methods used to demonstrate synovial inflammation in determining the indication for treatment in addition to clinical examination.

Direct radiography is also useful in determining joint degeneration and damage. MR imaging can give more information in the evaluation of soft tissues.

Since the frequency of target joint bleeding is important in patients who are candidates for radiosynovectomy due to hemophilic synovitis, factors such as the number of intraarticular bleeding in the last 6 months and whether they receive factor prophylaxis or not are evaluated. Patients with a history of bleeding of three or more in the last 6 months are the most beneficial group even though they receive secondary prophylaxis in the treatment of hemophilic synovitis. Radiosynovectomy should not be considered as first-line therapy in patients with rheumatoid arthritis. Patients should undergo a complete rheumatological evaluation and have tried standard anti-rheumatoid drug (DMARDs) therapy for at least 6 months before radiosynovectomy indication. The patient should be observed for 6 months after at least one intraarticular glucocorticoid injection in the osteoarthritis group, where there is no effective systemic pharmacological treatment [5].

17.2.1 Indications

- Rheumatoid arthritis, seronegative spondyloarthropathy (e.g., reactive or psoriatic arthritis).
- Other inflammatory joint diseases (e.g., Lyme disease, Behçet's disease).
- Unspecified arthritis characterized by synovitis, synovial thickening, or effusion.
- Resistant synovial effusion (e.g., after arthroscopic synovectomy or after joint prosthesis).
- Osteoarthritis.
- Pigmented villonodular synovitis.
- Hemophilic synovitis.

17.2.2 Contraindications

- Pregnancy.
- Breastfeeding.
- Localized skin infection.
- Acute rupture of popliteal cyst (Baker's cyst).

17.2.3 Relative Contraindications

- If the expected benefit of treatment in children and adolescents is greater than its potential risks, it should be administered.
- Common joint instability and bone destruction.
- Significant joint cartilage loss.

17.3 Patient Preparation and Radiosynovectomy

It is important that the penetration distance of the beta energy of radionuclide is compatible with the synovial thickness and that the half-life of radionuclide is important in radiopharmaceutical selection. Y-90 citrate for knee joint, Re-186 sulfide for shoulder and medium-sized joints such as the wrist and hip joint, and Er-169 citrate for small joints in hands and feet, as well as sternoclavicular and acromioclavicular joint and temporomandibular joint, are among the licensed radiopharmaceuticals used for radiosynovectomy treatment in Europe.

Radiosynovectomy is a local treatment that does not require special preparation (drug discontinuation, etc.) except for outpatient hemophilia patients. It is important to regulate the level of factor concentration by the hematologist in order to perform factor injection 1–2 h before the procedure and to continue on the following days after the procedure according to the clinical status of the patient in order to reduce the risk of bleeding as with all interventional procedures in hemophilic patients. The nuclear medicine specialist is responsible for the indication of radiosynovectomy, which is a radionuclide therapy after the clinical signs of the patients are evaluated together with the relevant clinicians. A detailed anamnesis and clinical examination should be performed before treatment. Patients or, in pediatric cases, their parents should be informed and their consent should be obtained before treatment.

Radiosynovectomy treatment should be performed in an area prepared in accordance with radiation safety rules and aseptic conditions for intervention. The use of appropriate equipment (such as syringe shield, transport container) to protect against beta radiation during the treatment process is particularly effective in reducing the finger dose of the personnel performing the administration. The radiation doses exposed to the personnel during the treatment are at low levels. Preoperative local anesthesia (cooling with 1% lidocaine solution or ethyl chloride in large joints) is recommended especially in hemophilic patients in the pediatric group in terms of patient comfort and compliance. Ensuring that the needle is positioned in the joint space during the intraarticular intervention and completing the procedure without traumatizing the joint integrity as much as possible is the most important stage in the prevention of complications (Fig. 17.2). For this purpose, intraarticular injection can be made with the guidance of ultrasonography or under fluoroscopy especially in small- and medium-sized joints where degeneration is evident [6]. Discharging all kinds of fluid (such as effusion, blood) in the joint space without radiopharmaceutical injection into the joint is important for reducing intraarticular pressure and ensuring homogeneous radiopharmaceutical distribution after the procedure. Successive injections of lidocaine or glucocorticosteroid after intraarticular injection of radiopharmaceutical are recommended by some researchers to reduce pain and possible inflammatory response due to radiation after the procedure. However, its usefulness and necessity are controversial [7]. After the radiopharmaceutical injection is completed, it is absolutely necessary to wash with saline solution before the needle is withdrawn from the joint space in order to prevent the escape of the radiopharmaceutical from the area where the needle passes to the skin surface and to prevent skin necrosis.

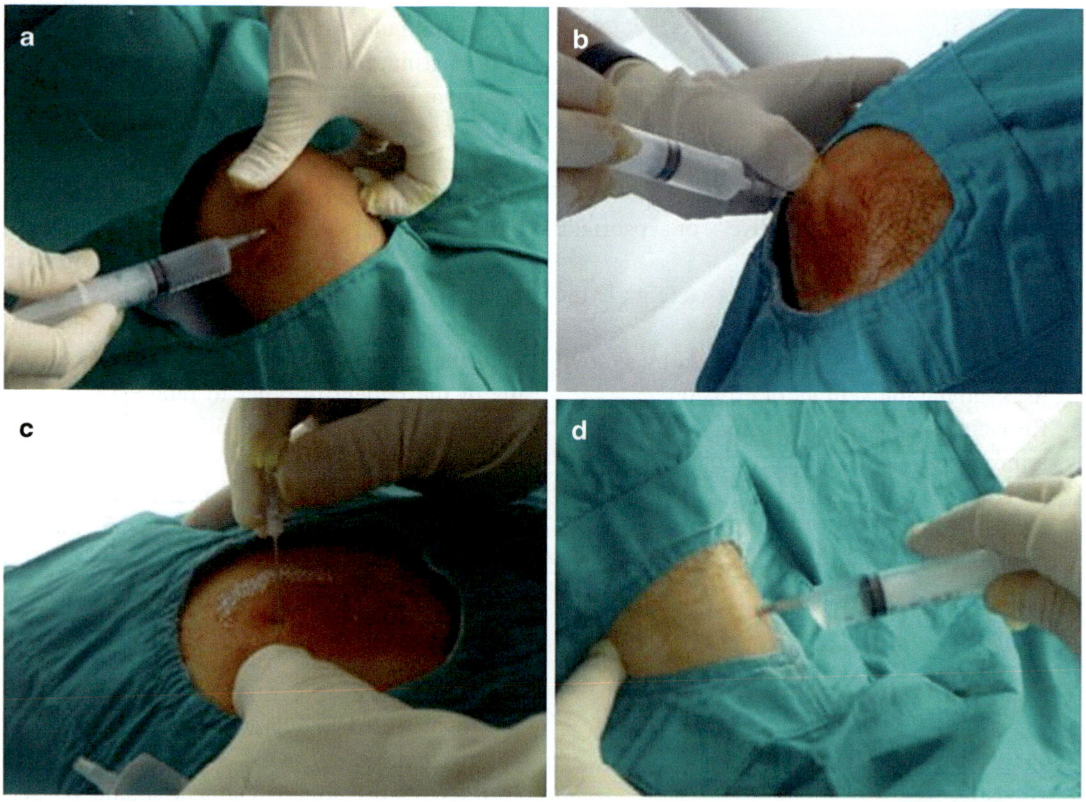

Fig. 17.2 Injection techniques to knee (**a**), elbow (**b**), shoulder (**c**), and ankle (**d**) joints in the treatment of radiosynovectomy

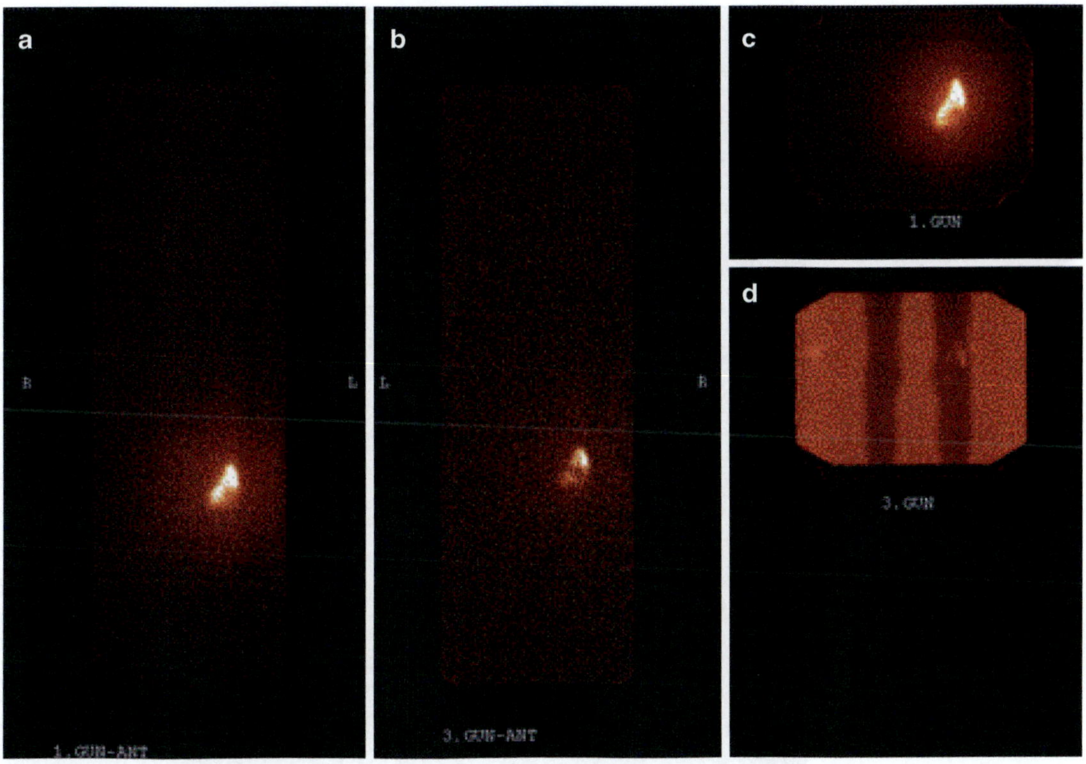

Fig. 17.3 It was observed that scintigraphic images showed homogeneous distribution of radiopharmaceutical in the joint and there was no leakage out of the joint in the Bremsstrahlung whole-body (**a** and **b**) and static (**c** and **d**) images of the patient who underwent Y-90 radiosynovectomy treatment to the left knee joint due to hemophilic synovitis

Immobilization of the joint for 48 h after radiosynovectomy is recommended to prevent systemic escape to the periarticular soft tissue and lymphatic system. Additional measures such as elastic bandages, splints, or restriction of stepping on lower extremity joints are also useful for this purpose. Intraarticular distribution and extraarticular escape of the radiopharmaceutical are evaluated by acquiring scintigraphic images with gamma camera or PET (Y-90) imaging devices. Forty-eight-hour images are more valuable in determining lymphatic escape (Figs. 17.3 and 17.4).

It is useful to evaluate the clinical complaints and local complications of the patient if the patient is seen 48 h after radiosynovectomy. Forceful activity or physical therapy should be avoided for 1 month after treatment.

17.4 Treatment Effectiveness

The onset of treatment effectiveness after radiosynovectomy may vary from a few weeks to several months. Three-phase bone scintigraphy or blood pool imaging is performed for scintigraphic evaluation as well as radiological imaging such as physical examination, hematological and biochemical parameters, ultrasonography, and MRI when necessary 6–8 weeks after treatment (Fig. 17.5).

If a positive response to treatment has not been achieved by 6 months, treatment can be repeated. Alternative treatment methods should be tried in cases where no results can be obtained although radiosynovectomy is performed twice in the same joint. The results of meta-analysis and prospective studies reveal that approximately

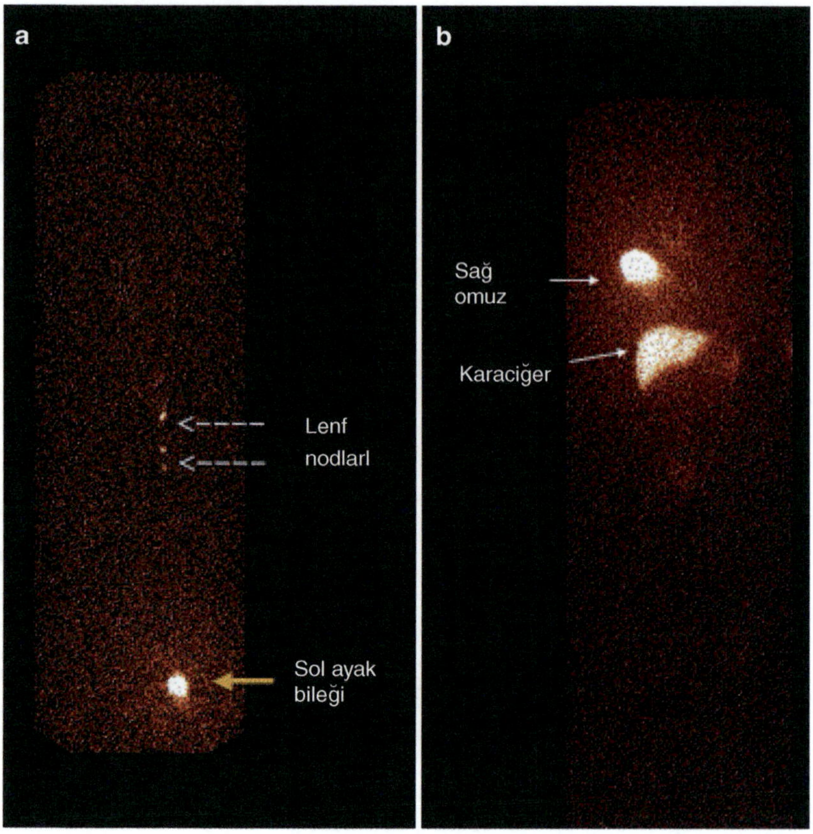

Fig. 17.4 Extraarticular uptake of radiopharmaceutical due to extraarticular leakage is observed in the lymph nodes (**a**) and liver (**b**) in whole-body images of two different patients who underwent Re-186 radiosynovectomy to the left ankle (**a**) and right shoulder (**b**) joint with the diagnosis of hemophilic synovitis

75% of patients have a good response to treatment and the response continues in varying periods from a few months to several years even though the effectiveness of treatment after radiosynovectomy with different indications and different radiopharmaceuticals varies in the literature [8–11]. The most important indicators of poor prognosis are joint damage and the presence of degeneration, advanced osteoarthritis, and long-term inflammation. Early treatment of arthritis is decisive for optimal treatment response. Treatment response varies between 73% ± 12% with radiosynovectomy in the early period, while this rate decreases to 52% ± 24% in the advanced stage in rheumatoid arthritis [8]. Treatment response rates in osteoarthritis were also low as 56% ± 11%. Joint type is also effective in treatment response. Deutsch et al. reported radiosynovectomy efficacy as 55–79% in small joints; 60–83% in medium-sized joints such as elbows, wrists, and shoulders; and 40–85% in the knee joint [12]. Studies comparing the effectiveness of radiosynovectomy with glucocorticoid injection show that the effectiveness of treatment with reduced pain and effusion when combined with radiosynovectomy is longer and 75–78% of patients who do not benefit from glucocorticoid injection alone benefit from radiosynovectomy [13, 14]. Radiosynovectomy administrations complementing surgical (open or arthroscopic) synovectomy also increase the effectiveness of treatment in cases of villonodular synovitis.

Hemophilic synovitis is the patient group with the highest and longest success rate due to the difference in etiology of the disease and treatment target. The success rate of radiosynovectomy in hemophilic synovitis is defined as at least 75% reduction in the development of hemarthrosis, reduction of pain, and preservation of joint mobility, and the success rate varies between 75 and 90% in publications including 6–40 months of follow-up [15–18]. The treatment effective-

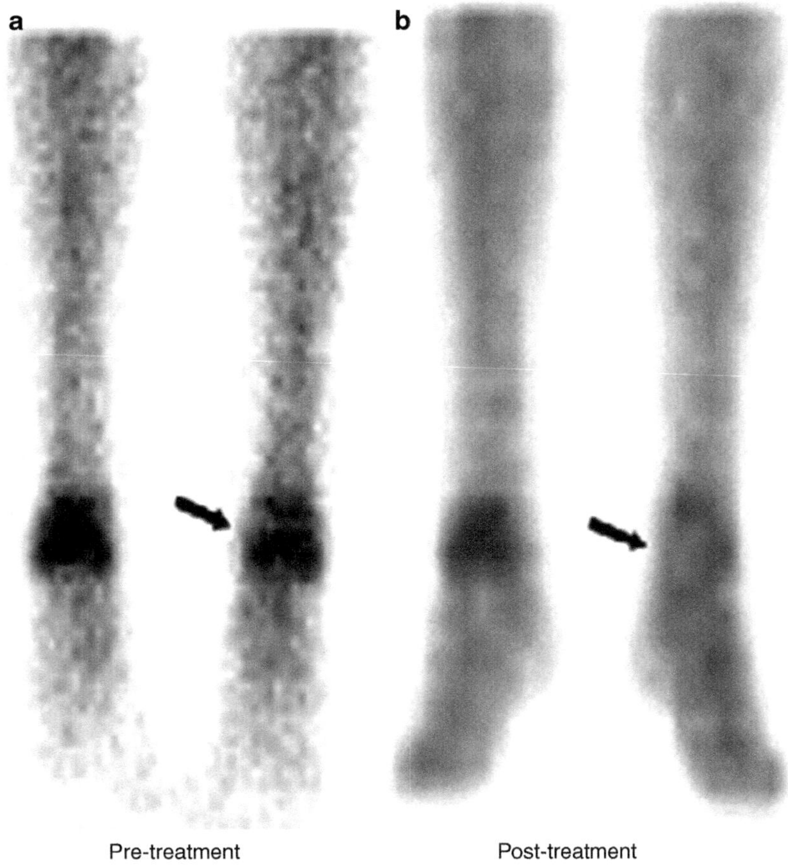

Fig. 17.5 Hypoactive appearance due to decrease in synovial blood supply in the left ankle is observed in the blood pool images of the patient who underwent Re-186 radiosynovectomy to the left ankle with the diagnosis of hemophilic synovitis

ness (progression-free survival) of radiosynovectomy, which was administered to target joint in the knee, ankle, and elbow in hemophilic synovitis treatment, was 72, 67, and 72 months, respectively, in studies involving the experience of Istanbul University, Istanbul Faculty of Medicine [19, 20]. Significant advantages of hemophilia patients are that it is a noninvasive procedure compared to surgical synovectomy and does not require hospitalization and the need for factor is low.

17.5 Side Effects and Complications

The incidence of side effects and complications after radiosynovectomy is fairly low. Possible side effects and complications include infections, inflammation due to radiation synovitis, pain, thrombosis due to immobilization, erythema due to extraarticular leakage of radiopharmaceuticals, and skin necrosis. The side effect rates reported in a survey study covering the 6-year follow-up data of 36 centers are fairly low in Germany, where approximately 40,000–60,000 radiosynovectomy therapies are administered annually in Europe [21]. No side effects were reported in 23 centers in this study. Three of the 20 insurance companies reported a total of 9 complications. Data from this survey reveal that the most important complication is skin necrosis with 28 cases. In addition, 13 cases of intraarticular infection and 12 cases of thrombosis were reported. It is possible to minimize these reported complications with an appropriate injection technique and some precautions. Joint infection was not observed in Istanbul University, Istanbul Faculty of Medicine's experience of more than a thousand radiosynovectomy therapies in approximately 20 years, skin necrosis was observed in only one case, Y-90-related radiation synovitis was observed in six cases, and erythema was observed in one case.

Patients should be closely monitored for side effects and complications after treatment, and their complaints should be seriously evaluated. It can be seen especially after radiosynovectomy with Y-90 due to its high energy even though radiation-related synovitis development after treatment is rare. The development of inflammation-related signs such as redness, swelling, and pain in the joint in the week after treatment should suggest radiation synovitis. Cold application, analgesics, and anti-inflammatory drugs are used in the acute period as in the treatment of synovitis due to other factors. Intraarticular corticosteroid administration during radiosynovectomy also reduces the risk of developing radiation synovitis. Wide surgical excision of necrotic tissue and hyperbaric oxygen therapy are recommended for the treatment and limitation of complications, especially in cases with periarticular or skin necrosis due to Y-90 leakage. Joint fluid aspiration and bacterial culture allow diagnosis in patients with symptoms of joint infections. Local antibiotic administration can be performed with joint lavage or endoscopy in cases where results cannot be obtained within 24–48 h with oral antibiotics. Prophylactic anticoagulant administration against the risk of developing thromboembolism due to immobilization after radiosynovectomy is recommended only in patients who are treated with symmetrical joints in the lower extremity and have at least two risk factors [22].

Whole-body radiation dose due to radiosynovectomy, which is a local radionuclide therapy, is at low levels. There is no clinical study revealing the relationship between radiosynovectomy and cancer that has been performed for more than 50 years. However, it should not be overlooked that epidemiological and bio-dosimetric studies in this area also have significant limitations. Results from epidemiological studies investigating the relationship between radiation exposure and cancer development reveal that there is no significant risk for cancer development at doses below 100 mSv [23]. The radiation doses exposed due to radiosynovectomy determined in dosimetric studies are below 50 mSv dose [4].

Two 9-year-old and 14-year-old patients with acute lymphoblastic leukemia (ALL) developed after radiosynovectomy with P-32 colloid with the diagnosis of hemophilic synovitis have been reported in the literature. ALL development occurs 1 year after uncomplicated radiosynovectomy in both cases [24]. The time interval between radiation exposure due to radiosynovectomy and malignancy development is much shorter than expected in these two cases with a history of autoimmune disease. No cancer development was observed in 577 patients who underwent 1027 radiosynovectomy therapies with P-32 colloid since 1988 in a survey study covering hemophilia centers in the United States. In an epidemiological study in Canada involving 2400 patients undergoing Y-90 radiosynovectomy, no significant difference was found in the incidence of cancer in the patient group than expected in the population [25].

The rate of leakage to the lymphatic system after radiosynovectomy with appropriate technique is reported to be 2–5% [19, 26]. The determination of dicentric chromosomal aberrations in peripheral lymphocytes in bio-dosimetric studies to investigate the association of radiosynovectomy with carcinogenesis is considered to be an indicator of ionizing radiation-induced cell damage. It was determined that high radiation doses that would cause genotoxic effects were not reached with radiosynovectomy in pediatric cases in our studies involving cytogenetic analyses such as chromosomal aberration, micronucleus, and sister chromatid exchange in patients undergoing radiosynovectomy with Y-90 and Re-186 [27, 28]. Similar results have been demonstrated in different studies [29–31]. It is recommended that the time interval between the recurrent treatments of these patients is 6 months or more in terms of repair of the possible damage and the spread of the cumulative radiation dose over time since the radiation dose exposed to the lymphatic system is higher in cases with lymphatic leakage detected by gamma camera imaging after radiosynovectomy.

17.6 Concluding Remarks

Radiosynovectomy is a preferred local radionuclide therapy method in the treatment of arthritic diseases accompanied by synovial inflammation, especially hemophilic synovitis and rheumatoid arthritis, as a low-risk and economical treatment method compared to surgical methods that are easy to perform and alternative.

References

1. Kresnik E. Radiosynovectomy: introduction and overview of literature. In: Kampen WU, Fischer M, editors. Local treatment of inflammatory joint diseases. Heidelberg, New York, Dordrecht, London: Springer; 2015. p. 81–93.
2. Ansell BM, Crook A, Mallard JR, Bywaters EG. Evaluation of intra-articular colloidal gold Au 198 in the treatment of persistent knee effusions. Ann Rheum Dis. 1963;22:435–9.
3. Fischer M, Mödder G. Radionuclide therapy of inflammatory joint diseases. Nucl Med Commun. 2002;23(9):829–31.
4. Turkmen C. Safety of radiosynovectomy in hemophilic synovitis: it is time to re-evaluate. J Coagul Dis. 2009;1:1–8.
5. Clunie G, Fischer M. EANM procedure guidelines for radiosynovectomy. Eur J Nucl Med Mol Imaging. 2003;30(3):BP12–6.
6. Modder G. Radionuclide therapy of inflammatory joint diseases (radiation synovectomy, radiosynoviorthesis). In: Baum RP, editor. Therapeutic nuclear medicine. Heidelberg, New York, Dordrecht, London: Springer; 2014. p. 459–92.
7. Ćwikła B, Żbikowski P, Kwiatkowska B. Radiosynovectomy in rheumatic diseases. J Ultrason. 2014;14:241–51.
8. Kresnik E, Mikosch P, Gallowitsch HJ, et al. Clinical outcome of radiosynoviorthesis: a meta- analysis including 2190 treated joints. Nucl Med Commun. 2002;23:683–8.
9. Liepe K. Efficacy of radiosynovectomy in rheumatoid arthritis. Rheumatol Int. 2012;32:3219–24.
10. Knut L. Radiosynovectomy in the therapeutic management of arthritis. World J Nucl Med. 2015;14:10–5.
11. Uğur O, Gedik GK, Atilla B, Rubello D. Radiosynovectomy: current status in the management of arthritic conditions. Nucl Med Commun. 2008;29(9):755–8.
12. Deutsch E, Brodack JW, Deutsch KF. Radiation synovectomy revisited. Eur J Nucl Med. 1993;20:1113–27.
13. Jahangier ZN, Moolenburgh JD, Jacobs JW, Serdijn H, Bijlsma JW. The effect of radiation synovectomy in patients with persistent arthritis: a prospective study. Clin Exp Rheumatol. 2001;19(4):417–24.
14. Liepe K, Zaknun JJ, Padhy A, Barrenechea E, Soroa V, Shrikant S, et al. Radiosynovectomy using yttrium-90, phosphorus-32 or rhenium-188 radiocolloids versus corticoid instillation for rheumatoid arthritis of the knee. Ann Nucl Med. 2011;25:317–23.
15. Ozcan Z. Radiosynovectomy in hemophilic synovitis. Mol Imaging Radionucl Ther. 2014;23(1):1–4.
16. Kavakli K, Aydogdu S, Taner M, et al. Radioisotope synovectomy with rhenium186 in haemophilic synovitis for elbows, ankles and shoulders. Haemophilia. 2008;14(3):518–23.
17. Kavakli K, Aydoğdu S, Omay SB, et al. Long-term evaluation of radioisotope synovectomy with Yttrium 90 for chronic synovitis in Turkish haemophiliacs: Izmir experience. Haemophilia. 2006;12(1):28–35.
18. Türkmen C, Zülfikar B, Taşer O, et al. Radiosynovectomy in hemophilic synovitis: correlation of therapeutic response and blood-pool changes. Cancer Biother Radiopharm. 2005;20(3):363–70.
19. Zulfikar B, Turkmen C, Kilicoglu O, et al. Long-term outcomes in haemophilic synovitis after radiosynovectomy using rhenium-186: a single-centre experience. Haemophilia. 2013;19(2):275–80.
20. Turkmen C, Kilicoglu O, Dikici F, et al. Survival analysis of Y-90 radiosynovectomy in the treatment of haemophilic synovitis of the knee: a 10-year retrospective review. Haemophilia. 2014;20(1):e45–50.
21. Kampen WU, Matis E, Czech N, Soti Z, Gratz S, Henze E. Serious complications after radiosynoviorthesis. Survey on frequency and treatment modalities. Nuklearmedizin. 2006;45:262–8.
22. Kampen WU. Local complications after radiosynovectomy and possible treatment strategies: a literature survey. In: Kampen WU, Fischer M, editors. Local treatment of inflammatory joint diseases: benefits and risks. Springer International Publishing Switzerland; 2015. p. 115–26.
23. UNSCLEAR. Sources, effects and risks of ionizing radiation. New York: United Nation Scientific Committee on the effect of Atomic Radiation. United Nations; 2006.
24. Dunn AL, Manco-Johnson M, Busch MT, Balark KL, Abshire TC. Leukemia and P32 radionuclide synovectomy for hemophilic arthropathy. J Thromb Haemost. 2005;3:1541–2.
25. Infante-Rivard C, Rivard GE, Derome F, Cusson A, Winikoff R, Chartrand R, et al. A retrospective cohort study of cancer incidence among patients treated with radiosynoviorthesis. Haemophilia. 2012;18:805–9.
26. Gedik GK, Uğur O, Atilla B, Pekmezci M, Yildirim M, Seven B, Varoğlu E. Comparison of extraarticular leakage values of radiopharmaceuticals used for radionuclide synovectomy. Ann Nucl Med. 2006;20(3):183–8.
27. Turkmen C, Ozturk S, Unal SN, et al. Monitoring the genotoxic effects of radiosynovectomy with Re-186 in paediatric age group undergoing therapy for haemophilic synovitis. Haemophilia. 2007;13(1):57–64.
28. Turkmen C, Ozturk S, Unal SN, et al. The genotoxic effects in lymphocyte cultures of children treated with

radiosynovectomy by using yttrium-90 citrate colloid. Cancer Biother Radiopharm. 2007;22(3):393–9.
29. Fernandez-Palazzi F, Caviglia H. On the safety of synoviorthesis in haemophilia. Haemophilia. 2001;7(Suppl. 2):50–3.
30. Kavakli K, Cogulu O, Aydogdu S, et al. Long-term evaluation of chromosomal breakages after radioisotope synovectomy for treatment of target joints in patients with haemophilia. Haemophilia. 2010;16(3):474–8.
31. Turkmen C. Risk of cancer induction. In: Kampen WU, Fischer M, editors. Local treatment of inflammatory joint diseases: benefits and risks. Springer International Publishing Switzerland; 2015. p. 127–34.

Radionuclide Pain Palliation Therapy

18

Bilge V. Salancı

18.1 Bone Metastases

Bone is a common metastatic site after the lung and liver for many cancer types, especially prostate cancer and breast cancer. Today, the "seed and soil" hypothesis is accepted for the formation of bone metastases. According to this hypothesis, cancer cells reach the bone marrow via circulation. Cells adapt to the microenvironment in the bone marrow and stay dormant for years. These dormant metastatic cells are stimulated and start to grow forming micrometastases and macrometastases. The stimulants for this activation process are still unknown [1].

Bone metabolism is an ongoing process of bone destruction and reconstruction. The continuity of bone reabsorption and new bone synthesis is ensured by a wide variety of growth factors that are continuously secreted from the bone matrix and bone marrow. These growth factors include vascular endothelial growth factors (VEGF), transforming growth factor-β (TGF-β), insulin-like growth factors (IGF-1, IGF-2), fibroblast growth factors (FGF), platelet-derived growth factors (PDGF), and bone morphogenetic proteins. They are necessary for bone development and metabolism, and they also form a favorable environment for the formation and development of bone metastases [2, 3].

Bone metastases can be grouped under two headings according to their radiological appearance and metastasis formation mechanisms: osteoblastic metastases and lytic bone metastases. Bone metastases are predominantly blastic in prostate cancer. Wnt secreted from metastatic cancer cells in osteoblastic metastases activates the Wnt/beta-catenin pathway and stimulates the division of osteoblasts and the increase in the number of blasts [2]. Cytokines such as endothelin-1, TGF-β, IGF-1, and FGF secreted by tumor cells stimulate osteoblasts and increase bone production (Fig. 18.1). Cytokines such as prostate-specific antigen (PSA) and urokinase-type plasminogen activator (uPA) also block osteoclasts and osteoclastic activity (Fig. 18.1) [3]. Thus, osteoblastic metastases are characterized by increased Tc-99 m MDP uptake in bone scintigraphy; and sclerosis in radiologically direct radiographs and computed tomography sections (CT).

18.1.1 Morbidity Factors of Bone Metastases

Bone metastases may present with pain or fractures; in advanced cases the patients may experience bone marrow suppression, extramedullary hematopoiesis, and nerve compression.

B. V. Salancı (✉)
Faculty of Medicine, Department of Nuclear Medicine, Hacettepe University, Ankara, Turkey
e-mail: bilgev@hacettepe.edu.tr

R. Bekiş et al. (eds.), *Radionuclide Therapy*, https://doi.org/10.1007/978-3-030-97220-2_18

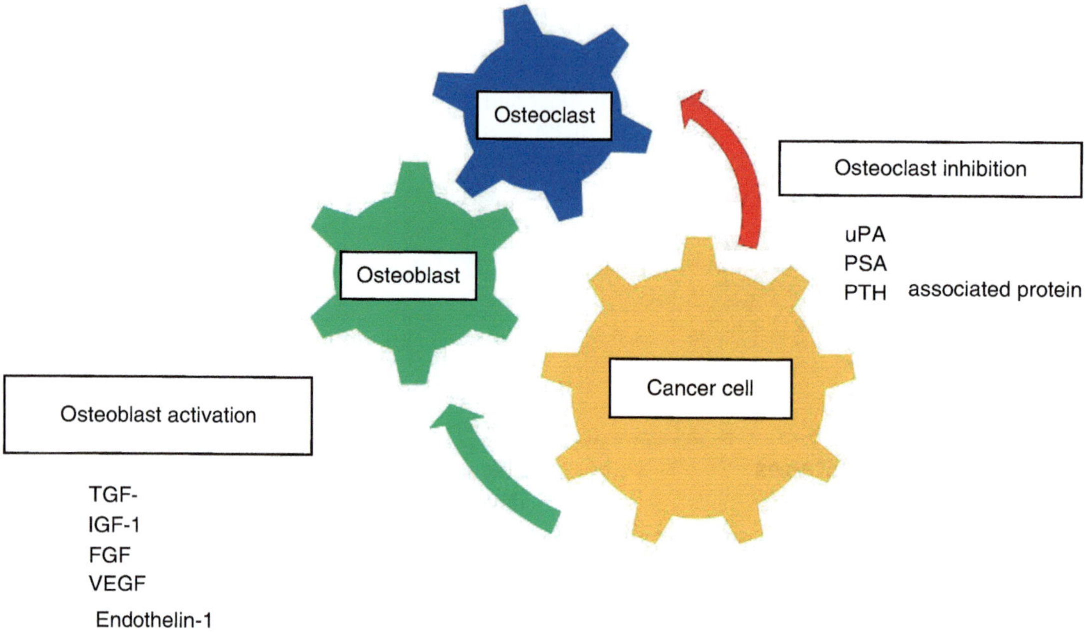

Fig. 18.1 Osteoblastic metastasis formation: Cancer cell activates osteoblasts by secreting TGF-β, IGF-1, FGF, VEGF, and endothelin-1. Osteoclasts are inhibited by the secretion of cytokines such as PSA and urokinase-type plasminogen activator (uPA) and PTH-associated protein. Bone destruction also decreases and contributes to the blastic reaction. Accordingly, the formation of osteoblastic metastases presents as sclerotic lesions in radiographs and shows increased Tc-99 m MDP uptake in bone

Table 18.1 Physical properties of bone-seeking radiopharmaceuticals used in the radionuclide pain palliation therapy

Radionuclide	Half-life (days)	Mean β energy (keV)	Maximum β energy (MeV)	Gamma ray (keV)	Maximum tissue penetration (mm)
P-32	14.3	695	1.71	–	8
Sr-89	50.5	584	1.49	909 (0.1%)	6
Sm-153	1.9	233	0.807	103 (28%)	2.5
Re-186	3.8	359	1.07	137 (9%)	4.5
Re-188	0.7	730	2.12	155 (15%)	10
Lu-177	6.2	149	0.497	208 (10%)	2
Ho-166	1.1	651	1.85	81 (6.4%)	3.8
Y-90-DOTA	2.67	267	2.27	–	11

Patients complain of regional pain and this symptom decreases both quality of life and performance status of the patients. In most of the patients, painful bone metastases have osteolytic character, and these often present with pathologic fractures which increase morbidity in patients [4]. Pathologic fractures occur frequently in weight-bearing bones such as lumbar vertebrae, femur, and pelvic bones even though it can be seen throughout the skeleton. Bone fractures also worsen the patient's performance status and cause additional complications such as thromboembolism. Pathological fractures are observed in 39% of breast cancers and 17% of prostate cancers, and the risk of death is increased in these patients [5]. Radiotherapy not only controls the regional pain but also decreases the risk of pathological fracture formation. Drugs such as zoledronic acid or pamidronate are similarly effective in controlling complaints [5, 6].

Hypercalcemia is seen in metastatic bone disease and is associated with increased bone resorption due to the secreted cytokines from the metastatic tumor cells. Hypercalcemia is often accompanied with bone pain, and it has been reported that skeletal system complications such as fracture and spinal cord compression are more likely to be observed in such patients [6].

Spinal cord compression is another factor that affects morbidity. It is most frequently observed in the thoracic vertebrae. Patients may have complaints such as weakness in lower extremities, bladder dysfunction, or changes in bowel functions. Pain is almost always present. Spinal cord compression is a clinical emergency. Complaints usually improve if diagnosed and treated early. Improvement in neurological complaints is observed in 20% of patients after surgery or radiotherapy.

Bone marrow has increased blood supply and high levels of cytokines are secreted in order to maintain hematopoiesis. For this reason, bone marrow is an important site of metastasis. Bone marrow metastases may recover with fibrosis after treatment, which may lead to a decrease in bone marrow reserve over time and results in extramedullary hematopoiesis. Hyperblastosis in peripheral blood is considered an indicator of extramedullary hematopoiesis.

18.2 Radionuclide Pain Therapy

Patients with bone metastases complain of pain at any stage of the disease. Bone pain may be resistant to painkillers and may restrict the movements of patients in daily life. Radionuclide pain therapy is used to relieve bone pain caused by osteoblastic metastases. The therapy generally aims for effective and long-term pain palliation and can be repeated when necessary. For this purpose, different bone-seeking radiopharmaceuticals that have high affinity to hydroxyapatite crystals of the bone are used. Phosphorus-32 (P-32) is the oldest of these radiopharmaceuticals and is currently used in myeloproliferative diseases rather than metastatic bone disease. Other major bone-seeking radiopharmaceuticals are beta emitters such as Strontium-89 chloride (Sr-89), Samarium-153 lexidronam (Sm-153), Rhenium-186 HEDP (Re-186), and Rhenium-188 HEDP (Re-188) (Table 18.1). Radium-223 (Ra-223) is an alpha-emitter radionuclide and is used to treat metastatic bone disease rather than pain palliation. Beta-emitter bone-seeking radiopharmaceuticals that are commonly used for pain palliation will be discussed in this chapter.

Patients are selected for radionuclide pain palliation therapy if they have chronic bone pain in multiple sites and if this chronic bone pain is resistant to use of standard painkillers and disease-specific chemotherapeutic agents. The candidates should have osteoblastic metastases that show increased radioactivity uptake on bone scintigraphy. Although this therapy is used predominantly for established indications such as prostate cancer and breast cancer, it is not cancer specific and can be used for pain palliation in the presence of pure osteoblastic or mixed blastic metastases of any cancer type. Radionuclide pain palliation therapy can be planned if pain is associated with osteoblastic foci on bone scintigraphy.

18.2.1 Indications

This therapy can be applied to the patients with chronic, resistant bone pain due to osteoblastic or mixed blastic metastases. Osteoblastic metastasis should be documented by bone scintigraphy, and it should be in the bones where the chronic pain was described by the patients. Since the pain palliation starts relatively late, patients should have a life expectancy preferably longer than 3 months. Therapy is not administered in the presence of pure lytic metastases, i.e., without the osteoblastic component.

18.2.2 Contraindications

Pregnancy is an absolute contraindication for therapy. Effective contraception should be used at least for 6 months after therapy. Breastfeeding is also an absolute contraindication. Breastfeeding should be discontinued before therapy. The kidney is the route of excretion of therapeutic bone-seeking radiopharmaceuticals. Therefore, renal function should be monitored during therapy decision-making. Therapy cannot be administered if the glomerular filtration rate falls below 30 mL/min. Dose reduction should be considered if the patients have glomerular filtration values below 50 mL/min [7].

Bone marrow reserve should be taken into account when therapy using bone-seeking radiopharmaceuticals is considered, since the therapy has a suppressive effect on bone marrow. It is preferred that the hemoglobin is at least 9 mg/dL, the white blood cell count is at least 3.5 10^9/L, the platelet count is over 100 10^9/L, and total blood counts should be stable [7]. Superscan appearance on bone scintigraphy also corresponds to low bone marrow reserve and is considered among the contraindications.

Radionuclide pain palliation therapy is not effective and therefore cannot be applied in the presence of neurogenic pain, in the presence of known pathological fracture or vertebral collapse, or in the presence of metastasis causing spinal cord compression or nerve root entrapment.

18.2.3 Dosimetry

A possible mechanism of pain palliation using beta-emitter bone-seeking radiopharmaceuticals is that they prevent the growth of metastases and reduce the pressure on the surrounding cells [8]. Another possible mechanism is the decrease in the levels of regional growth factors and cytokines that are synthesized from tumor and surrounding tissues [8]. The radiopharmaceuticals used have different energies and different physical half-lives. Therefore, effects and timing of these effects and the side effects vary among these radiopharmaceuticals. Ho-166 was reported to give the highest dose to the bone marrow in a dosimetry study when compared to Sm-153 and Lu-177 [9].

Today, weight-adjusted or fixed doses are used for each radiopharmaceutical that is used for radionuclide pain palliation therapy. However, it is possible to give more accurate doses by individual dosimetry applications. Dosimetry calculations were made based on posttreatment images. The doses given to metastatic foci were similar for both Lu-177 EDTMP and Sm-153 EDTMP, and an average radiation dose of 14 mGy/MBq should be given [10]. For Re-188 HEDP, it has been reported that the biological half-life of radionuclide is longer in metastatic foci and an average radiation dose of 12 mGy/MBq should be administered [11].

18.2.4 Therapy Administration

The radionuclide pain palliation therapy should be applied in centers where the proper infrastructure and an experienced team are present. Candidate patients for radionuclide pain palliation therapy should be evaluated by a medical oncologist and radiation oncologist for the risk of fractures due to bone metastases since therapy requires a multidisciplinary approach. In addition, radiation safety experts who can respond quickly to possible contamination and radiation accidents during the administration of the treatment should be available.

Detailed patient history should be present including previous therapies and potential comorbidities. The presence of sclerotic bone metastases in CT images is not sufficient for treatment planning. The bone scintigraphy should be evaluated in detail, and the bone scintigraphy should be performed within a maximum of 8 weeks of the treatment. Older examinations should be renewed.

Bone PET (F-18 NaF) shows more lesions when compared to bone scintigraphy (Fig. 18.2). However, the vast majority of studies and administration guidelines consider that bone scintigraphy images are sufficient for patient selection [7].

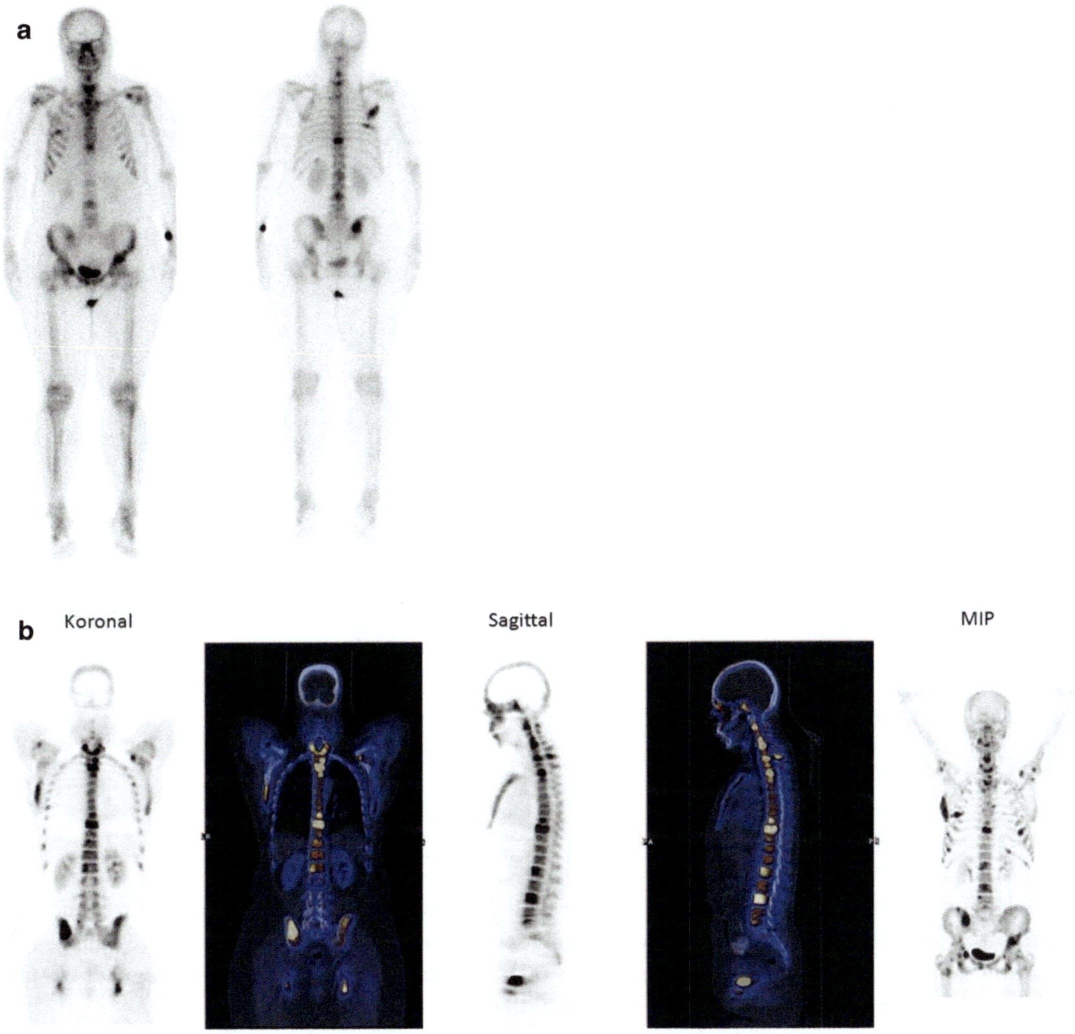

Fig. 18.2 A 40-year-old female patient with metastatic breast cancer. She complains of diffuse bone pain, more prominently on her back and right shoulder. She received external radiotherapy to L5-S2 and right iliac bone region (3780 Gy), left sixth rib (3000 Gy), T4-T6 vertebrae, and T7-L4 vertebrae (3000 Gy). After radiotherapy, the pain complaint decreased for a while but still continued. (**a**) Increased Tc-99 m HDP uptake is observed in the cervical vertebrae; T1, T3, T6, L1 vertebrae; lateral edge of the right scapula; posterolateral of the right seventh rib; right iliac bone; left acetabulum superior; and right femur. (**b**) Bone PET image showed increased F-18 NaF uptake in many foci in the calvarial bones, vertebrae, pelvis, and ribs, right scapula, bilateral humerus, and bilateral femur. On corresponding CT images, lytic-sclerotic lesions were detected. (**c**) 85 mCi Sm-153 EDTMP therapy was administered to the patient, and post-therapy whole-body images revealed radioactivity uptake in the vertebral column, scapula, pelvic bones, and ribs. The patient's baseline kidney function tests were normal, and complete blood count values were as follows: hemoglobin, 13.1 g/dL; leukocyte, 4.3 × 10^3/μL; and platelets, 249 × 10^3/μL. Complete blood count at 1 month after treatment was obtained as follows: hemoglobin, 12 g/dL; leukocyte, 4.1 × 10^3/μL; and platelets, 256 × 10^3/μL. The patient's pain complaint decreased significantly after a month. (**d**) Bone scintigraphy of the patient, who was readmitted with diffuse bone pain 8 months after treatment, showed increased Tc-99 m HDP uptake consistent with diffuse progressive bone metastasis. The patient received radiotherapy to the left hemipelvis and surgery was performed to both femurs to prevent fractures. She was reevaluated at 15 months after the first Sm-153 EDTMP treatment, due to diffuse bone pain. However, she also had hypercalcemia and diffuse liver metastases. The patient was deceased in the following month later due to pneumonia and cardiopulmonary arrest

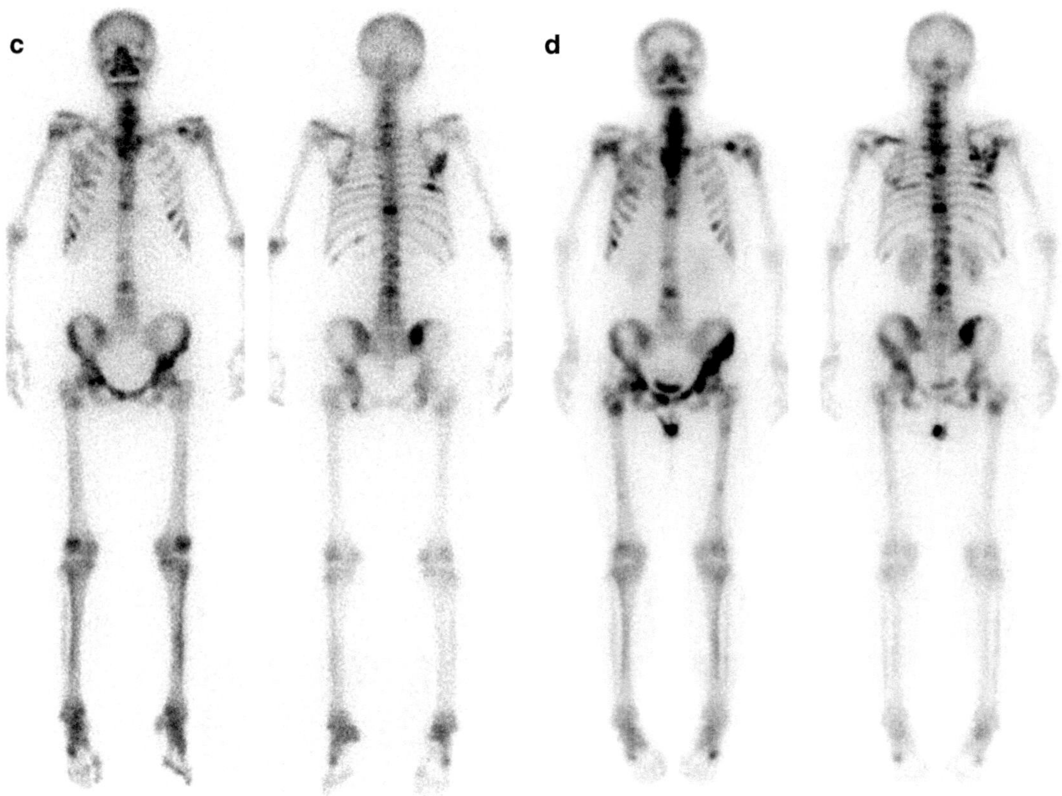

Fig. 18.2 (continued)

A detailed history should be taken from the patients that are referred for radionuclide bone palliation therapy. A patient with the complaint of worsening pain at the sites of osteoblastic metastases on the bone scintigraphy is a good candidate for the therapy. A multidisciplinary approach is necessary to diagnose the metastatic sites prone to any complication such as fractures or spinal cord injury. Early diagnosis could provide prevention of such complications. Renal function tests and complete blood count results should be seen at the time of bone scan. Complete blood counts should be repeated a week before the treatment because these patients generally have low bone marrow reserve due to both metastases and prior treatments such as radiotherapy and chemotherapy.

The patients should be informed about the treatment and should give informed consent. No patient preparation is required before treatment. Complete blood count and kidney function tests are generally repeated on the day of treatment to set a baseline for follow-up. A pregnancy test should be obtained on the day of treatment in fertile women.

The administered dose differs among the used bone-seeking radiopharmaceuticals and is listed in Table 18.2. Intravenous line should be ready. To ensure a functional intravenous line, it should be washed with saline solution before infusion. Bone-seeking radiopharmaceutical should be administered as a slow infusion and should be checked regularly to prevent extravasation. During Sr-89 administrations, the patients may experience flushing as seen in calcium infusions. Patients should be informed about this symptom before the infusion and the infusion should be given slowly.

In case of extravasation, the infusion should be terminated immediately, and the remaining amount of the radiopharmaceutical should be administered via a new intravascular line. Cold

Table 18.2 Clinical information of radionuclides used for radionuclide pain palliation

RF	Treatment dose	Time to treatment effect (day)	Treatment response (%)	Thrombocytopenia and leukocyte decline (%)	Pain palliation time (week)	Time to retreatment (months) (min)
P-32	185–370 MBq (IV) 370–444 MBq (Oral)	14	50–87	14 and 34	10	Not recommended
Sr-89	148 MBq	14–28	65–90	37 and 61	12–26	3
Sa-153 EDTMP	37 MBq/kg	2–7	55–83	15 and 25	4–35	2
Re-186 HEDP	1.3 GBq	2.7	55–85	17 and 25	8–10	2
Re-188 HEDP	1.3–4.4 GBq	2–7	64–77	20 and 25	8	N.A.

application to the extravasation site could prevent excessive spread of radiopharmaceuticals in the tissue [12]. It is recommended to elevate the injection site and apply warm compression for 24 hours during follow-up. Overdose may result in tissue necrosis and compartment syndrome, as rarely reported in the literature, and such cases may require surgical intervention. In most of the cases, necrosis is self-limiting and resolves on its own. Antibiotics and topical steroids are recommended in case of ulcerations and tissue damage [12].

Bone-seeking radiopharmaceuticals are excreted via urine; therefore, the patients should be informed about the risk of contamination that may occur while urinating.

18.2.5 Side Effects

Analgesic effects of the treatment may not start within the first week after treatment. Patients should be ensured to continue their analgesics during and after treatment. Some patients may experience an increase in pain within the first 3 days of treatment. This is an expected finding and is defined as "flare effect." The increase in pain is usually self-limiting and can be controlled with analgesic drugs. The flare effect, observed after radionuclide therapies, is associated with good treatment response [7].

A decrease in platelet and leukocyte levels may be observed after treatment. The intensity and timing varies according to the energy and half-life of the radiopharmaceuticals used (Table 18.2). It is usually a grade 2 toxicity and self-limiting [13]. Severe bone marrow suppression is one of the most serious side effects, seen rarely. It is often associated with prior use of chemotherapeutics or extended radiotherapy, extent of metastatic disease, and energy of bone-seeking radiopharmaceutical.

In a meta-analysis that compared various bone-seeking radiopharmaceuticals, grade 3 or more thrombocytopenia and leukopenia were reported more after treatment with Sr-89 [13]. Pain flare and nausea were also associated with Sr-89 treatment early after treatment. Grade 3 and above leukopenia has been reported as acute toxicity after Sm-153 EDTMP treatment in the same meta-analysis [13].

18.2.6 Posttreatment Follow-Up

Pain palliation success is one of the most important treatment goals and evaluated by a decrease in the need for analgesics or a decrease in pain complaints. The onset of pain control and duration of control also vary depending on the half-life and energy of the bone-seeking radiopharmaceutical used in treatment (Table 18.2). Other measures of treatment effectiveness include decreased symptomatic skeletal system complaints, increased quality of life, and increased patient mobility.

In a meta-analysis evaluating 57 studies using Sr-89 and Sm-153 EDTMP, pain palliation was reported to be 70% and increases to 74% when combined treatments were used [14]. Another meta-analysis of a total of 1877 patients showed that radionuclide pain therapy using bone-seeking pharmaceuticals showed that pain palliation therapy was effective in the control of skeletal system complaints [13]. The increase in the overall quality of life was found to be significant regardless of the radiopharmaceutical used, and it was stated that no advantage could be obtained in terms of overall survival in the same study [13].

Complete blood count monitoring of the patients after treatment is valuable in terms of follow-up of side effects. It would be appropriate to change the follow-up time according to the radiopharmaceutical used (Table 18.2).

18.3 Radiopharmaceuticals Used in Radionuclide Pain Therapy

18.3.1 Phosphorus-32

P-32, which is produced in nuclear reactors, is the first radionuclide used in the treatment of bone metastases. Its half-life is 14.3 days with an average energy of 1.71 MeV and its maximum range in the tissue is 8 mm. It binds to other intracellular molecules containing phosphorus other than hydroxyapatite. Therefore, it is primarily used to treat myeloproliferative diseases. However, it had been used in the treatment of bone metastases (Table 18.1).

The biological half-life of P-32 in the bone marrow is 7–9 days. The highest radiation exposure is to the bone marrow, spleen, and liver. The radiation dose of P-32 to the bone and bone marrow was calculated as 11 mGy/MBq [15]. The radiation exposure of the soft tissue is 0.74 mGy/MBq as it is rapidly retained in bone tissue. Grade 4 pancytopenia has rarely been reported even though it is more likely to cause bone marrow toxicity due to its high energy and wide range than other radionuclides used [16]. It can be administered orally or intravenously, but its absorption is variable in oral administration, and close monitoring of radiation exposure of caregivers and strict contamination control are recommended.

18.3.2 Strontium-89 Chloride

Strontium-89 is a radioactive element from the group of alkaline earth metals as calcium. It is a pure beta-emitter radionuclide with a half-life of 50.5 days (Table 18.1). Gamma-ray emission is less than 0.01%, so it cannot be used for imaging. It mimics calcium, enters the structure of hydroxyapatite crystals, and is retained at a high rate in osteoblastic metastases where high bone metabolism exists [17]. It is retained 2–25 times more in bones than normal bone marrow when administered intravenously [17, 18]. Sr-89 has a range of approximately 3 mm in bone tissue with a maximum range of 7 mm [17]. The radiation dose of Sr-89 to the normal bone tissue and bone marrow was determined as 17 mGy/MBq and 11 mGy/MBq, respectively [15]. Thirty to 35% of the administered dose remains in the bones. The route of excretion is mostly via the kidneys and less commonly via the intestines (excretion rate: kidney/intestine = 4:1) [15].

The pain palliation effect of Sr-89 treatment begins about 2–3 weeks, at the earliest on the ninth day post-administration, and lasts for 3–6 months [19, 20]. Finlay et al. reported in their meta-analysis that pain palliation could last up to 15 months [20]. Significant pain palliation was reported in 70%–79% of the patients; analgesic use decreased in 71–81%; and quality of life improved in 65% of the patients [14, 20, 21]. The flare effect was reported in 5–15% of patients within 24–48 hours of administration, and the effect was associated with the volume of bone metastases [17, 22, 23]. Systematic reviews did not confirm this relationship, while the flare effect was reported to predict good treatment response [21, 24]. The standard administered dose is 148–150 MBq (4 mCi), and although no survival advantage has been reported at higher doses, it has been reported that pain palliation and reduction in the number of skeletal system-related symptomatic events were more pronounced, but the bone marrow suppression also increases with higher administered doses [13].

A 30% decrease in leukocyte and platelet counts was reported after treatment and was mostly associated with grade 2–3 hematological toxicity. However, this effect is more prolonged compared to other bone-seeking radiopharmaceuticals due to its long half-life. This limits the use of Sr-89 in repeated treatments and in combination with chemotherapies. Grade 3 and above hematological toxicity was reported with Sr-89 compared to other beta-emitting bone-seeking radiopharmaceuticals in a meta-analysis published by Tunio et al. [13]. The flare effect and nausea were also reported more frequently after treatment. There was no difference in therapy effectiveness between Sr-89 and Ra-223 in terms of pain palliation [13].

An increase in pain was reported in 39% of patients within the first 3 days after Sr-89 treatment in a multicenter study in prostate cancer patients [25]. A decrease in PSA of more than 50% was observed in 37% of patients, and pain palliation and an increase in quality of life were reported in 63% of patients in the first 4 months after treatment [25].

In a double-blind study comparing Sr-89 injection at 75 MBq 3 times monthly versus placebo in prostate cancer patients, the 2-year survival was 46% in the treated group when compared to 4% in the placebo group [26]. On multivariate analysis, tumor grade had an effect on survival in addition to Sr-89 treatment [26]. It was reported in another multicenter study that pretreatment performance status and bone metastasis affected quality of life in prostate cancer patients. Therefore, it is possible to obtain a better therapy response when bone-seeking radiopharmaceuticals are used at an early stage in patients with diffuse bone pain [25].

In a phase III clinical study, investigating the effect of zoledronic acid in combination with Sr-89 treatment, the patients receiving Sr-89 treatment received less radiotherapy and needed less concomitant treatment, and therefore the authors concluded that Sr-89 treatment might provide a cost advantage [27]. In addition, combination therapy with zoledronic acid and Sr-89 has been reported to be more effective in pain palliation [28].

In a randomized phase II study on 105 castration-resistant prostate cancer patients who received induction chemotherapy followed by doxorubicin consolidation chemotherapy with or without additional Sr-89 bone pain therapy, neutropenia was observed at a higher rate in patients treated with Sr-89 and consolidation chemotherapy [29]. Progression-free survival (7 months versus 13.7 months) and overall survival (27.7 months versus 16.8 months) were found to be significantly better in patients receiving additional Sr-89 therapy [29].

The tumoricidal effect of Sr-89 treatment in combination with zoledronic acid was evaluated through CT images at the earliest 2 months after treatment in a study conducted by Baba et al. on 51 patients [28]. They reported that in addition to pain relief, 36% of the patients had a partial response and 50% of the patients had stable disease after therapy [28].

18.3.3 Samarium-153 Lexidronam

Samarium-153 is a radionuclide from the group of lanthanide metals that emit beta particles. It has a half-life of 46.2 hours (1.9 days) and is one of the shortest half-lives among other bone-seeking radiopharmaceuticals (Table 18.1). A 103 keV gamma ray emitted with 28% abundance during Sm-153 decay is used for imaging in addition to a maximum beta energy of 0.810 MeV. Sm-153 can form stable complexes with different bisphosphonate derivatives.

Among the bisphosphonate derivatives used, the most widespread administration was made with ethylenediaminetetramethylenephosphonate (EDTMP). Sm-153 EDTMP is a radiopharmaceutical that accumulates by chemo-adsorption in hydroxyapatite crystals in bones.

Sm-153 EDTMP is cleared from blood at a high rate after intravenous injection. After injection 50% of the administered dose is excreted from the kidneys in the first 8 hours [30]. Its uptake in bone was found to be very similar to Tc-99 m HDP and is retained at a higher (approximately fivefold) rate in osteoblastic metastases compared to normal bone tissue [30, 31].

The recommended treatment dose is between 37 and 55 MBq/kg. However, higher doses (111 MBq/kg) have been administered in the literature [32, 33]. In a study with escalating doses of Sm-153 EDTMP, pain palliation was reported in 65% of patients treated at 18.5–37 MBq/kg (0.5–1 mCi/kg); grade 2 bone marrow toxicity was observed regardless of the dose [34]. Bone marrow toxicity has been reported to depend on bone marrow reserve and disease type; it was also associated with previous treatment schemes [34]. In another dose-escalation study, 18.5 and 37 MBq/kg Sm-153 EDTMP doses were reported to be effective in pain palliation in patients with metastatic bone disease of different cancer types [35]. Low levels of bone marrow suppression were reported at 37 MBq/kg doses, which were shown to be effective pain palliation in this study. A phase I–II study in 52 prostate cancer patients reported a statistically significant decrease in platelet and neutrophil counts accompanied with patients anemia at doses of 92.5 MBq/kg compared to 37 MBq/kg.

Sm-153 EDTMP was also used for treatment of osteosarcomas. Doses up to 1.11 GBq/kg have been given in combination with autologous bone marrow transplantation, and transient hypocalcemia has been reported in primary bone tumors [36]. Consecutive administration of first low dose (37–51.8 MBq/kg) followed by 222 MBq/kg was applied in osteosarcomas with autologous bone marrow support [37]. This study was conducted for the treatment of osteosarcoma, not for pain palliation, and 44% of the patients were reported to have radiologically stable disease, and some patients had a treatment response in the soft-tissue component [37]. Similarly, the treatment response was compared with 3D radiation dosimetry in another study performed with tandem Sm-153 EDTMP in osteosarcoma patients, and it was reported that disease progression was observed in all patients receiving low-dose treatment, and treatment response was obtained when the radiation dose administered to the tumor was 21Gy and above [38].

The radiation doses to the normal bone, bone marrow, and bone tumors have been reported to be 6.8 mGy/MBq, 1.5 mGy/MBq, and 11.3 mGy/MBq, respectively [39]. It has been reported that the radiation dose exposure of hospital personnel during treatment is negligible, but the cumulative estimated radiation dose to be received by the patient's caregivers was 0.4 mGy after 19 days [40].

After Sm-153 EDTMP administration, white blood cell levels decrease at the second week, and platelet counts decrease at sixth week [41, 42]. Thrombocytopenia and lymphopenia have been reported after consecutive low-dose administrations; neutropenia and infectious complications have been reported after high doses [37]. However, no significant relation was found between treatment doses and bone marrow suppression [37, 42]. It has been reported that, among other dosimetric markers, the radiation dose received by the red bone marrow can be evaluated by trabecular volume correction obtained from CT images [42]. Grade 1 toxicity could be observed when the dose given to the red bone marrow was 2–2.5 Gy [42]. Sm-153 EDTMP had less bone marrow toxicity with a shorter half-life compared to Sr-89 treatment [41]. Bone marrow toxicity observed in patients resolves spontaneously without requiring intervention. Grade 4 toxicity such as infection and spontaneous bleeding have rarely been reported in Sm-153 EDTMP administrations for pain palliation.

Pain palliation begins 2 weeks after treatment and maximum pain palliation is achieved within 4–6 weeks (Fig. 18.2). Pain palliation was observed in 70–83% of prostate and breast cancer patients even though there was no correlation between the administered doses [33, 35, 41]. In a multivariate analysis in prostate cancer patients, better pain palliation and decrease in opiate use were reported within the first week in patients receiving 92.5 MBq/kg compared to the standard dose of 37 MBq/kg [33]. Pain palliation has been shown to continue for up to 3 months in patients receiving Sm-153 EDTMP [43].

It has been reported that Sm-153 EDTMP treatment in combination with low-dose capecitabine or mitoxantrone provides higher rates of pain palliation compared to Sm-153 EDTMP alone with no significant difference in bone marrow toxicity [44]. Sm-153 EDTMP was also administered in combination with docetaxel in patients with castration-resistant prostate cancer with bone metastases, and pain palliation was achieved in 77% of patients without an increase in bone marrow toxicity [45]. It has also been reported that three consecutive Sm-153 EDTMP administrations in combination with docetaxel can be performed with acceptable bone marrow toxicity [46].

18.3.4 Rhenium-186 HEDP

Rhenium-186 is a radionuclide from group VII metals in the periodic table with technetium-like chemical properties. It is a beta emitter with a maximum energy of 1.07 MeV and an average beta energy of 350 keV. The half-life of Re-186 (90 hours) is shorter than other bone-seeking radionuclides used for therapy (Table 18.1). Gamma rays with 137 keV energy are formed at a rate of 9% during decay and used in scintigraphic imaging after treatment. Re-186 HEDP complex has an effective half-life of approximately 32 hours in bone and approximately 9–10 days in osteoblastic metastases [47].

Re-186 HEDP is administered at doses of 1110–1295 MBq. It is excreted 70% in the urine in the first 72 hours after injection [16]. It is retained 22 times longer in bone when compared to bone marrow [48].In a phase II study, after 1295 MBq Re-186 HEDP administration, pain palliation and decreased analgesic use was reported in 38% and 46% of the patients, respectively [49]. Objective responses were reported in 75% of patients with prostate cancer and 80% of patients with breast cancer [49]. Leukocyte nadir was seen on the 45th day and returned spontaneously to normal at the end of the third month, and grade 2 leukocytosis and grade 3 thrombocytosis were detected in this study [49]. Short-term treatment response was 80%; prolonged pain palliation after 60 days was reported in 45% of patients in another study [50]. In patients with extended disease and decreased performance score, the treatment response duration was shorter [50]. It was suggested that Re-186 HEDP treatment could prevent disease progression [50]. Re-186 HEDP treatment compared to placebo has been reported to provide pain palliation in 80% of patients, and no side effects were reported in these patients [48]. In 38 patients with prostate cancer who received a high-dose (5000 MBq) Re-186 HEDP with autologous bone marrow support, PSA response was observed in 29%, and pain palliation was observed in 74% of the patients [47]. The therapeutic effect of Re-186 HEDP was found to be more effective when compared to placebo [47]. Although no significant PSA response was found in another study, RE-186 etidronate resulted in significantly longer pain palliation, patients required less radiotherapy, but no survival advantage was achieved [51].

Re-186 HEDP in combination with chemotherapy was also administered. In a dose-escalation study combined with six courses of docetaxel, the treatment protocol was well tolerated by patients, thrombocytopenia was of low grade and resolved spontaneously, and combined therapy provided a statistically significant survival advantage compared to patients receiving docetaxel alone [52].

18.3.5 Rhenium-188 HEDP

Rhenium-188 HEDP can be obtained more easily than other radionuclides because it is obtained from a tungsten (W-188)/Re-188 generator [53]. Re-188 with a half-life of 16.9 hours has a maximum beta energy of 2.12 MeV and an average beta energy of 760 keV (Table 18.1). It is chemically very similar to Technetium and therefore tends to bind to compounds bound by Tc-99 m. It emits gamma rays of 155 keV energy at 15% rate and is suitable for acquiring images with gamma cameras.

In a dose-escalation study conducted on 22 patients, hematological toxicities are seen at doses greater than 2.6 GBq; grade 3 thrombocytopenia was observed in 2 patients and grade 4 leukopenia was observed in 1 patient when the dose is 4.4 GBq [54]. Pain palliation lasted for an average of 7.5 weeks in 64% of patients and the maximum tolerated dose was 3.3 GBq [54].

18.3.6 Lutetium-177 Macrocyclic Biphosphonates

Lutetium-177, a lanthanide group metal, allows scintigraphic imaging after treatment as it contains gamma rays in addition to a 6.7-day half-life and 497 keV maximum beta energy (Table 18.1). Nowadays, Lu-177 is frequently used in the treatment of neuroendocrine tumors (Lu-177-DOTA peptide) and prostate cancers (Lu-177-PSMA). Lu-177 has been conjugated with EDTMP and used in pain palliation of bone metastases in recent years. It has high affinity to hydroxyapatite crystals as with other phosphonate-containing radionuclides. However, it is fairly stable at physiological pH because it is smaller than other lanthanide group metals [55]. Sodium pyrophosphate and methylene diphosphate compounds labeled with Lu-177 were also used aside from EDTMP [56, 57].

18.3.7 Holmium-166-Labeled Agents

Holmium belongs to the lanthanide metals group. Holmium-185 can be produced by neutron bombardment, but it can adversely affect patient dose exposure by being present in the mixture at long half-life Ho-166 m in this case. Ho-166 is formed by dysprosium-166 (Dy-166) beta decay, and it was possible to produce Ho-166 with 99% purity without any radio-contaminant with Dy-166/Ho-166 generator using this feature [58]. It is used by chelating with molecules from the Ho-166 phosphonate group. It is retained in the bones as Sm-153 EDTMP and shows a similar bio-distribution. It has been shown that treatment can also be administered using Dy-166/Ho-166-EDTMP mixture [59]. Ho-166 was also chelated with 1,2-propylene di-amino tetra (methyl-1-enephosphonic acid) (DOTMP) [60]. Both DOTMP and EDTMP radiopharmaceuticals have been shown to be retained at a high rate in bones similar to Sm-153 EDTMP in animal studies. No information could be obtained about the treatment effectiveness at the time of writing this chapter because there were no prospective randomized studies conducted with Ho-166 even though it is a potential treatment agent.

18.4 Concluding Remarks

The literature on radionuclide pain therapy using bone-seeking radiopharmaceuticals consists predominantly of randomized controlled trials and mostly evaluates early posttreatment outcomes. The treatment effectiveness, as summarized above, was predominantly obtained from patients with prostate cancer and was projected to other cancer types. Publications on patients with breast cancer are limited as emphasized in a systematic review article conducted in 2012 [61]. This gap in the literature has rapidly begun to be replaced by beta-emitting radionuclides used for radionuclide pain treatment after the results of a placebo-controlled double-blind ALSYMPCA phase III study with Ra-223 showed a survival advantage over the placebo group [62]. Low bone marrow toxicity has an effect on this behavior since alpha particles have rather short range. However, Ra-223 treatment has not been reported to provide a survival advantage over abiraterone [63]. Radionuclide pain treatment using bone-seeking radiopharmaceuticals is recommended for pain palliation and improves quality of life; however, the treatment is not expected to contribute to the life expectancy of patients.

References

1. Kan C, et al. Cancer cell colonisation in the bone microenvironment. Int J Mol Sci. 2016;17(10):1674.
2. Hauschka PV, et al. Growth factors in bone matrix. Isolation of multiple types by affinity chroma-

tography on heparin-Sepharose. J Biol Chem. 1986;261(27):12665–74.
3. Wu MY, et al. Molecular regulation of bone metastasis pathogenesis. Cell Physiol Biochem. 2018;46(4):1423–38.
4. Vassiliou V, et al. Clinical and radiological evaluation of patients with lytic, mixed and sclerotic bone metastases from solid tumors: is there a correlation between clinical status of patients and type of bone metastases? Clin Exp Metastasis. 2007;24(1):49–56.
5. Saad F, et al. Pathologic fractures correlate with reduced survival in patients with malignant bone disease. Cancer. 2007;110(8):1860–7.
6. Tanaka R, et al. Risk factors for developing skeletal-related events in breast cancer patients with bone metastases undergoing treatment with bone-modifying agents. Oncologist. 2016;21(4):508–13.
7. Handkiewicz-Junak D, et al. EANM guidelines for radionuclide therapy of bone metastases with beta-emitting radionuclides. Eur J Nucl Med Mol Imaging. 2018;45(5):846–59.
8. McEwan AJ. Use of radionuclides for the palliation of bone metastases. Semin Radiat Oncol. 2000;10(2):103–14.
9. Ranjbar H, Ghannadi-Maragheh M, Bahrami-Samani A, Beiki D. Dosimetric evaluation of 153Sm-EDTMP, 177Lu-EDTMP and 166Ho-EDTMP for systemic radiation therapy: Influence of type and energy of radiation and half-life of radionuclides. Radiat Phys Chem. 2015;108:60–4.
10. Sharma S, et al. Comparative Therapeutic Efficacy of (153)Sm-EDTMP and (177)Lu-EDTMP for Bone Pain Palliation in Patients with Skeletal Metastases: Patients' Pain Score Analysis and Personalized Dosimetry. Front Med (Lausanne). 2017;4:46.
11. Liepe K, et al. Dosimetry of 188Re-hydroxyethylidene diphosphonate in human prostate cancer skeletal metastases. J Nucl Med. 2003;44(6):953–60.
12. van der Pol J, et al. Consequences of radiopharmaceutical extravasation and therapeutic interventions: a systematic review. Eur J Nucl Med Mol Imaging. 2017;44(7):1234–43.
13. Tunio M, et al. Comparative efficacy, tolerability, and survival outcomes of various radiopharmaceuticals in castration-resistant prostate cancer with bone metastasis: a meta- analysis of randomized controlled trials. Drug Des Devel Ther. 2015;9:5291–9.
14. D'Angelo G, et al. Targeted "bone-seeking" radiopharmaceuticals for palliative treatment of bone metastases: a systematic review and meta-analysis. Q J Nucl Med Mol Imaging. 2012;56(6):538–43.
15. Radiation dose to patients from radiopharmaceuticals. ICRP Publication 53. vol. 18. 1988: Pergamon Press, pp. 1-4.
16. Silberstein EB. The treatment of painful osseous metastases with phosphorus-32-labeled phosphates. Semin Oncol. 1993;20(3 Suppl. 2):10–21.
17. Blake GM, et al. Strontium-89 therapy: measurement of absorbed dose to skeletal metastases. J Nucl Med. 1988;29(4):549–57.
18. Robinson RG, et al. Strontium-89: treatment results and kinetics in patients with painful metastatic prostate and breast cancer in bone. Radiographics. 1989;9(2):271–81.
19. Baziotis N, et al. Strontium-89 chloride in the treatment of bone metastases from breast cancer. Oncology. 1998;55(5):377–81.
20. Finlay IG, Mason MD, Shelley M. Radioisotopes for the palliation of metastatic bone cancer: a systematic review. Lancet Oncol. 2005;6(6):392–400.
21. Kraeber-Bodere F, et al. Treatment of bone metastases of prostate cancer with strontium- 89 chloride: efficacy in relation to the degree of bone involvement. Eur J Nucl Med. 2000;27(10):1487–93.
22. Zenda S, et al. Strontium-89 (Sr-89) chloride in the treatment of various cancer patients with multiple bone metastases. Int J Clin Oncol. 2014;19(4):739–43.
23. Robinson RG. Strontium-89--precursor targeted therapy for pain relief of blastic metastatic disease. Cancer. 1993;72(Suppl. 11):3433–5.
24. Jong JM, et al. Radiopharmaceuticals for palliation of bone pain in patients with castration-resistant prostate cancer metastatic to bone: a systematic review. Eur Urol. 2016;70(3):416–26.
25. Turner SL, et al. Less pain does equal better quality of life following strontium-89 therapy for metastatic prostate cancer. Br J Cancer. 2001;84(3):297–302.
26. Buchali K, et al. Results of a double blind study of 89-strontium therapy of skeletal metastases of prostatic carcinoma. Eur J Nucl Med. 1988;14(7-8):349–51.
27. James ND, et al. Clinical outcomes and survival following treatment of metastatic castrate-refractory prostate cancer with docetaxel alone or with Strontium-89, Zoledronic Acid, or both: the TRAPEZE Randomized Clinical Trial. JAMA Oncol. 2016;2(4):493–9.
28. Baba K, et al. Tumoricidal effect and pain relief after concurrent therapy by strontium-89 chloride and zoledronic acid for bone metastases. Hell J Nucl Med. 2018;21(1):15–23.
29. Tu SM, et al. Bone-targeted therapy for advanced androgen-independent carcinoma of the prostate: a randomised phase II trial. Lancet. 2001;357(9253):336–41.
30. Singh A, et al. Human pharmacokinetics of samarium-153 EDTMP in metastatic cancer. J Nucl Med. 1989;30(11):1814–8.
31. Paes FM, Serafini AN. Systemic metabolic radiopharmaceutical therapy in the treatment of metastatic bone pain. Semin Nucl Med. 2010;40(2):89–104.
32. Alberts AS, et al. Dose response relationship and multiple dose efficacy and toxicity of samarium-153-EDTMP in metastatic cancer to bone. Radiother Oncol. 1997;43(2):175–9.
33. Collins C, et al. Samarium-153-EDTMP in bone metastases of hormone refractory prostate carcinoma: a phase I/II trial. J Nucl Med. 1993;34(11):1839–44.
34. Farhanghi M, et al. Samarium-153-EDTMP: pharmacokinetic, toxicity and pain response using an esca-

lating dose schedule in treatment of metastatic bone cancer. J Nucl Med. 1992;33(8):1451–8.
35. Resche I, et al. A dose-controlled study of 153 Sm-ethylene diamine tetramethylene phosphonate (EDTMP) in the treatment of patients with painful bone metastases. Eur J Cancer. 1997;33(10):1583–91.
36. Anderson PM, et al. High-dose samarium-153 ethylene diamine tetramethylene phosphonate: low toxicity of skeletal irradiation in patients with osteosarcoma and bone metastases. J Clin Oncol. 2002;20(1):189–96.
37. Loeb DM, et al. Tandem dosing of samarium-153 ethylenediamine tetramethylene phosphoric acid with stem cell support for patients with high-risk osteosarcoma. Cancer. 2010;116(23):5470–8.
38. Senthamizhchelvan S, et al. Tumor dosimetry and response for 153Sm-ethylenediamine tetramethylene phosphonic acid therapy of high-risk osteosarcoma. J Nucl Med. 2012;53(2):215–24.
39. Eary JF, et al. Samarium-153-EDTMP biodistribution and dosimetry estimation. J Nucl Med. 1993;34(7):1031–6.
40. Wrzesien M, Napolska K, Olszewski J. Exposure of personnel and public due to using 153Sm-labelled EDTMP-Quadramet(R) in nuclear medicine procedures. Radiat Prot Dosim. 2016;168(3):396–400.
41. Lange R, et al. Pharmaceutical and clinical development of phosphonate-based radiopharmaceuticals for the targeted treatment of bone metastases. Bone. 2016;91:159–79.
42. Pacilio M, et al. Improving the dose-myelotoxicity correlation in radiometabolic therapy of bone metastases with 153Sm-EDTMP. Eur J Nucl Med Mol Imaging. 2014;41(2):238–52.
43. Dolezal J. Efficacy and toxicity of 153samarium-EDTMP in painful breast cancer bone metastases. Onkologie. 2009;32(1-2):35–9.
44. Ricci S, et al. Clinical benefit of bone-targeted radiometabolic therapy with 153Sm-EDTMP combined with chemotherapy in patients with metastatic hormone-refractory prostate cancer. Eur J Nucl Med Mol Imaging. 2007;34(7):1023–30.
45. Fizazi K, et al. Phase II trial of consolidation docetaxel and samarium-153 in patients with bone metastases from castration-resistant prostate cancer. J Clin Oncol. 2009;27(15):2429–35.
46. Tu SM, et al. Phase I study of concurrent weekly docetaxel and repeated samarium-153 lexidronam in patients with castration-resistant metastatic prostate cancer. J Clin Oncol. 2009;27(20):3319–24.
47. O'Sullivan JM, et al. A phase 2 study of high-activity 186Re-HEDP with autologous peripheral blood stem cell transplant in progressive hormone-refractory prostate cancer metastatic to bone. Eur J Nucl Med Mol Imaging. 2006;33(9):1055–61.
48. Maxon HR 3rd, et al. Rhenium-186(Sn)HEDP for treatment of painful osseous metastases: results of a double-blind crossover comparison with placebo. J Nucl Med. 1991;32(10):1877–81.
49. Kolesnikov-Gauthier H, et al. Evaluation of toxicity and efficacy of 186Re-hydroxyethylidene diphosphonate in patients with painful bone metastases of prostate or breast cancer. J Nucl Med. 2000;41(10):1689–94.
50. Sciuto R, et al. Short- and long-term effects of 186Re-1,1-hydroxyethylidene diphosphonate in the treatment of painful bone metastases. J Nucl Med. 2000;41(4):647–54.
51. Han SH, et al. The PLACORHEN study: a double-blind, placebo-controlled, randomized radionuclide study with (186)Re-etidronate in hormone-resistant prostate cancer patients with painful bone metastases. Placebo Controlled Rhenium Study. J Nucl Med. 2002;43(9):1150–6.
52. van Dodewaard-de Jong JM, et al. A phase I study of combined docetaxel and repeated high activity 186Re-HEDP in castration-resistant prostate cancer (CRPC) metastatic to bone (the TAXIUM trial). Eur J Nucl Med Mol Imaging. 2011;38(11):1990–8.
53. Argyrou M, et al. Rhenium-188 production in hospitals, by w-188/re-188 generator, for easy use in radionuclide therapy. Int J Mol Imaging. 2013;2013:290750.
54. Palmedo H, et al. Dose escalation study with rhenium-188 hydroxyethylidene diphosphonate in prostate cancer patients with osseous metastases. Eur J Nucl Med. 2000;27(2):123–30.
55. Sepini LJ. D; Jarvis, N; Zeevaart, JR, Complexation studies of 177Lu with ethylenediaminetetramethylene phosphonic acid (EDTMP) as a bone pain palliative therapeutic radiopharmaceutical. Polyhedron. 2016;106:101–5.
56. Abbasi IA. Studies on 177Lu-labeled methylene diphosphonate as potential bone-seeking radiopharmaceutical for bone pain palliation. Nucl Med Biol. 2011;38(3):417–25.
57. Abbasi IA. Preliminary studies on (177)Lu-labeled sodium pyrophosphate (177Lu-PYP) as a potential bone-seeking radiopharmaceutical for bone pain palliation. Nucl Med Biol. 2012;39(6):763–9.
58. Guerra Liberal FDC, Tavares AAS, Tavares J. Palliative treatment of metastatic bone pain with radiopharmaceuticals: a perspective beyond Strontium-89 and Samarium-153. Appl Radiat Isot. 2016;110:87–99.
59. Pedraza-Lopez M, et al. Preparation of (166)Dy/(166)Ho-EDTMP: a potential in vivo generator system for bone marrow ablation. Nucl Med Commun. 2004;25(6):615–21.
60. Zolghadri S, et al. Development of (166) Holmium-1,2 Propylene Di-amino Tetra (Methylenephosphonicacid) as a possible bone palliation agent. World J Nucl Med. 2014;13(1):28–33.
61. Christensen MH, Petersen LJ. Radionuclide treatment of painful bone metastases in patients with breast cancer: a systematic review. Cancer Treat Rev. 2012;38(2):164–71.

62. Parker C, et al. Alpha emitter radium-223 and survival in metastatic prostate cancer. N Engl J Med. 2013;369(3):213–23.
63. Smith MR, Parker CC, Saad F, Miller K, Tombal B, Ng QS, Bögemann M, Matveev V, Piulats JM, Zucca LE, Heidenreich A, Kakehi Y, Zhang A, Krissel H, Shen J, Wagner V, Higano C. A phase III trial of radium-223 (Ra-223) in combination with abiraterone acetate and prednisone/prednisolone for the treatment of asymptomatic or mildly symptomatic chemotherapy-naïve patients (pts) with bone-predominant metastatic castration-resistant prostate cancer (mCRPC). Ann Oncol. 2018;29(Suppl):8.

19 Radionuclide Therapy with Alpha-Emitting Agents in Bone Metastasis

Çiğdem Soydal and Nuriye Özlem Küçük

Radium-223 (Ra-223 dichloride) is an alpha-emitting radiopharmaceutical used to treat bone metastases. Ra-223 has a physical half-life of 11.4 days. Ra-223, a heavy metal, acts similarly to calcium and forms a complex with hydroxyapatite in sites where bone turnover increases [1–3]. It causes breaks in double-helix DNA, leading to the death of cancer cells [4–6]. Alpha particles have less than 100 micrometers of penetration distance within the tissue and radiate 2–10 cell distance around them [7]. Therefore, its effect on bone marrow and surrounding healthy tissues is minimal [8].

In the phase 2 study, a significant change in bone turnover parameters was reported after 4 weeks following Ra-223 treatment of 31 patients in the comparison of 33 patients in placebo arm [9].

19.1 Indications

It is indicated for the treatment of bone metastases in prostate cancer patients without castration-resistant visceral organ metastases [10]. Many clinical studies also included patients with lymph node metastasis with a short axis less than 3 cm even though visceral organ metastasis is considered a contraindication [11, 12].

Ç. Soydal (✉) · N. Ö. Küçük
Department of Nuclear Medicine, Ankara University, School of Medicine, Ankara, Turkey
e-mail: csoydal@ankara.edu.tr; okucuk@medicine.ankara.edu.tr

19.2 Contraindications

Even though the most important contraindication is pregnancy, it is insignificant in clinical practice since there is no approved indication available in female patients. Pregnancy category is X. It is not recommended for men of reproductive age to have children for 6 months after treatment due to its potential effect on spermatogenesis. The necessary treatment for cord compression should be completed before Ra-223 treatment in patients with spinal cord compression. Orthopedic stabilization should be performed before Ra-223 treatment in patients with pathological bone fracture [10].

19.3 Therapy Administration

Ra-223 treatment should be administered by nuclear medicine physicians authorized to administer radionuclide treatments, in clinics with imaging and treatment facilities that are necessary for radionuclide treatments and their possible complications. The procurement, transfer, storage, and administration of the radiopharmaceutical must be carried out by licensed persons in accordance with the radiation safety rules of national organizations. The radiation dose of the patient and radiation workers should be reduced as much as possible as with all radionuclide therapies. Ra-223 is supplied as 6 mL vials containing 1100 kBq radionuclide per mL. It is

R. Bekiş et al. (eds.), *Radionuclide Therapy*, https://doi.org/10.1007/978-3-030-97220-2_19

administered intravenously. 55 kBq/kg activity is administered as a 1-minute IV infusion by washing the vascular tract with saline before and after. It is recommended to administer a total of six cycles at 4-week intervals. It is quickly cleaned from the blood after administration. Eighty percent of the activity is cleared from the vascular bed at the 15 min after injection. The part that is not trapped by the bone is quickly excreted through the gastrointestinal tract. It does not undergo metabolism in the liver. Renal excretion is fairly minimal. No significant uptake is observed in the heart, liver, kidney, bladder, and spleen at the fourth hour after injection. Blood pool activity drops below 1% at 24 h.

No dose reduction is required in the geriatric group. No difference was found in terms of safety or effectiveness in patients under 65 years of age and above in the phase 3 study of 600 patients [11]. There is no information about its administration in the children.

19.4 Complications

Common side effects are transient anemia, lymphocytopenia, leukopenia, thrombocytopenia, nausea, diarrhea, vomiting, and peripheral edema. Less rarely, impaired renal function, dehydration, pancytopenia, edema, and erythema at the injection site may be observed. Evaluation should be performed before initiation of therapy, especially for myelosuppression, and after each cycle. Neutrophil count should be $>1.5 \times 10^9$/L, platelets $>100 \times 10^9$/L, and hemoglobin >10.0 g/dL before starting treatment. The neutrophil count must be $>1.0 \times 10^9$/L and the platelet count must be $>500 \times 10^9$/L in the evaluation made between cycles. Treatment should be discontinued if the desired levels are not reached despite the necessary supportive treatment at the sixth week after cycle. There are no reported side effects on liver and kidney function. It can be safely administered in patients with mild impaired hepatic and renal function. Dose reduction is also not recommended in patients with moderate or advanced liver and kidney dysfunction. No effect on liver and kidney functions is expected since the main route of elimination is the gastrointestinal tract [10].

There are no data on the effectiveness and safety of concurrent administration with chemotherapy. However, it is not recommended in routine practice due to potential myelosuppression. Side effects of around 1% were observed in both patient groups in a phase 3 study comparing Ra-223 with placebo. There are no reported data on drug interaction. Co-administration with other systemic radionuclide therapies or semi-body radiotherapy may also increase the risk of myelosuppression apart from chemotherapeutics.

19.5 Clinical Trials

Ra-223 has been shown to have a safe profile with minimal myelosuppressive effect in patients with bone metastasis in the phase 1 study [13]. Nilsson et al. observed a decrease in serum alkaline phosphatase levels in the Ra-223 group in a multicenter placebo-controlled phase 2 study [14]. Parker et al. showed a dose-dependent decrease in serum markers indicating that it may be associated with disease control in patients treated with Ra-223 [15].

The most common grade 3 side effect was anemia with 5%, followed by thrombocytopenia with 2%, neutropenia with 1%, and leukopenia with 1% in the safety studies. All side effects could be controlled with supportive and symptomatic therapy [9].

The clinical effectiveness and safety of Ra-223 in patients with castration-resistant symptomatic bone metastasis with prostate cancer were evaluated in a phase 3, double-blind, placebo-controlled, multicenter study (ALSYMPCA). Patients with visceral organ metastasis or lymph node metastasis greater than 3 cm were excluded. The primary endpoint was determined as overall survival. The study enrolled 921 (614 in the Ra-223 group, 307 in the placebo group) patients. Patients were grouped according to baseline ALP level, biphosphonate, or docetaxel usage. Median OS was 3.6 months longer (14.9 months vs. 11.3 months) in the Ra-223 group compared to the placebo group. Moreover, the risk of death was calculated to be 30% (HR, 0.70; 95% CI 0.58–0.83; $p < 0.001$) less in the Ra-223 group.

The frequency of side effects in the Ra-223 group was also found to be lower compared to the placebo group in this study [16]. Ra-223 did not interact with the timing and duration of chemotherapy compared to placebo [17]. This result showed that the safe profile of Ra-223 is likely to be administered sequentially or in combination with other treatment agents. Therefore, the phase 1–2 study of Ra-223 in combination with docetaxel completed patient recruitment, and the results will be reported soon [18]. 696 patients received at least 1 dose and 403 patients received 6 doses of Ra-223 treatment; patients were followed for a median duration of 7.5 months in a phase 3 study involving 839 castration-resistant prostate cancer patients. Median duration of OS was reported as 16 months. Longer OS durations have been reported in patients with a baseline ALP level below the upper limit of normal, a high Hb level of 10 g/dL, an ECOG performance score of 0, and no pain before treatment. Longer median survival was found among those receiving Ra-223 treatment with denosumab compared to those receiving it alone [12].

Sartor et al. reported the results of 44 patients who were re-treated with Ra-223 in patients who had previously received 6 doses of Ra-223 treatment. Sixty-six percent of the patients completed six doses of adjunctive therapy, and no serious hematological effects were observed in this study. The median total survival and the time to progression in the skeletal system could not be reached during this study [19].

Recently, there have been reports that Ra-223 can be administered in patients with a limited number of soft tissue metastases and even response can be observed in soft tissue lesions with abscopal effect even though it is indicated for patients without visceral metastases [20]. However, further studies are required on this subject.

It was reported that only 12% of specialist clinicians would prefer Ra-223 in first-line treatment in the final report from the Advanced Prostate Cancer Consensus Conference held in St. Gallen. However, it is predicted that Ra-223 will have a synergistic effect with other treatments and will provide not only pain palliation but also biochemical response and prolonged survival [12]. Following all these developments, Ra-223 entered the current ASCO, ESMO, NCCN, and EAU guidelines at level 1 evidence level for the treatment of bone metastases in patients with metastatic castration-resistant prostate cancer.

19.6 The Place of Nuclear Medicine Imaging in Ra-223 Treatment

Bone scintigraphy is the most commonly used and cheapest method to evaluate bone metastases in patients with prostate cancer. Bone scintigraphy is considered visually in clinical practice. However, it is possible to quantitatively calculate osteoblastic activity by bone scintigraphy index (BSI) using special software from bone scintigraphy images. Fosbol et al. found that BSI showed a significant correlation with OS in 88 castration-resistant prostate cancer patients undergoing Ra-223 treatment. Median OS in patients with a BSI greater than 5 was calculated as 8.2 months, while median OS in patients with a BSI greater than 5 and less was calculated as 15 months in this study. Moreover, baseline BSI was found to be prognostic in predicting hematological toxicity. The risk of hematological toxicity was calculated to be 3 times higher in patients with more than 5 BSI. However, there was no relationship between OS and changes observed during and after treatment in BSI. As a result, it was concluded that BSI can be used in the prognosis determination and prediction of hematological toxicity of patients to be treated with Ra-223 [21].

Another imaging method showing osteoblastic activity is F-18 NaF PET/CT. The quantification of F-18 NaF PET/CT images is easier compared to bone scintigraphy. Rohren et al. showed that there was a relationship between OS and volumetric parameters calculated by accepting ten threshold values for SUVmax for bone lesions in F-18 NaF PET/CT performed before

Ra-223 treatment [22]. Similarly, Etchebehere et al. reported the results of 42 patients who underwent Ra-223 treatment using tumor burden TLF10 and FTV10 values. They found a very strong relationship between baseline TLF10 and FTV10 values and OS ($p = 0.02$, HR = 5.99) [23].

18F-FDG PET/CT, which is frequently applied in oncological diseases, is very successful in detecting bone metastases considering all malignancies. Osteolytic metastases are known to have higher SUV values [24]. However, prostate cancer metastases are usually of osteoblastic nature and have also been reported to exhibit low glycolytic activity, especially during hormone-sensitive periods [25]. Therefore, prostate cancer has a lower sensitivity in bone metastases compared to bone scintigraphy [26, 27]. Ga-68 PSMA PET/CT, which has become widely used in recent years, has a high sensitivity in detecting bone metastasis of prostate cancer [28, 29]. Brauer et al. performed Ga-68 PSMA PET/CT Ra-223 before treatment and detected visceral metastasis in 15% of patients and changed the treatment approach [30]. Similarly, Ga-68 PSMA PET/CT performed before Ra-223 has been shown to be more successful compared to bone scintigraphy in selecting appropriate patients for Ra-223 treatment [31].

Bone scintigraphy is likely to have a flare effect in the first trimester after Ra-223 treatment. Therefore, it should take at least 4–6 months to evaluate the response [32]. Gayed et al. reported bone scintigraphy results performed before and after Ra-223 treatment in prostate cancer patients. One patient had mixed response and one patient had progression, whereas the number of lesions in the scintigraphy performed after treatment decreased in five of the seven patients with symptomatic and biochemically acceptable responses. On the other hand, flare phenomenon was observed in three of the five patients with no significant response, while progression was observed in one patient and decreased signs in one patient [33]. Ga-868 PSMA PET/CT seems to be a more appropriate method in follow-up. However, consensus could not be reached on the timing [34, 35].

References

1. Brechbiel MW. Targeted alpha-therapy: past, present, future? Dalton Trans. 2007;21(43):4918–28.
2. Bruland OS, Nilsson S, Fisher DR, et al. High-linear energy transfer irradiation targeted to skeletal metastases by the alpha-emitter 223Ra: adjuvant or alternative to conventional modalities? Clin Cancer Res. 2006;12(20 Pt 2):6250s–7s.
3. Henriksen G, Fisher DR, Roeske JC, et al. Targeting of osseous sites with alpha-emitting 223Ra: comparison with the beta-emitter 89Sr in mice. J Nucl Med. 2003 Feb;44(2):252–9.
4. Kassis AI, Adelstein SJ. Radiobiologic principles in radionuclide therapy. J Nucl Med. 2005;46(Suppl. 1):4S–12S.
5. Ritter MA, Cleaver JE, Tobias CA. High-LET radiations induce a large proportion of non-rejoining DNA breaks. Nature. 1977;266(5603):653–5.
6. Sgouros G. Alpha-particles for targeted therapy. Adv Drug Deliv Rev. 2008;60(12):1402–6.
7. Hall EJ. Radiobiology for the radiologist. 4th ed. Philadelphia: Lippincott, Williams &Wilkins; 1994.
8. Larsen RH, Murud KM, Akabani G, et al. 211At- and 131I-labeled bisphosphonates with high in vivo stability and bone accumulation. J Nucl Med. 1999;40(7):1197–203.
9. Nilsson S, Franzen L, Parker C, et al. Bone-targeted radium-223 in symptomatic, hormone- refractory prostate cancer: a randomised, multi centre, placebo-controlled phase II study. Lancet Oncol. 2007;8(7):587–94.
10. https://omr.bayer.ca/omr/online/xofigo-pm-en.pdf
11. Vogel Zang NJ, Coleman RE, Michalski JM, et al. Hematologic safety of Radium-223 dichloride: baseline prognostic factors associated with myelosuppression in the ALSYMPCA trial. Clin Genitourin Cancer. 2017;15(1):42–52.
12. Saad F, Carles J, Gillessen S, et al. Radium-223 and concomitant therapies in patients with meta- static castration-resistant prostate cancer: an international, early access, open-label, single-arm phase 3b trial. Lancet Oncol. 2016;17:1306–16.
13. Chittenden SJ, Hindorf C, Parker CC, et al. A Phase 1, open-label study of the biodistribution, pharmacokinetics, and dosimetry of 223RA-dichloride in patients with hormone-refractory prostate cancer and skeletal metastases. J Nucl Med. 2015;56(9):1304–9. Available from http://www.ncbi.nlm.nih.gov/pubmed/26182965
14. Nilsson S, Franzén L, Parker C, et al. Bone-targeted radium-223 in symptomatic, hormone- refractory prostate cancer: a randomised, multicentre, placebo-controlled phase II study. Lancet Oncol. 2007;8(7):587–94.
15. Parker CC, Pascoe S, Chodacki A, et al. A randomized, double-blind, dose-finding, multicenter, phase 2 study of radium chloride (Ra 223) in patients with

bone metastases and castration- resistant prostate cancer. Eur Urol. 2013;63(2):189–97.
16. Parker C, Nilsson S, Heinrich D, et al. Alpha emitter radium-223 and survival in metastatic prostate cancer. N Engl J Med. 2013;369(3):213–23.
17. Sartor O, Coleman RE, Nilsson S, et al. 2510 3-year follow-up of chemotherapy following radium-223 dichloride (Ra-223) in castration-resistant prostate cancer (CRPC) patients (Pts) with symptomatic bone metastases (Mets) from ALSYMPCA. Eur J Cancer. 2015;51:S477. Elsevier[cited 2017 Mar 24]
18. (Clinical-Trials.gov number, NCT 01106352 https://clinicaltrials.gov/ct2/show/results/NCT01106352?sect=X01256#all).
19. Sartor O, Heinrich D, Mariados N, et al. Re-treatment with radium-223: first experience from an international, open-label, phase I/II study in patients with castration-resistant prostate cancer and bone metastases. Ann Oncol. 2017;28:2464–71.
20. Kwee SA, Lim J, Coel MN. Soft tissue response on 18F-Fluorocholine PET/CT in metastatic castrate-resistant prostate cancer treated with 223Ra-dichloride: a possible abscopal effect? Clin Nucl Med. 2017;42(11):868–71.
21. Fosbol MO, Petersen PM, Kjaer A, et al. Radium-223 therapy of advanced metastatic castration- resistant prostate cancer: quantitative assessment of skeletal tumor burden for prognostication of clinical outcome and hematological toxicity. Nucl Med. 2018;59(4):596–602.
22. Rohren EM, Etchebehere EC, Araujo JC, et al. Determination of skeletal tumor burden on 18F-Fluoride PET/CT. J Nucl Med. 2015;56:1507–12.
23. Etchebehere EC, Araujo JC, Fox PS, et al. Prognostic factors in patients treated with 223Ra: the role of skeletal tumor burden on baseline 18F-Fluo- ride PET/CT in predicting overall survival. J Nucl Med. 2015;56:1177–84.
24. Cook GJ, Houston S, Rubens R, et al. Detection of bone metastases in breast cancer by 18FDG PET: differing metabolic activity in osteoblastic and osteolytic lesions. J Clin Oncol. 1998;16:3375–9.
25. Morris MJ, Akhurst T, Osman I, et al. Fluorinated deoxy glucose positron emission tomography imaging in progressive metastatic prostate cancer. Urology. 2002;59:913–8.
26. Shreve PD, Grossman HB, Gross MD, et al. Metastatic prostate cancer: initial findings of PET with 2-deoxy-2-[F-18]fluoro-D-glucose. Radiology. 1996;199:751–6.
27. Yeh SD, Imbriaco M, Larson SM, et al. Detection of bony metastases of androgen-independent prostate cancer by PET-FDG. Nucl Med Biol. 1996;23:693–7.
28. Afshar-Oromieh A, Avtzi E, Giesel FL, et al. The diagnostic value of PET/CT imaging with the (68) Ga-labelled PSMA ligand HBED-CC in the diagnosis of recurrent prostate cancer. Eur J Nucl Med Mol Imaging. 2015;42:197–209.
29. Afshar-Oromieh A, Haberkorn U, Eder M, et al. [68Ga]Gallium-labelled PSMA ligand as superior PET tracer for the diagnosis of prostate cancer: comparison with 18F-FECH. Eur J Nucl Med Mol Imaging. 2012;39:1085–6.
30. Bräuer A, Rahbar K, Konnert J, et al. Diagnostic value of additional 68Ga-PSMA-PET before 223 Ra-dichloride therapy in patients with metastatic prostate carcinoma. Nukl Med. 2017;56:14–22.
31. Ahmadzadehfar H, Azgomi K, Hauser S, et al. 68Ga-PSMA-11 PET as a gate keeper for the treatment of metastatic prostate cancer with 223Ra: proof of concept. J Nucl Med. 2017;58:438–44.
32. Azad GK, Taylor B, Rubello D, et al. Molecular and functional imaging of bone metastases in breast and prostate cancers: an overview. Clin Nucl Med. 2016;41:e44–50.
33. Gayed I, Salama V, Dawood L, et al. Can bone scans guide therapy with radium-223 dichloride for prostate cancer bone metastases? Cancer Manag Res. 2018;10:3317–24.
34. Ahmadzadehfar H, Schlenkhoff CD, Rogenhofer S, et al. 68Ga-PSMA-11 PET represents the tumoricidal effect of 223Ra in a patient with castrate-resistant metastatic prostate cancer. Clin Nucl Med. 2016;41:695–6.
35. Hama Y. Antitumor effect of 89Sr for multiple bone metastases of breast cancer: diagnosis by 18F-FDG PET/CT. Clin Nucl Med. 2014;39:e290–1.

Part VIII

Clinical Information: Lymphoproliferative Diseases

20 Radionuclide Therapy in Lymphoproliferative Diseases

Ümit Özgür Akdemir and Lütfiye Özlem Atay

Lymphoproliferative diseases are the general name given to different disease conditions with monoclonally overproliferated lymphocytes. Non-Hodgkin's lymphoma (NHL) originating from B-lymphocytes, polycythemia vera (PV) which is one of the myeloproliferative diseases, essential thrombocytosis (ET), and multiple myeloma (MM) originating from plasma cells are important lymphoproliferative diseases in which radionuclide therapy is administered. The place of radionuclide therapy in these diseases in the clinic, the method of administration, and the clinical results of the administrations are mentioned in this chapter.

20.1 Radioimmunotherapy in NHL

NHL includes a group of lymphoproliferative diseases that exhibit clinically and biologically heterogeneous features and originate from B-lymphocytes, T-lymphocytes, or natural killer (NK) cells [1, 2]. NHL may contain indolent species such as follicular lymphoma (FL) with a slow clinical course, but it also has clinically aggressive species. NHL has a 3% rate among all cancer types in Turkey as of 2014 [3]. Disease-related mortality rates have decreased even though the incidence of NHL has increased in the last 20–30 years worldwide [4]. This decrease occurred largely as a result of targeted therapies with new chemoimmunological treatment regimens, monoclonal antibodies, radioimmunotherapy (RIT), and small molecular inhibitors [4].

FL, defined as the primary indication of RIT, is the second most common type of NHL with a rate of 22% (Table 20.1) [1, 5]. The most common type of NHL is diffuse large B-cell lymphoma with a rate of 31% [1]. FL is a type of slow-course B-cell lymphoma and is typically seen in the seventh decade [6]. The disease is usually diagnosed at an advanced clinical stage and the median survival after diagnosis is 10 years [6]. Current treatment options are rarely curative, mostly aimed at delaying disease progression and improving survival. Rituximab (Mabthera®), a CD20 monoclonal antibody, targets B-cells that express CD20 surface protein [2, 4–6]. Rituximab is involved in many treatment regimens since it contributes to survival when administered with chemotherapy and used as consolidation therapy [2, 4–6]. An alternative treatment that is used less frequently is RIT administration. Tositumomab and ibritumomab, which are monoclonal CD20 antibodies, bind with iodine-131 (I-131) and yttrium-90 (Y-90), respectively, for this treatment [5].

Because NHL is a widespread multifocal disease and has a high sensitivity to radiation, RIT is a rational approach in the treatment of these

Ü. Ö. Akdemir (✉) · L. Ö. Atay
Faculty of Medicine, Department of Nuclear Medicine, Gazi University, Ankara, Turkey
e-mail: uoakdemir@gazi.edu.tr; ozlematay@gazi.edu.tr

R. Bekiş et al. (eds.), *Radionuclide Therapy*, https://doi.org/10.1007/978-3-030-97220-2_20

Table 20.1 NHL World Health Organization Classification

	Frequency (%)
Mature B-cell NHL types	
Diffuse large B-cell lymphoma	31
Follicular lymphoma	22
Small lymphocytic lymphoma/chronic lymphocytic leukemia	6
Mantle cell lymphoma	6
Extranodal marginal zone MALT-type lymphoma	5
Primary mediastinal (thymic) large cell lymphoma	2
Marginal zone nodal-type lymphoma	1
Lymphoplasmacytic lymphoma	1
Burkitt lymphoma	1
Other types	<1
Mature T-cell NHL types	
Peripheral T-cell lymphoma	6
Anaplastic large cell lymphoma	2
Angioimmunoblastic T-cell lymphoma	2
Lymphoblastic lymphoma	2
Other types	<1

patients. RIT allows malignant cells to be continuously exposed to low doses of radiation unlike conventional radiotherapy [4]. Apart from this, RIT has several advantages over treatments with cold (non-radiolabeled) monoclonal antibodies; firstly, it is not an absolute necessity for the patient to have a functional immune system to kill malignant cells in RIT administration. Secondly, beta radiation emitted by radioisotopes is effective on 100–200 cell diameters [4]. In this way, other malignant cells near the cells targeted by monoclonal antibodies are also destroyed by radiation. This feature of RIT is known as crossfire effect [4]. RIT also has various superior aspects compared to radiotherapy; high radiation exposure of normal tissues and organs around the target tumor can be avoided, thanks to RIT. In addition, because RIT is a systemic treatment, other unknown tumor foci and unexpected involvement sites in the body are also treated in addition to the known tumor foci [4].

Several clinical studies have shown that a high rate of treatment response with RIT can be achieved in patients with recurrent or treatment-resistant NHL and FL patients who respond to first-line chemotherapy as a consolidation treatment [7–14]. In addition, there are studies showing the clinical benefit of RIT in FL as a first-line treatment option and in stem cell transplantation treatment [14–20]. Longer-term responses can be obtained in RIT administration compared to standard chemotherapy regimens containing rituximab regarding the high sensitivity of NHL tissues to radiation [7–14, 21]. RIT use as a treatment option in FL treatment is included in NCCN (National Comprehensive Cancer Network) and European Society for Medical Oncology (ESMO) practice guidelines prepared for NHL [2, 22]. Unfortunately, RIT is often used as a last choice treatment method in the late stages of the disease, where treatment effectiveness is lower [8, 13, 22, 23].

RIT is not sufficiently utilized in clinical practice today despite all its superior aspects in terms of effectiveness and side effects. The causes of this condition include various concerns and prejudices that clinicians have about RIT administration in NHL. These include clinicians thinking that RIT is economically costly, that they do not know how to access treatment or think that it is difficult, that there are not enough randomized studies, that treatment will damage bone marrow and prevent autologous stem cell transplantation to be performed later, that treatment has possible side effects for the late period, and that there are other non-radioactive treatment options [24]. However, RIT is a treatment that can be administered without affecting the daily life activities of patients [5]. Various early and late side effects caused by multiple chemotherapy regimens administered as standard treatment can be avoided with RIT administration [5, 23, 25].

RIT demonstrates high treatment effectiveness and safety compared to standard treatments in patients with recurrent or treatment-resistant B-cell NHL. For this indication, it was shown that the treatment response rate was 80% in 143 patients with 30% achieving complete response, while the treatment rate remained at 56% (16% complete response rate) in the group receiving rituximab treatment in a phase 3 study with Y-90-ibritumomab tiuxetan (Zevalin®) [7]. The data of this study provided grounds for FDA approval for RIT in 2002 in recurrent or treatment-resistant low-grade FL. Then, the FDA approved RIT as consolidation therapy in FL patients who responded partially and fully to first-line chemotherapy in 2009. I-131-tositumomab (Bexxar®), another radiopharmaceutical similar to Y-90-ibritumomab tiuxetan approved for this indication, has not been produced since 2014 [20]. Therefore, this section mainly includes RIT administration with Y-90-ibritumomab tiuxetan.

RIT is administered as consolidation therapy after initial treatment in FL. However, different results were obtained from clinical trials conducted with this indication. Median progression-free survival time with FIT (first-line indolent lymphoma), an international randomized controlled phase 3 study, was 36.5 months in the group in which Y-90-ibritumomab tiuxetan administration was added to treatment and 13.3 months in the group in which it was not added ($p < 0.001$) [11]. However, no significant difference was found between the two groups given RIT or rituximab as consolidation therapy after CHOP (cyclophosphamide, doxorubicin, vincristine, and prednisone) in terms of 2-year progression-free and overall survival rates in another phase 3 study called SWOG S0016 using I-131-tositumomab [12, 21]. Consolidation RIT administration after induction chemotherapy was well tolerated in previously untreated FL patient groups in both studies. It was observed that the rate of complete response with RIT consolidation therapy was 82.7% and the overall response rate was 96.2% in a meta-analysis study evaluating a total of 8 studies and 783 patient data for this indication [6]. Two-year progression-free survival and overall survival were 76.8% and 94.2%, respectively, as a result of this meta-analysis [6]. Although the studies included in the analysis showed high to moderate variability in response to treatment and survival rates, the results of these studies suggest that adding consolidation RIT to induction chemotherapy generally increases response rates to treatment.

RIT is also used as consolidation therapy in patients diagnosed with aggressive NHL apart from FL. A multicenter study involving a total of 215 aggressive B-cell NHL patients showed that RIT administered as consolidation therapy after multiple chemotherapy steps provided 63.3% treatment response (44.3% complete response) [10]. Neutropenia and thrombocytopenia at grade 4 and anemia at grade 3 were observed; it was stated that the median time required for improvement of blood counts was 81 days in this study. Therefore, RIT is a treatment that provides satisfactory response rates with acceptable toxicity in recurrent aggressive B-cell NHL.

Y-90-ibritumomab tiuxetan has also shown promising results in first-line treatment of untreated FL patients. Eighty-seven percent treatment response (41% complete response) and 25.9-month median progression-free survival were achieved at 6 months post-RIT in 59 patients with low-grade, stage 2–4 diagnosed CD20+, in a multicenter clinical study using Y-90-ibritumomab tiuxetan alone as first-line treatment in FL [26]. Forty-eight percent of patients had thrombocytopenia at 3 or 4°, 34% had leukopenia, 32% had neutropenia, and 20% had lymphopenia, most notably at 6 and 8 weeks after RIT [26]. Side effects other than hematological toxicities never exceeded grade 2. RIT is an important alternative to first-line therapy, especially for elderly FL patients with significant comorbidities or who refuse chemotherapy.

It is possible to achieve long-term treatment responses with high-dose chemotherapy followed by autologous stem cell transplantation in patients with recurrent or treatment-resistant B-cell aggressive NHL. Preparation prior to cell transplantation usually involves total-body irradiation with chemotherapy. Recently, researchers have begun to include RIT in this preparation phase [16–20, 27]. In this indication, RIT is combined with chemotherapy and used either instead of whole-body irradiation or in addition to standard radiotherapy applications. Data from phase 1 and 2 studies have shown that Y-90-ibritumomab tiuxetan administration in high-risk B-cell NHL can be safely added to preparation regimens for stem cell transplantation and improve survival [16–20, 27].

20.1.1 Y-90-Ibritumomab Tiuxetan

Y-90-ibritumomab tiuxetan was approved by the European Medicines Agency (EMA) in January 2004 for the treatment of treatment-resistant or recurrent CD20+ follicular B-cell NHL in adult patients [28]. Y-90-ibritumomab tiuxetan treatment for the same indication in Turkey is within the scope of reimbursement by the Social Security Institution. Contraindications for RIT with Y-90-ibritumomab tiuxetan are summarized in Table 20.2 [28].

Y-90-chloride is formed by strontium-90 (Sr-90) decay, a radioactive precursor nuclide. Y-90 decay occurs by beta radiation release with a maximum energy of 2.281 MeV (99.98%), resulting in stable zirconium-90 (Zr-90). Y-90 has a half-life of 64 h (2.7 days). Y-90 emits high-energy beta radiation with an average soft tissue range of 5.3 mm. A range of this width corresponds to 100–200 cell diameters. Ibritumomab tiuxetan consists of a tiuxetan compound that binds radionuclide metal with ibritumomab, a murine monoclonal antibody (Fig. 20.1).

Ibritumomab tiuxetan targets normal (excluding pre-B cells and secretory B cells) and malignant B lymphocytes that express CD20 surface antigen. The immunospecific portion of this antibody in the IgG structure that recognizes the CD20 antigen is located at the tips of the "Y"-shaped arms. Since the antibody structure (approximately 70–90% of IgG) outside this immunospecific portion obtained from the murine antibody is derived from humans, ibritu-

Table 20.2 Contraindications for 90Y-ibritumomab tiuxetan

Pregnancy and ongoing breastfeeding
Known hypersensitivity for radiopharmaceutical components
Children and adolescents younger than 18 years of age
Bone marrow suppression (leukocyte <1,500/m^3; platelet <100,000/m^3)[a]
>25% bone marrow infiltration on bone marrow biopsy
Previously administered radiotherapy to more than 25% of the active bone marrow
Previous bone marrow or stem cell transplant
Human "anti-mouse" antibody (HAMA) positivity

[a]Peripheral blood cell count shouldn't be lower than the specified limits above. While low blood count does not constitute an absolute contraindication, it increases the risk of severe and long-term bone marrow suppression and thus infection and/or bleeding. In such a case, 90Y-ibritumomab tiuxetan indication can be decided by weighing the benefits and disadvantages of all local and systemic available alternative treatments

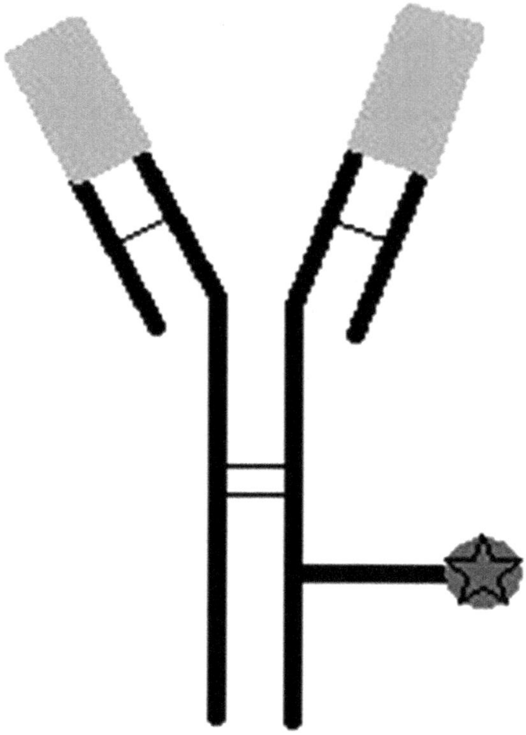

Fig. 20.1 The structure of Y-90-ibritumomab tiuxetan. Y-90-ibritumomab tiuxetan is obtained as a result of stable binding of Y-90 radioisotope (indicated by a star-containing circle) with ibritumomab, a murine monoclonal antibody, via tiuxetan. Ibritumomab is chimeric because the portion of this antibody in the IgG structure that provides specific binding to the CD20 antigen (gray region at the end of the "Y"-shaped arms) is derived from the murine antibody obtained from the mouse gene and the antibody structure (black portions of the "Y"-shaped arms) outside this portion is obtained from the human gene

momab is chimeric [29]. Chimeric monoclonal rituximab antibody commonly used for clinical treatment is also derived from ibritumomab antibody [29].

Pharmacokinetic studies have shown that Y-90-ibritumomab tiuxetan is retained almost entirely in the body after injection. The mean effective half-life of Y-90-ibritumomab tiuxetan in the blood is 27 h, provided that rituximab infusion is performed beforehand and the human "anti-mouse" antibody (HAMA) is negative. Expression occurs primarily via the urinary system, and only 7.3% (±3.2%) of the administered activity is excreted in the urine during the 7 days after injection [28].

Rituximab administered prior to Y-90-ibritumomab tiuxetan dose improves Y-90-ibritumomab tiuxetan biodistribution by clearing circulating peripheral B-lymphocytes as a preliminary stage of RIT. Rituximab administration prevents Y-90-ibritumomab tiuxetan from binding to sites other than the tumor (normal B-lymphocytes, spleen) and allows it to penetrate the tumor better and its distribution in tumor tissues to be more homogeneous. Moreover, rituximab itself kills tumor cells through various mechanisms, such as antibody-dependent cellular cytotoxicity, complement-dependent cytotoxicity, direct stimulation of apoptosis, and cell-cycle blockade. Biological effects caused by monoclonal antibody and radiation strengthen each other during RIT.

20.1.2 Preparation for RIT Practice

RIT should only be performed in centers that can meet the standards of radionuclide therapy administration and are licensed for this. Receipt, storage, administration to the patient, and waste management of the radiopharmaceutical can be done by persons authorized in accordance with national regulations and in designated environments. The relevant nuclear medicine specialist is responsible for conducting all preliminary procedures and treatment steps for RIT in harmony with the hematology/oncology ward that directs the patient.

Age, gender, height, weight, diagnosis, and clinical indication information of the patient as well as detailed information about previous treatments (chemotherapy, radiotherapy, stem cell transplantation) and medications used (especially affecting coagulation and blood counts) should be collected during the preparation phase of the patient. Recent chemotherapy in particular and radiotherapy affecting active bone marrow may worsen RIT-related bone marrow suppression. It should be demonstrated that the rate of tumor infiltration is less than 25% with an adequate bone marrow biopsy no more than 3 months prior to the planned treatment. In addition, the density of cells showing normal hematopoiesis on biopsy should also be assessed to predict adequate hematopoietic recovery after treatment. Pregnancy should be excluded before RIT and breastfeeding should be discontinued in breastfeeding patients. Blood count, prothrombin time (INR), serum creatinine, and bilirubin levels should be checked within 1 week prior to treatment. It is recommended not to treat if these values are 2.5 times the normal limit even though there is not enough experience with RIT in patients with high creatinine or bilirubin levels. The life expectancy of the patient should be >3 months and Karnofsky index should be >70%. RIT will not be of any benefit in a patient with a life expectancy of less than 3–4 weeks. Similarly, RIT is not appropriate in patients with rapidly progressing disease as the effectiveness of treatment will be delayed.

Dosimetry studies have not shown a relationship between the doses absorbed and the clinical response possibly due to methodological problems. Therefore, neither therapeutic effectiveness nor therapeutic toxicity can be predicted for RIT with current dose calculations. Therefore, EMA considered that a dosimetry study prior to treatment was not necessary. The activity to be given to the patient is determined by the patient's body weight and platelet count. However, imaging with indium-111 (In-111)-labeled ibritumomab tiuxetan is mandatory prior to treatment in Switzerland and the United States of America. However, this imaging is not done for dosimetric purposes, but as an additional security measure to confirm the expected biodistribution. In addition, a dosimetric study before treatment is required in other clinical conditions other than the indication approved by the EMA and in investigational RIT administrations.

20.1.3 Instructions for Patients

RIT should be performed in close cooperation with the physician(s) performing the treatment and follow-up of the patient. The nuclear medicine specialist responsible for RIT administration prior to treatment should verify the patient's fitness for treatment criteria and discuss all technical and clinical aspects of RIT with the patient. Patients should be provided with written instructions for radiation safety and expected side effects, including telephone numbers that they can access when necessary. Oral or written consent of the patient should be obtained depending on the national legislation after informing the patient verbally and in writing.

The precautions to be followed during the first week after RIT and the situations in which patients should be informed are listed below [28]:

- The radiation dose that people in contact with the patient are exposed to is minimal. Therefore, it is not necessary to limit the patient's interaction with their family and other people.
- Patients do not need to change their daily life habits when treatment is administered. Special precautions such as the use of separate toilets and the separation of food containers are not required.
- Male patients should urinate squatting/sitting down; if urine splashes, this urine should be cleaned using absorbent toilet paper and discarded in the trash or toilet drain.
- All patients should wash their hands after urinating.
- Patients should use condoms if they engage in sexual activity.
- Pregnancy prevention is recommended for 1 year after treatment, as with other anticancer treatments. Male patients may experience temporary infertility or even permanent infertility at a low risk. It may be recommended to preserve sperm in male patients even though there are no studies confirming this risk. Fertility is not expected to be affected in female patients.
- Low incidence (1.4%) of secondary malignancies observed after Y-90-ibritumomab tiuxetan treatment may be associated with chemotherapy previously experienced by patients. Indeed, the reported incidence of secondary malignancy after chemotherapies containing alkylating agents alone ranges from 1 to 8%.
- Secondary malignancy has not been reported in patients using RIT as first-line therapy.

20.1.4 Preparing the Radiopharmaceutical

Ibritumomab tiuxetan cold kit contains the non-radioactive components necessary to produce a dose of Y-90-ibritumomab tiuxetan. This kit contains 3.2 mg (1.6 mg/ml) ibritumomab tiuxetan, 2 ml sodium acetate solution, 10 ml formulated buffer solution, and an empty 10 ml reaction bottle in individual bottles. This kit should be stored at 2 °C–8 °C and it should not be frozen. The radioactive component Y-90 is also supplied. Only carrier-free Y-90 should be used in labeling of the antibody since metal contamination may reduce labeling effectiveness.

Y-90-ibritumomab tiuxetan preparation is performed at room temperature. The final formulation obtained by radiolabeling contains 2.08 mg Y-90-ibritumomab tiuxetan in a total volume of 10 ml. The prepared dose should then be stored in a refrigerator at a temperature of 2 °C–8 °C in a way that does not see light and used within a maximum of 8 h.

Preparation of Y-90-ibritumomab tiuxetan should be performed by experienced people in centers with appropriate radiation safety, measurement, and quality control facilities, providing aseptic conditions at all stages of labeling. Syringes and other carrier bottles should have plexiglass shield at least 1 cm thick, and forceps and tongs should be used to hold them; plastic gloves, preferably disposable waterproof apron, and plexiglass eye protection should be used during radiolabeling and administration of the treatment dose. Detailed information on radioactive labeling and treatment preparation can be found in the text contained in the product content.

It is very unlikely that labeling will fail if attention is paid to the radioactive labeling method. It should be confirmed that the binding efficiency is 95% or more by performing quality control of the prepared dose. Thin-layer chromatography is the recommended method for quality control, in which a gamma counter is sufficient for measurements. Attention should be paid to drop size, which is the most common source of error in the quality control process, and dead time errors that may occur during the measurement of thin-layer chromatography strips.

Activity in a 10 mL syringe should be measured in a dose calibrator before Y-90-ibritumomab tiuxetan is injected. The dose calibrator must have been calibrated using a known Y-90 source of activity and volume before preparing the first patient dose. The same equipment (in terms of geometric shape, volume, and material) used in this first measurement should also be used in subsequent activity measurements. Otherwise, recalibration will be required.

20.1.5 RIT Administration Protocol

The patient does not need to fast before treatment, but it is necessary to ensure adequate hydration. Rituximab infusions should be performed twice by the patient's hematologist or oncologist experienced in rituximab before Y-90-ibritumomab tiuxetan treatment.

250 mg/m^2 rituximab infusion is administered on day 1 according to the recommended administration protocol (Fig. 20.2). This infusion is followed by an In-111-ibritumomab tiuxetan (180 MBq) IV infusion lasting 10 min in Switzerland and the United States of America. In-111-ibritumomab tiuxetan distribution is evaluated by a complete body scan performed twice 24 h and 7–9 days after infusion. Y-90-ibritumomab tiuxetan is administered after the second 250 mg/m^2 rituximab dose is administered between the seventh and ninth days of the protocol. Y-90-ibritumomab tiuxetan dose should be administered as a slow IV infusion lasting 10 min and not as an IV bolus. Y-90-ibritumomab tiuxetan infusion should preferably be performed within 4 h after the second rituximab infusion, but may be delayed up to 48 h without further rituximab administration if necessary.

Y-90-ibritumomab tiuxetan activity is 15 MBq/kg (0.4 mCi/kg), and maximum activity is 1184 MBq (32 mCi) for patients with

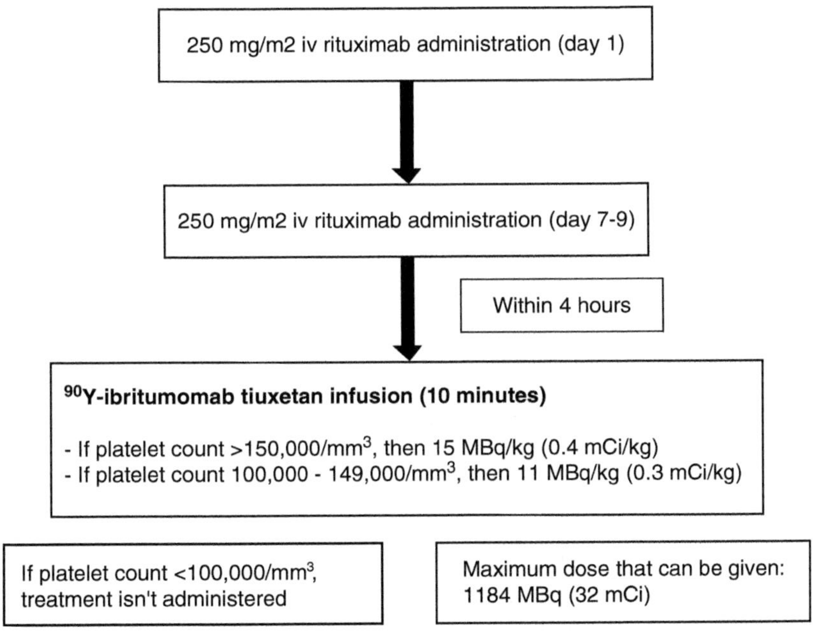

Fig. 20.2 Y-90-ibritumomab tiuxetan administration protocol. The first rituximab administration (250 mg/m^2) is administered approximately 1 week before Y-90-ibritumomab tiuxetan treatment. Y-90-ibritumomab tiuxetan is preferably administered within 4 h after the second rituximab dose (250 mg/m^2) is administered between the seventh and ninth days after the first rituximab administration. Y-90-ibritumomab tiuxetan dose is administered as a slow IV infusion lasting 10 min. Y-90-ibritumomab tiuxetan activity recommended for patients with platelet count ≥150,000/mm^3 is 15 MBq/kg (0.4 mCi/kg), and maximum activity is 1184 MBq (32 mCi). 11 MBq/kg (0.3 mCi/kg) activity is given to patients with platelet count of 100,000–149,000/mm^3

platelet count ≥150,000/mm³. 11 MBq/kg (0.3 mCi/kg) activity is given to patients with platelet count of 100,000–149,000/mm³. There is not enough data on re-treatment of patients with Y-90-ibritumomab tiuxetan. However, the maximum tolerated dose may be lower in terms of hematological toxicity in re-treatment.

This preparation should not be administered to the patient if the mean radiochemical purity rate of the prepared Y-90-ibritumomab tiuxetan dose is less than 95%. This dose should be stored at 2–8 °C and protected from light and administered to the patient within 8 h. Infusion of the radiopharmaceutical agent is via the venous catheter. The vascular tract can be controlled by a rapid physiological infusion of saline in order to prevent paravascular leakage. Y-90-ibritumomab tiuxetan is administered directly from a three-way tap line or using a separate infusion system with a perspex shield. In addition, a line filter is used. The system is washed with at least 10 ml saline, and the radiopharmaceutical dose is fully administered after the infusion. The remaining activity in the catheter should be measured with a needle and/or infusion kit to accurately calculate the activity administered.

The infusion should be discontinued from the arm of administration immediately in case of extravasation during infusion. The remaining dose can be continued from the other arm and the treatment can be completed. Extravasation can lead to radionecrosis, and unfortunately, there is no specific treatment for it. Approaches such as local hyperthermia, the elevation of the extremity, and mild massage, which support regional lymphatic drainage and thus reduce the local radiation dose, are used in the case of extravasation.

The incidence of anaphylaxis and other hypersensitivity reactions is below 1%. Blood pressure and pulse should be monitored during administration, as with other monoclonal antibodies. An emergency kit containing glucocorticoids and antihistamines should be available for possible allergic reactions.

Hospitalization may not be necessary after Y-90-ibritumomab tiuxetan administration depending on national regulations. The patient is discharged after being retained under observation for side effects for 30–120 min after completion of the infusion in this case. Healthcare professionals and their relatives should wear plastic gloves to prevent skin contact with the patient's excretions (such as urine). There is no risk of the patient being together with relatives or other patients apart from this.

20.1.6 Dosimetry

Absorbed radiation doses were obtained from pretreatment imaging with In-111-ibritumomab tiuxetan in studies that formed the basis for Y-90-ibritumomab tiuxetan approval. These data should not be used prospectively to predict toxicity in any patient. Y-90-ibritumomab tiuxetan treatment was calculated as radiation doses (mGy/MBq) absorbed for the spleen, liver, lungs, bone marrow (according to blood activity), bone surface, bladder wall, other organs (including the ovary and testicle), and whole body as 7.35, 4.32, 2.05, 0.59, 0.53, 0.89, 0.41, and 0.54, respectively [28]. In particular, the bone marrow dose is strongly dependent on the quantification method used. In addition, the dose to the testicles has been reported to be higher for male patients in some publications.

20.1.7 Posttreatment Follow-Up and Side Effects

Recurrent treatments may trigger HAMA and human anti-chimeric antibody (HACA) formation in the patient since ibritumomab is a chimeric (mouse/human) monoclonal antibody [28, 30]. The presence of these antibodies may reduce the benefit of treatment by affecting the pharmacokinetics of Y-90-ibritumomab tiuxetan [29]. In addition, it is recommended that patients be premedicated with antihistamines, monitored in the clinic for 30–120 min after the infusion, and that the necessary drugs and equipment for emergency intervention be kept in the clinic since the presence of antibodies may cause allergic side effects during RIT administration [29]. Generally, the development of HAMA or HACA antibodies after RIT is a rare and transient side effect. HAMA or HACA antibodies were reported to develop in 1–2% of patients treated with Y-90-ibritumomab tiuxetan [28]. Low incidence of HAMA positivity may be associated with immunodeficiency status in lymphoma patients, rituximab administration before Y-90-ibritumomab tiuxetan, or other treatments previously administered [28].

The nuclear medicine specialist should participate in the patient follow-up as a member of the patient management team. There may be a 30–70% reduction in leukocyte and platelet counts compared to baseline values, sometimes very rapidly. The lowest values usually occur at weeks 7–9 after treatment (median, 60 days). Weekly blood tests are recommended starting from the second week after treatment, for at least 3 months, or until blood count values increase to baseline levels. Checks should be performed at shorter intervals if there is a more rapid decrease than expected in blood count values. Blood counts should be checked at least three times a week if the platelet count falls below 30,000/m^3 [28]. Platelet transfusion should be performed and growth factors should be given to the patient when necessary. Bone marrow involvement before RIT administration is a risk factor for hematological toxicity in patients. The incidence of grade 4 neutropenia was significantly higher in patients with bone marrow involvement compared to patients without bone marrow involvement ($P = 0.001$). The incidence of neutropenia, thrombocytopenia, and anemia in patients with ≥20% involvement in bone marrow was reported as 53%, 13%, and 25%, respectively [28]. Patients should be informed of the increased risk of infection and of bleeding. In addition, other frequently observed non-hematologic side effects (WHO grades 1–2) and their incidence (in %) within the first 12 weeks after treatment are as follows: fatigue (35%), nausea (25%), tremor (21%), fever (13%), headache (9%), sore throat (9%), abdominal pain (8%), dizziness (8%), vomiting (7%), shortness of breath (7%), itching (7%), rash (7%), cough (6%), and ecchymosis (6%). Evaluation of response to treatment should be performed according to the criteria specified in the international guidelines 3 months after RIT administration [2, 22].

RIT administration is thought to cause secondary malignancies in the long term apart from this. It has been reported that 5.2% of patients treated with RIT with recurrent or treatment-resistant B-cell NHL develop myelodysplastic syndrome and/or acute myeloid leukemia in clinical trials [4]. Myelodysplastic syndrome and/or acute myeloid leukemia were observed in 19 patients (2.5%) during the median 4.4-year follow-up period in the analysis of a total of 746 patients with NHL treated with RIT from different studies [31]. These malignancies developed after a median of 5.6 years (range, 1.4–13.9 years) after the diagnosis of NHL and a median of 1.9 years (range, 0.4–6.3 years) after RIT administration. It has been emphasized that multiple cytogenetic changes observed in these patients are associated with chemotherapy previously experienced by patients, and the secondary malignancy rate observed in the RIT group is similar to the overall secondary malignancy rates in NHL patients; therefore, RIT administration does not pose a risk for the development of myelodysplastic syndrome and acute myeloid leukemia [28].

Fifty-three elderly NHL patients treated with RIT at a myeloablative dose developed myelodysplastic syndrome or acute myeloid leukemia in four patients during the median 49-month follow-up [32]. The 5-year cumulative risk (8.3%) reported for myelodysplastic syndrome and acute myeloid leukemia is similar to the 5-year cumulative risk (8.0%) after myeloablation with chemotherapy in this study [32]. Therefore, RIT administration is not considered to pose an additional risk for the development of myelodysplastic syndrome and acute myeloid leukemia [4, 28, 31, 32].

20.2 Treatment of Myeloproliferative Diseases with Phosphate-32

Phosphate-32 (P-32) has been an accepted treatment method in myeloproliferative diseases for more than 40 years [33]. However, P-32 is currently only used as an optimal treatment option in a limited group of patients, elderly PV patients, and ET as a result of the development of new treatment agents [34].

P-32 is a radionuclide produced in a nuclear reactor that emits pure beta and has a physical half-life of 14.3 days. The maximum and average beta particle energies are 1.71 MeV and 0.695 MeV, respectively, and have an average and maximum particle range of 3 and 8 mm in tissue, respectively. The biological half-life of P-32 in the bone marrow after intravenous administration of P-32 phosphate in the form of a liquid solution is 7–9 days. The highest radiation exposure during treatment occurs in the bone marrow, liver, and spleen [34]. P-32 causes in particular the destruction of myeloproliferative cells and suppression of increased proliferative activity since it is actively incorporated into the nucleic acids of rapidly proliferating cells. It improves symptoms, normalizes, or decreases blood count values in patients without causing myelosuppressive complications in this way [33].

Indications for P-32 therapy include PV, a chronic progressive myeloproliferative disease characterized by an increase in red blood cell counts. Leukocytosis, thrombocytosis, and splenomegaly are also commonly seen in PV patients. The diagnosis of PV should be confirmed by excluding secondary causes of polycythemia before starting treatment. The incidence of PV is between 1 and 2/100,000 per year and increases with age. Treatment varies depending on the patient's age. The development of bone marrow with scar tissue (spent phase) and acute myeloid leukemia (AML) are the primary clinical problems in patients under the age of 50. The most important problem in older patients (older than 60 years) is the development of thrombosis. Therefore, the clinical risk associated with PV in elderly patients is mainly vascular. There are serious risks such as the development of sequelae that impair quality of life due to thrombosis and that may cause mortality. In contrast, P-32 treatment is well tolerated in elderly (>65 years) patients and provides excellent quality of life and long survival [34]. The recurrence of the disease in a short time after P-32-induced remission provides information on the degree of the disease. Five-year survival with P-32 treatment after life-threatening vascular diseases are excluded in elderly PV patients is not different from matched controls in terms of age and gender [34]. There is no significant difference in survival or AML frequency compared to busulfan or hydroxyurea treatments [34]. The incidence of AML was reported to be approximately 10% 10 years after P-32 treatment [34]. Therefore, P-32 treatment is usually administered in elderly (>65–70 years) patients.

ET is a chronic myeloproliferative disease characterized by persistent platelet elevation. Secondary causes of thrombocytosis should be excluded for diagnosis. It is a rare disease. The clinical risk associated with vascular diseases is the same as PV, and treatment with P-32 is generally preferred in patients over 65 years of age [34].

20.2.1 Contraindications

Pregnancy and breastfeeding are absolute contraindications. P-32 treatment is not recommended in fertile women even though not necessarily contraindicated. Other relative contraindications include rapid worsening of renal function, total white blood cell count <2000/mm^3, and hemoglobin <90 g/dL in ET patients [34].

20.2.2 Procedure

P-32 treatment should be performed in an approved facility that complies with applicable national legislation for treatments with pure beta-emitting radionuclides. P-32 treatment can be given by trained healthcare personnel in a center with the necessary equipment and guidelines for handling radiation safety, waste management, and possible contamination. The nuclear medicine physician responsible for the treatment of the patient should know the clinical pathophysiology, natural course, and alternative forms of treatment of the disease and should be able to establish close contact with other physicians involved in the clinical follow-up and treatment of the patient.

The hematocrit is reduced to 42–47% by phlebotomy before P-32 treatment in PV patients. Chemotherapy should be discontinued within 1 week after administration of P-32. The patient's latest blood count values, renal function, and weight information should be learned. Patients should be informed about the treatment and administration both in writing and verbally, and written consent should be obtained from the patient before treatment.

20.2.3 Administration

P-32 is administered by oral route or by intravenous injection. It is generally calculated as 74–111 MBq/m2 (2–3 mCi/m^2) with an upper limit of 185 MBq (5 mCi) or 3.7 MBq/kg (0.1 mCi/kg) with a slightly higher upper limit of 260 MBq (7 mCi). This calculation practically means giving a constant activity over 70 kg of body weight. Some researchers recommend a 25% reduction in activity in patients over 80 years of age.

Alternatively, a gradual dose escalation approach can be adopted: Initially, the patient is administered 111 MBq (3 mCi) P-32. A sufficient response (e.g., if the hematocrit value for PV is <47%, platelet and leukocyte levels are >25%; platelet count for ET is <450,000/mm^3), a second treatment is administered after 3 months, this time with an increase of 25% in dose. The dose is increased every 3 months until an adequate response is obtained in this method. The maximum dose that can be administered in a single administration is 260 MBq (7 mCi). The treatment response is maintained for several months or years. Re-treatment can be administered in progressive disease [34].

20.2.4 Measures, Follow-Up, and Side Effects

The nuclear medicine physician administering the treatment should inform the patient about radiation safety. P-32 excretion will occur especially in the urine on the first 2 days after administration. Patients should be reminded that people sharing the same toilet should pay attention to toilet cleaning so that they are not exposed to unnecessary radiation. Hospital personnel who will take care of the patient should also be informed about radiation safety if the patient needs to take this treatment inpatient. Concerns about radiation exposure should not interfere with treatment and medical interventions that the patient may need. Blood counts are performed at 4–6-week intervals to determine myelosuppression and to plan subsequent treatment cycles. It should be kept in mind that the use of estrogen or androgen can change the biological distribution of P-32. Leukopenia and thrombocytopenia, which are early side effects, are usually observed in 4–6 weeks and resolve spontaneously within 4 months.

PV is associated with an increased risk for acute leukemia. Chlorambucil, busulfan, and P-32 treatments have been shown to be associated with leukemia [34]. In contrast, there is no data showing that hydroxyurea, interferon-alpha, and anagrelide treatments used in PV and ET treatments are associated with leukemic transformation. The incidence of leukemia observed after 10 years in patients treated with P-32 varies between 2% and 15% [34]. This incidence is close to the incidence of leukemia associated with chemotherapeutic regimens.

Radiopharmaceutical sodium phosphate [P-32] is provided ready-to-use in the form of orthophosphate [PO43] in liquid solution. Organs exposed to the highest radiation dose are the bone surface, red bone marrow, and breast. The effective dose is 2.4 mSv/MBq [34]. The amount of activity to be administered to the patient should be checked using a dose calibrator.

20.3 Radionuclide Therapy in Multiple Myeloma

Multiple myeloma is a disease characterized by proliferation of bone marrow clonal plasma cells, representing approximately 15% of hematological cancers. It results in increased monoclonal immunoglobulins in the blood. These immunoglobulins may be detected in serum or urine. Organ damage in MM occurs in the form of lytic bone lesions, renal failure, hypercalcemia, and anemia. The average survival of patients has increased from 3 years to 6 years in the last two decades, thanks to the increased use of autologous stem cell transplantation and immunomodulatory drugs (e.g., thalidomide, lenalidomide, pomalidomide) and proteasome inhibitors (e.g., bortezomib, carfilzomib) [35]. The disease recurs in the majority of patients despite these treatment strategies.

The fact that external radiotherapy is effective in the treatment of plasmacytomas indicates that MM cells are highly sensitive to radiation [35]. Therefore, MM can be a good administration site for targeted radionuclide therapies. Some new radiolabeled peptides have been shown to be able to view MM lesions specifically in recent years [35]. Among these, the peptide called Ga-68-pentixafor shows the most hope [35]. This peptide has a high affinity for CXCR4 (chemokine receptor-4), which is highly expressed in MM cells. Whole-body PET imaging with Ga-68-Pentixafor has shown that lesions can be visualized with an excellent tumor/background ratio in MM patients. This peptide can also be used for treatment purposes by binding with beta- or alpha-emitting radionuclides [35–37]. Indeed, the treatment responses provided in MM patients with Y-90-pentixather bound to CXCR4 are promising [36]. In addition, treatment responses with cold CD38 antibodies in recurrent and treatment-resistant MM patients indicate that these antibodies can be used for RIT just as in NHL as a result of radioactive labeling [35].

Preclinical studies have shown that CD38 antibodies bound with radionuclides such as Y-90 or alpha-emitting bismuth-213 and actinium-225 are effective in plasmacytoma treatment [35]. In addition, many other molecules such as CD138, CD40, CD54, CD74, SLAMF7, and IL-6 receptors, which are highly expressed in MM cells, can also be used as RIT targets [35]. Studies are ongoing to develop treatment for these targets.

20.4 Concluding Remarks

Nuclear medicine methods offer effective and low-side-effect treatment options that contribute to survival in lymphoproliferative diseases with high radiation sensitivity in general. RIT applications targeting CD20 antigen, especially in B-cell NHL, are the most commonly used area in the treatment of radiolabeled antibodies. Although these administrations have gained especially popularity in the past years, they are unfortunately not used sufficiently today. Nuclear medicine offers promising options for the treatment of lymphoproliferative diseases with the identification of new treatment goals and the production of radiopharmaceuticals for these. Communication between nuclear medicine physicians and hematologists and oncologists should be increased in order for radionuclide therapies to be more involved in clinical management of patients with lymphoproliferative diseases.

References

1. Fisher RI, Miller TP, Grogan TM. New REAL clinical entities. Cancer J Sci Am. 1998;4:S5–S12.
2. NCCN clinical practice guidelines in oncology: non-Hodgkin lymphoma Version 4.2014.
3. 2014-yılı-türkiye-kanser-istatistikleri. https://hsgm.saglik.gov.tr/tr/kansistatistikleri/yillar/495-2014-yili-türkiye-kanser-istatistikleri.html.
4. Rizzieri D. Zevalin((R)) (ibritumomab tiuxetan): After more than a decade of treatment experience, what have we learned? Crit Rev Oncol Hematol. 2016;105:5–17.
5. EANM procedure guideline of radio-immunotherapy for B-cell lymphoma with 90Y- radiolabeled ibritumomab tiuxetan (Zevalin®).
6. Rose AC, Shenoy PJ, Garrett G, et al. A systematic literature review and meta-analysis of radioimmunotherapy consolidation for patients with untreated follicular lymphoma. Cl Lymph Myelom Leuk. 2012;12(6):393–9.
7. Witzig TE, Gordon LI, Cabanillas F, et al. Randomized controlled trial of yttrium-90-labeled ibritumomab tiuxetan radioimmunotherapy versus rituximab immunotherapy for patients with relapsed or refractory low-grade, follicular, or transformed B-cell non-Hodgkin's lymphoma. J Clin Oncol. 2002;20(10):2453–63.
8. Gordon LI, Molina A, Witzig T, et al. Durable responses after ibritumomab tiuxetan radioimmunotherapy for

CD20(+) B-cell lymphoma: long-term follow-up of a phase 1/2 study. Blood. 2004;103(12):4429–31.
9. Gordon LI, Witzig T, Molina A, et al. Yttrium 90-labeled ibritumomab tiuxetan radioimmunotherapy produces high response rates and durable remissions in patients with previously treated B-cell lymphoma. Clin Lymphoma. 2004;5(2):98–101.
10. Hohloch K, Lankeit HK, Zinzani PL, et al. Radioimmunotherapy for first-line and relapse treatment of aggressive B-cell non-Hodgkin lymphoma: an analysis of 215 patients registered in the international RIT-Network. Eur J Nucl Med Mol I. 2014;41(8):1585–92.
11. Morschhauser F, Radford J, Van Hoof A, et al. (90) Yttrium-ibritumomab tiuxetan consolidation of first remission in advanced-stage follicular non-Hodgkin lymphoma: updated results after a median follow-up of 7.3 years from the International, Randomized, Phase III First-Line Indolent Trial. J Clin Oncol 2013;31(16):1977−+.
12. Press OW, Unger JM, Rimsza LM, et al. Phase III randomized intergroup trial of CHOP Plus rituximab compared with CHOP chemotherapy Plus (131) Iodine-tositumomab for previously untreated follicular Non-Hodgkin lymphoma: SWOG S0016. J Clin Oncol. 2013;31(3):314–20.
13. Witzig TE, Hong F, Micallef IN, et al. A phase II trial of RCHOP followed by radioimmunotherapy for early stage (stages I/II) diffuse large B-cell non-Hodgkin lymphoma: ECOG3402. Brit J Haematol. 2015;170(5):679–86.
14. Wondergem MJ, Zijlstra JM, de Rooij M, et al. Improving survival in patients with transformed B cell non Hodgkin lymphoma: consolidation with 90Yttrium ibritumomab tiuxetan-BEAM and autologous stem cell transplantation. Brit J Haematol. 2012;157(3):395–7.
15. Illidge TM, Pettengell R, Bayne M, et al. Fractionated (90)y Ibritumomab Tiuxetan (Zevalin TM) radioimmunotherapy as an initial therapy of follicular lymphoma first results from a phase ii study in patients requiring treatment according to GELF/BNLI criteria. Blood. 2011;118(21):49–50.
16. Berinstein NL, Bhella S, Pennell NM, et al. Prolonged clinical remissions in patients with relapsed or refractory follicular lymphoma treated with autologous stem cell transplantation incorporating rituximab. Ann Hematol. 2015;94(5):813–23.
17. Briones J, Novelli S, Garcia-Marco JA, et al. Autologous stem cell transplantation after conditioning with yttrium-90 ibritumomab tiuxetan plus BEAM in refractory non-Hodgkin diffuse large B-cell lymphoma: results of a prospective, multicenter, phase II clinical trial. Haematologica. 2014;99(3):505–10.
18. Hermet E, Cabrespine A, Guieze R, et al. Autologous hematopoietic stem cell transplantation in elderly patients (>= 70 years) with non-Hodgkin's lymphoma: A French Society of Bone Marrow Transplantation and Cellular Therapy retrospective study. J Geriatr Oncol. 2015;6(5):346–52.
19. Siddiqi T, Tsai NC, Palmer J, Forman SJ, Krishnan AY. Effect of radioimmunotherapy-based conditioning for autologous stem cell transplantation on poor-risk molecular profiling in diffuse large B-cell lymphoma. J Clin Oncol. 2012;30(15)
20. Shimoni A, Zwas ST. radioimmunotherapy and autologous stem-cell transplantation in the treatment of b-cell non Hodgkin lymphoma. Semin Nucl Med. 2016;46(2):119–25.
21. Press OW, Unger JM, Rimsza LM, et al. A Phase III randomized intergroup trial (SWOG S0016) of CHOP chemotherapy plus rituximab vs. CHOP chemotherapy plus Iodine-131-tositumomab for the treatment of newly diagnosed follicular non-Hodgkin's lymphoma. Blood. 2011;118(21):48.
22. Buske C, Hutchings M, Ladetto M, et al. ESMO Consensus Conference on malignant lymphoma: general perspectives and recommendations for the clinical management of the elderly patient with malignant lymphoma. Ann Oncol. 2018;29(3):544–62.
23. Illidge T, Morschhauser F. Radioimmunotherapy in follicular lymphoma. Best Pract Res Cl Ha. 2011;24(2):279–93.
24. Schaefer NG, Huang P, Buchanan JW, Wahl RL. Radioimmunotherapy in non-Hodgkin lymphoma: opinions of nuclear medicine physicians and radiation oncologists. J Nucl Med. 2011;52(5):830–8.
25. Emmanouilides C. Radioimmunotherapy for non-Hodgkin lymphoma: historical perspective and current status. J Clin Exp Hematop. 2007;47(2):43–60.
26. Scholz CW, Pinto A, Linkesch W, et al. (90)Yttrium-ibritumomab-tiuxetan as first-line treatment for follicular lymphoma: 30 months of follow-up data from an international multicenter phase II clinical trial. J Clin Oncol. 2013;31(3):308–13.
27. Krishnan A, Palmer JM, Tsai NC, et al. Matched-cohort analysis of autologous hematopoietic cell transplantation with radioimmunotherapy versus total body irradiation-based conditioning for poor-risk diffuse large cell lymphoma. Biol Blood Marrow Tranplant. 2012;18(3):441–50.
28. Tennvall J, Fischer M, Delaloye AB, et al. EANM procedure guideline for radio-immunotherapy for B-cell lymphoma with Y-90-radiolabelled ibritumomab tiuxetan (Zevalin). Eur J Nucl Med Mol I. 2007;34(4):616–22.
29. Goldsmith SJ. Radioimmunotherapy of Lymphoma: Bexxar and Zevalin. Semin Nucl Med. 2010;40(2):122–35.
30. Kersten MJ. Radioimmunotherapy in follicular lymphoma: some like it hot. Transfus Apher Sci. 2011;44(2):173–8.
31. Czuczman MS, Emmanouilides C, Darif M, et al. Treatment-related myelodysplastic syndrome and acute myelogenous leukemia in patients treated with ibritumomab tiuxetan radioimmunotherapy. J Clin Oncol. 2007;25(27):4285–92.
32. Guidetti A, Carlo-Stella C, Ruella M, et al. Myeloablative doses of Yttrium-90-Ibritumomab tiuxetan and the risk of secondary myelodysplasia/

acute myelogenous leukemia. Cancer- Am Cancer Soc. 2011;117(22):5074–84.
33. Berlin NI. Treatment of the myeloproliferative disorders with P-32. Eur J Haematol. 2000;65(1):1–7.
34. Tennvall J, Brans B. EANM procedure guideline for 32P phosphate treatment of myeloproliferative diseases. Eur J Nucl Med Mol Imaging. 2007;34(8):1324–7.
35. Mesguich C, Zanotti-Fregonara P, Hindie E. New perspectives offered by nuclear medicine for the imaging and therapy of multiple myeloma. Theranostics. 2016;6(2):287–90.
36. Herrmann K, Schottelius M, Lapa C, et al. First-in-human experience of CXCR4-directed endoradiotherapy with Lu-177- and Y-90-labeled pentixather in advanced-stage multiple myeloma with extensive intra- and extramedullary disease. J Nucl Med. 2016;57(2):248–51.
37. Schottelius M, Osl T, Poschenrieder A, et al. [Lu-177] pentixather: comprehensive preclinical characterization of a first CXCR4-directed endoradiotherapeutic agent. Theranostics. 2017;7(9):2350–62.

Part IX

Radioimmunotherapy

Basics and Clinical Applications of Radioimmunotherapy

21

Murat Tuncel and Pınar Ö. Kıratlı

The most commonly used modalities in the treatment of cancer patients include radiation therapy and immunotherapy. Radiation therapy is performed externally, via devices outside the patient or by administering radiopharmaceuticals targeted to a specific receptor or antigen used in nuclear medicine. Unlike external radiotherapy (ERTx), radiation given in nuclear medicine is administered systemically via the intravenous or oral route. However, ERTx delivers radiation to limited areas and causes radiation to healthy, off-target areas on its way to the target. Radiation in nuclear medicine is transmitted through radiolabeled targeted molecules. Unfortunately, radiopharmaceuticals used in radionuclide therapy may also retain in healthy tissues leading to radiation toxicity. Therefore, specific targeting methods are needed. Specific molecules used in immunotherapy are ideal for this method. Radioimmunotherapy (RIT) has been developed using the tumoricidal effect of radiation and targeted immunotherapy molecules in the light of this knowledge [1].

Radioimmunotherapy benefits from the compounds that the immune system develops against cancer. Antibodies (Abs) are glycoproteins secreted from plasma B cells. They fight against pathogens such as bacteria and viruses. They can also destroy malignant tumors due to their cytotoxic potential. Immunotherapy alone significantly increases the survival rate of the patients [2]. In order to improve this effect, cytotoxic radioisotopes (or particle emitters) are conjugated to Abs or fragments. This strategy uses target-specific guidance of immunotherapy to provide targeted tumor-specific radiation therapy. The antibody fragments that bind to the target provide high radiation to that region.

The first molecules used for RIT started with the binding of I-131 to protein, due to its easy binding and accessibility [3, 4]. Today, this treatment has become commercialized as Y-90-labeled ibritumomab tiuxetan (Zevalin®) and I-131-labeled tositumomab (Bexxar®) which are used in patients with CD20-positive lymphoma. Improved overall (60–80%) and complete response (15–40%) in recurrent non-Hodgkin's lymphoma were reported in studies with these therapies [5, 6]. These radioimmunoconjugates were superior to non-radioactive antibodies and were accepted in the current guidelines [7]. However, the success of RIT is lower in solid cancers. It is generally used as adjuvant therapy after surgery or in combination with chemotherapy, not as a single treatment in these tumors [8]. The main critical points and clinical developments in RIT are discussed in this chapter.

M. Tuncel (✉) · P. Ö. Kıratlı
Faculty of Medicine, Department of Nuclear Medicine, Hacettepe University, Ankara, Turkey
e-mail: murat.tuncel@hacettepe.edu.tr; pkiratli@hacettepe.edu.tr

R. Bekiş et al. (eds.), *Radionuclide Therapy*, https://doi.org/10.1007/978-3-030-97220-2_21

21.1 Basic Principles in Radioimmunotherapy

The main factor that determines the damage given to the tissue by radiation is the energy given per unit length (LET, linear energy transfer) [9]. The most commonly used radionuclides in radionuclide therapies are auger-, beta-, and alpha-emitting agents that damage tissue due to their ionization properties (Table 21.1).

Beta emitters (I-131, Y-90, Lu-177, Re-188, Re-186, and Cu-67) have a relatively low LET (0.2 keV/μm). The distance these emissions penetrate in the tissue ranges from 0.5 to 12 mm, and their energies range from 30 keV to 2.3 MeV. Some of these radionuclides (e.g., Lu-177) emit gamma and X-rays in addition to beta rays, which can be used in imaging. The beta emission travels several millimeters in the tissue, so radiation affects the cells to which the radiopharmaceutical binds and the adjacent cells along the passage in the tissue. This effect is called the cross-fire effect, which also provides radiation to tumor cells that do not retain therapeutic RIT agents. However, cells other than tumor cells are also exposed to radiation and get affected from this toxicity [8, 10]. Most beta emitters used in clinical trials are I-131, Y-90, Lu-177, and Re-186. These radionuclides are relatively easy to access and have radiochemistry which allows them to bind antibodies. For example, the main advantage of I-131 is its relatively cheap cost and detection with gamma cameras. It is used to treat various malignancies, including thyroid cancer, NHL, and AML [11, 12].

Apart from the energy of the radionuclide, retention time in the cell, penetration, and dissociation from the main molecule is important. The disadvantage of I-131 is that it undergoes rapid deiodination after endocytosis. This may lead to release of I-131 tyrosine and free I-131 to the environment, causing exposure to nontarget and undesired radiation [13]. In addition, by its beta ray emission with high-energy gamma rays, I-131 brings additional radiation exposure to the patient and their relatives. Alternative radiochemistry methods are being studied to reduce this drawback.

Y-90 is another high-energy beta emitter used in treatment. It damages the tissue due to its high energy. However, radiation emitted by radionuclides such as Y-90 is high at the end of the particle range, where the beta particle slows down. This phenomenon, "Bragg ionization peak," causes lower absorbed radiation where the particle originates. This reduces the success of these

Table 21.1 Radionuclides used in radioimmunotherapy

Radionuclide	Half-life (T1/2)	Maximum energy (keV)	Maximum range (mm)	Emission type
β-Emitters (LET, 0.2 keV/μm)				
Y-90	2.67 days	2280	11.3	β−
I-131	8.02 days	606.31	2.3	β−, γ
Lu-177	6.65 days	498.3	1.8	β−, γ
Cu-67	61.83 h	577	2.1	β−, γ
Re-186	3.72 days	1069.5	4.8	β−, γ
Re-188	17 h	2120.4	10.4	β−, γ
α-Emitters (LET, 50–230 keV/μm)				
Bi-213	45.59 min	8400	90	α, β−, γ
Bi-212	60.54 min	7800	100	α, β−, γ
At-211	7.21 h	7500	80	α, EC
Ac-225	9.92 days	8400	90	α, β−, γ
Auger-emitters (LET, 4–26 keV/μm)				
In-111	2.80 days	26	17	Auger, γ
Pt-195	4 days	64	76	Auger

radionuclide-labeled RIT agents in small tumors where particle range exceeds tumor size. It is recommended to use radionuclides with a lower particle range in such tumors. The advantage of Y-90 is its endurance in cells longer after endocytosis. However, free Y-90 leakage can still occur, which can increase the radiation dose of the bone marrow. Y-90 is an alternative β-emitter suitable for therapeutic administrations and emits almost only β-particles, which do not radiate outside the patient. Therefore caregivers are exposed to lower radiation compared to both beta- and gamma-emitting radionuclides (e.g., I-131). However, with pure β-emitter radionuclides, it is impossible to obtain adequate images from the patients, which makes evaluation of radiotracer uptake after treatment impossible, even though this provides an advantage in radiation safety terms [14].

Damage caused by beta particles (DNA fractures, etc.) is mostly caused by free oxygen radicals. Adequate oxygenation is required in the area where the radiopharmaceutical retains. Both the penetration of the radiopharmaceutical and the amount of free radicals formed are reduced in hypoxic tumors. High-energy alpha emitters may be more effective due to decreased oxygenation in large solid tumors [15]. These radioisotopes (Ac-225, At-211, Bi-212, Bi-213, and Pb-212) have high-LET radiation (50–230 keV/μm), and their energy varies between 5 and 9 MeV. The distance these particles travel through the tissue is short (typically 50–100 μm) and leaves high energy per unit distance.

Alpha rays act directly on DNA, causing double DNA fractures that are difficult to repair without oxygenation. This feature gives alpha emitters the advantage of inflicting more tumor cell damage than beta emitters. Short particle range reduces damage to surrounding tissues, but success rate is low in heterogeneous tumors, especially when it is not well retained [16].

Rarely auger-electron emitters (I-125, In-111, Ga-67, and Pt-195m) are also used in RIT. These radionuclides have moderate LET radiation (4–26 keV/μm). The energy of these agents is 1 eV–1 keV and the particle range is less than 1 μm. These radionuclides give high radiation at nanometer level and have low cross-fire effects. In order to have high effect, these radionuclides should be internalized and localized near the nucleus [17, 18].

In summary, optimum radionuclide selection for RIT depends on intended usage (tumor type, etc.) and practical evaluations (transportation possibilities, etc.). I-131 and Y-90 with high beta energies are frequently used in the studies.

21.2 Special Situations in Radioimmunotherapy

RIT has been administered in the most radiosensitive tumors, hematological malignancies (leukemia and lymphoma). The α/β ratios indicate the radiobiology of the cells. Tissues with high α/β ratios are tissues with low repair capacity and are easy to destroy. Low ratios are moderate radiosensitive tissues (solid tumors). Solid tumors are more radioresistant and require approximately five times the radiation needed for other tumors for effective treatment. For example, Y-90 panitumumab treatment did not provide an advantage in survival in ovarian cancer. The reason for this was thought to be the low radiation dose given to the tumor cell during the treatment. In addition, RIT is a nonuniform and low-dose rate radiation treatment, unlike ERTx. Conventional ERTx exposes at least 50 Gy for response in tumors such as breast, lung, and colon. Doses given with RIT are typically in 1.8–33 Gy range [8, 19]. These doses alone do not possibly destroy the tumor. Besides RIT doses are nonuniform. Some cells may have less uptake either due to penetration or due to receptors on the cell. Therefore, the tumor dosimetry is critical and this value varies with each repeated dose. Dosimetry algorithms developed in recent years in nuclear medicine enable this treatment to be given more optimally.

One of the most problematic parts of RIT is the cost. Special antibodies and radionuclides used in treatment are expensive and are not produced in many places around the world. Cost constraints and difficulties in accessing this treatment kept the studies only in phase 1/2.

21.3 RIT Administration Routes

21.3.1 Intracompartmental Approach

Intrathecal and intraventricular 131-I-81C6 (tenascin monoclonal antibody) administration provides objective response and prolonged survival in the treatment of leptomeningeal carcinomatosis and malignant brain tumors [20]. It also provides long-term remission for patients with recurrent brain metastasis and leptomeningeal carcinomatosis from neuroblastoma with intraventricular 131-I-3F8 (anti-GD2; NCT00445965) and 131-I-8H9 (anti-B7-H3; NCT00089245). This intracompartmental injection method leads to higher doses compared to systemic treatment. The radiation doses administered to the tumor range from 5000 to 10,000 cGy and are 10 times higher compared to intravenous administration.

The absence of immune system cells to prevent antibody binding in cerebrospinal fluid and the one-way renewal of the current in a certain cycle provides an advantage [21].

21.3.2 RIT Administered Systemically

Slow removal of the unbound radiopharmaceutical from the blood circulation causes high background activity, which limits the administered dose. Small fragments of antibodies are used to solve this problem and speed up the cleaning of the radiopharmaceutical. These particles enter the tumor faster but lead to lower intratumoral concentrations. Therefore, it should be noted that each changing molecule has different kinetics and dosimetry, although its target is the same.

Retained radiopharmaceutical in normal tissue after treatment may cause side effects such as bone marrow suppression. Dose fractionation is performed to reduce this side effect, and in some patients, treatment is interrupted for the recovery of bone marrow. The success of systemic RIT in solid tumors is low due to relatively high resistance to radiation and the difficulty of penetrating large antibody fragments into solid tumors.

21.4 Methods Used to Increase RIT Effectiveness and Utilization

Radionuclides that emit both beta and gamma rays which allow dosimetry calculation were tried to increase RIT success in solid tumors. Scandium-47 (Sc-47) was used as both gamma- and β-emitter (T1/2, 3.35 days; Eβ−, 162 keV; Eγ, 159 keV), and Lu-177 (T1/2, 6.65 days; Eβ−, 134 keV; E<UNK>, 113, 208 keV) with similar properties [22]. Alpha-emitting radionuclides such as Pb-212 and Ac-225/Bi-213 are produced by generators. These radionuclides are used for RIT accompanied by alpha emitter [23].

One of the methods used to increase RIT effectiveness is "pretargeting" method. In this method, first target-specific mAb and then small molecules carrying radionuclides to bind antibody are given into the system. Various preclinical and clinical studies have shown that this method increases tumor involvement. This treatment approach was used with PC3 xenograft with prostate cancer. The median survival after administration of trivalent bispecific antibody TF12 (anti-TROP2 × anti-HSG [histamine-succinyl-glycine]) was >150 days in mice receiving two or three courses of pretargeted 177-Lu-labeled diHSG peptide (IMP288), while this duration was 76 days in untreated mice [24]. Anti-CEA pretargeted RIT has been used in rapidly progressing medullary thyroid cancer. Forty-two patients received I-131 bivalent pills (1.8 Gb/m2) 4–6 days after anti-CEA mAb. This treatment provided disease control in 76.2% of patients [25].

21.5 Radioimmunotherapy in Hematological Malignancies

Radioimmunotherapy has been widely used in hematological malignancies. The presence of cell surface antigens in hematological malignancies, the presence of many antibodies against these malignancies, the sensitivity of leukemia and lymphoma to radiation therapy, and the low incidence of HAMA (human anti-mouse antibody) in hematological malignancies are the most important reasons that enable the therapeutic success.

The collection of the patient's own cells before high-dose RIT (autologous transplantation or stem cell collection) is routinely performed in many oncology centers before high-dose chemotherapy. This development provides an advantage over hematological toxicity, which is the main limiting factor in RIT, thus allowing for higher doses of radiation [26, 27]. High myeloablative doses of RIT and subsequent bone marrow transplantation in B-cell malignancies resulted in complete remission of over 80% for approximately 5 years in initial studies [2]. However, it reduced the chance of finding a routine clinical administration due to the difficulties encountered in bone marrow collection and high-dose I-131 labeling. I-131 tositumomab and Y-90 ibritumomab tiuxetan (Zevalin), developed by targeting CD20 and giving lower radiation dose without patient hospitalization, were used with acceptable non-myeloablative toxicity in B-cell lymphomas.

RIT clinical trial studies are mostly labeled with CD20 antibodies in hematopoietic tumors. Both I-131 and Y-90 have significantly higher overall response and complete response rates compared to non-labeled antibody therapies (rituximab) in relapsed non-Hodgkin's lymphomas (NHL). The complete response ranged from 15% to 38%, and the overall response rate was 74% and 83% in studies with Y-90 ibritumomab tiuxetan. These rates were 18% and 55% for rituximab, respectively [5, 28–30]. Zevalin, a radiotherapeutic antibody targeted to CD20, has entered into use with FDA approval in patients with (1) relapsed or refractory low-grade or follicular B-cell NHL and (2) previously untreated NHL and who had partial or complete response to initial serial chemotherapy. These patients must meet certain criteria before treatment (Table 21.2).

In this therapy, 250 mg/m^2 rituximab is administered intravenously on the first day of treatment. On the seventh, eighth, or ninth day, 0.4 mCi/kg (14.8 MBq/kg) in patients with platelets ≥150,000/mm^3 and 0.3 mCi/kg (11.1 MBq/kg) in patients with platelets ≥100,000 and ≤149,000/mm^3 in combination with Y-90-labeled ibritumomab tiuxetan (Zevalin) are administered intravenously 4 h after 250 mg/m^2 rituximab administration. Treatment is not given in those patients with <100,000/mm^3. Patients are administered acetaminophen 650 mg and diphenhydramine 50 mg orally before rituximab infusion. It is recommended that the maximum dose of Y-90 Zevalin should not exceed 32 mCi (1184 MBq). Zevalin comes to the nuclear medicine departments with 3.2 mg ibritumomab tiuxetan, Y-90 chloride solution, sodium acetate, and buffer solution in 2 ml 0.9% sodium chloride. It is added to Y-90 chloride labeling vial with special lead and plastic protection (Fig. 21.1).

Table 21.2 Treatment and exclusion criteria

Treatment criteria	Exclusion criteria
CD20 expression in the biopsy	Pregnancy and breastfeeding
Less than 25% involvement in bone marrow within 6–8 weeks	Hypersensitivity and allergy
Complete blood values within normal limits within 1 week	Significant bone marrow suppression (leukocyte <1.5 × 10^9/L; platelet <100 × 10^9/L)
No allergy history	>25% bone marrow infiltration
Life expectancy >3 months	>25% active bone marrow site radiotherapy
Karnofsky index >70%	Previous bone marrow or stem cell transplantation
	HAMA reaction

It is critical that there is no radioactive material contamination at this time. After labeling, 2.08 mg ibritumomab tiuxetan is administered in 10 ml volume, and this solution should be administered to the patient slowly after quality control. After synthesis, the product should be stored at 2–8 °C and administered to the patient as a slow infusion within 8 h of synthesis (Fig. 21.2). Radiation safety rules must be observed during this preparation.

Myelosuppression is the most serious side effect in patients receiving treatment. All grades of thrombocytopenia, neutropenia, and anemia

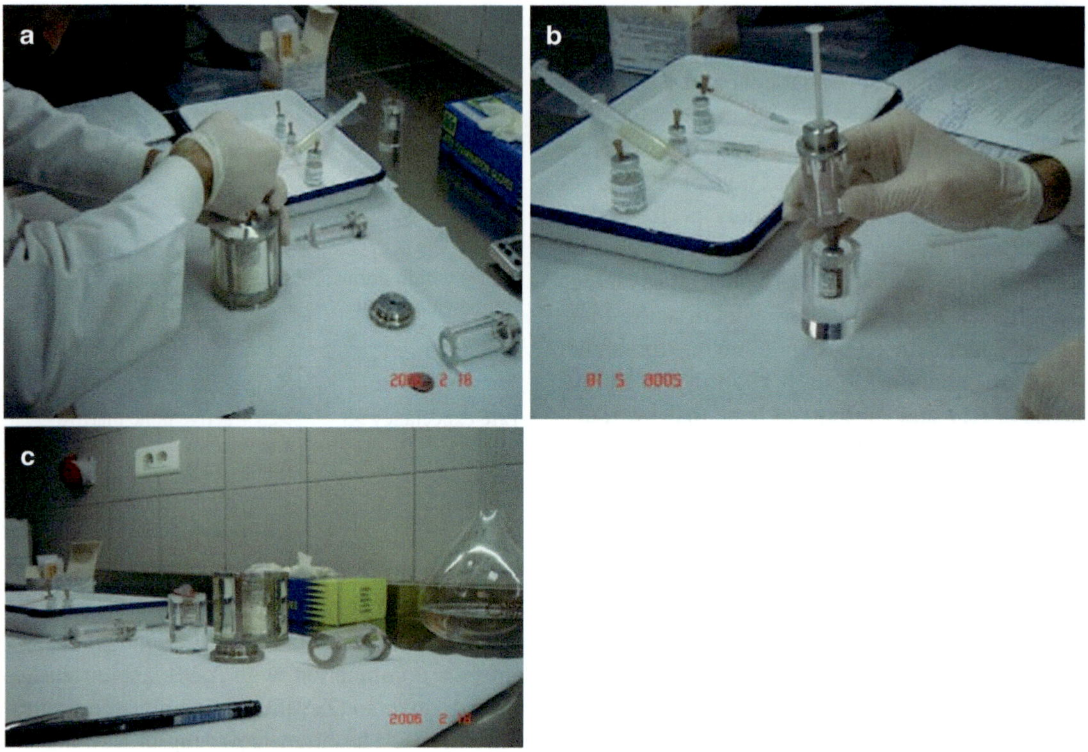

Fig. 21.1 Preparation of Y-90 ibritumomab tiuxetan. Placement of radiopharmaceutical in reaction vial with special lead and plastic shield (**a**, **b**). Quality control of synthesized radiopharmaceutical (**c**)

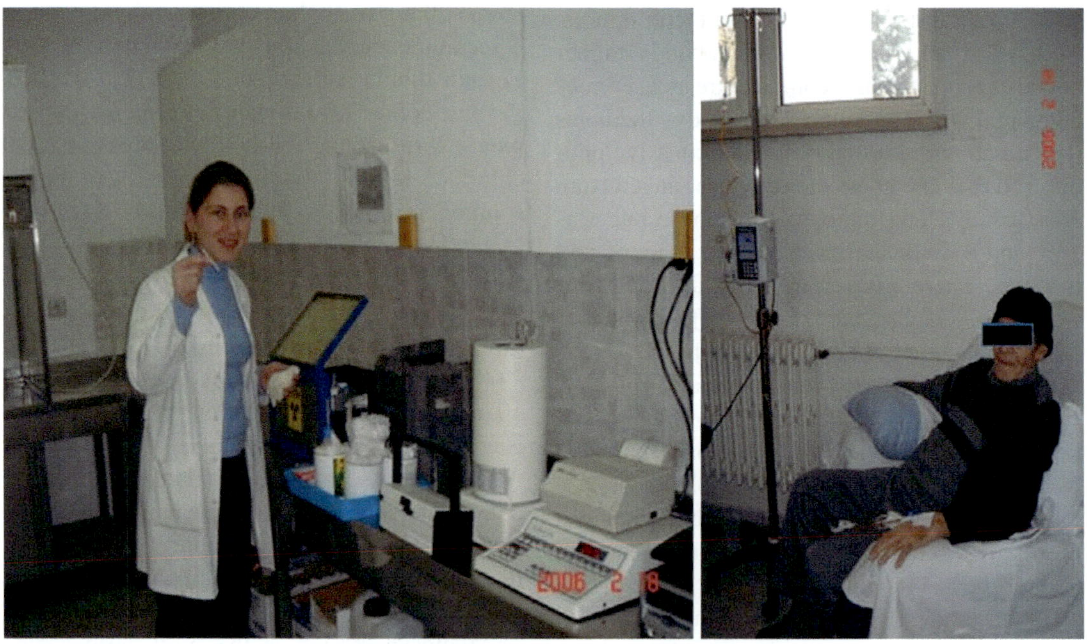

Fig. 21.2 Administration of synthesized Y-90 ibritumomab tiuxetan to the patient

occur in 95%, 77%, and 61% of the patients, respectively. Grade 3–4 toxicity appears as 63%, 60%, and 17%, respectively. These side effects are mostly temporary, but some patients may require supportive treatment [31]. Some studies suggest reducing the dosage in patients with more than 25% bone marrow involvement and with limited bone marrow reserve [32].

Temporary and treatable side effects such as asthenia, nausea, and fever are also seen in 5–35% of patients receiving Zevalin treatment. The incidence of secondary MDS and acute leukemia in patients receiving this treatment is <1%.

In this treatment the spleen, liver, and intestines receive the highest radiation doses. The dose received by healthcare personnel is low (0.00295 mSv/h) since pure beta-emitting Y-90 is used. The patients do not need to wait in the isolation room. The radiation dose to the patient's family is 0.04–0.15 mSv in the first week [31].

Y-90 Zevalin treatment developed against CD20 antibody was administered to 11 NHL patients aged 24–72 years, F/M: 5/6 at Hacettepe University Faculty of Medicine in accordance with the guidelines [33]. Five of the patients had diffuse B-cell lymphoma. All patients had refractory and/or relapsed NHL. Among these, seven patients had stage IV, and four patients had stage III disease. Different levels of hematological toxicity were observed in all but one patient. Progression was observed in four patients, complete response in four patients, partial response in two patients, while one patient had stable disease. Four patients died due to infection and hematological causes at the end of the 30-month follow-up (Figs. 21.3 and 21.4).

Studies like the combination of RIT with autologous hematopoietic stem cell transplantation, using pretargeting protocols and several monoclonal antibodies labeled with different B-cell antigens, have been conducted to increase the effectiveness of RIT [34]. RIT has been shown to be 90–100% effective in ORR and 60–100% effective in CR in various phase 2 and phase 3 studies conducted as early-stage use of RIT in NHL or as consolidation therapy after chemotherapy [28].

Studies with RIT are not limited to B-cell lymphoma. Promising studies are also carried out in other hematological malignancies. Labeling targets such as CD33, CD45, and CD66 and using alpha emitters such as Bi-212 and Ac-225

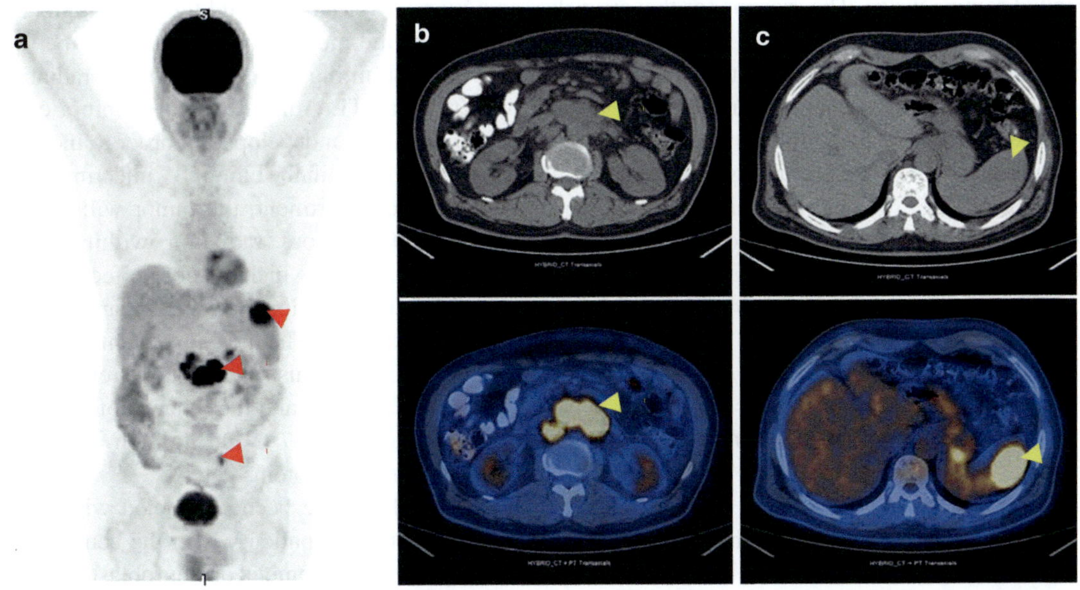

Fig. 21.3 A 55-year-old male patient was referred with recurrent follicular B-cell NHL diagnosis. Pretreatment FDG PET-CT images show increased FDG uptake (SUV max, 13) in the paraceliac, paracaval, paraaortic, and left main iliac enlarged lymph nodes (**a**, **b**: arrows) and spleen (**c**: arrowhead) in the abdomen

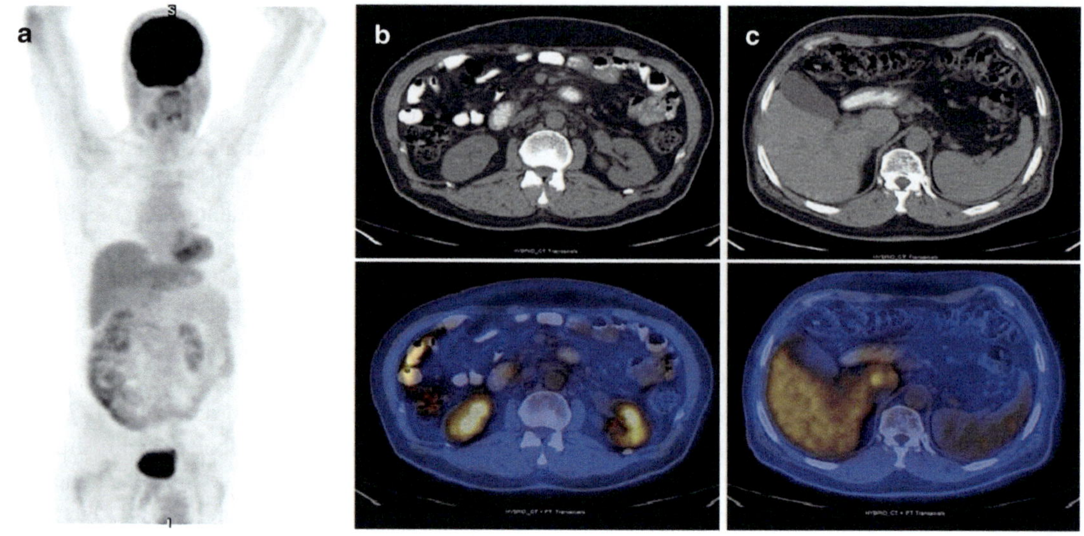

Fig. 21.4 FDG PET-CT images obtained at the third month after 0.4 mCi/kg Zevalin treatment are consistent with complete metabolic response (**a**). The images show that the lymph nodes in the abdomen (**b**) and the lesion in the spleen have significantly shrunk and lost FDG uptake (**c**)

have been shown to be more effective compared to beta emitters in other hematological tumors such as AML [35].

Although effectiveness and safety issues have been proven in many studies and approved by FDA, these radioimmunoconjugates have not found routine usage. The reasons for this are risk of bone marrow suppression, myelodysplasia, and suboptimal radiation doses to tumoral tissue. However, pretargeting administrations and alpha emitters can solve the problems and increase the utilization of RIT by providing safer and more effective RIT. The communication between nuclear medicine and medical oncology departments is also critical to increase usage in the presence of several alternative chemotherapy protocols.

21.6 Radioimmunotherapy in Solid Tumors

Successful results have been obtained with RIT in hematological malignancies; however the efficacy is lower in solid tumors. This can be explained by their lower radiosensitivity than hematological tumors due to low vascularization, weak lymphatic flow, and limited diffusion for radioimmunoconjugates [36]. Besides the biological half-life of antibody-labeled radioimmunoconjugate due to intravenous route of administration is long, which may limit the radiation dose.

It is important that the target/background activity ratio for RIT in solid tumors is high, and the therapeutic index is sufficient. Bone marrow is the dose-limiting organ, due to high radiation burden after RIT. Administration within a compartment has been developed in order to increase RIT effectiveness in the clinic. By injecting to the intrathecal compartment, the tumor will receive almost tenfold more radiation within 5000–10,000 cGy range, which is more effective than systemic administration. Every compartment has its own biokinetics. The most important factor for the intrathecal administration is the circulation of 150 ml of CSF fluid and the renewal of CSF in a one-way flow every 7 h and its high affinity to antibody-binding proteins [1].

RIT studies have been conducted with intrathecal injection in patients with the central nervous system involvement of neuroblastoma and high-risk metastatic central nervous system tumors. Phase 1 studies have given promising results [21, 37]. In fact, the risk of radiation necrosis observed in external radiotherapy in the pediatric patient group is minimal with RIT and neurological deficits do not develop in patients for a long time [38].

Similarly, there are studies on administering this treatment method to other cavities in the body region where tumor tissue is present. Studies have been conducted to administer RIT intraperitoneally in cases with peritoneal carcinomatosis of ovarian and gastric tumors, but different responses have been obtained [39]. The development of hematological toxicity due to systemic absorption has always been a limiting factor despite providing antitumor effect and prolonged overall survival in cases with low tumor burden.

A pretreatment preventive chelation agent is used to eliminate this problem [40]. It is thought that RIT may be effective in different responses obtained from phase 1 and 2 studies, at least in radiosensitive tumors where tumor burden is not high, with and/or after surgery.

21.7 Neoadjuvant/Combination Therapies

Combining other treatment options such as surgery, chemotherapy, and/or external radiotherapy to increase the efficacy of RIT is on the agenda. Pharmacological agents are tried in combination treatment to improve the therapeutic index by setting different goals. Progress in the treatments of melanoma, non-small cell lung cancer, and renal cancers have been observed by blocking immune checkpoints with monoclonal antibodies in recent years. Phase 1/2 studies in head and neck tumors started with the combination of immune checkpoint blockade and radiotherapy; thus, a safe downstaging evaluation will be performed in preoperative resection [41].

21.8 "Pretargeted" Therapies

Even though RIT has been successful in hematological malignancies, it has not found widespread application in other tumors. This is partly due to the prolonged circulation of radiolabeled antibodies leading to high radiation exposure to bone marrow. Therefore, the radiation dose required for effective treatment cannot be administered due to toxicity concerns. A "pretargeting" method has been developed in order to reduce this problem. Unlike the conventional radioimmunoconjugate method, monoclonal antibodies (mAb) are not used for labeling. mAb is administered in advance and is expected to be localized in tumoral tissue, and then the radioactivity is given into circulation with a molecule having suitable pharmacokinetics. Many methods have been developed for this purpose. Avidin/streptavidin approach seems promising in glioblastoma treatment with Y-90 biotin [42]. Another approach is the use of bispecific mAb. In this method, one arm of the compound binds to the antigen monitored on the tumor, while the other arm specifically binds to the small radioactive molecule. Bispecific mAb has been developed for selective binding of gamma-ray complexes such as In-111(DTPA). Even though this method is successful when used for diagnostic purposes, it failed in therapeutic administrations with agents such as Y-90 and Lu-177, because DTPA is not a good chelator for both metal cations.

More appropriate methods that enable the use of radioactive metal isotopes in pretargeting are being investigated for this reason. Sharkey et al. developed a histamine derivative, using anti-pill antibodies against succinyl glycine (HSG). Pretargeting approach is used in clinical phase 1/2 studies in colorectal cancer and non-small cell lung cancer [43, 44]. The circulation of unbound RIT particles and high-dose radioactivity in background activity are important in terms of pharmacokinetics and are dose-limiting properties of this treatment [45].

21.9 Concluding Remarks

RIT is a treatment method that has proven its effectiveness, especially in hematological malignancies. This treatment will continue to have its potential place in the future, with advances in immunotherapy and increased access/use of radioisotopes. We believe that "pretargeting" method, intracompartmental administration, and dosimetry studies will increase the effectiveness of this treatment.

References

1. Larson SM, Carrasquillo JA, Cheung NK, Press OW. Radioimmunotherapy of human tumours. Nat Rev Cancer. 2015;15(6):347–60.
2. Scott AM, Wolchok JD, Old LJ. Antibody therapy of cancer. Nat Rev Cancer. 2012;12(4):278–87.
3. Eisen HN, Keston AS. The immunologic reactivity of bovine serum albumin labeled with trace-amounts of radioactive iodine (I131). J Immunol. 1949;63(1):71–80.
4. Sharkey RM, Goldenberg DM. Cancer radioimmunotherapy. Immunotherapy. 2011;3(3):349–70.
5. Witzig TE, Gordon LI, Cabanillas F, et al. Randomized controlled trial of yttrium-90-labeled ibritumomab tiuxetan radioimmunotherapy versus rituximab immunotherapy for patients with relapsed or refractory low-grade, follicular, or transformed B-cell non-Hodgkin's lymphoma. J Clin Oncol. 2002;20(10):2453–63.
6. Postema EJ, Oyen WJ, Boerman OC, Corstens FH. Administration guidelines for radioimmunotherapy of non-Hodgkin's lymphoma with 90Y-labeled anti-CD20 monoclonal antibody. J Nucl Med. 2003;44(5):853.
7. Horwitz SM, Zelenetz AD, Gordon LI, et al. NCCN Guidelines Insights: Non-Hodgkin's lymphomas, version 3.2016. J Natl Compr Canc Netw. 2016;14(9):1067–79.
8. Martins CD, Kramer-Marek G, Oyen WJG. Radioimmunotherapy for delivery of cytotoxic radioisotopes: current status and challenges. Expert Opin Drug Deliv. 2018;15(2):185–96.
9. Goodhead DT. The initial physical damage produced by ionizing radiations. Int J Radiat Biol. 1989;56(5):623–34.
10. Pouget JP, Navarro-Teulon I, Bardies M, et al. Clinical radioimmunotherapy—the role of radiobiology. Nat Rev Clin Oncol. 2011;8(12):720–34.
11. Rajendran JG, Gopal AK, Fisher DR, Durack LD, Gooley TA, Press OW. Myeloablative 131I-tositumomab radioimmunotherapy in treating non-Hodgkin's lymphoma: comparison of dosimetry based on whole- body retention and dose to critical organ receiving the highest dose. J Nucl Med. 2008;49(5):837–44.
12. Pagel JM, Gooley TA, Rajendran J, et al. Allogeneic hematopoietic cell transplantation after conditioning with 131I-anti-CD45 antibody plus fludarabine and low-dose total body irradiation for elderly patients with advanced acute myeloid leukemia or high-risk myelodysplastic syndrome. Blood. 2009;114(27):5444–53.
13. Geissler F, Anderson SK, Press O. Intracellular catabolism of radiolabeled anti-CD3 antibodies by leukemic T cells. Cell Immunol. 1991;137(1):96–110.
14. Koppe MJ, Postema EJ, Aarts F, Oyen WJ, Bleichrodt RP, Boerman OC. Antibody-guided radiation therapy of cancer. Cancer Metastasis Rev. 2005;24(4):539–67.
15. Wulbrand C, Seidl C, Gaertner FC, et al. Alpha-particle emitting 213Bi-anti-EGFR immunoconjugates eradicate tumor cells independent of oxygenation. PLoS One. 2013;8(5):e64730.
16. Kim YS, Brechbiel MW. An overview of targeted alpha therapy. Tumour Biol. 2012;33(3):573–90.
17. Jackson MR, Falzone N, Vallis KA. Advances in anticancer radiopharmaceuticals. Clin Oncol (R Coll Radiol). 2013;25(10):604–9.
18. Kassis AI. Molecular and cellular radiobiological effects of Auger emitting radionuclides. Radiat Prot Dosimetry. 2011;143(2-4):241–7.
19. Tempero M, Leichner P, Baranowska-Kortylewicz J, et al. High-dose therapy with 90Yttrium-labeled monoclonal antibody CC49: a phase I trial. Clin Cancer Res. 2000;6(8):3095–102.
20. Reardon DA, Akabani G, Coleman RE, et al. Salvage radioimmunotherapy with murine iodine-131- labeled antitenascin monoclonal antibody 81C6 for patients with recurrent primary and metastatic malignant brain tumors: phase II study results. J Clin Oncol. 2006;24(1):115–22.
21. Kramer K, Kushner BH, Modak S, et al. Compartmental intrathecal radioimmunotherapy: results for treatment for metastatic CNS neuroblastoma. J Neurooncol. 2010;97(3):409–18.
22. Muller C, Bunka M, Haller S, et al. Promising prospects for 44Sc-/47Sc-based theragnostics: application of 47Sc for radionuclide tumor therapy in mice. J Nucl Med. 2014;55(10):1658–64.
23. Ma D, McDevitt MR, Finn RD, Scheinberg DA. Breakthrough of 225Ac and its radionuclide daughters from an 225Ac/213Bi generator: development of new methods, quantitative characterization, and implications for clinical use. Appl Radiat Isot. 2001;55(5):667–78.
24. van Rij CM, Frielink C, Goldenberg DM, et al. Pretargeted radioimmunotherapy of prostate cancer with an anti-TROP-2xAnti-HSG bispecific antibody and a (177)Lu-labeled peptide. Cancer Biother Radiopharm. 2014;29(8):323–9.
25. Salaun PY, Campion L, Bournaud C, et al. Phase II trial of anticarcinoembryonic antigen pretargeted radioimmunotherapy in progressive metastatic medullary thyroid carcinoma: biomarker response and survival improvement. J Nucl Med. 2012;53(8):1185–92.
26. Press OW, Eary JF, Appelbaum FR, et al. Radiolabeled-antibody therapy of B-cell lymphoma with autologous bone marrow support. N Engl J Med. 1993;329(17):1219–24.
27. Press OW, Eary JF, Appelbaum FR, et al. Phase II trial of 131I-B1 (anti-CD20) antibody therapy with autologous stem cell transplantation for relapsed B cell lymphomas. Lancet. 1995;346(8971):336–40.
28. Kaminski MS, Tuck M, Estes J, et al. 131I-tositumomab therapy as initial treatment for follicular lymphoma. N Engl J Med. 2005;352(5):441–9.

29. Witzig TE, Flinn IW, Gordon LI, et al. Treatment with ibritumomab tiuxetan radioimmunotherapy in patients with rituximab-refractory follicular non-Hodgkin's lymphoma. J Clin Oncol. 2002;20(15):3262–9.
30. Davis TA, Kaminski MS, Leonard JP, et al. The radioisotope contributes significantly to the activity of radioimmunotherapy. Clin Cancer Res. 2004;10(23):7792–8.
31. Bennett JM, Kaminski MS, Leonard JP, et al. Assessment of treatment-related myelodysplastic syndromes and acute myeloid leukemia in patients with non-Hodgkin lymphoma treated with tositumomab and iodine I131 tositumomab. Blood. 2005;105(12):4576–82.
32. Mones JV, Coleman M, Kostakoglu L, et al. Dose-attenuated radioimmunotherapy with tositumomab and iodine 131 tositumomab in patients with recurrent non-Hodgkin's lymphoma (NHL) and extensive bone marrow involvement. Leuk Lymphoma. 2007;48(2):342–8.
33. Tennvall J, Fischer M, Bischof Delaloye A, et al. EANM procedure guideline for radio-immunotherapy for B-cell lymphoma with 90Y-radiolabelled ibritumomab tiuxetan (Zevalin). Eur J Nucl Med Mol Imaging. 2007;34(4):616–22.
34. Sharkey RM, Press OW, Goldenberg DM. A re-examination of radioimmunotherapy in the treatment of non-Hodgkin lymphoma: prospects for dual-targeted antibody/radioantibody therapy. Blood. 2009;113(17):3891–5.
35. Mulford DA, Scheinberg DA, Jurcic JG. The promise of targeted {alpha}-particle therapy. J Nucl Med. 2005;46(Suppl. 1):199S–204S.
36. Bartholoma MD. Radioimmunotherapy of solid tumors: Approaches on the verge of clinical application. J Labelled Comp Radiopharm. 2018;61(9):715–26.
37. He P, Kramer K, Smith-Jones P, et al. Two-compartment model of radioimmunotherapy delivered through cerebrospinal fluid. Eur J Nucl Med Mol Imaging. 2011;38(2):334–42.
38. Kramer K, Pandit-Taskar N, Zanzonico P, et al. Low incidence of radionecrosis in children treated with conventional radiation therapy and intrathecal radioimmunotherapy. J Neurooncol. 2015;123(2):245–9.
39. Zeltsman M, Mayor M, Jones DR, Adusumilli PS. Surgical immune interventions for solid malignancies. Am J Surg. 2016;212(4):682–90 e5.
40. Rosenblum MG, Verschraegen CF, Murray JL, et al. Phase I study of 90Y-labeled B72.3 intraperitoneal administration in patients with ovarian cancer: effect of dose and EDTA coadministration on pharmacokinetics and toxicity. Clin Cancer Res. 1999;5(5):953–61.
41. Seyedin SN, Schoenhals JE, Lee DA, et al. Strategies for combining immunotherapy with radiation for anticancer therapy. Immunotherapy. 2015;7(9):967–80.
42. Paganelli G, Grana C, Chinol M, et al. Antibody-guided three-step therapy for high grade glioma with yttrium-90 biotin. Eur J Nucl Med. 1999;26(4):348–57.
43. Schoffelen R, Boerman OC, Goldenberg DM, et al. Development of an imaging-guided CEA-pretargeted radionuclide therapy of advanced colorectal cancer: first clinical results. Br J Cancer. 2013;109(4):934–42.
44. Schoffelen R, Woliner-van der Weg W, Visser EP, et al. Predictive patient-specific dosimetry and individualized dosing of pretargeted radioimmunotherapy in patients with advanced colorectal cancer. Eur J Nucl Med Mol Imaging. 2014;41(8):1593–602.
45. Goodwin DA, Meares CF, Osen M. Biological properties of biotin-chelate conjugates for pretargeted diagnosis and therapy with the avidin/biotin system. J Nucl Med. 1998;39(10):1813–8.

Part X

Intracavitary Radionuclide Therapy

Intracavitary Radionuclide Applications

22

Handan Tokmak

Radiopharmaceuticals are prepared by radioactive atoms entering or displacing the molecular structure. Today, they are mostly used for diagnostic purposes, while they are used to a lesser extent for treatment. The main principle of its use in treatment is to benefit from the cytotoxic effect of the radioactive substance applied locally to the organ or tissue or directed to the target tissue through metabolic carriers caused by radiation in the target cells [1, 2]. This treatment administration, which is defined as internal radiotherapy, is different from external radiotherapy (Fig. 22.1).

Therapeutic nuclear medicine involves a theranostic approach that combines targeted diagnosis and treatment of the disease with the use of a radionuclide or a pair of radionuclides. It was aimed in the theranostic approach to detect the tumor using unique biological pathways and then to irradiate the tumor cellularly with radionuclide administered for treatment [3].

Diagnostic imaging guides the use of specific treatment agents by determining the presence and intensity of the receptor/molecule on the target tissue.

It is also possible to evaluate the posttreatment response in the therapeutic approach. Theranostic radiopharmaceuticals, when properly administered, have the potential to make a significant contribution to personalized administrations that will provide better-targeted diagnoses and treatments. Treatments planned using this approach can be adapted to specific disease parameters, imaging data at the time of treatment can be analyzed in real time, and it may be possible to predict the possible effectiveness of treatment [4].

The objectives of radionuclide therapy are maximum destruction of target tissues, high effectiveness, and the least secondary damage to other organs as well as low toxicity. Systemic radionuclide therapy requires molecular targeting mechanisms in which carrier cells, receptors, and/or enzymes use the vascular system along biological barriers to transmit cytotoxic radionuclide agents to target cells. The association with the vascular structure in systemic therapy inevitably results in damage to all organs in proportion to the intensity of interstitial vascularization and radionuclide accumulation. Local radionuclide therapy, unlike systemic treatment, requires geometric proximity only to the target tissues. Toxicity or secondary damage caused by topical radionuclide therapy depends on body fluid flow along the biological barrier, the intensity of collateral microvascularity, lymphatic flow, and diffusion. Because diffusion along biological barriers is generally slow, the essential element in the treatment of locoregional radionuclide is

H. Tokmak (✉)
Mehmet Ali Aydınlar University, Acıbadem Maslak Hospital, Istanbul, Turkey
e-mail: handantokmak@gmail.com

R. Bekiş et al. (eds.), *Radionuclide Therapy*, https://doi.org/10.1007/978-3-030-97220-2_22

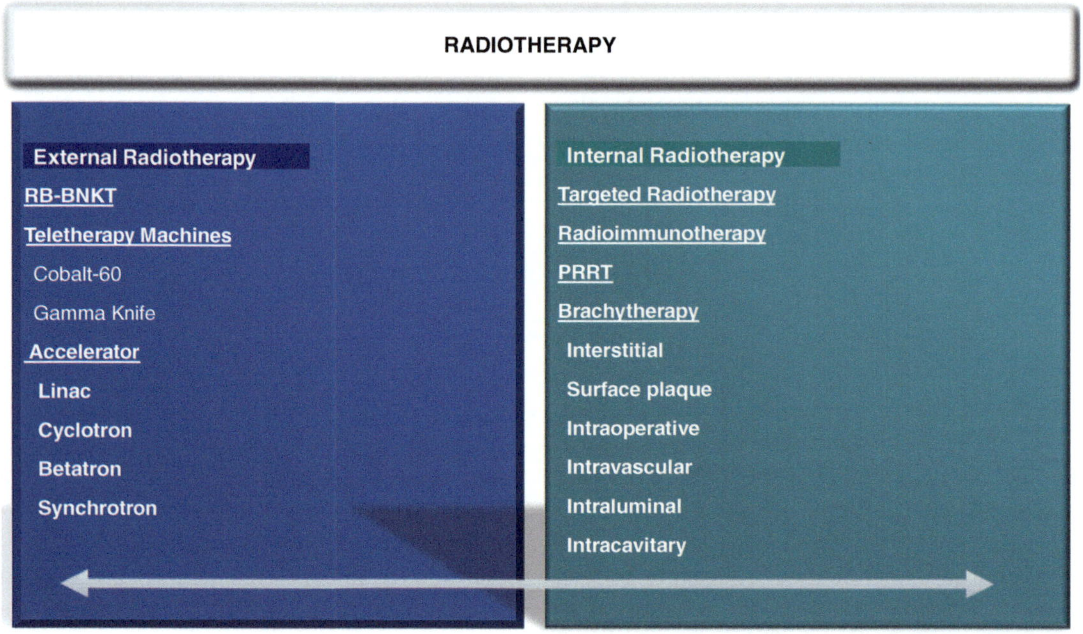

Fig. 22.1 External and internal radiotherapy methods

based on the capillary-lymphatic return physiology of the hydraulic radionuclide of the respective body fluid flow.

22.1 Selection of Appropriate Agents in Radionuclide Therapy

Radionuclides to be used in targeted treatment are expected to cause significant damage to cancer cells during radioactive decay. The rate of damage to biomolecules caused by particulate radiation during radionuclide decay is fairly low compared to the total damage mediated by reactive oxygen species (ROS) formed as a result of radiolysis of water. Alpha-emitters, β-emitters, and Auger electron emitters are assumed to have the highest therapeutic efficacy due to their higher biological activity compared to ionizing electromagnetic radiation types (X-rays and γ-radiation). However, Auger electron emitters appear to be less effective in clinical trials than α- or β-emitters [5, 6].

22.2 Regional Radionuclide Therapy of Primary and Metastatic Cancers

A better evaluation of the localization and biodistribution of radiopharmaceuticals has shown that locoregional radionuclide cancer therapy (LRCT) may be possible in cancer treatment and its more intensive use has come to the fore. It is possible to determine the radiation dose and distribution by simulation and to calculate the dosimetry almost completely with current administration protocols.

Theoretical advantages of LRCT include higher effectiveness, larger therapeutic windows, less radioactivity, lower systemic toxicity, and simpler radiation dosimetry models. In addition to the identified advantages, it can be considered that localized radiation can trigger systemic antitumor mechanisms by preventing recurrences by increasing awareness of the immune system by suppressing immunological resistance locally, immune recognition amplification (similar to the abscopal effect). The chemical specificity requirement of LRCT is less since the tumor is ablated by radioactive radiation by radionuclide due to the proximity of the radiopharmaceutical to the tumor. The disadvantage of this is that distant metastases cannot be treated due to the shorter emission level compared to what is necessary to destroy large tumors [7, 8].

22.3 Methods of Intracavitary Administration

Administration can be performed by intraarterial injection catheter or interstitial injection into the tumor bed. Imaging studies are required before treatment administration in these procedures where intervention and/or surgical procedures are required. Only radionuclides with imaging feature are used in localization, distribution pattern of activity, and dosimetry calculations for this purpose. Intracavitary injection often requires the placement of a catheter to provide reliable and reproducible access to the space to be administered. For example, an intraventricular catheter attached to the reservoir on the scalp is placed for intrathecal radionuclide therapy. 0.5–1 mCi In-111 DTPA is used to determine that this apparatus is successfully inserted and open in areas with cerebrospinal flow in order to evaluate the circulation of cerebrospinal fluid (CFS). The 3-day physical half-life of In-111 allows long-term observation of possible blockage or delayed rotation in the general circulation. It is possible to display In-111 DTPA distribution on the entire CFS circulation trace by obtaining follow-up images. This helps to identify spinal fluid leakage and to evaluate ventriculoperitoneal shunts [9] (Fig. 22.2). Other carriers such as Tc-99m DTPA can serve the same purpose even though In-111 DTPA is the only FDA-approved intrathecal radiopharmaceutical in the United States. Studies are ongoing regarding the use of radiopharmaceuticals with or without tumor affinity in intrathecal local treatment administrations.

An example of intracavitary radionuclide therapy is Y-90-DOTA-TOC administration in the treatment of postoperative cavities in patients diagnosed with glioma [9]. Good responses were reported with Y-90-DOTA-TOC for treatment purposes used after demonstrating the activity of In-111-octreotide in the tumor bed area without leakage in serial imaging performed after In-111-octreotide administration for imaging purposes. This shows that interstitial/intracavitary treatment of brain tumors is possible using radiopharmaceuticals.

Pleural, peritoneal areas and/or postoperative tumor bed require radiographic and/or scinti-

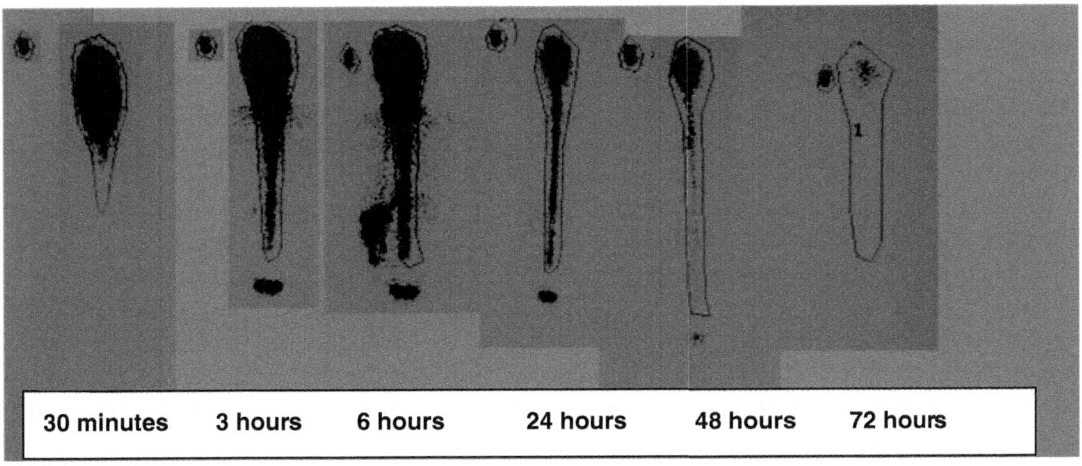

Fig. 22.2 Evaluation of the CFS flow in the patient who underwent Ommaya shunt. Patient injected with 0.5 mCi In-111 DTPA via an Ommaya chamber connected by a ventriculoperitoneal shunt through an on-off valve. No valve closed leakage until the sixth hour. Abdominal activity is seen when the valve in the peritoneal area is opened in 6 h. The ventriculoperitoneal shunt is functioning smoothly

graphic confirmation of adequate injection distribution, typically using Tc-99m-MAA or sulfur colloids in other intracavitary LRCT used in the treatment of primary and metastatic cancer. Intracavitary radiopharmaceuticals may be effective in the remaining micrometastases after surgery. Interstitial injection of particulate radiopharmaceuticals into the tumor bed is usually limited to a controlled site around the injection site. Other surrounding tissues are not affected by radiation.

22.4 Intracavitary Radionuclide Therapy in High-Grade Gliomas

Primary brain tumors such as astrocytoma, oligodendroglioma, glioblastoma multiforme (GBM) caused by craniopharyngiomas, and glial elements originating from epithelial elements are difficult to treat. High-grade malignant glioma treatment is still among the unresolved clinical problems despite years of intensive research and progression in advanced technology and treatment. Glioblastoma accounts for 23% of multiforme malignant primary brain tumors. External radiotherapy, as well as systemic chemotherapy, is often the key to tumor control due to extensive microscopic involvement. If there are sufficient structural or vascular changes after the identification of the tumor mass with contrast-enhanced MRI, surgery can be planned for the resection of the local disease.

However, if the microscopic tumor implants surrounding the surgical cavity are left untreated, it will often cause local recurrence after surgery. Therefore, radiotherapy of the locoregional cavity has come to the forefront in order to prevent local recurrence. However, although approved by the FDA, in a liquid I-125 (Iotrex) locoregional radionuclide therapy study conducted via balloon catheter to provide efficacy of 60 Gy at a surgical margin of 1 cm, BCNU (1,3-bis(2-chloroethyl)-1-nitrosourea), a total of 60 Gy (in fractions divided by 1.7 Gy), was found to fail to provide additional benefit compared to an alkylating chemotherapy agent [10]. New therapeutic strategies, such as the use of monoclonal antibodies (MoAbs) in combination with radioisotopes, are therefore needed to achieve a better response and better prognosis. The increased specificity created by the irradiation of the tumor cell by radioisotopes such as radioimmunotherapy (RIT), for example, is exciting. RIT, which is administered both systemically and locoregionally, is recommended to be used as a modality combined with surgery, radiotherapy, and chemotherapy [11, 12]. For example, such administrations may be an impressive alternative in the strategic approach for the treatment of locally recurrent or progressive glioblastoma after it has been shown that receptor-mediated local radionuclide therapy can be administered with Y-90-DOTA-TOC and well-tolerated. It has been found that locally injected Y-90-DOTA-TOC may be effective in the treatment of recurrent or progressive glioblastoma after confirmation of somatostatin receptor using Ga-68 DOTA-TOC in three patients with stage IV recurrent glioblastoma (a 23-year-old woman and two men aged 61–62) based on similar results in the literature [9]. A cumulative dose of 1.7–2.2 GBq of Y-90-labeled [1,4,7,10-tetraazacyclododecane-*N*,*N*′,*N*″,*N*″-tetraacetic acid(0)-d-Phe [1],Tyr [3]] octreotide (DOTA-TOC) reached in three or four administrations targeting somatostatin receptor was injected locally into a pre-implanted catheter system in the study. Treatment was successful in all three patients and only minimal side effects were reported. MRI and PET-CT evaluation results showed complete remission in one patient and partial remission in other patients after treatment. Moreover, these results were found to be well correlated with clinical improvement and improved quality of life [9].

Patient survival was reported to be 46 months in anaplastic astrocytoma (AA) patients and 19 months in GBM patients, respectively, in studies using I-131-induced monoclonal antibodies administered directly to the postoperative cavities in patients with AA or GBM [13–21]. Studies reported that mAb-labeled Y-90 reached 85 mCi in three to five cycles and reported patient survival as 90 and 20 months, respectively [10]. It was shown in the study where 30 mCi Y-90-labeled biotin was administered by using the three-step pretargeted adjuvant radioimmunotherapy (PARIT) approach locally that this dose could be tolerated with steroid use in patients considering the maximum tolerated dose level that creates the risk of repeated injections creating neurotoxicity [14]. Forty-two percent prolonged survival was reported with the local injection of 4 mg mitoxantrone every 20 days and the approach using local regional PARIT biotin Y-90 up to 27 mCi in 10-week cycles in another study [22]. In a study by Reulen et al. showing that fractional locoregional radiotherapy administered to patients diagnosed with World Health Organization grade III and IV glioma using iodine-131- or yitrium-90-labeled anti-tenascin monoclonal antibodies (I-131-mAb or Y-90-mAb) prolonged the average life expectancy in GBM and AA patients, in addition to reporting the median life expectancy as 77.2 months in AA patients (15 patients) within the study group, 11 years and longer follow-ups of 5 patients (33%) in this group were reported [23].

22.5 Intracavitary Radionuclide Therapy for Recurrent Cystic Brain Tumors

Intracranial cystic lesions can be caused by tumor-induced cysts, such as craniopharyngiomas or cystic astrocytomas, or by postoperative cavities. Intracranial cystic lesions may be good candidates for treatment of locoregional radionuclide with relatively short radiation access, as the risk of damage to normal tissue outside the wall surrounding the cyst is low. The most important factor is the determination of the most effective radiation dose with minimum access outside the wall of the cyst of varying thickness in the treatment of these cysts using locoregional radionuclide. There is no standard algorithm for the selection of injected radioactivity. However, more precise dosimetry estimation requires comprehensive calculations such as Monte Carlo simulation [24]. Validation of the methodology and the effects of heterogeneous intracystic radionuclide distribution on estimation and dosimetry should be evaluated. However, good responses have been reported when a planar source providing homogeneous distribution of 200–250 Gy doses to the cyst wall using P-32 colloids is used [25–31]. A follow-up study conducted after injecting 0.2–7.8 mCi Y-90 colloids into the cyst during the follow-up of craniopharyngiomas showed that tumors shrunk in most patients. Temporary visual field defects, third nerve paralysis, hypothalamic injury, increased intracranial pressure, and blindness in tumors close to optic chiasm have been observed very rarely due to the longer access distance of Y-90 [32].

Usually, the cyst is first accessed with an Ommaya reservoir catheter and then the volume is evaluated by CT. The radioactivity required for the ablation of tumor cells depends on the intrinsic sensitivity of tumor cells, the geometry of the cyst, and the distribution of radionuclide within the cyst. 400–600 mCi I-125 Iotrex, which is also a surgically implanted inflatable balloon catheter, was used to provide 60 Gy administration of 1 cm in length from the cavity surface for 100 h through closed administration in one study [33, 34]. Direct dripping of radiopharmaceuticals by stereotactic injection or through an externally accessible reservoir catheter surgically attached to the cavity is one of the methods used as an alternative to the described methods of administration. Au-198, P-32, Re-186, or Y-90 nonspecific radiocolloids were used with variable activity in regional internal administrations [32, 35]. Holmium-166 has ideal properties with a half-life of 27 h and a beta emission of 94% among the various isotopes used for internal irradiation. It also has a high energy release of 1.85 MeV and a maximum penetration of 8.5 mm.

Holmium-166, colloid carrier radioisotopes have the characteristics of an ideal radioisotope for internal radiation treatment with an appropriate half-life (26.8 h), high beta energy suitable for treatment, gamma radiation providing imaging, and monitoring. However, preclinical studies have shown its effectiveness in solid tumors in subjects; systemic involvement in systemic liver, spleen, lungs, and bones has significantly limited its clinical use since it causes leakage problems from membranes due to its low molecular weight and the possibility of foreign body reaction. The addition of chitosan, a polymer of 2-deoxy-2-amino-D-glucose, to keep radionuclide in the target region and prevent systemic absorption with the holmium-166-chitosan complex (Ho-166-chico) developed by the Korea Atomic Energy Research Institute (KAERI) has produced successful results.

Chitosan, obtained by deacetylation of natural chitin, has been shown to cause almost no absorption when biocompatible, bioaffinitive, and biodegradable holmium-166 forms chelate complex with chitosan. However, the preparation condition of this complex at −23 °C and the low yield rate (36%) prevent the widespread use of this composition. Chitosan is a deacetylated polymer of chitin [poly-β(1-4)-N-acetyl-D-glucosamine], an amino-polysaccharide naturally found in crab shell, shrimp, and squid bones. Commercially available chitosan (SamcheonRiPharm. Co.) is a 98% deacetylated form of 500,000 Da molecular weight. The free amino group of chitosan can be complexed by Ho-166 (NO_3) 3 · $5H_2O$ through chelate formation at room temperature. This biocompatible Ho-166-chitosan complex remained completely in the in vivo cystic cavity for more than 48 h (99.7% of the amount injected) and was completely biodegraded without provoking any foreign body reaction. The safety and effective measurement of the procedure were also evaluated in a study evaluating the treatment and response of cystic brain tumor patients with the holmium-166-chitosan complex (Ho-166-chico) consisting of a beta-emitting radionuclide holmium-166 and a biodegradable polymer. Clinical improvement and long-term tumor control in both benign tumors and low-grade astrocytomas for recurrent cystic brain tumors were demonstrated in 70% of cases with radiological response to intracavitary radiation using Ho-166-chico in this study. Furthermore, the measurement of the radioactivity of the cystic fluid (>92%) showed that Ho-166-chico was bound to the cyst wall at 12 h and systemic absorption and blood sample at 24 h were negligible. Repeated intracavitary radiation of low doses of Ho-166-chico can be considered as one of the useful methods for the treatment of clinically difficult cystic brain tumors. Twenty-two patients with recurrent cystic brain tumors and/or located in a favorable deep location were included in the pilot study. Evaluation was performed using cyst volume and wall thickness on CT or MRI to evaluate the radiological response. Ho-166-chico activity injected through the Ommaya reservoir was calculated as 10–25 Gy to the cyst wall at a depth of 4 mm [36]. Oculomotor paresis was observed in two patients with recurrent craniopharyngioma. Of the 20 images from the other 20 patients, 14 had radiological response (70%). Seven patients with significant radiological response experienced more than 25% reduction in both cyst volume and wall thickness. The other seven patients were shown to have decreased cyst volume without significant change in wall thickness. It provided symptomatic improvement in all patients with benign tumors or low-grade gliomas. Ho-166-chico intracavitary radiation therapy for cystic tumor is a safe palliation method without serious complications.

The reservoir/catheter system is installed in all patients to evaluate the repeatable injection of the isotope 3 weeks before Ho-166-chico injection, to aspirate the cystic fluid to eliminate pressure-related symptoms when needed, to test for injection leakage using the reservoir, to prevent this leakage if any, and to evaluate the results of the studies conducted. 1 cc of diluted metrizamide solution or Omnipaque 300 is performed using CT scanning after injection for leakage testing. The system is used and useful for detecting possible minimal leakages and measuring the exact cyst volume just before injection. Ho-166-chico activity used in injections was in the range of 4–20 mCi for each injection. It was decided to administer 10–25 Gy per 4 mm of the internal cyst wall considering the patient's expected survival, the degree of histological malignancy, or the presence of adjacent critical structure.

The dose injected per volume ranged from 0.17 to 3.95 mCi/mL since the dose per injection is intended to be less than 5 mCi/mL. The number of repetitions of Ho-166-chico injection was determined based on radiological evaluation and clinical response at least 1 month apart. The number of injections administered to patients in the study ranged from 1 to 5 (average 1.4 per patient). Lower complication rates were interpreted to be associated with precautionary dosimetry and careful precautionary assessment of leakage prevention compared to previous studies. It was reported that both patients with complications were recurrent craniopharyngioma and adhesion of the thin-walled cyst to the oculomotor nerve was responsible for radiation injuries. It was emphasized that minimal-dose radioisotope injection via subcutaneous reservoir and close follow-up are important to avoid intracavitary radiation complications during treatment in patients with thin-walled cyst structures in very close proximity to critical neural structures [37, 38].

22.6 Local Intracavitary Therapy of Secondary GBM with Bi-213-Dota-SP

GBM has been shown to oversuppress NK-1 receptor, and substance P has been reported to be used as a ligand for targeted therapy. Radionuclides acting with alpha rays such as high-energy Bi-213 with a short reach allow selective irradiation of tumor cells while maintaining adjacent neuronal structures.

Nine patients with recurrent GBM who were selected from 50 glioma patients of different subtypes treated with target alpha therapy at Warsaw University Faculty of Medicine, who underwent postoperative chemoradiotherapy, were injected with therapeutic doses of one to six doses, 0.9–2.3 GBq Bi-213-DOTA-[Thi8,Met(O2)11]-substance P (Bi-213-DOTA-SP) at 2-month intervals. Biodistribution was evaluated by PET/CT study by injecting Ga-68-DOTA-[Thi8,Met(O2)11]-substance P (Ga-68-DOTA-SP) for simultaneous imaging with therapeutic injections. Treatment response evaluation was performed with MRI [39]. Treatment responses other than transient adverse reactions such as mild headache due to transient peripheral edema reactions at activity doses ranging from 1.4 to 9.7 (median 5.8) GBq Bi-213-DOTA-SP were well-tolerated, and median progression-free survival after initiation of alpha therapy was reported as 5.8 months and overall survival as 16.4 months. It was reported among the patients with a median overall survival time of 52.3 months in the first diagnosis that the patient was successful in reaching this time after the initiation of radionuclide therapy [39].

Targeted alpha therapy of secondary GBM with Bi-213-DOTA-SP is safe and well-tolerated and presented as a promising new therapeutic option for secondary GBM [39, 40].

22.7 Dosimetry in Intracavitary Radionuclide Therapy

The most important factor is the determination of the minimum effective radiation dose outside the wall of the cyst of varying thickness in internal radiotherapy. The main factors determining the radiation dose to the cyst wall at a certain isotope dose are cyst volume, degree of isotope dispersion, and proportion of the attached form. Cyst volume and isotope density are decisive factors in treatment [41]. It has been reported that it would be appropriate to include cyst wall thickness as one of the parameters in dosimetry formulas for dose calculation in cystic lesions [42]. However, wall thickness is usually very thin (<10 mm), and changes in thickness make a significant difference [43]. Cyst aspiration was performed at random intervals according to clinical requirement in the study of Kim J. H. et al. Researchers evaluated symptomatic improvement, recurrence, survival, reduction in cystic fluid accumulation, or reduction in cyst size in response to treatment in many studies. However, these parameters are difficult to consider as a direct effect of radiation on the tumor cyst. Half of the treated cases showed measurable changes even though it was not easy to measure the thickness change in the thin-walled cyst. Sometimes the expected results secondary to treatment in malignant tumors can be seen even in early imaging after a short follow-up period of 1 month. Radiation response is monitored earlier in malignant tumors compared to benign slow-growing tumors. As a matter of fact, Taasan et al. showed that most malignant tumors that responded in the early period recurred later and that repeated injections at fixed intervals were necessary to prevent progression [44]. The effectiveness of intracavitary radiation has gained importance especially for benign cystic tumor (cystic craniopharyngioma) considering that conventional external radiation treatment for craniopharyngioma carries a high risk of pituitary insufficiency in long-term follow-up. Studies have shown significant clinical response to intracavitary radionuclide therapy in all benign cystic tumors, including low-grade glioma.

22.8 Intracavitary Radionuclide Use in the Treatment of Peritoneal Carcinomatosis

The use of radionuclide therapy agents for postoperative residual micrometastases of ovarian and other gynecological malignancies, intraperitoneal prophylaxis, and palliation of malignant acids has been investigated since the 1960s in peritoneal metastasis. The widely preferred radiocolloid in the first studies is P-32. Intraperitoneal radiocolloid administration is performed either during surgery or through a peritoneal catheter placed postoperatively in the abdomen.

Malignant acids occur as a result of increased peritoneal fluid production due to peritoneal irritation and/or decreased drainage of peritoneal fluids due to lymphatic obstruction. It can be exacerbated by low plasma oncotic pressure. The most common type of malignant acids is large implants on the viscera resulting from the loss of tumor cells and solid tumor implants. The number of tumor cells in peritoneal fluid ranges from 50 to 1000 cells/microliter. Intracavitary radionuclide therapy can treat free circulating tumor cells and induce serosal fibrosis, but it can rarely be effective in controlling visceral metastases due to limited emission ranges.

The group with the best response to intravitreal radionuclide therapy was malignant acid and the group with high tumor cell counts (microliters/more than 4000 cells). The type of peritoneal acid, which is less frequent, is caused by large tumor mass and venous return or lymphatic obstruction. The number of tumor cells in the peritoneal fluid is low, and the response to intracavitary treatment is very low in this group. Malignant acid is common in metastatic ovary, renal, gastrointestinal cancer, mesothelioma, and lymphoma. FDA limits intracavitary radiocolloid therapy to acids caused by metastases in the United States. Intracavitary radionuclide therapy is indicated for palliation when systemic disease occurs. Treatment and paracentesis reduce symptoms such as abdominal distension, shortness of breath, cough, or hiccups caused by diaphragmatic irritation [45].

The peritoneal dialysis catheter with fenestration is typically administered under aseptic conditions with visual guidance, and the catheter is fixed to the abdominal surface in radionuclide administration. After the acid liquid is removed, 1 mCi Tc-99m sulfur colloid is injected for imaging purposes and washed with 250 mL of liquid. The patient is allowed to turn right and left to distribute the activity before scintigraphy is performed to confirm the distribution to the peritoneal cavity. Then, 15–25 mCi P-32 chronic phosphate in 500 mL of saline is injected into the catheter before removal. The patient is then positioned to extend to the left side; the right side is tilted upside down, each with a foot tilt for 5 min; and Bremsstrahlung imaging is performed to verify the distribution.

P-32 colloids are rapidly cleared from the peritoneal fluid with only 5% retention within 24 h, and the remaining portion is coated on the serosal surface. Radiocolloids are also cleared by macrophages and diaphragmatic lymphatics [46–48]. Potential side effects are nausea, vomiting, diarrhea, and abdominal pain associated with radiation peritonitis. It has been reported that up to 9% of patients may develop small bowel obstruction due to simultaneous radiation effect [49]. Cessation of peritoneal fluid production over 3 months is considered excellent, and significantly reduced peritoneal fluid accumulation is a good response even though there is no universal definition of response criteria.

Radionuclide-linked antibodies, mucin (MUC16/CA125, MUC1) and glycoproteins (TAG72, aFR/gp38, or folate receptors), have been applied to target tumor surface markers in different studies [50, 51]. Prior to systemic radioimmunotherapy, the biodistribution of antibodies is confirmed by radionuclide (such as low-dose I-131 or indium) labeling and subsequent visualization of an antibody such as anti-CD20.

A large-scale phase III study of 447 patients using Y-90 mycin IgG HMFG1 achieved complete remission in patients with epithelial ovarian cancer (stage IC-IV) after surgical resection. However, no advantage was shown in survival. Strategies to improve locoregional radioimmunotherapy include selection of radionuclide (Lu-177 over Y-90), use of systemic evaluation agents such as DTPA to reduce systemic toxicity, pretargeting, and in combination with other treatment modalities.

Results suggest that the use of bi-213-16F12 and BIP-RIT may be an effective solution for adjuvant RIT immediately after cytoreduction to eliminate microscopic disease after resection. This approach should be recommended to selected patients as with HIPEC administrations. In addition, the first clinical trial using anti-MISRII GM102 mAb in ovarian cancers is ongoing (NCT02978755/March 2020 is planned to be completed). Lu-177- or Bi-213-labeled antibodies may be advantageous for treatment purposes in eligible patients after pre-trial evaluation by diagnostic imaging (when labeled with Zr-89) of a radiolabeled anti-MISRII mAb when standard antibody treatments are compared. Specifically, radiolabeled antibodies can kill tumor cells that cannot be directly accessed by the naked antibody through cross-fire radiation and bystander effects (unpublished data). The use of Lu-177-16F12 is theoretically most advantageous when administered systemically to patients treated by the BIP-RIT standard method.

Monoclonal antibodies that recognize the B7-H3 epitope expressed on ovarian cancer cells and cancer-inducing cells (CICs) as a carrier molecule for targeted alpha-particle radioimmunotherapy (RIT) have been studied in ovarian cancer preclinical models to develop new therapies that effectively kill differentiated cancer cells and CICs that cause chemotherapy resistance and disease relapse in order to reduce morbidity and mortality of ovarian cancer treatment (mAb) (376.96), and positive results have been reported [52].

22.9 Concluding Remarks

Radionuclide-mediated radiation can be used locally without damaging the surrounding tissue and provides theoretical and practical pharmacokinetic advantages in cancer therapy, unlike standard radiotherapy applications. Today, safer use has become possible with advances in radiochemistry, imaging technology, and dosimetry algorithms. Locoregional radionuclide therapy will play a greater role in the fight against cancer, in the personalized approach with more theoretical and clinical research.

The purpose of radionuclide therapy is to destroy diseased tissue by causing destruction in target tissues as a result of local or systemic administration of radionuclides. The target tissue is irradiated and the surrounding tissue is minimally damaged in this sense, unlike external radiotherapy. Correct calculation of the amount of radiation received in the targeted tissue for treatment purposes constitutes the main point in the treatment approach. As a result of the increase in the use of radionuclide therapy administrations in current personalized therapy administrations, personalized dosimetric administrations are of great importance in order to increase the therapy effectiveness and also to ensure radiation safety. Radionuclide therapeutic dosimetry should be considered as a standard component of radionuclide therapeutic administrations as in radiation oncology studies where therapeutic administrations are performed.

It is important to predict pretreatment tumor response and normal tissue toxicity in order to perform individual patient dosimetry. It is important to know the dose-response relationship, to determine the individual maximum safe radiation absorption dose and minimum effective dose for each patient, to compare the individual radionuclide dose-response relationship for each radiopharmaceutical, and to increase knowledge and experience in radiobiology in line with the purpose of new administrations and approaches in order to calculate the tumor's treatment response and normal tissue toxicity.

References

1. Pouget JP, Lozza C, Deshayes E, Boudousq V, Navarro-Teulon I. Introduction to radiobiology of targeted radionuclide therapy. Front Med. 2015;2:12.
2. Curcio CG, Vasile C, Gianciotta A, Casali A, Gionfra T, Rinaldi M, Guadagni A, LePera V, Sega E. Short-term results of combined radioimmunotherapy in inoperable lung cancer. Tumori. 1976;62:587–98.
3. Sfakianakis GN, DeLand FH. Radioimmuno diagnosis and radioimmunotherapy, 1982. J Nucl Med. 1982;23:840–50.
4. Goldenberg DM, Chang CH, Rossi EA, McBride JW, Sharkey RM. Pretargeted molecular imaging and radioimmunotherapy. Theranostics. 2012;2:523–40.
5. Jackson MR, Falzone N, Vallis KA. Advances in anticancer radiopharmaceuticals. Clin Oncol. 2013;25:604–9.
6. Kassis AI, Adelstein SJ. Radiobiologic principles in radionuclide therapy. J Nucl Med. 2005;46:4S–12S.
7. McCready VR. A different approach to the use of unsealed radionuclides for cancer therapy. Eur J Nucl Med. 1995;22(1):1–3.
8. McCready VR, Cornes P. The potential of intratumoural unsealed radioactive source therapy. Eur J Nucl Med. 2001;28(5):567–9.
9. Heute D, et al. Response of recurrent high-grade glioma to treatment with (90)Y-DOTATOC. J Nucl Med. 2010;51(3):397–400.
10. Tatter SB, et al. An inflatable balloon catheter and liquid 125I radiation source (GliaSite Radiation Therapy System) for treatment of recurrent malignant glioma: multicenter safety and feasibility trial. J Neurosurg. 2003;99(2):297–303.
11. Hopkins K, et al. Direct injection of 90Y MoAbs into glioma tumor resection cavities leads to limited diffusion of the radioimmunoconjugates into normal brain parenchyma: a model to estimate absorbed radiation dose. Int J Radiat Oncol Biol Phys. 1998;40(4):835–44.
12. Wernicke AG, et al. The role of dose escalation with intracavitary brachytherapy in the treatment of localized CNS malignancies: outcomes and toxicities of a prospective study. Brachytherapy. 2010;9(1):91–9.
13. Paganelli G, et al. Radioimmunotherapy of brain tumor. Neurol Res. 2006;28(5):518–22.
14. Paganelli G, et al. Pre-targeted locoregional radioimmunotherapy with 90Y-biotin in glioma patients: phase I study and preliminary therapeutic results. Cancer Biother Radiopharm. 2001;16(3):227–35.
15. Reardon DA, et al. A pilot study: 131I-antitenascin monoclonal antibody 81c6 to deliver a 44-Gy resection cavity boost. Neuro Oncol. 2008;10(2):182–9.
16. Riva P, et al. Treatment of intracranial human glioblastoma by direct intratumoral administration of 131I-labelled anti-tenascin monoclonal antibody BC-2. Int J Cancer. 1992;51(1):7–13.
17. Riva P, et al. Intralesional radioimmunotherapy of malignant gliomas. An effective treatment in recurrent tumors. Cancer. 1994a;73(Suppl. 3):1076–82.
18. Riva P, et al. Glioblastoma therapy by direct intralesional administration of I-131 radioiodine labeled antitenascin antibodies. Cell Biophys. 1994b;24–25:37–43.
19. Riva P, et al. Local treatment of malignant gliomas by direct infusion of specific monoclonal antibodies labeled with 131I: comparison of the results obtained in recurrent and newly diagnosed tumors. Cancer Res. 1995;55(Suppl. 23):5952s–6s.
20. Riva P, et al. Loco-regional radioimmunotherapy of high-grade malignant gliomas using specific monoclonal antibodies labeled with 90Y: a phase I study. Clin Cancer Res. 1999;5(10 Suppl):3275s–80s.
21. Riva P, et al. Role of nuclear medicine in the treatment of malignant gliomas: the locoregional radioimmunotherapy approach. Eur J Nucl Med. 2000;27(5):601–9.
22. Boiardi A, et al. Intratumoral delivery of mitoxantrone in association with 90-Y radioimmunotherapy (RIT) in recurrent glioblastoma. J Neurooncol. 2005;72(2):125–31.
23. Reulen HJ, Poepperl G, Goetz C, Gildehaus JF, Schmidt M, Tatsch K, Pietsch T, Kraus T, Rachinger W. Long-term outcome of patients with WHO Grade III and IV gliomas treated by fractionated intracavitary radioimmunotherapy. J Neurosurg. 2015;123(3):760–70.
24. Bond WH, Richards D, Turner E. Experiences with radioactive gold in the treatment of craniopharyngioma. J Neurol Neurosurg Psychiatry. 1965;28:30–8.
25. Sadeghi M, et al. Dosimetry of (32)P radiocolloid for treatment of cystic craniopharyngioma. Appl Radiat Isot. 2007;65(5):519–23.
26. Zhao R, et al. Treatment of cystic craniopharyngioma with phosphorus-32 intracavitary irradiation. Childs Nerv Syst. 2010;26(5):669–74.
27. Hasegawa T, et al. Management of cystic craniopharyngiomas with phosphorus-32 intracavitary irradiation. Neurosurgery. 2004;54(4):813–20. Discussion 820–822
28. Shapiro B, Fig LM, Gross MD. Intracavitary therapy of craniopharyngiomas. Q J Nucl Med. 1999;43(4):367–74.
29. Liu Z, et al. Stereotactic intratumour irradiation with nuclide for craniopharyngiomas. Chin Med J (Engl). 1996;109(3):219–22.
30. Pollock BE, et al. Phosphorus-32 intracavitary irradiation of cystic craniopharyngiomas: current technique and long-term results. Int J Radiat Oncol Biol Phys. 1995;33(2):437–46.
31. Julow J, et al. Stereotactic intracavitary irradiation of cystic craniopharyngiomas with yttrium-90 isotope. Prog Neurol Surg. 2007;20:289–96.

32. Sadeghi M, Karimi E, Sardari D. Monte Carlo and analytical calculations of dose distributions in craniopharyngioma cysts treated with radiocolloids containing 32P or 186Re. Appl Radiat Isot. 2009b;67(9):1697–701.
33. Lanka VK. Balloon brachytherapy for brain tumor-radiation safety experiences at the University of Medicine and Dentistry of New Jersey. Health Phys. 2006;91(Suppl. 5):S83–6.
34. Chan TA, et al. Treatment of recurrent glioblastoma multiforme with Glia Site brachytherapy. Int J Radiat Oncol Biol Phys. 2005;62(4):1133–9.
35. Lin LL, et al. Long-term outcome in children treated for craniopharyngioma with and without radiotherapy. J Neurosurg Pediatr. 2008;1(2):126–30.
36. Ha EJ, Gwak HS, Rhee CH, Youn SM, Choi CW, Cheon GJ. Intracavitary radiation therapy for recurrent cystic brain tumors with holmium-166-chico: a pilot study. J Korean Neurosurg Soc. 2013;54(3):175–82.
37. Kobayashi T, Kageyama N, Ohara K. Internal irradiation for cystic craniopharyngioma. J Neurosurg. 1981;55:896–903.
38. Rogers LR, Barnett G. Percutaneous aspiration of brain tumor cysts via the Ommaya reservoir system. Neurology. 1991;41(Pt 1):279–82.
39. Krolicki L, Bruchertseifer F, Kunikowska J, Koziara H, Królicki B, Jakuciński M, Pawlak D, Apostolidis C, Mirzadeh S, Rola R, Merlo A, Morgenstern A. Prolonged survival in secondary glioblastoma following local injection of targeted alpha therapy with 213Bi- substance P analogue. Eur J Nucl Med. 2018; https://doi.org/10.1007/s00259-018-4015-2.
40. Cordier D, Forrer F, Bruchertseifer F, et al. Targeted alpha-radionuclide therapy of functionally critically located gliomas with 213Bi-DOTA-[Thi8,Met(O2)11]-substance P: a pilot trial. Eur J Nucl Med Mol Imaging. 2010;37:1335–44.
41. Wen PY, Macdonald DR, Reardon DA, Cloughesy TF, Sorensen AG, Galanis E, et al. Updated response assessment criteria for high-grade gliomas: response assessment in neuro-oncology working group. J Clin Oncol. 2010;28:1963–72.
42. Henson JW, Ulmer S, Harris GJ. Brain tumor imaging in clinical trials. AJNR Am J Neuroradiol. 2008;29:419–24.
43. Kim JH, Lec JT, Kim EK, Won JY, Kim MJ, Lee JD, et al. Percutaneous sclerotherapy of renal cysts with a beta-emitting radionuclide, holmium-166-chitosan complex. Korean J Radiol. 2004;5:128–33.
44. Taasan V, Shapiro B, Taren JA, Beierwaltes WH, McKeever P, Wahl RL, et al. Phosphorus-32 therapy of cystic Grade IV astrocytomas: technique and preliminary application. J Nucl Med. 1985;26:1335–8.
45. Kasten BB, Arend RC, Katre AA, Kim H, Fan J, Ferrone S, Zinn KR, Buchsbaum DJ. B7-H3-targeted 212Pb radioimmunotherapy of ovarian cancer in preclinical models. Nucl Med Biol. 2017;47:23–30.
46. Tharp M, Hornback NB. Complications associated with intraperitoneal 32P. Gynecol Oncol. 1994;53(2):170–5.
47. Verheijen RH, et al. Phase III trial of intraperitoneal therapy with yttrium-90-labeled HMFG1 murine monoclonal antibody in patients with epithelial ovarian cancer after a surgically defined complete remission. J Clin Oncol. 2006;24(4):571–8.
48. Meredith RF, et al. Intra peritoneal radioimmunochemotherapy of ovarian cancer: a phase I study. Cancer Biother Radiopharm. 2001;16(4):305–15.
49. Meredith RF, et al. Brief overview of preclinical and clinical studies in the development of intraperitoneal radioimmunotherapy for ovarian cancer. Clin Cancer Res. 2007;13(18 Pt 2):5643s–5s.
50. Wilkinson RH Jr. Pleuroperitoneal migration of intraperitoneal phosphorus-32-chromic phosphate therapy for stage I ovarian carcinoma. J Nucl Med. 1996;37(4):636–9.
51. Oei AL. Decreased intraperitoneal disease recurrence in epithelial ovarian cancer patients receiving intraperitoneal consolidation treatment with yttrium-90-labeled murine HMFG1 without improvement in overall survival. Int J Cancer. 2007;120(12):2710–4.
52. Fauci JM, Sabbatino F, Wang Y, Londoño-Joshi AI, Straughn JM Jr, Landen CN, Ferrone S. Monoclonal antibody- based immunotherapy of ovarian cancer: targeting ovarian cancer cells with the B7-H3-specific mAb 376.96. Gynecol Oncol. 2014;132(1):203–10.

GPSR Compliance

The European Union's (EU) General Product Safety Regulation (GPSR) is a set of rules that requires consumer products to be safe and our obligations to ensure this.

If you have any concerns about our products, you can contact us on ProductSafety@springernature.com

In case Publisher is established outside the EU, the EU authorized representative is:

Springer Nature Customer Service Center GmbH
Europaplatz 3
69115 Heidelberg, Germany

Batch number: 10732799

Printed by Printforce, the Netherlands